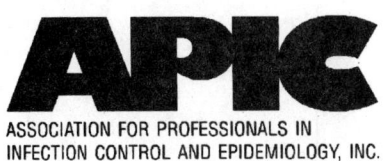

ASSOCIATION FOR PROFESSIONALS IN
INFECTION CONTROL AND EPIDEMIOLOGY, INC.

CW01511535

APIC Text of Infection Control and Epidemiology

2nd Edition

January 2005

Copyrighted © 2005 by the Association for Professionals in Infection Control and
Epidemiology, Inc. (APIC)
1275 K Street, NW, Suite 1000
Washington, DC 20005-4006
Tel.: 202-789-1890
Fax: 202-789-1899
e-mail: apicinfo@apic.org
internet: www.apic.org

All rights reserved. No part of this publication may be reproduced, stored in a retrieval
system, or transmitted, in any form or by any means, electronic, mechanical,
photocopied, recorded, or otherwise, without written permission from the publisher.

ISBN paper: 1-933013-00-1
ISBN looseleaf: 1-933013-01-X

TABLE OF CONTENTS

Copyright © 2005, Association for Professionals in Infection Control and Epidemiology, Inc.

APIC Text of Infection Control and Epidemiology

Copyright © 2005, Association for Professionals in Infection Control and Epidemiology, Inc.

Association for Professionals in Infection Control and Epidemiology, Inc.

Text Program

Chair:
Ruth Carrico, Ph.D., RN, CIC
Infection Control Director
University of Louisville Hospital
Louisville, Kentucky

Joan Heath RN, BSN, CIC
Manager, Infection Control Department
Children's Hospital and Regional Medical Center
Seattle, Washington

Jaime Ritter BS, MT(ASCP), MPH, CIC
Infection Control Specialist
CR Bard, Inc.
Atlanta, Georgia

**Joan M. Wideman, MS, MS,
    MT(ASCP)SLS, CIC**
Consultant
JMW Consulting, LLC
Clawson, Michigan

Linda Adam, RN, BScN, CIC
Infection Control Practitioner
Vancouver/Richmond Health Board
Richmond, British Columbia
Canada

Ruth Curchoe, RN, MSN, CIC
Infection Control Director
Unity Health System
Rochester, New York

Linda Griffin Kean, Managing Editor
APIC
Washington, DC

Copyright © 2005, Association for Professionals in Infection Control and Epidemiology, Inc.

2004 APIC Board of Directors

President
Jeanne A. Pfeiffer, RN, MPH, CIC
Infection Control
Hennepin City Medical Center
Minneapolis, Minnesota

President Elect
Sue Sebazco, RN, BS, CIC
Arlington Memorial Hospital
Arlington, Texas

Secretary
Patti Grant, RN, BSN, MS, CIC
RHD & TMC Tenet Health System
Dallas, Texas

Treasurer
Janet E. Frain, RN, CIC, CPHQ
Sutter Medical Center, Sacramento
Sacramento, California

Immediate Past President
Barbara M. Soule, RN, MPA, CIC
Olympia, Washington

Kathleen Meehan Arias, MS, MT, SM, CIC
Arias Infection Control Consulting, LLC
Crownsville, Maryland

Mary L. Andrus, RN, BA, CIC
Centers for Disease Control and Prevention
Atlanta, Georgia

Bonnie M. Barnard, MPH, CIC
St. Peters Hospital
Helena, Montana

Kathy L. Brooks, RN, PhD, CIC
Infection Control Program Manager
Overton Brooks VA Medical Center
Shreveport, Louisiana

Loretta L. Fauerbach, MS, CIC
Shands Hospital at the University of Florida/
    Shands Healthcare
Gainesville, Florida

Gail E. Harris, RN, MS, MA, CIC
Las Vegas, Nevada

Marie A. Kassai, RN, BSN, MPH, CIC
Elmwood Park, New Jersey

Denise Murphy, RN, BSN, MPH, CIC
Barnes-Jewish Hospital at Washington Univ.
Saint Louis, Missouri

Christine J. Nutty, RN, MSN, CIC
Western Baptist Hospital
Paducah, Kentucky

Board Advisors
AJIC Editor
Elaine Larson, RN, PhD, FAAN, CIC
Columbia University School of Nursing
New York, New York

Auditor
Leonard G. Pepe, CPA
BDO Seidman, LLP
Boston, Massachusetts

Legal Counsel
Ralph J. Rivkind, JD, LLM
Rackemann Sawyer & Brewster, P.C.
Boston, Massachusetts

Executive Director
Kathy Warye, CAE
Association for Professionals in Infection Control
    and Epidemiology
Washington, DC

Copyright © 2005, Association for Professionals in Infection Control and Epidemiology, Inc.

Preface

The *APIC Text of Infection Control and Epidemiology* is an infection control professional's best tool for lifelong learning. The *APIC Text* is a dynamic document, under constant review and revision to ensure that it contains the most up-to-date practice standards for professionals across the spectrum of healthcare settings.

This 2005 revision has become especially important as a result of several important events. First, the U.S. Centers for Disease Control and Prevention (CDC) led the way through its Healthcare Infection Control Practices Advisory Committee (HICPAC) and revised a number of essential guidelines that are fundamental for infection prevention and control practice. (These guidelines are included on the CD bundled with this revised edition of the *APIC Text*.) Second, both APIC and SHEA (Society for Healthcare Epidemiology of America) released position papers that are important to specific areas of practice. Third, the terrorism events of September 2001 and the anthrax-related events of October 2001 spawned monumental efforts in the realm of emergency preparedness. Finally, new and emerging infectious diseases have challenged many of our traditional infection control strategies and exposed our vulnerabilities in both knowledge and application of infection prevention. Throughout these challenges, APIC members have partnered with individuals and organizations to plow new ground and truly impact our healthcare landscape.

During the ongoing review of the *APIC Text,* it became apparent that these many events resulted in the need to completely revise the chapters and add several new ones so that this text could continue to be our profession's primary body of fundamental knowledge. Chapters were revised using a specific template that supported inclusion of information regarding future trends and international perspectives. In addition, our organization has continued to develop partnerships with other healthcare disciplines that have need of basic infection prevention and control information relevant to their respective practices. To this end, the APIC Text Program committee led a team of hundreds of authors and reviewers to fully update the APIC Text, now published as this revised edition. (The members of the APIC Text Program committee are listed on page v. The authors and reviewers are listed in the index to this APIC Text.)

This 2005 revised edition includes 121 chapters and is easier to manage in many ways than the 2002 edition. This edition continues to comprise two volumes, but the first volume is more compact and includes only 27 "essential" chapters. This first volume of "Essential Elements" will be useful to new and developing infection control professionals, and will also be beneficial to those in many other healthcare disciplines. Volume 2, Scientific and Practice Elements, contains the remaining 94 chapters organized into the following sections: Advanced Program Management, Patient Populations, Practice Settings, Clinical and Support Services, Organisms and Presentations, Clinical Syndromes, Care Environment, Advanced Occupational Health, and Local and International Community. A separate booklet includes the index and a full listing of authors and reviewers, as well as the interactive CD version of this *APIC Text*. In addition to the full contents of the print edition, the CD includes hyperlinks to the index and to external Internet resources and also includes dozens of additional resources (educational pamphlets, official APIC documents, and guidelines).

At the request of APIC members, the print edition of this revised edition is available in two formats: paperback and on looseleaf sheets that are three-hole punched to be inserted into two binders for quick reference.

This revision has been an amazing endeavor for the Text Program committee and for the hundreds of APIC members and others involved in its development and production. I personally thank the members of the Text Program committee for their devotion to this process: Joan Wideman, Ruth Curchoe, Joan Heath, Jaime Ritter, and Linda Adam our representative from CHICA (Community and

Copyright © 2005, Association for Professionals in Infection Control and Epidemiology, Inc.

Hospital Infection Control Association-Canada). Special thanks go to Linda Griffin Kean, the Managing Editor, for her outstanding leadership and support throughout this process.

As always, it is essential to remember that this document has been produced for our members and is charged with meeting the needs of those members. In an effort to continue to be responsive, your comments and suggestions are encouraged. Please forward comments to info@apic.org or contact me directly at ruthca@ulh.org.

Ruth Carrico, PhD, RN, CIC
Editor, *APIC Text of Infection Control and Epidemiology*
Chair, APIC Text Program

Copyright © 2005, Association for Professionals in Infection Control and Epidemiology, Inc.

Association for Professionals in Infection Control and Epidemiology

Code of Ethics

APIC believes strongly that its members must uphold the highest standards of ethical and professional behavior. All members agree to abide by the following principles:

1. To hold paramount the safety, health and welfare of the public and healthcare workers in the performance of professional duties.
2. To assist colleagues in their professional development and support them in following this code of ethics.
3. To treat all persons fairly, without regard to race, religion, gender, abilities, age or national origin.
4. To act in such a manner as to uphold and enhance personal and professional honor, integrity and the dignity of the profession.
5. To avoid real or perceived conflicts of interest whenever possible, and to disclose them to affected parties when they do exist.
6. To support and comply with APIC bylaws and any laws and regulations, domestic or foreign, that are applicable to APIC.
7. To engage in infection control and epidemiologic research in a professional manner and to strive at all times to assure that analysis and report preparation meet high standards of excellence.
8. To honestly represent professional credentials, academic degrees and research experience in all circumstances.
9. To refuse to accept gratuities, gifts or favors that might impair or appear to impair professional judgment, to offer any favor, service or thing of value to obtain special advantage.

Copyright © 2005, Association for Professionals in Infection Control and Epidemiology, Inc.

Infection Control and Prevention Programs

Candace Friedman, MPH, CIC
Manager, Infection Control and Epidemiology
University of Michigan Hospitals and Health
Centers
Ann Arbor, Michigan

ABSTRACT

Infection control and prevention (IC) programs in the United States have changed greatly since the mid-20th century. Much of this change was due to the influence of professional organizations; government, regulatory, and accrediting agencies; and scientific research and publications. There are various models outlined for IC programs and standards developed for IC professionals.

I.   BACKGROUND

The first hospital IC efforts in the United States began in the 1950s concurrent with the growth of intensive care and increasing staphylococcal infections.[1] IC programs extended into thousands of hospitals in the late 1960s and 1970s in response to urging from various organizations (e.g., American Hospital Association [AHA], Joint Commission on Accreditation of Healthcare Organizations [JCAHO], then the Joint Commission on Accreditation of Hospitals). In the decades since the 1970s, changes to these programs have occurred as a result of state and federal agencies, professional organizations, and scientific information published in journals. The modern concept of IC also includes areas other than healthcare-associated infections (HAI) (e.g., risk to employees, maintenance of the physical environment, and use of increasingly complex medical devices).[2]

IC professionals need to be alert to changing recommendations, scientific literature, and guidelines and make appropriate modifications to IC programs. In addition, local and state requirements must be followed. This chapter outlines the specific agencies and organizations that have a major impact on IC programs and the general issues to consider in the organization and function of IC programs.

II.   BASIC PRINCIPLES

American Hospital Association

The AHA's Advisory Committee on Infections within Hospitals published its first edition of *Infection Control in the Hospital* in 1968. The purpose of this manual was to describe the elements of an IC program that an AHA advisory committee "considers essential to the reduction and elimination of the human and economic wastage that results

Copyright © 2005, Association for Professionals in Infection Control and Epidemiology, Inc.

from our failure to prevent those nosocomial infections that are preventable . . . . "Three editions of the manual were printed, the last published in 1979.[3] The AHA affected IC practice through educational programs and conferences, journals and other publications, briefings, and consultants. The AHA dissolved its IC section in 1995 and began a collaboration with the Association for Professionals in Infection Control and Epidemiology (APIC) to meet the IC needs of AHA members.

Association for Professionals in Infection Control and Epidemiology

APIC was established in 1972 to provide education and science-based information to strengthen and improve the practice of IC. Its mission is to improve health and promote safety by reducing risks of infection and other adverse outcomes.

APIC's major influences on IC activities are its development of professional and practice and standards, education and training programs, a scientific journal, and governmental affairs activities. It established the Certification Board of Infection Control and Epidemiology in 1981 to administer an IC certification program. In 1993, the Research Foundation for Prevention of Complications Associated with Health Care was created to facilitate funding of priority-driven research projects.[2] APIC partnered with other professional organizations to produce two consensus documents outlining infrastructure requirements for IC programs in hospitals and nonhospital settings and a document defining practice and professional standards for the field.[4-6]

Centers for Disease Control and Prevention

In the 1960s, the Centers for Disease Control and Prevention (CDC) began recommending that hospitals conduct surveillance for the occurrence of nosocomial infections. Training programs in IC surveillance were started at the CDC in the early 1970s. The programs stressed surveillance for infections, developing and implementing policies for prevention of infections, and reducing wasteful activities (e.g., environmental culturing). Because of increasing training opportunities available in the United States, the CDC discontinued these programs in 1983.

The Division of Healthcare Quality Promotion (DHQP) of the National Center for Infectious Diseases is the CDC's focus for information, surveillance, investigation, prevention, and control of HAI. The division has set seven goals for the reduction of adverse outcomes:

1. Reduce catheter-associated adverse events by 50% among patients in healthcare settings.

2. Reduce targeted surgical adverse events by 50%.

3. Reduce hospitalizations and mortality from respiratory tract infections among long-term-care patients by 50%.

4. Reduce targeted antimicrobial-resistant bacterial infections by 50%.

5. Eliminate laboratory errors leading to adverse patient outcomes.

6. Eliminate occupational needlestick injuries among healthcare personnel.

7. Achieve 100% adherence to Advisory Committee on Immunization Practices guidelines for immunization of healthcare personnel.

In January 1970, the CDC began the National Nosocomial Infections Surveillance (NNIS) system. One purpose of this program is to monitor trends in nosocomial infection rates, pathogens, and antibiotic susceptibility patterns in the United States. National surveillance of hospital nosocomial infections is coordinated and analyzed by NNIS. The NNIS program publishes hospital nosocomial infection rate data. CDC is transitioning the NNIS program into a web-based knowledge system— the National Healthcare Safety Network (NHSN). The NHSN will also include the National Surveillance System for Healthcare Workers and the Dialysis Surveillance Network. The NHSN can be used by institutions in performance improvement activities.[7]

In 1974, the CDC initiated a study to determine the efficacy of IC activities in reducing the risks of nosocomial infections in hospitals, the Study on the Efficacy of Nosocomial Infection Control (SENIC) project. The SENIC project defined an infection surveillance and control program as one containing three main elements:

1. Epidemiological surveillance for the occurrence of infections in patients within the hospital

2. Formulation of policies and procedures to control infections based on data generated by surveillance and other sources

3. Personnel specially trained in hospital epidemiology to collect the surveillance data and coordinate intervention activities

The SENIC Project compared nosocomial infection rates that occurred in 1970 and 1976 in a stratified random sample of U.S. hospitals.[8] The project found that compared with hospitals that had no program activities, hospitals that established infection surveillance and control programs with a full-time-equivalent IC professional per 250 occupied beds, an effectual IC physician with special interest in IC, and a program for reporting wound infection rates to surgeons reduced

Copyright © 2005, Association for Professionals in Infection Control and Epidemiology, Inc.

their nosocomial infection rates by approximately 32%.[9]

The DHQP began a nosocomial infection guidelines and recommendation process in 1981. Several documents were developed for specific IC practices. This process was discontinued in the mid-1980s.

The Healthcare Infection Control Practices Advisory Committee (HICPAC) was established in 1991 to provide advice and guidance to the CDC and others regarding the practice of healthcare IC and strategies for surveillance, prevention, and control of HAI. The committee influences IC programs through its periodic updating of guidelines and other policy statements regarding prevention of HAIs. These guidelines are developed in partnership with various affiliated professional organizations.

Centers for Medicare and Medicaid Services

As part of CMS's required conditions for certification and participation in Medicare and Medicaid programs, healthcare facilities must comply with federal standards that include specific requirements for an active IC program.[10] A program to investigate, control, and prevent infections in long-term-care facilities accepting Medicare and Medicaid patients is mandated by CMS.[11]

Food and Drug Administration

The Food and Drug Administration (FDA) is responsible for implementing, monitoring, and enforcing standards for the safety, efficacy, and labeling of all drugs and biologicals for human use. Of particular interest to the IC team are its activities related to food, blood, medical devices (especially single-use devices), and antimicrobial products and chemical germicides used with medical devices.[1] The Environmental Protection Agency also is involved in testing and use of hospital germicide products.

Joint Commission on Accreditation of Healthcare Organizations

JCAHO started publishing minimal IC standards for hospitals in 1953. In 1976, IC programs became a specific requirement for accreditation by JCAHO.[1] JCAHO's standards for IC have been used by many institutions, including hospitals, long-term-care facilities, behavioral-health facilities, and home health agencies, to establish a framework for an IC program.

These standards have undergone many revisions over the years. In general, the standards state that the goal of the surveillance, prevention, and control of infection function is for the healthcare organization to identify and reduce the risks of infections in patients and healthcare workers (HCWs). There must be a func-tioning program, coordinating all activities related to the surveillance, prevention, and control of infections. The program should be doing the right things, doing these things well, be supported, and be focused toward improvement of processes and outcomes.[12,13] As part of its Shared Vision–New Pathways program begun in 2002, JCAHO began a project to review, revise, and coordinate all of its standards.[14] Revised Surveillance, Prevention, and Control of Infection standards become effective January 1, 2005.

National Institute for Occupational Safety and Health

NIOSH was established in 1970 and became part of the CDC in 1973. It is responsible for conducting laboratory and epidemiological research on occupational hazards.[15] Decisions regarding types of devices used for employee protection (e.g., respirators and sharps containers) are part of NIOSH's mandate.

Occupational Safety and Health Administration

OSHA began its IC activities in 1987 with the draft publication of bloodborne pathogens rules. These rules were finalized in 1991.[16] In 2001, a revision to the bloodborne pathogens rules was published to clarify issues related to sharps safety.[17] OSHA may enforce other IC issues (e.g., tuberculosis) under the General Duty Clause of the Occupational Safety and Health Act. OSHA standards focus on determining employees' health risks as the result of exposure to communicable diseases.

Society for Healthcare Epidemiology of America

SHEA was founded in 1980 to foster the development and application of the science of healthcare epidemiology.[18] The organization provides educational programs, develops position papers, and produces a scientific journal. SHEA cosponsors a training course in healthcare epidemiology with the CDC. SHEA was a partner in the development of two consensus documents outlining infrastructure requirements for IC programs.[4,5]

III. OVERALL STRUCTURE AND FUNCTION

Each institution is unique, and its specific needs must be considered when developing or reorganizing an IC program. Factors include size, case-mix, and types of care provided. The principal functions are generally similar, however, and include the following:[4,5]

Copyright © 2005, Association for Professionals in Infection Control and Epidemiology, Inc.

1. To obtain and manage critical data and information, including surveillance for infections

2. To develop and recommend policies and procedures

3. To intervene directly to prevent infections

4. To educate and train HCWs, patients, and nonmedical caregivers

Because of differing needs, there may be various groups, individuals, and functions within the organization that are responsible for the IC program. The following sections outline various persons and activities essential to an IC program.

Infection Control Team

Often the core of the IC program is the infection control practitioner (ICP), chair of the IC committee, and the healthcare epidemiologist. An individual responsible for employee health or administration also may be a part of the team. The team is responsible for carrying out all aspects of the IC program. There should be one person, however, who is designated as having responsibility for the program.[4,5] Team members must be qualified and guided by sound principles and current information.

A facility may have an infection control committee (ICC) that functions as the central decision-making and policy-making body for IC. The ICC chair reports either to the medical staff or to the administration. The ICC acts as the advocate for prevention and control of infections in the facility, formulates and monitors patient care policies, educates staff, and provides political support that empowers the team.[19]

The ICC must be multidisciplinary, composed of representatives from most departments. It should meet regularly, usually monthly or quarterly. Representation typically includes members of administration and clinical and ancillary staff. Because IC issues and measures often cross departmental lines, a multidisciplinary ICC is crucial.

The ICC often refines and ratifies the ideas of the IC team. Its members disseminate the information discussed in the meeting. The ICC gives political and administrative support to the IC program.[20]

An ICC is not required by JCAHO; however, some states do require an ICC. Institutions also may support a committee structure for the reasons outlined earlier. If a committee is not used, the IC team needs to develop other mechanisms (e.g., use of continuous quality improvement [CQI] models) to obtain multidisciplinary support for changes and actions. CQI models use a collaborative approach, including use of multidisciplinary teams. These teams meet regularly, usually

weekly or biweekly. Teams are responsible for planning, policy development, interventions, and decision-making. The team leader may be the IC professional.

Dissemination of IC information is a crucial component of an IC program. Surveillance data and policy decisions should be communicated throughout the organization. This communication may be accomplished through routine reports to clinicians or department heads and through various electronic methods.

Infectcion Control Professionals

The role of IC professionals includes numerous responsibilities, as follows:[4-6,21,22]

1. Collection and analysis of infection data

2. Evaluation of products and procedures

3. Development and review of policies

4. Consultation on infection risk assessment, prevention, and control strategies

5. Education efforts directed at interventions to reduce infection risks

6. Implementation of changes mandated by regulatory and licensing agencies

7. Application of epidemiological principles, including activities directed at improving patient outcomes

8. Provision of high-quality services in a cost-efficient manner

9. Participation in research projects

Some IC professionals work less than full-time on IC. They also may be involved in such areas as employee health, quality improvement, and risk management. In non–acute care facilities, IC professionals typically have multiple roles to fill and usually have only a few hours per week available to devote to IC activities.[23]

Many training courses exist for IC professionals. Local and national APIC organizations, SHEA, state organizations, academic institutions, and private firms offer training courses. Various courses are available for beginning and experienced individuals.

An IC professional's time is split among data management, policy and procedure development, education, employee health, quality improvement, consulting, and investigating potential outbreaks. They also may take part in research activities.[6] Task and job analyses have been performed to specify what the IC professional's day-to-day work may entail. The IC professional also may be involved in investigations related to adverse outcomes other than infections.[24,25] Certification for IC professionals is available through the Certification Board of Infection Control and Epidemiology (CBIC).

Copyright © 2005, Association for Professionals in Infection Control and Epidemiology, Inc.

There are two key IC professionals—the IC practitioner and the healthcare epidemiologist. The IC practitioner (ICP) predominately has such backgrounds as nursing, medical technology, microbiology, or public health.[26] Titles used by ICPs include *infection control nurse, infection control coordinator, nurse epidemiologist, infection control officer,* and *infection control practitioner.* The ICP role involves the daily collaborative efforts within all facets of healthcare,[27] and the ICP typically functions as a consultant, educator, role model, researcher, and change agent. Responsibilities include education, surveillance, prevention and control, and quality improvement.[6]

The healthcare epidemiologist may be the chair of the ICC or may occupy a separate position as either a technical advisor or a member of the committee. This person may be a physician with special training in healthcare epidemiology and IC; often the position is filled by an infectious diseases physician who works closely with the medical staff. Specific training courses in healthcare epidemiology are offered throughout the United States cosponsored by SHEA and the CDC.

Depending on the institution, IC professionals may report to administration, nursing or medical services, or quality improvement departments. Other reporting relationships also exist. In some institutions, IC is integrated with other departments (e.g., risk management, utilization management, or quality improvement).

Staffing

On the basis of pilot studies in eight community hospitals in which different staffing levels were evaluated, in 1969 the CDC recommended one full-time ICP for every 250 occupied beds.[28] The SENIC project strongly supported the 250-bed recommendation.[9] Because the CDC recommendation is more than 30 years old, staffing requirements may be outdated. This is especially true because there have been dramatically increased demands on the IC professional's time for surveillance, education, and consultation in addition to many changes in healthcare.

A more recent study compared staffing at University HealthSystem Consortium's hospitals using various parameters such as bed census, outpatient visits, intensive care unit beds, and personnel.[29,30] Another innovative method uses workload units to develop staffing requirements.[31] A point system for staffing was adopted by a working group of the Belgian Department of Health. The number of IC professionals is based on the number of points obtained by multiplying the number of beds of each patient-care unit by a factor that is specific for the patient population treated in the unit.[32] Some innovative methods have been designed to extend the reach of an IC professional

through computers,[33,34] nurse-advisors,[35] unit-based programs,[36] liaisons,[37] and clerical positions.[38]

APIC initiated a Delphi project on staffing that was published in 2002.[39] It noted that staffing recommendations must consider the number of occupied beds, scope of the program, complexity of the healthcare facility, characteristics of the patient population, and unique needs of the facility. This study recommends a ratio of 0.8 to 1.0 ICP for every 100 occupied acute care beds.

IV. DOCUMENTING IMPACT OF HEALTHCARE-ASSOCIATED INFECTIONS ON OUTCOMES AND COSTS

The SENIC project found that one third of nosocomial infections could be prevented by effective IC programs, including surveillance and practice activities. In addition, prevention of approximately 6% of HAIs offset the cost of a program in a 250-bed hospital.[9]

Part of a program's effectiveness is a reflection of the influence of IC professionals. They must be visible, provide a resource for staff, and use their scientific expertise when making specific recommendations. Effectiveness also depends on commitment to IC by administration.[40]

Decision analysis can be used to compare costs with outcomes.[41] Cost-effectiveness studies and cost-benefit studies are examples of decision analysis. *Effectiveness* refers to the outcome of care. It can be expressed as the number of cases of disease prevented, the number of lives saved, or the number of life-years saved. Cost-benefit analysis looks at outcome in terms of cost. Benefits other than direct costs also are important in evaluating the impact of infection prevention activities. These include decreasing malpractice claims, protecting employees from injury, assisting in patient safety efforts, and enhancing the organization's image.[42]

Various methods can be used to estimate how much HAIs cost an institution. The cost of the IC program itself consists of salaries, employee benefits, education, and commodity expenses. Cost-benefit estimates also can be developed for mortality and morbidity in patients. A crude estimate of cost can be obtained by multiplying the estimated numbers of HAIs at various sites by the site-specific cost weights (cost per infection) derived from the SENIC project and adjusted for time. Other methods use actual cost weights or costs determined through prospective, randomized studies. Prevalence surveys also can be used to assess the costs of HAIs.[43-46]

Copyright © 2005, Association for Professionals in Infection Control and Epidemiology, Inc.

It is important to outline the cost-benefit of an IC program.[47] Targeted surveillance should be tied to specific interventions to decrease HAIs. Appropriate interventions to decrease infections will then result in documentation of cost savings.

V.   INFLUENCING PRACTICE

Characteristics of the Organization

The ability of the IC program to influence practices that affect quality patient care depends on certain characteristics of the patient population and patients' risk of infection and characteristics of personnel. These characteristics include number of beds, professional school affiliation, geography, volume of patient encounters, patient population served, clinical focus, numbers of employees, and administrative philosophy. It is important to understand these characteristics when developing a program to meet optimally the IC needs of the organization and the patients it serves.

The IC program influences practice through direct actions (e.g., review and evaluation of products, policy and procedure review and development, and observations). Training and education of staff can assist in skill development and increase employees' knowledge base.[48]

Written IC policies are often developed that relate to staff and patient-care practices, construction/renovation, employee health, and sterilization/disinfection. General policies are applicable to staff in the whole facility. These policies may form the basis of an IC manual. Specific policies may be developed for each unit or area. These policies must be supported scientifically and address IC needs for the institution.

Providers of direct patient care must implement these policies consistently to benefit patients and protect staff. IC professionals usually attempt to affect patient care outcomes by influencing these practices of patient care and other healthcare personnel. Teaching personnel to increase their knowledge and skills of appropriate infection prevention practices is one method to influence quality patient care and protection of employees. Education of staff is crucial to the success of any IC program.

Patient Safety

IC personnel play a crucial role in preventing infections and other adverse events.[1,49,50] Because of their expertise in epidemiological methods, ICPs can support IC, quality improvement, and adverse health event reduction programs.[49] IC professionals can use basic healthcare epidemiology (e.g., surveillance, outbreak investigation, and special studies) and other quality improvement tools (e.g., root cause analysis) to improve patient safety.

Administrative Support

It is important that the administrative leaders of the organization approve and support its IC activities. IC professionals should schedule regular meetings with the administrator to whom they are responsible. This practice helps to maintain liaison between the program and administration and increase the awareness of the institution's leaders of IC program activities.

VI.   QUALITY OF AN INFECTION CONTROL AND PREVENTION PROGRAM

Every year, goals and objectives for the IC program should be determined. These should be based on the institution's strategic goals and on institutional data and findings from the previous year's activities. IC resources and data systems need should be evaluated in the context of these goals and objectives.

An annual evaluation of the IC program is important to outline achievements and activities of the program and to describe support requirements. The value of the IC program to the organization should be emphasized, along with patient outcomes and cost savings. This evaluation report should be widely disseminated to leaders throughout the organization, in particular to the chief executive officer, chief medical and nursing executive, and board members.

Another method to explain the importance of the program to others is through a mission statement, a description of the vision for the program, and an outline of core values. These governing ideas answer three critical questions: What? Why? How?

1. *Vision* is the *what*—the picture of the desired future of the IC program. A vision needs to focus on the IC program's strategic advantage in the organization.[51]

2. *Mission* is the *why*—the answer to the question, "Why does the IC program exist?" The mission helps to communicate the purpose of the program and sets general parameters for accomplishing its goals.[52] A mission statement defines the common purpose, focus, and context for all departmental activities. Mission statements enable a group to know what is and is not within their jurisdiction and understand where they fit in the organization's overall improvement efforts.[53] The IC mission must support the overall institutional mission.

3. *Core values* are the *what*—they answer the question, "How does the IC program want to act, consis-

Copyright © 2005, Association for Professionals in Infection Control and Epidemiology, Inc.

tent with our mission, along the path toward achieving our vision?" Values describe how the program functions on a day-to-day basis.[54]

Customer Identification

A customer is anyone to whom the IC program provides service. A customer is defined more broadly than a patient. Internal customers of IC professionals may include nurses, physicians, administrators, technologists, and ancillary staff. External customers may include IC staff at other institutions, health department staff, and regulatory agency personnel. It is important that IC professionals know what is expected of them by the people they serve. IC professionals usually are able to negotiate changes in requirements of internal customers if those requested are unrealistic. Every work process should be studied and constantly improved so that the final product or service exceeds customer expectations.[51,55,56]

Multidisciplinary Activities

Major gains in quality and productivity most often result from collaborative teams—a group of people pooling their skills, talents, and knowledge to achieve a common goal. Teams identify processes or problems needing improvement and work together to find solutions. Teams developed to work on IC issues should include individuals from multiple functional areas integral to the specific issue being studied. Flowcharting the process is one way to determine which areas should be involved in the team.[53,57]

Epidemiological Method

IC professionals must be able to demonstrate their ability to apply the epidemiological method and must be familiar with basic statistical techniques. Using epidemiological principles, data can be analyzed for trends, assist in solving problems, and evaluate processes. The application of epidemiological tools and principles to the problems of HAIs is strongly connected to the quality improvement concept of using dependable data to improve processes.[58]

Performance Improvement

IC professionals have been active in various quality aspects of medical care since the 1960s; the IC program is an essential component of quality patient care. The IC program must be coordinated with the facility's process for assessing and improving organizational performance.[59-62]

Quality improvement provides the means for tracking and identifying clinical problems and providing information to clinicians that helps determine opportunities for

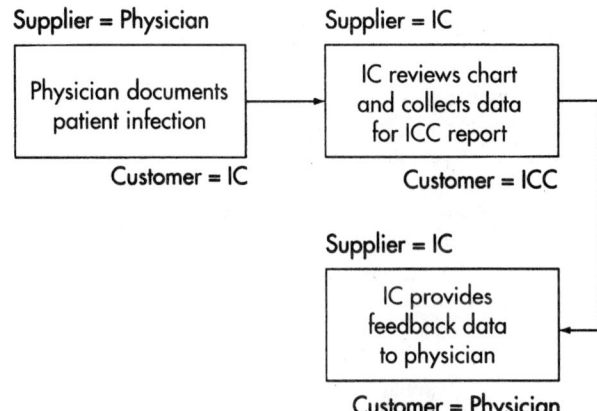

Figure 1–1 Two types of variation in processes.

improvement in patient care. There should be an ongoing study of ways to improve prevention and control processes to reduce HAI rates to the lowest possible levels. It is important to incorporate the principles of continuous quality improvement in the IC program. These methods include root cause analysis, human factors research, hazards analysis, and economic assessment. Likewise, the core activities in IC are tools with broad applicability to healthcare quality. These include cluster and outbreak investigations, case-control studies, surveillance, and efficacy and effectiveness studies.[63-68]

Variation is inherent in healthcare practices and outcomes. There are two types of variation in processes (see Figure 1–1). An unexpected, significant deviation outside predicted control limits is considered to represent a special cause of variation. Special causes tend to cluster by person, place, and time (i.e., epidemiological). Special-cause variation represents changes that can be investigated and assigned to an identifiable source.[56,58] IC has routinely examined special causes; however, common causes also must be evaluated to make improvement in infection rates.

Common-cause variation results from chance events that occur without a specific cause and from the inherent design of the process. Rates of specific processes and outcomes (e.g., HAIs) fluctuate within statistically predictable bounds over time. The success of improvements can be ascertained by determining whether they improve the rate of a process or outcome significantly compared with the predicted rate based on previous experience.[69]

Outcomes and processes should be evaluated—outcomes to understand the results and processes to understand what has been done to cause those results. Performance measurement data can be used to

---

Copyright © 2005, Association for Professionals in Infection Control and Epidemiology, Inc.

improve processes and to verify the effectiveness of actions and improvement initiatives.[70-73]

Processes can be categorized as clinical, structural, or decision-making.[62] Clinical processes are processes that directly influence patient care, such as skin care and intravascular practices. Structural processes involve the environment, such as needle disposal systems or regulated medical waste management. Decision-making processes involve various departments and issues, such as implementation of standard precautions. Controlled trials to determine efficacy in reducing rates of infections are of interest to the IC team. An example of this type of study showed the efficacy of proper timing of perioperative antibiotics.[74]

VII. SET PRIORITIES FOR INFECTION CONTROL AND PREVENTION PROGRAMS

Setting priorities helps focus on appropriate allocation of IC program resources. Realistic strategies for surveillance and intervention should be developed. Steps to use in this process include the following:[75]

1. Establishing a reliable, focused surveillance program

2. Streamlining data management activities

3. Analyzing HAI rates

4. Aiming for a benchmark

5. Educating staff regarding prevention techniques

6. Identifying opportunities for performance improvement

7. Taking a leadership role on performance improvement teams

8. Developing and implementing action plans that outline the steps needed to accomplish each objective[76,77]

The quality of the IC program should be assessed routinely by evaluating customer satisfaction,[78] appropriateness, efficacy, timeliness, availability, effectiveness, and efficiency.

REFERENCES

1. McDonald LL: Health policy for infection control and epidemiology in critical care, *Crit Care Nurs Clin* 7:727–732, 1995.
2. Lynch P, Jackson M, Saint S: Research Priorities Project, year 2000: establishing a direction for infection control and hospital epidemiology, *Am J Infect Control* 29:73–78, 2001.
3. American Hospital Association: *Infection control in the hospital,* Chicago, 1979, American Hospital Association.
4. Scheckler WE, Brimhall D, Buck AS, et al: Requirements for infrastructure and essential activities of infection control and epidemiology in hospitals: a consensus panel report, *Am J Infect Control* 26:47–60, 1998.
5. Friedman C, Barnette M, Buck AS, et al: Requirements for infrastructure and essential activities of infection control and epide-
miology in out-of-hospital settings: a consensus panel report, *Am J Infect Control* 27:418–430, 1999.
6. APIC/CHICA-Canada Professional and Practice Standards Task Force: APIC/CHICA-Canada infection control and epidemiology: professional and practice standards, *Am J Infect Control* 27:47–51, 1999.
7. National Nosocomial Infections Surveillance (NNIS) System Report: data summary from January 1992 to June 2003, issued August 2003, *Am J Infect Control* 31:481–498, 2003.
8. Haley RW, Quade D, Freeman HE, et al: Study on the efficacy of nosocomial infection control (SENIC Project): summary of study design, *Am J Epidemiol* 111:472–485, 1980.
9. Haley RW, Culver DH, White JW, et al: The efficacy of infection surveillance and control programs in preventing nosocomial infections in US hospitals, *Am J Epidemiol* 121:182–205, 1985.
10. Conditions of Participation for Hospitals: *CMS, Code of Federal Regulations 42CFR482, 2000*; available online: *http://www.access.gpo.gov/nara/cfr/waisidx_04/42cfr482_04.html.*
11. Requirements for long-term care facilities, CMS. Code of Federal Regulations 42CFR483, 2003.
12. Joint Commission on Accreditation of Healthcare Organizations: Standards: surveillance, prevention and control of infection. In JCAHO: *2004 hospital accreditation standards,* Chicago, 2003, Joint Commission on Accreditation of Healthcare Organizations.
13. Kobs A: Infection control, *Nurs Manage* 28:17–19, 1997.
14. Shared visions—new pathways, *Perspectives* 22:1–15, 2002.
15. Request for comment on the proposed NIOSH document on guidelines for protecting the safety and health of health care workers, *Fed Reg* 61:66281–66282, 1996.
16. Department of Labor, Occupational Safety and Health Administration: Occupational exposure to bloodborne pathogens: final rule, *Fed Reg* 56:64004–64182, 1991.
17. Occupational Exposure to Bloodborne Pathogens: Needlestick and other sharps injuries: final rule, *Fed Reg* 66:5317–5325, 2001.
18. Larson E: A retrospective on infection control: Part 2: twentieth century—the flame burns, *Am J Infect Control* 25:340–349, 1997.
19. Wiblin RT, Wenzel RP: The infection control committee, *Infect Control Hosp Epidemiol* 17:44–46, 1996.
20. Wenzel RP: Leadership and management for health-care epidemiology. In Wenzel RP, editor: *Prevention and control of nosocomial infections,* ed 4, Philadelphia, 2003, Lippincott Williams & Wilkins, pp 609–618.
21. Schollenberger D: The infection control forum: where do we go from here? *Asepsis* 12:11, 1990.
22. Osguthorpe SG, Ormond L: Management constraints in infection control, *Crit Care Nurs Clin* 7:703–712, 1995.
23. Smith PW, Rusnak PG: Infection prevention and control in the long-term care facility, *Am J Infect Control* 25:488–512, 1997.
24. Goldrick BA, Dingle DA, Gilmore GK, et al: Practice analysis for infection control and epidemiology in the new millennium, *Am J Infect Control* 30:437–448, 2002.
25. Rhinehart E: Watching the bottom line: Enhancing the role and impact of infection control in a managed care environment, *Am J Infect Control* 28:25–29, 2000.
26. Jackson MM, Soule BM, Tweeten SS: APIC strategic planning member survey, 1997, *Am J Infect Control* 26:113–125, 1998.
27. The role of the infection control practitioner, *Can J Infect Control* 11:36–37, 1996.
28. Eickhoff TC, Brachman PS, Bennett JV, et al: Surveillance of nosocomial infections in community hospitals: I. surveillance methods, effectiveness, and initial results, *J Infect Dis* 120:305–317, 1969.
29. Friedman C, Chenoweth C: A survey of infection control professionals staffing patterns at University HealthSystem Consortium institutions, *Am J Infect Control* 26:239–244, 1998.
30. Friedman C, Chenoweth C: Infection control staffing patterns, *Am J Infect Control* 29:130–132, 2001.
31. Kuwaki-Chuman I, Becker L, Hardy, MJ, et al: Development and application of infection control workload unit tool to determine staffing needs, *Am J Infect Control* 22:117, 1993.
32. Reybrouck G: Scoring system suggested to determine staffing level, *Am J Infect Control* 14:148, 1986.
33. Wenzel RP, Streed SA: Surveillance and use of computers in hospital infection control, *J Hosp Infect* 13:217–229, 1989.

Copyright © 2005, Association for Professionals in Infection Control and Epidemiology, Inc.

34. Gransden WR: Information, computers and infection control, *J Hosp Infect* 15:1–5, 1990.

35. Amundsen J, Drennan DP: An infection control nurse-advisor program, *Am J Infect Control* 11:20–23, 1983.

36. Colletti MA, Kasey C, Fellencer C: Unit-based infection control: it makes a difference, *Am J Infect Control* 15:32A-34A, 1987.

37. Ross KA: A program for infection surveillance utilizing an infection control liaison nurse, *Am J Infect Control* 10:24–28, 1982.

38. Haim L, Booth JH, Greaney K: Recommendations for optimizing an infection control practitioner's effectiveness in an ambulatory care setting, *J Health Care Q* 16:31–34, 1994.

39. O'Boyle C, Jackson M, Henly SJ: Staffing requirements for infection control programs in US health care facilities: Delphi project, *Am J Infect Control* 30:321–333, 2002.

40. Mehtar S: Infection control programmes—are they cost-effective? *J Hosp Infect* 30:26–34, 1995.

41. Nettleman MD: Cost and cost benefit of infection control. In Wenzel RP, editor. *Prevention and control of nosocomial infections,* ed 4, Philadelphia, 2003, Lippincott Williams & Wilkins, pp 33–41.

42. Dunagan WC, Murphy DM, Hollenbeak CS, et al: Making the business case for infection control: pitfalls and opportunities, *Am J Infect Control* 30:86–92, 2002.

43. Wenzel RP: The economics of nosocomial infections, *J Hosp Infect* 31:79–87, 1995.

44. Haley RW: *Managing hospital infection control for cost-effectiveness,* Chicago, 1986, American Hospital Association.

45. Wakefield DS, Pfaller MA, Hammons GT, et al: Use of the appropriate evaluation protocol for estimating the incremental costs associated with nosocomial infections, *Med Care* 25:481–488, 1987.

46. French GL, Cheng AFB: Measurement of the costs of hospital infection by prevalence surveys, *J Hosp Infect* 18(Suppl A): 65–72, 1991.

47. Fraser VJ, Olsen MA: The business of health care epidemiology: creating a vision for service excellence, *Am J Infect Control* 30: 77–85, 2002.

48. Haley RW: The development of infection surveillance and control programs. In Bennett JV, Brachman JS, editors: *Hospital infections,* ed 4, Philadelphia, 1998, Lippincott-Raven Publishers.

49. Jarvis WR: Infection control and changing health-care delivery systems, *Emerg Infect Dis* 7:170–173, 2001.

50. Burke JP: Infection control—a problem for patient safety, *N Engl J Med* 348:651–656, 2003.

51. Belasco JA: *Teaching the elephant to dance: the manager's guide to empowering change,* New York, 1991, Crown Publishers, pp 99–103.

52. Soule BM: From vision to reality: strategic agility in complex times, *Am J Infect Control* 30:107–119, 2002.

53. Scholtes PR: *The team handbook: how to use teams to improve quality,* Madison, WI, 1988, Joiner Associates.

54. Senge PM: *The fifth discipline: the art and practice of the learning organization,* New York, 1990, Doubleday, pp 223–235.

55. Marszalek-Gaucher E, Coffey RJ: *Transforming healthcare organizations: how to achieve and sustain organizational excellence,* San Francisco, 1990, Jossey-Bass, p 85.

56. Gabor A: *The man who discovered quality,* New York, 1990, Random House, p 82.

57. Vander Hyde K, Friedman C: Using a quality improvement team for determining strategies to reduce body substance exposures, *Am J Infect Control* 22:108, 1994.

58. Brewer JH, Gasser CS: The affinity between continuous quality improvement and epidemic surveillance, *Infect Control Hosp Epidemiol* 14:95, 1993.

59. Nystrom B: The role of hospital infection control in the quality system of hospitals, *J Hosp Infect* 21:169–177, 1992.

60. Post BA, Kreutzer-Baraglia L: Infection control. In Spicer JG, Robinson MA, editors: *Managing the environment in critical care nursing,* Baltimore, 1990, Williams & Wilkins, p 42.

61. Johnson J, Bonadonna L, Webster B: Integrating infection control practices into unit-based quality improvement, *Am J Infect Control* 21:106, 1993.

62. Atkins PM: Reducing risks through quality improvement, infection control, and risk management, *Crit Care Nurs Clin* 7:733–741, 1995.

63. Donabedian A: Contributions of epidemiology to quality assessment and monitoring, *Infect Control Hosp Epidemiol* 11: 117–121, 1990.

64. Karanfil L, Josephson A, Alonzo H: An infection control quality improvement (QI) approach to nosocomial bacteremia in neonates, *Am J Infect Control* 19:108, 1991.

65. Kelleghan S, Salemi C, Padilla S, et al: An effective quality improvement program for prevention of nosocomial ventilator pneumonia, *Am J Infect Control* 19:122, 1991.

66. McKenzie M, Taylor G: Infection control in an environment of continuous quality improvement, *Am J Infect Control* 20:96, 1992.

67. Cook JD, Lewis L, Thomassen K: Using total quality management to achieve proper isolation, *Am J Infect Control* 22:123, 1994.

68. Gerberding JL: Health-care quality promotion through infection prevention: beyond 2000, *Emerg Infect Dis* 7:363–366, 2001.

69. Kritchevsky SB, Simmons BP: Continuous quality improvement, *JAMA* 266:1817–1823, 1991.

70. Joint Commission on Accreditation of Healthcare Organizations: Standards: improving organizational performance. In JCAHO: *2004 hospital accreditation standards,* Chicago, 2003, Joint Commission on Accreditation of Healthcare Organizations.

71. Friedman C, Richter D, Skylis T, et al: Process surveillance: auditing infection control policies and procedures, *Am J Infect Control* 12:228–232, 1984.

72. Baker OG: Process surveillance: an epidemiologic challenge for all health care organizations, *Am J Infect Control* 25:96–101, 1997.

73. Nadzam DM, Loeb JM: Measuring and improving the performance of health care providers: accreditation in the 21st century, *Am J Infect Control* 26:126–135, 1998.

74. Classen DC, Evans RS, Pestotnik SL, et al: The timing of prophylactic administration of antibiotics and the risk of surgical-wound infection, *N Engl J Med* 326:281–286, 1992.

75. Murphy DM: From expert data collectors to interventionists: changing the focus of infection control professionals, *Am J Infect Control* 30:120–132, 2002.

76. Bennett G, Baker O: Developing an integrated quality improvement program, *Am J Infect Control* 18:118–125, 1990.

77. Haley RW: Surveillance by objective: a new priority-directed approach to the control of nosocomial infections, *Am J Infect Control* 13:78–89, 1985.

78. Friedman C, Baker CA, Mowry-Hanley, et al: Use of the total quality process in an infection control program: a surprising customer-needs assessment, *Am J Infect Control* 21:155–159, 1993.

SUPPLEMENTAL RESOURCES

Farr BM: Organization of infection control programs. In Abrutyn E, Goldmann DA, Scheckler WE, editors: *Saunders infection control reference service,* ed 2, Philadelphia, 2001, WB Saunders, pp 13–21.

Friedman C, et al: Requirement for infrastructure and essential activities of infection control and epidemiology in out-of-hospital settings: A Concensus Panel report. *Am J Infect Control* 27:418–430.

Friedman C, Chenoweth C: Infection control. In Schmele JA, editor. *Quality management in nursing and health care,* Albany, NY, 1996, Delmar Publishers, pp 507–519.

Garner JS: The CDC Hospital Infection Control Practices Advisory Committee, *Am J Infect Control* 21:160–162, 1993.

Haley RW: The development of infection surveillance and control programs. In Bennett JV, Brachman PS, editors: *Hospital infections,* ed 4. Philadelphia, 1998, Lippincott-Raven, pp 53–64.

Horan-Murphy E, et al: APIC/CHICA-Canada infection control and epidemiology: Professional and practice standards. *Am J Infect Control* 27:47–51

Jackson MM: Infection prevention and control in the managed care era: dinosaur, dragon, or dark horse? *Am J Infect Control* 25: 38–43, 1997.

Mehtar S: *Hospital infection control: setting up with minimal resources,* London, 1992, Oxford University Press.

Copyright © 2005, Association for Professionals in Infection Control and Epidemiology, Inc.

Mehtar S: How to cost and fund an infection control programme, *J Hosp Infect* 25:57–69, 1993.

O'Boyle C: The expanded role of the nurse in hospital epidemiology. In Wenzel RP, editor: *Prevention and control of nosocomial infections,* ed 4, Philadelphia, 2003, Lippincott Williams & Wilkins, pp 55–65.

Organizing for infection control in home care. In Rhinehart E, Friedman MM, editors: *Infection control in home care,* Gaithersburg, MD, 1999, Aspen Publishers, pp 171–176.

Organizing for infection prevention, surveillance, and control. In Friedman C, Petersen KH, editors: *Infection control in ambulatory care,* Sudbury, MA, 2004, Jones & Bartlett, pp 189–191.

Pugliese G, Kroc KA: Development and implementation of infection control policies and procedures. In Mayhall CG, editor: *Hospital epidemiology and infection control,* Baltimore, 1996, Williams & Wilkins, pp 1068–1079.

Scheckler WE, et al: Requirements for Infrastructure and essential activities of infection control and epidemiology in hospitals: A Consensus Panel report. *Am J Infect Control* 28:47–60.

Selwyn S: Hospital infection: the first 2500 years, *J Hosp Infect* 18(Suppl A):5–64, 1991.

Wenzel RP, Pfaller MA: Feasible and desirable future targets for reducing the costs of hospital infections, *J Hosp Infect* 18(Suppl A): 94–98, 1991.

WEB BASED RESOURCES

Association for Professionals in Infection Control and Epidemiology (APIC): *www.apic.org*

Center for Disease Control and Prevention (CDC): *www.cdc.gov*

Joint Commission on Accreditation of Healthcare Organizations (JCAHO): *www.jcaho.org*

Copyright © 2005, Association for Professionals in Infection Control and Epidemiology, Inc.

General Principles of Epidemiology

Samantha M. Tweeten, PhD, MPH
Graduate School of Public Health
San Diego State University
San Diego, California

ABSTRACT

Epidemiology, the study of the frequency, distribution, cause, and control of disease in populations, forms the basis of all health-related studies. It provides the background for interventions to reduce transmission of infecting organisms, reduce the number of nosocomial infections, and protect healthcare providers from infection. Understanding the relationships of host, environment, and organism will aid the infection control professional (ICP) in designing studies to determine the cause of nosocomial infections and design interventions.

KEY CONCEPTS

- Chain of infection
- Study design
- Koch's postulates
- Primary, secondary, tertiary prevention
- Association
- Causation
- Hill's criteria
- Data presentation

I. BACKGROUND

The purpose of this chapter is to provide information about the epidemiological principles and methods used in the practice of infection surveillance, prevention, and control, and that they are an important part of the discipline also known as epidemiology.

The infectious disease process is a set of complex interrelationships of agent, host, and environment that has been studied by epidemiologists for well over a century. One goal of epidemiology is to understand the natural history of diseases and conditions to develop strategies for their prevention and control. Three closely interrelated components—distribution, determinants, and frequency—are integral to the principles and methods of epidemiology. By becoming familiar with these concepts, the ICP will begin to develop and expand a knowledge base for interpreting data gathered within and outside the healthcare facility, and for understanding the associations between risk factors and infection in different settings and how these findings can be used to reduce

Copyright © 2005, Association for Professionals in Infection Control and Epidemiology, Inc.

infection risks for patients and healthcare workers. The bibliography cited at the end of this chapter reflects the breadth and depth of the discipline.

Epidemiology as a discipline incorporates the use of statistics to determine associations and test hypotheses. Examples used to explain formulas and calculations are drawn from familiar settings, yet the ICP with little or no background in statistics is not expected to master the materials in this chapter without additional study. An expanded discussion about the statistics used in epidemiology is beyond the scope of this chapter.

Although information is provided about the theoretical basis for epidemiology and statistics, the principal goal of this chapter is to present practical information that will allow the ICP to use epidemiological skills in day-to-day practice. Following completion of this chapter, it is hoped that the learner will have a better understanding of nosocomial infections within the total discipline of epidemiology and how principles of epidemiology can be applied to many practice issues.

II. BASIC PRINCIPLES

Epidemiology is the study of the distribution and determinants of disease and other conditions in human populations; both a body of knowledge and a method of study. Epidemiology encompasses the study of many factors that are detrimental to human health, including infectious diseases; chronic diseases, such as cancer or heart disease; drug or alcohol abuse and their sequelae; violence; injury; and others.

Epidemiology, unlike clinical medicine, is population-based and is useful for describing health-related phenomena in groups of people. Epidemiological methods are used in the measurement of a disease and its determinants and its distribution in a particular population in question before, during, and after an intervention. Therefore, epidemiology can be used in determining whether there is a problem in a population, risk factors for a disease, and whether there has been a change in disease outcome after an intervention. Although epidemiology studies groups of people rather than an individual patient, its principles are used widely in all areas of healthcare. Epidemiology provides information for community and preventive medicine, analysis of health assessments, safety programs, utilization review and management of resources, and health planning and forecasting. As an applied science, epidemiology is a professional discipline that encompasses all academic fields of study.

The primary purpose of epidemiology is to aid in the understanding of the cause of a disease by knowing its distribution, its determinants in terms of person, place, and time, and its natural history. This information is also used in epidemiology to plan and to evaluate inter-

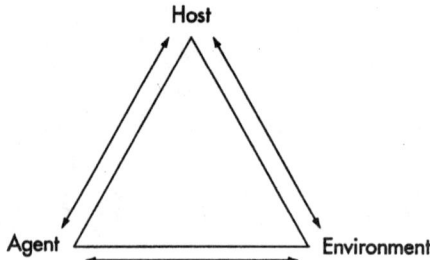

Figure 2–1 Epidemiologic triangle model of disease causation.

ventions and prevention efforts more effectively. To this end, several approaches, or methodologies, are used in obtaining epidemiological information. These include observational studies, in which the natural course of events is observed; and experimental studies, in which the investigator actively intervenes to modify one or more factors. Observational studies may be either descriptive, in which events are described in terms of person, place, or time; or they may be analytical, in which risk factors and trends are observed and compared. These methodologies will be described in greater detail later.

To understand the interactions between risk factors and the development of disease, it is first important to understand the elements that cause disease. The "epidemiological triangle" model of disease (see Fig. 2–1) consists of three elements: host, agent, and environment. The host is the human, whereas the environment consists of all external factors associated with the host. The agent may be a bacteria, virus, fungus, protozoan, helminth, or prion. In this model of dynamic interaction, change in any component alters the existing equilibrium. Change may increase or decrease the frequency of disease. Although this model is particularly useful in the study of infectious diseases, it is also applicable to other conditions.

The "wheel" model (see Fig. 2–2) consists of a hub (the host or human) with an inner core of genetic

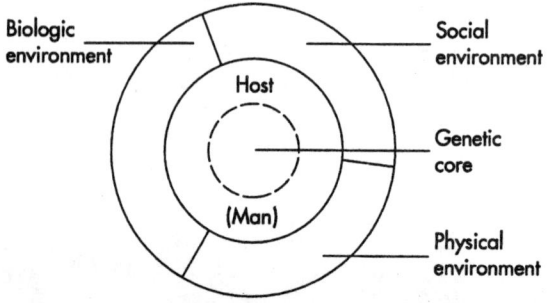

Figure 2–2 "Wheel" model of disease causation.

APIC Text of Infection Control and Epidemiology

Copyright © 2005, Association for Professionals in Infection Control and Epidemiology, Inc.

information. The environment surrounding the host is divided into three parts: physical, biological, and social. The size of each component is related to the disease process under consideration. For example, the genetic core is large for hereditary disease, small for childhood viral diseases. The emphasis in this model is not the agent per se but on the interaction between the host and the environment and the agent and the environment.

Association and Causation

Association occurs if, as one variable changes, there is a concomitant or resultant change in the quantity or quality of another variable. When a statistical association between a factor and a disease has been demonstrated, it may be of three types: artifactual (or spurious), indirect or noncausal, or causal. Artifactual associations are false associations that occur because of error in study design or analysis. A certain number of associations will simply occur by chance, with the number of associations rising as a greater number of factors or variables are studied. This is known as *random error*. Artifactual associations may also be caused by bias in study methods. *Bias* is systematic error and may occur in information gathering when one fails to measure what is thought to be measured. This may result from instrument, observer, or data collection method biases. Classification, or *selection*, bias occurs when an error is made in the classification or selection of cases or controls and results in noncomparability of groups under study. Failure to control for confounding variables in the study design or analysis may also result in artifactual associations. Bias and random error may also result in no association being seen when one actually exists.

Indirect or noncausal associations may result from the mixing of effects between the exposure, the disease and a third factor, or confounding variable, that may be associated with the exposure and independently affect the outcome of interest. Confounding can lead to the assumption that there are differences that do not really exist or to the observation that there is no difference when one truly exists. Causal associations exist whenever evidence indicates that one factor is clearly shown to increase the probability of the occurrence of a disease. In a causal relationship, the reduction, or diminution, of a factor decreases the frequency of the disease being studied. This should not be confused with causality, which requires a number of conditions to be met, one of which is the presence of causal associations.

The scientific criteria for disease causation have their roots in Koch's postulates (Robert Koch, 1843–1910). Koch's postulates consist of four points:

1. The organism must always be found with the disease, in accordance with the clinical stage observed.

2. The organism must then be grown up in pure culture from a diseased host.

3. The same disease must be reproduced when a pure culture of the organism is inoculated into a healthy susceptible host.

4. The organism must then be recovered from the experimentally infected host.

These postulates were originally accepted as an attempt to establish a causal relationship between microorganisms and disease processes. Although historically significant, as we have learned more about disease causation, it has become apparent that Koch's postulates cannot always be fulfilled (e.g., multicausal diseases, chronic diseases, some viral diseases). Koch himself accepted that not all of his criteria would be met in each case.

The currently used criteria for causality were developed by Austin Bradford Hill (1897–1991) and are known as Hill's criteria. These criteria use modern epidemiological methods to determine whether a factor is causal for a given disease and are listed in Table 2–1. These criteria are equally applicable to infectious and noninfectious diseases.

1. *Strength* of association is the first criterion: The incidence of disease should be higher in those who are exposed to the factor under consideration than in those who are not exposed; that is, the stronger the association between an exposure and a disease, the more likely the exposure is to be causal. For example, lung cancer is common in those who smoke.

2. *Consistency* means that the association should be observed in numerous studies, preferably by different researchers using different research methodologies. If the association is particular to one factor and to one disease, the relationship is said to be

Table 2-1. Hill's Criteria for Causation

Strength
Consistency
Specificity
Temporality
Biological gradient
Plausibility
Coherence
Experiment
Analogy

General Principles of Epidemiology

Copyright © 2005, Association for Professionals in Infection Control and Epidemiology, Inc.

specific, and the association is more likely to be causal. This criterion also refers to the extent to which the occurrence of one factor can be used to predict the occurrence of another (disease). In reality, such a one-to-one relationship is rare due to the multifactorial causes of most diseases and because, sometimes, the same factor(s) can cause more than one disease.

3. *Temporality* must also be addressed when determining cause of disease. Essentially, exposure to the hypothesized causal factor must precede the onset of disease. The *biological gradient* is a dose-response relationship between increased exposure to a factor and increased likelihood of disease. For example, the longer one smokes, the more likely one is to develop lung cancer. If the association demonstrates a biological gradient between the factor (exposure) and effect (disease), the relationship is more likely to be causal. The association in question should also be *biologically plausible* in light of current knowledge. This criterion may be the most elusive and variable of the nine. Because biological knowledge is ever expanding, lack of biological plausibility does not necessarily disprove a theoretical association.

4. In addition, the association should be in accordance with other facts known about the natural history of the disease; that is, there should be *coherence* between known information about the biological spectrum of the disease and the associated factor.

5. Associations derived from *experiments* add considerable weight to evidence supporting causal associations. These experiments can be animal model studies or clinical trials; however, although animal models may be helpful, many diseases do not manifest the same way in animals and humans.

6. Finally, if similar associations have been shown to be causal, by *analogy* the association is more likely to be causal. Determining causality may also help to determine at which points the natural history of a disease may be interrupted, so that prevention and control efforts are effective. It can also add information on the natural history of a disease.

The association between *Shigella sonnei* and gastroenteritis provides an example of applying Hill's criteria to an infectious disease. Strength is demonstrated by disease occurrence among those exposed to the organism. The association between ingestion of *S. sonnei* and gastroenteritis has been demonstrated consistently in numerous studies by different investigators, and results specifically in gastroenteritis, although this may not be true 100% of the time. Temporality is demonstrated because exposure to the organism precedes development of gastroenteritis and occurs within the

correct incubation period. The biological gradient is evident because larger doses of *S. sonnei* are more likely to result in disease. *S. sonnei* is a biologically plausible cause of gastroenteritis, based on knowledge of its toxin production, and disease caused by *S. sonnei* is coherent with other facts known about gastroenteritis. Additionally, experiments have shown that *S. sonnei* causes gastroenteritis and that other species of *Shigella* cause, analogously, similar disease. All this leads to the conclusion that there is a causal association between *S. sonnei* and gastroenteritis.

Applying the criteria for causality is not as straightforward when the etiology is not clear. The associations between toxic shock syndrome (TSS), *Staphylococcus aureus*, and tampon use pose such a problem. Strength is demonstrated by the increased risk of disease in females who use tampons, and most studies (consistency) have shown a relationship between *S. aureus* and TSS. Although other organisms can cause TSS, in no case has TSS associated with tampon use been associated with any other organism (specificity), although in the initial stages of the investigation, the role of many other vaginal organisms was studied. The presence of *S. aureus* alone or tampons alone does not cause disease; a number of other factors are involved. No specific phage has been found that induces the production of the toxin implicated in TSS associated with tampon use. Temporally, colonization with *S. aureus* probably precedes TSS disease and also cases of TSS in patients with postoperative wounds. It is postulated that continuous, more than intermittent (biological gradient) use of superabsorbent tampons allows a large number of organisms to persist in the vaginal canal. Plausibility and coherence is demonstrated by the knowledge that some *S. aureus* strains produce toxins that can cause toxic poisoning and a shock syndrome. Experiments with *S. aureus* toxins have shown that these toxins produce disease. Toxic shock syndrome is consistent with a toxin-induced illness, and the disease is consistent with our knowledge of *S. aureus* diseases, such as staphylococcal food poisoning and scalded skin syndrome, both of which are caused by *S. aureus* toxins (analogy). Based on Hill's criteria, the conclusion is reached that a causal association exists between *S. aureus* and TSS, however, a simple causal relationship does not exist between superabsorbent tampons and TSS. Superabsorbent tampons are one of many risk factors for TSS.

There are difficulties associated with the use of criteria for causality. Although certain study designs (e.g., random-allocation clinical trials) produce data that are used to prove causality, in fact, even with all criteria met, it is rarely possible to explain all the factors contributing to a specific disease entity. For example, tuberculosis has been classically viewed as meeting all

Copyright © 2005, Association for Professionals in Infection Control and Epidemiology, Inc.

of the criteria to satisfy Koch's postulates. Yet recent approaches to the study of this disease clearly indicate that socialization and lifestyle, and coinfection with human immunodeficiency virus (HIV), have an impact on the risk for development of tuberculosis. Additionally, if a well-described disease with a clearly defined etiological agent is subject to a "third cause" (i.e., an unmeasurable factor), it follows that diseases that are less well described or lack clearly defined etiological agents will frequently be subjected to challenges about undetermined contributing factors. An example is the challenge to the causal association of smoking and lung cancer. The tobacco industry maintains that the association between smoking and lung cancer is the result of some yet to be defined variable and that the association with smoking is only a spurious result. The tobacco industry uses the argument that not all people who develop lung cancer are smokers. (However, epidemiological research and analyses of many studies by Doll and Peto have demonstrated that smoking meets Hill's criteria for causality of lung cancer and a number of other diseases.)

III. Uses of Epidemiology in Healthcare

One of the uses of epidemiology is to apply information gathered to various forms of disease prevention. There are three categories of prevention, which are sometimes referred to as *Leavell's levels*: primary, secondary, and tertiary. Primary prevention includes health promotion programs like wellness programs and specific protections, such as immunization. The goal is the complete prevention of a disease before any manifestation of that disease occurs, preferably before the occurrence of any preclinical changes that may lead to disease. Secondary prevention refers to early diagnosis and treatment and includes skin testing in tuberculosis and breast self-exam and mammograms for early detection of breast cancer. Secondary prevention also involves methods that may limit disability, such as stopping smoking in people with chronic bronchitis. The emphasis is on preventing further deterioration by intervention as early in the disease course as possible. Tertiary prevention occurs after disease is well established and deals with sequelae of disease. Examples of tertiary prevention include rehabilitation and organ transplantations.

Applications of disease prevention, using information gathered with epidemiological studies, are wide-ranging. Prevention efforts occur in community and healthcare facility-based healthcare delivery systems. Forecasting for future needs in both treating illness and promoting health is important in healthcare planning. Prevention forms a part of occupational and environmental programs in the workplace, the ambient environment, and in the reduction of worker's risk. Noninfectious events, both acute (e.g., auto accidents,

poisonings) and chronic (e.g., heart diseases, malignant neoplasms) have had many prevention programs developed around them.

Prevention programs also have a place in infectious diseases. Acute infections with the potential for spread into the community, such as measles, rubella or other childhood diseases, are addressed with vaccine programs. Infections that may become chronic, such as tuberculosis, are prevented by limiting exposure to those who are contagious and by treatment of those who have active disease. Prevention of nosocomial infections requires intensive staff education. It is also important to understand the stages of the natural history of disease and the relationship to primary, secondary, and tertiary levels of prevention (Fig. 2–3). Decisions about prevention will, in part, be dependent on the stage of a given disease at which interventions can be made. Ideally, primary prevention should be carried out, but this is not necessarily practical or possible.

Prevention strategies in hospital infection control depend on the disease in question and what information is available to the practitioner. Prevention strategies to reduce the risk of transmission, including barrier precautions; immunizations of healthcare workers; and cleaning, sterilization, and disinfection, are designed to prevent the occurrence of disease and, therefore, form primary prevention measures. Forecasting for future health needs as the general population ages must lead to infection control practices that deal with health problems of the elderly. Occupational and environmental health exposures may be prevented in hospital workers through programs and training, such as the use of barrier methods to prevent transmission of bloodborne pathogens or appropriate barriers to prevent tuberculosis transmission. Prevention of nosocomial infections also requires an understanding of the impact that chronic diseases and underlying conditions (e.g., immunosuppression, chronic obstructive pulmonary disease) have on increasing the risk of nosocomial infections.

Useful Terms in Infectious Disease Epidemiology

A basic knowledge of terminology used in infectious disease epidemiology makes both understanding and communication easier. Listed below are a number of terms and their definitions that will be useful to the infection control practitioner.

Incidence: the number of new cases of a given disease in a given time period. For example, the number of newly diagnosed cases of active tuberculosis in a calendar year in a given county is the incidence of tuberculosis in that county.

Copyright © 2005, Association for Professionals in Infection Control and Epidemiology, Inc.

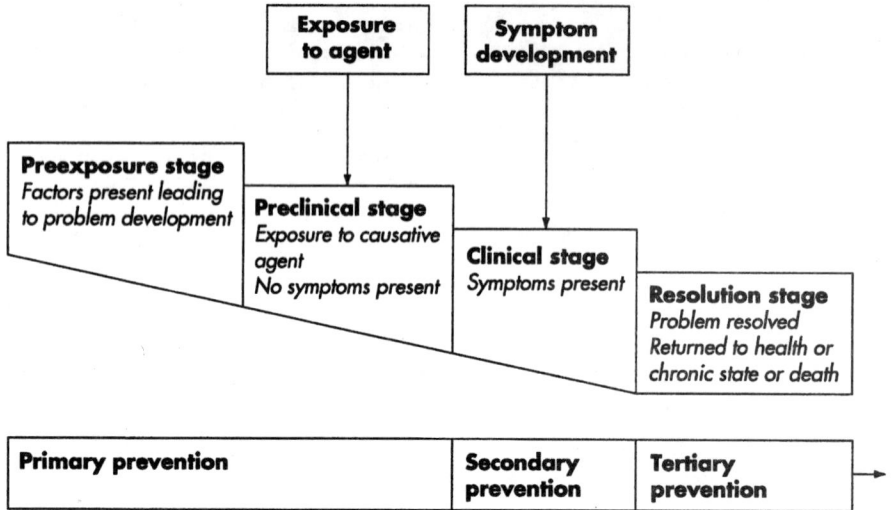

Figure 2–3 Stages of the natural history of a condition and their relationship to primary, secondary, and tertiary levels of prevention. (Redrawn from Clark MJ. *Nursing in the Community*, Norwalk, CT: Appleton & Lange; 1992.)

Prevalence: the number of existent cases of a given disease at a given time, for example, the number of active tuberculosis cases in the same county, at the midpoint of the calendar year.

Endemic: the usual incidence of a given disease within a geographical area during a specified time period.

Epidemic: an excess over the expected incidence of disease within a given geographical area during a specified time period. If the expected number of cases of a disease in a county is eight per year, and sixteen occur in one year, this indicates an epidemic. It should be noted that an epidemic is not defined on the absolute number of cases but on the number of cases in comparison to what is expected.

Pandemic: an epidemic spread over a wide geographical area, across countries or continents.

Outbreak: synonymous with epidemic but a term often preferred when dealing with the public. It may not evoke the same fearful response as the term *epidemic.*

Enzootic: the usual presence of disease among animals within a geographical area. The animals may serve as a reservoir for a zoonotic disease.

Epizootic: an excess over the expected extent of disease within an animal population in a geographical area during a specified time period.

Zoonosis: a disease transmitted from animals to humans (e.g., cat scratch fever, psittocosis).

Reservoir: place in which an infectious agent can survive but may or may not multiply, for example, *Pseudomonas* in nebulizers and hepatitis B on the surface of a hemodialysis machine. Healthcare workers may also be reservoirs for a number of nosocomial organisms.

Fomite: an inanimate object on which organisms may exist for some period of time, for example, the hemodialysis machine in the previous example.

Herd immunity: the resistance of a group to invasion and to spread of an infectious agent, based on the immunity of a high proportion of individual members of the group.

Risk: the probability or likelihood of an event occurring.

Risk factor: a characteristic, behavior, or experience that increases the probability of developing a negative health status (e.g., disease, infection).

Infection is the entry into and multiplication of an infectious agent in the tissues of the host and tissue damage, resulting in apparent or inapparent changes in the host (Fig. 2–4). Inapparent, asymptomatic, or subclinical infections run a course similar to that of clinical disease but below the threshold of discernable clinical symptoms. Apparent, clinical, or symptomatic infections result in clinical signs and symptoms of a recognizable disease process.

Nosocomial infections are those that are not present or incubating at the time of admission to the hospital but are temporally associated with admission to or a

APIC Text of Infection Control and Epidemiology

Copyright © 2005, Association for Professionals in Infection Control and Epidemiology, Inc.

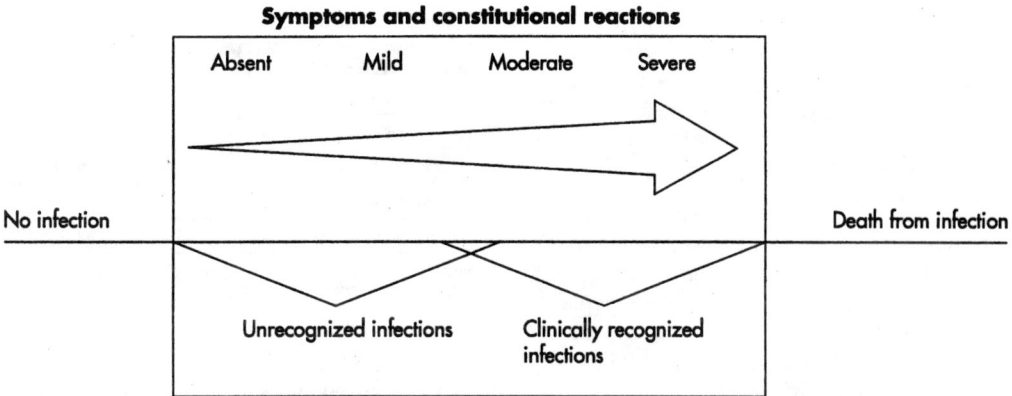

Symptoms and constitutional reactions

Absent   Mild   Moderate   Severe

No infection

Death from infection

Unrecognized infections   Clinically recognized infections

Figure 2-4   Infectious disease spectrum: various host responses to infection by an infectious agent. (Redrawn from Centers for Disease and Prevention. *Principles of Disease Control—A Three-Day Training Course*. Atlanta, GA; 1992).

procedure performed in a healthcare facility. An infection present or incubating at the time of admission may also be nosocomial, if it is related to a recent hospitalization.

In contrast to nosocomial infections are community-acquired infections, infections present or incubating on admission, or infections incubating at the time of admission and with no association to a recent hospitalization.

In addition to understanding the concepts of nosocomial and community-acquired infection, it is important that the infection control practitioner understand the concept of colonization. Colonization is the presence of microorganisms in or on a host with growth and multiplication but without tissue invasion or damage. A thorough understanding of this concept is essential in the planning and implantation of epidemiological studies in a hospital infection control program. Confusing colonization with infection can lead to spurious associations that may lead to expensive, ineffective, and time-consuming interventions. However, the infection control practitioner must also realize that colonization may become infection when changes in the host occur and that, for some disease entities, a colonized host may spread organisms to other patients.

The Chain of Infection

The infection process can be described as a chain of infection (Fig. 2–5). Understanding this chain must precede the breaking of its links, which leads to prevention of infection. Each component, or link, in this chain is connected to another link in the chain.

The causative agent of infection can be thought of as the first link in the chain. A causative agent is a biological, physical, or chemical entity capable of causing disease. Biological agents may be bacteria, viruses,

fungi, protozoa, helminthes, or prions. Some biological agents have characteristics that make them more successful in causing infection. To cause disease, these agents must be invasive enough to enter tissues, multiply, and cause some amount of damage. They must be sufficiently virulent to be pathogenic. The infectious dose, the number of organisms required to cause disease, and how viable an organism is in the free state also determines whether infection will develop. Host specificity impacts organism success as well. An organism causing disease only in marmosets will probably not have success in causing infection in humans. Organisms may also have high rates of antigenic variation that help to circumvent host-immune responses. This is the case with influenza, in which the outer

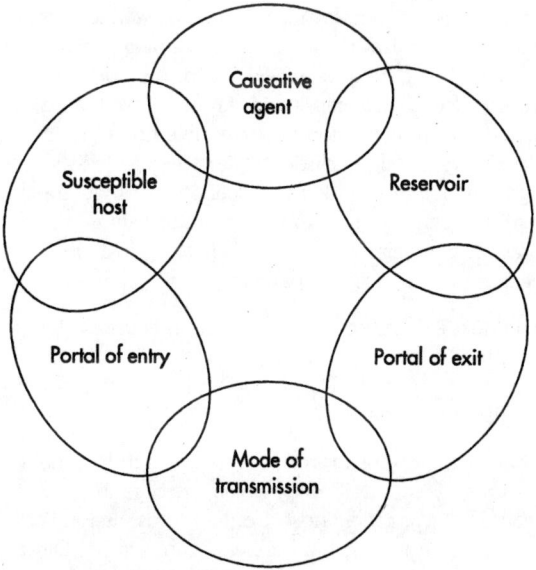

Figure 2-5   The chain of infection. Components of the infectious disease process.

Copyright © 2005, Association for Professionals in Infection Control and Epidemiology, Inc.

protein antigens change from year to year, necessitating the yearly development of a new influenza vaccine. The ability to develop antimicrobial resistance also provides the organism with an advantage to continue causing infection, despite what was previously appropriate treatment.

The next link in the chain is the reservoir, that is, a place in which an infectious agent can survive but may or may not multiply. There are three common reservoirs of interest: humans, animals, and environmental. Common reservoirs associated with nosocomial infections include patients, healthcare personnel, and healthcare equipment and environment. Human reservoirs are generally cases with the disease in question, either acute clinical cases or subclinical (asymptomatic) cases, or carriers. A carrier is a person who shows no recognizable signs or symptoms of a disease but is capable of spreading disease to others, such as persons in the prodromal period of an infectious disease or a healthcare worker with *S. aureus* nasal colonization. During the prodromal phase of some diseases, the organism is multiplying but has not yet caused signs and symptoms of the disease. Convalescent carriers are those who have recovered from the disease but still have organisms present that can be transmitted. For example, a patient with cholera may continue to shed bacteria in the stool for several weeks after diarrhea has subsided. Chronic or sustained carriers may continue to have organisms present for very long periods of time. "Typhoid" Mary Malone is an example of a chronic carrier: *Salmonella typhi* may continue to exist in the gall bladder of a significant number of persons who have recovered from typhoid. From the gall bladder it is shed through the gastrointestinal tract and may infect those who come in contact with the carrier's feces. Carriers can live long and healthy lives with the organism present. There are also intermittent carriers who periodically shed organisms, such as *S. aureus*. Subclinical cases and carriers present a particular risk of transmission to susceptible hosts in the healthcare setting because they are less likely to be recognized. There may be no indication that they are ill or that they may be infectious. Precautionary measures to prevent transmission are less likely to be instituted because illness is not apparent.

The next link in the chain of infection is the portal of exit, that is, the path by which an infectious agent leaves the reservoir. Portals of exit and portals of entry are listed in Table 2–2.

The mode of transmission, the next link in the chain of infection, is the method by which the organism reaches a susceptible host. Contact transmission is of particular importance in the healthcare setting. Direct contact is person-to-person spread with actual physical contact occurring between a source and a susceptible

Table 2-2. Portals of Entry and Exit

Portals of Exit	Portals of Entry
respiratory tract	respiratory tract
genitourinary tract	genitourinary tract
gastrointestinal tract	gastrointestinal tract
skin/mucous membrane	skin/mucous membrane
transplacental (mother to fetus)	transplacental (fetus to mother)
blood	parenteral (percutaneous via blood)

host (e.g., fecal-oral spread of hepatitis A virus). Indirect contact may occur when a patient comes in contact with a contaminated intermediate object or fomite. An example in the healthcare setting would be a bedrail contaminated with small particles of stool. Droplet transmission occurs when the infectious agent spends only a brief period passing through air and can be inhaled at that time. Droplets may arise from speaking, coughing, or sneezing. Because heavy droplets only travel a short distance, generally a meter (about 3 feet) or less, the infected person and susceptible host need to be relatively close to each other for efficient transmission to occur.

Common vehicles, such as food and water, may also transmit infectious agents. In active direct transmission with a common source, the organism first replicates in the vehicle, producing a larger dose of the organism, which is then ingested, that is, salmonella in raw chicken. Passive or indirect transmission may occur, if the organism is simply present. No increase in loading dose is necessary. An example of passive transmission by common vehicle is food contaminated with hepatitis A virus. The virus does not replicate in the food, but when ingested it may cause infection.

Airborne spread is an efficient mode of transmission and may involve varying distances between the source and host. The most efficient means of airborne transmission is by droplet nuclei. Droplet nuclei are very small, about 1 to 5 μm, and can be suspended in air for extended periods of time. The size of the particle makes it ideal for inhalation because it is small enough to reach the respiratory tree without being swept up by cilia. The small size of the particle and its ability to remain suspended in air also means that droplet nuclei may spread through ventilation systems. Tuberculosis is the classic example of a disease spread by droplet nuclei.

Vectors, such as insects, may also transmit infectious organisms, although this method of transmission is of less importance in the hospital setting in most industrialized nations. External vector-borne transmission is the mechanical transfer of microorganisms by a vector, such as a fly on food. Internal vector-borne transmis-

Copyright © 2005, Association for Professionals in Infection Control and Epidemiology, Inc.

sion involves transfer of infectious material directly from the vector into the new host, such that occurs in mosquitoes and malaria, fleas and plague, and louse-borne typhus. The vector may simply harbor the infectious organism, with no biological interaction taking place, or the agent may actually undergo changes within the vector (e.g., malaria parasites require that part of their life cycle take place within a mosquito).

The portal of entry is the means by which an infectious agent enters the susceptible host. Portals of entry associated with human hosts are listed in Table 2-2. The susceptible host is the next link in the chain of infection. In addition to the characteristics of the susceptible host shown in Table 2-3, the susceptible host has several nonspecific defense mechanisms that may modify the risks of becoming infected and developing disease. Normal (endogenous) flora in the host may protect it from other infectious organisms, and the host's natural antibodies attack some invading organ-

isms. Natural barriers to the entry of organisms include (1) skin and mucous membranes, which provide mechanical barriers; (2) cilia of the respiratory tract and cough mechanism that clear material from the respiratory structures; (3) gastric acid of the stomach that helps destroy ingested pathogens; (4) mechanical flushing that protects the genitourinary tract; and (5) tear flushing that helps to protect the eye. Finally, good nutritional status protects the host overall.

Salmonellosis can be studied in terms of the chain of infection. The causative agent of salmonellosis is *Salmonella*, a bacterium that can survive in the free-state and generally has an infective dose of 10^6 organisms or greater, if the host has normal gastric acidity. Some strains of *Salmonella typhi* have much smaller infective doses. The reservoirs for *Salmonella* include humans, both carriers and active cases, and animals (including poultry, cattle, reptiles, and others). There are also environmental reservoirs for *Salmonella*, including contaminated food products, untreated sewage, and biological waste products (e.g., fertilizers, bone meal). The portals of exit are the gastrointestinal tract and, to a lesser extent, the genitourinary tract. Modes of transmission include both contact and common vehicles. Direct contact with the organism may occur while changing diapers or while handling raw poultry. Indirect contact by the hands of personnel may happen after handling an incontinent patient and then tube feeding the next patient without washing hands. Use of gloves should never replace hand hygiene because although the gloves may reduce the likelihood of transmission, they may have microtears and contaminated matter may get under the wrist area of the glove. Common vehicle transmission, in this case contaminated food, is a well-known mode of transmission for *Salmonella*. The portal of entry is the gastrointestinal tract, and, although everyone is susceptible at some level, the elderly, the young, and those with decreased stomach acid are especially vulnerable.

Control of infectious diseases involves breaking the chain of infection by altering the host, the environment, or the agent. In the *Salmonella* example, measures directed at the agent and reservoir include proper storage, handling and cooking of food, and properly treating sewage to inactivate the organism. Educating cases and carriers about hygiene may also break the transmission of disease at the reservoir link in the chain of infection. The susceptible host breaks the chain through caution in cooking, eating, and hygiene habits. Environmental measures include restricting food handlers with disease, treatment of carriers (reservoir link), wearing of gloves when contact with stool or contaminated items is likely, and proper handwashing for patients and personnel providing care (transmission link).

Table 2-3. Host Characteristics Influencing Susceptibility to and Severity of Disease

Characteristic	Example
Age	"Childhood diseases" are seen more frequently in children, whereas chronic diseases, such as heart disease or COPD, occur more frequently in older patients.
Sex	Reproductive diseases are sex-specific.
Ethnicity	Tay-Sachs disease in Jews of European descent
Socioeconomic status	Ability to purchase healthcare services, food purchasing
Marital status	Some studies of stress-related diseases have shown marital status to be a factor influencing susceptibility.
Medical history	Individuals with diabetes are at increased risk of infection.
Lifestyle	Homelessness increases susceptibility due to poor nutrition and exposure.
Heredity	Sickle cell anemia influences susceptibility.
Nutritional status	Inadequate nutrition reduces immune function.
Occupation	Coal miners are at risk for black lung.
Immunization status	Those who have not been vaccinated for measles are at risk for the disease.
Diagnostic/therapeutic Procedures	Transplant patients have increased risk of infection.
Medications	Steroid use increases risk of infection.
Pregnancy	Tuberculosis-positive women who are pregnant are more likely to reactivate.
Trauma	Injury may provide portal of entry for organisms and triggers inflammatory response that may increase risk of infection.

Copyright © 2005, Association for Professionals in Infection Control and Epidemiology, Inc.

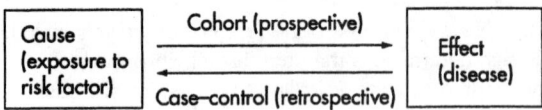

Figure 2-6 Contrasting prospective and retrospective investigation.

Interrupting the Chain of Infection: Epidemiological Study Design

Epidemiology uses tools to determine risk factors for disease, and these may help to identify links in the chain of infection that may be interrupted or broken. Primary study designs used in the healthcare setting are described as prospective or retrospective. These studies are commonly used in relation to cohort and case-control studies, respectively.

In prospective or cohort studies data are gathered over time. In this study design, a group of subjects, with a known exposure status for the risk factor(s) of interest, are followed over time to determine which of the subjects develops disease. These subjects form a cohort going through time together. Experimental studies are also prospective in nature: data are gathered as subjects move from the present into the future, while being followed by the researcher. In contrast, case-control studies are referred to as retrospective, moving backward from disease state to risk factor, by first identifying persons with the disease and then measuring their degree of exposure to the risk factor(s) of interest (see Fig. 2-6). Sometimes the terms *prospective* and *retrospective* are used in a temporal rather than conceptual sense. A cohort study that measures disease frequency in the present and among persons with a known exposure in the past is commonly called a "retrospective cohort study" (see Fig. 2-7).

Advantages and Disadvantages

Both cohort and case-control studies have relative advantages and disadvantages. Retrospective studies use data already available, such as patient charts or laboratory databases. They also require relatively small numbers of subjects relative to cohort studies because a sufficient number of cases are already included in the study, that is, the researcher does not have to wait for enough cases to develop to carry out an analysis. This makes the case-control method useful for disease states that occur rarely. It also makes retrospective studies less expensive because fewer total subjects may be required for analysis, and data are already available. These studies also take less time than prospective studies because the cases are already identified. However, case-control studies are dependent on the completeness of records, and it may be difficult to select an appropriate control group. Retrospective studies are used to get information about past events and are subject to recall bias because they rely on the memory of subjects and others for information on exposure.

Prospective, or cohort, studies are usually more expensive than case-control studies, in part, because they take longer. Long follow-up periods may be required while waiting for disease to occur in sufficient numbers for analysis. Attrition may result from long follow-up periods reducing the sample size of a study. Traditionally, cohort studies are considered to have fewer bias issues than case-control studies because they avoid the subjectivity involved in collecting after-the-fact exposure data from persons already affected by disease. They also yield incidence rates because the population at risk has already been identified and can yield associations between risk factors and disease that were not anticipated. Cohort studies generally carry more weight and tend to be used when controversial retrospective findings need to be verified.

Epidemiological studies can also be divided by levels of data and analysis. The first level of distinction is between observational and experimental studies. As discussed earlier, observational studies involve gathering data on existing subjects with no intervention. In experimental studies, the researcher provides one or more interventions and determines differences before and after the intervention. The simplest type of observational study is the descriptive study. This type of study seeks to describe a population in terms of person, place, and time: who gets disease, when, and in what kind of geographical location. Examples of "person"

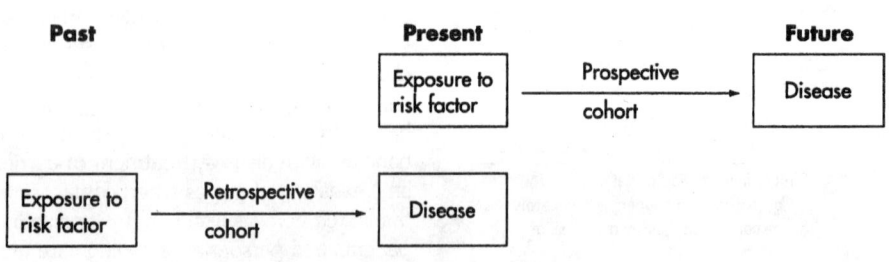

Figure 2-7 Retrospective and prospective cohort.

APIC Text of Infection Control and Epidemiology

Copyright © 2005, Association for Professionals in Infection Control and Epidemiology, Inc.

variables include age, sex or gender, occupation, marital status, ethnicity, and health status. These studies also describe "place" variables, such as urban/rural differences, socioeconomic differences across areas, interfacility locations, and others. Time, for these studies, may involve an epidemic period, month, quarter, season, or periods of consecutive years or months. Descriptive studies can be used to generate rates and identify populations at risk but cannot be used to show causality.

Analytic studies also fall under the observational umbrella. The simplest of these is the cross-sectional study. This method provides a snapshot of a population at one point in time. For this reason this type of study is sometimes referred to as a "prevalence study." The cross-sectional study is conducted at a specific point in time or for a specific period of time and measures previously and newly identified cases of disease. This study format can be used to examine relationships between some possible predisposing risk factor and disease, but it cannot generate incidence rates. Serial cross-sectional studies can generate data to determine trends over time.

Case-control studies are somewhat more complicated than cross-sectional studies and, as discussed earlier, are retrospective in nature. These studies start with a number of identified cases with the disease of interest and compares them in terms of past exposures to a group of control subjects without the disease of interest. For this reason, choice of control group is particularly important. If the control group is not comparable to the cases, the study will be invalid. This methodology is especially useful for the study of nosocomial infections and is frequently used for outbreak investigations. Case-control studies may show associations but cannot prove causality.

Cohort studies are next in the hierarchy of observational studies. At the beginning of this type of study, the population is free of the disease under study and is followed for exposure to risk factors and appearance of disease. Correlations are made between the presence and absence of disease and the presence and absence of the exposure. Cohort studies provide stronger evidence for a direct causal association because collection of risk factor information (i.e., exposure) occurs before the presence of disease is established. This is a relatively easy study methodology if the incubation period for the disease under study is relatively short, but it may be very difficult if there is a long latency period. It is difficult to conduct cohort studies when looking at rare diseases because insufficient number of cases may develop during a reasonable study period. For this reason, rare diseases are most often studied using a case-control study design.

Experimental studies are always prospective. In an experimental study, the investigator varies or manipulates one or more factors (variables), while the others remain constant. These studies require follow-up observation to determine outcome (effect of intervention). Strict control over choice of subject selection is required. Experimental studies can establish association and may establish causality, whereas other factors are strictly controlled. In true experiments, random assignment of subjects is used. Examples of experimental studies include (1) clinical trials in which new drugs or treatment modalities are compared to current practices; (2) community trials studying larger numbers of people, as is done in vaccine trials; and (3) experimental investigations using animal models. Experimental studies may be applied in infection control to determine whether changes in practice (interventions) actually lead to lower nosocomial infection rates. Examples include comparisons of systems of IV medication delivery, comparing the rates of hand cleansing before and after installation of hand sanitizer dispensers, and use of sterile water in nebulizers compared to unsterile water.

Recognizing Outcome-Related Events

Once epidemiological studies have been carried out, it is important to recognize the outcomes of those studies to apply knowledge gained. Outcome events are useful in evaluation of an infection control program. Modification of behaviors by healthcare personnel and learned skills by personnel can be measured by looking at outcomes. Changes in nosocomial infection rates can be determined (although extreme caution must be used in the interpretation of results because many nosocomial infections are not preventable by known interventions). Changes in policies and procedures may result in changes in outcomes or may result from outcome differences. Being able to show outcomes from studies may result in priority modifications in the future for the infection control and prevention program and/or the facility.

Data Presentation

Once data have been gathered and analyzed, they must be presented clearly and concisely, greatly helping others to understand the study, why it was done, and the outcomes. Data are generally presented graphically in one of three forms: tables, graphs, or charts. All well-constructed tables, graphs, and charts present a limited amount of information that is easily understood, and, ideally, each can stand alone. Too much information simply becomes confusing, defeating the purpose of graphically presenting the data. Each presentation graphic must have a complete title that describes the contents in terms of the event being

Copyright © 2005, Association for Professionals in Infection Control and Epidemiology, Inc.

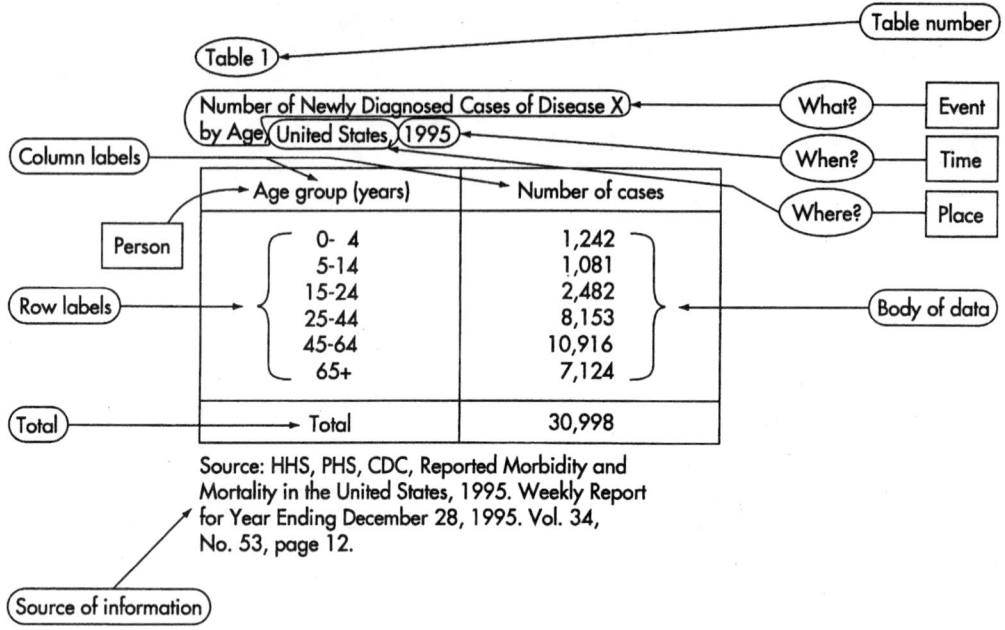

Figure 2-8 Elements of a well-constructed table.

studied, the population being studied, and the place and time of study. For example, a complete title might be, "Reported cases of bacteremia in surgical intensive care unit patients, in Hospital X, in March, 2004." This title tells the reader much more than the alternative "Bacteremia in the SICU." When preparing tables, graphs, or charts, it is helpful to indicate the date they were prepared. This may be important because data often change over the course of an outbreak investigation, and dating graphics will help the researcher keep current and to track changes. The source of data must be identified if data from an outside source are used in the table, graph, or chart.

A few definitions of terms used to describe the components of tables, graphs, and charts may be helpful. A *cell* is the space in a table, graph, or chart in which data are entered. The *class interval* is the subgrouping of values for any given epidemiological variable, such as age or sex. For example, "age" may be grouped into two class intervals: "less than 15 years old" and "15 years and older." *Continuous data* are data for which there is an infinite number of possible values between the minimum and maximum values. Examples include age, weight, and temperature This is in contrast to *discrete data*, which can only be counted in whole numbers, such as number of children. A *coordinate* is one of a pair of locators used to specify a particular point, for example, the x and y coordinates on a graph.

Tables

A table is a set of data arranged in rows and columns (see Fig. 2–8). Tables are used to present the frequency with which some event occurs and to present this information in different categories or subdivisions of a variable. Well-constructed tables are simple; ideally, they do not try to present more than three factors at a time. Readable tables have a clear concise title that answers who, what, where, when, and how questions, that is, they provide information about person, place, and time. Each column and row should be labeled and the column and row totals shown, if they are used. Codes, abbreviations, and symbols should be explained in a footnote. Sources of information, gathered from outside the institution or used for comparison, should be cited.

Graphs

Graphs are a method of showing quantitative data using a system of coordinates (see Fig. 2–9). A well-constructed graph consists of two sets of lines that intersect at right angles. Each axis (line) has a scale measurement and a label. By convention, the horizontal (x) axis reflects the variable time in whatever interval is being used (year, month, quarter, day, etc.) when time is to be presented. The vertical (y) axis usually reflects the frequency of occurrence of an event (e.g., the number of cases of disease) or the proportion (e.g., percent, cases per 1,000 patient days) with the event. More than one factor or variable can be shown on a graph, but each should be clearly differentiated by

Copyright © 2005, Association for Professionals in Infection Control and Epidemiology, Inc.

Arithmetic Line Graph

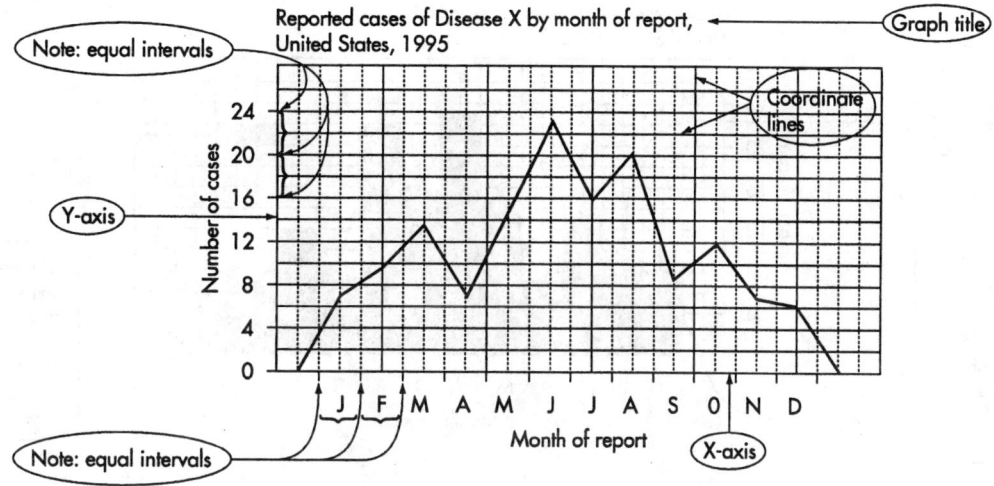

Figure 2–9 Elements of a well-constructed graph.

a legend or key. It is important to remember that each graph should be simple and self-explanatory.

There are several forms of graphs used in the presentation of epidemiological data. The arithmetic line graph uses equal distances along the y-axis to represent equal quantities anywhere on that axis (see Fig. 2–9). The semilogarithmic scale line graph uses a y-axis measured in logarithms of units. This is often used when examining a series of data over long periods of time to compress what would be very large spaces between data points or to normalize the appearance of data, but use of "semilog" must always be acknowledged both in the graph itself and in the text regarding the graph. A histogram is a graphic of a frequency distribution in which one bar is used for each time interval and there is no space between the intervals (see Fig. 2–10). This type of graph is used to depict an epi-

demic curve. A frequency polygon is similar to a line graph, but each coordinate point is represented by a point displayed on the graph with straight lines connecting them. A frequency polygon will provide the same data information as a histogram.

Charts

A chart is a method of illustrating information using only one coordinate. Charts are used to compare magnitudes of different events and to compare parts of a total picture. Types of charts include bar charts, geographical coordinate charts, pictograms, and pie charts. Bar charts use bars to depict the event being studied (see Fig. 2–11). The bars are the same column width and, unlike histograms, are separated by spaces. Bar charts can be used to compare magnitudes, show frequency distributions, and show time-series data. The

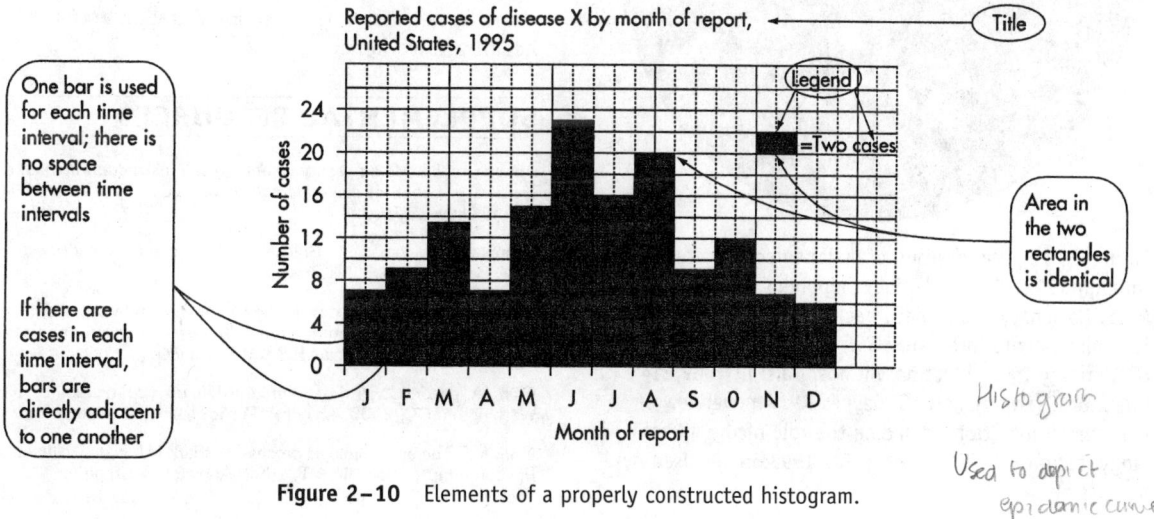

Figure 2–10 Elements of a properly constructed histogram.

Histogram

Used to depict
epidemic curve

General Principles of Epidemiology

Copyright © 2005, Association for Professionals in Infection Control and Epidemiology, Inc.

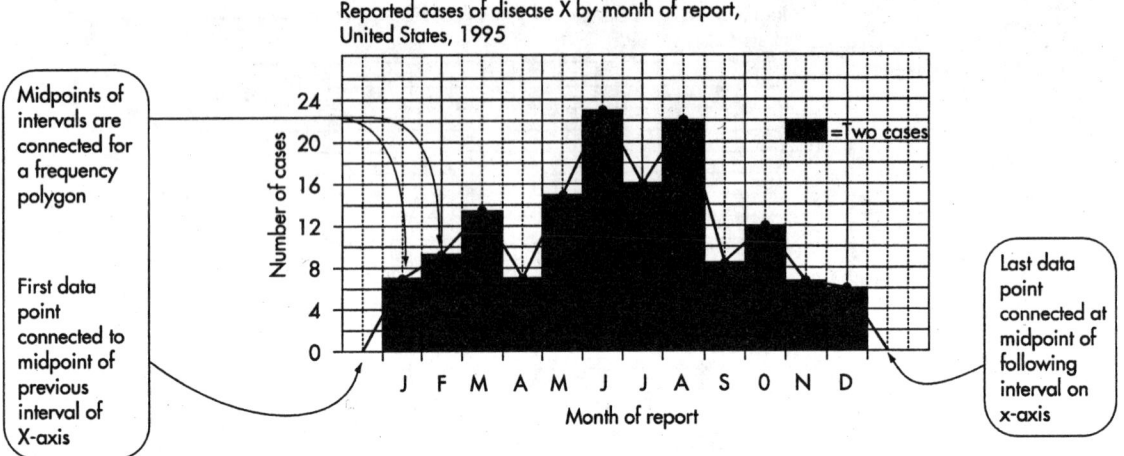

Figure 2–11 Comparision of a histogram and its corresponding frequency distribution.

pictogram is a variation of a bar chart that uses a series of small identifying symbols to represent the data. Geographical coordinate charts represent the occurrence of events using maps. Spot maps use dots or symbols at each location where an event took place (e.g., patient rooms with a dot for each patient with a disease). An area map uses shaded or coded areas to show the distributions of some conditions (e.g., color codes of wards based on the number of patients in the area with a given condition). The pie chart is used to represent proportions by assigning them to wedge-shaped proportions of a circle for comparison (see Fig. 2–12).

III. SUMMARY AND CONCLUSIONS

In summary, an ICP's basic understanding of epidemiological methods is crucial for a well-functioning infection control program. These methods form the basis of all studies and outbreak investigations conducted and in the assessment of programs developed. Understanding basic epidemiological methods will lead to better study design and studies that are more likely to provide accurate and comparable information for creating change to reduce nosocomial infection rates and clear and concise data presentation so that changes in rates, causes of outbreaks, and so forth, can be easily understood by healthcare facility administration and healthcare workers.

SUPPLEMENTAL RESOURCES

Abramsom JH: *Making sense of data: a self-instruction manual on the interpretation of epidemiological data*, ed 2, New York, 1994, Oxford University Press.

Bennet JV, Brachman PS, Brachman W, editors: *Hospital infections*, ed 4, Boston, 1998, Little Brown.

Cassells HB: Nursing process in the community. In Swanson JM, Albrrecht M, editors: *Community health nursing: promoting health of aggregates*, Philadelphia, 1993, WB Saunders.

Chin JA, editor: *Control of communicable disease manual*, ed 17, Washington, DC, 2000, American Public Health Association.

Clark MJ: The epidemiologic process. In Clark MJ, editor: *Nursing in the community*, Norwalk, CT, 1992, Appleton & Lange.

Figure 2–12 Distribution of major infection sites (1990 through 1992), hospital-wide component, NNIS system. *NNIS*, National Nosocomial Infection Surveillance System; *SSI*, surgical site infections; *BSI*, Bloodstream infections; *UTI*, urinary tract infection. All hospitals: *n* = 62,214 infections. (From Emori TG, Gaynes RP. An overview of nosocomial infection, including the role of the microbiology laboratory. *Clin Microbiol Rev* 1993;6:430. Used by permission.)

APIC Text of Infection Control and Epidemiology

Copyright © 2005, Association for Professionals in Infection Control and Epidemiology, Inc.

Evans AS: *Causation and disease: a chronological journey*, New York, 1993, Plenum Medical Book.

Friedman GD: *Primer of epidemiology*, ed 4, New York, 1994, McGraw-Hill.

Hennekens CH, Burning JE: *Epidemiology in medicine*, Boston, 1987, Little Brown.

Kahn HA, Sempos CT: *Statistical methods in epidemiology*, New York, 1989, Oxford University Press.

Kleinbaum DG, Jupper LL, Morgenstern H: *Epidemiologic research: principles and quantitative methods*, New York, 1982, John Wiley & Sons.

Last JM, Spasoff RA, Harris SS, et al: *Dictionary of epidemiology*, ed 4, New York, 2000, Oxford University Press.

Lillenfeld DE, Stolley PD: *Foundations of epidemiology*, ed 3, New York, 1994, Oxford University Press.

Mayhall CG, editor: *Hospital epidemiology and infection control*, ed 2, Baltimore, 1999, Williams & Wilkins.

Norman GR, Streiner DL: *Biostatistics: the bare essentials*, ed 2, Toronto, 2000, BC Decker.

Norman GR, Streiner DL: *PDQ epidemiology*, ed 2, Toronto, 1996, BC Decker.

Rothman KJ, Greenland S: *Modern epidemiology*, ed 2, Philadelphia, 1998, Lippincott-Raven.

Selvin S: *Statistical analysis of epidemiologic data*, ed 2, New York, 1996, Oxford University Press.

Vilanis B: *Epidemiology in nursing and health care*, ed 2, Norwalk, CT, 1992, Appleton & Lange.

Weiss NS: *Clinical epidemiology*, ed 2, New York, 1996, Oxford University Press.

Wenzel RP, editor: *Prevention and control of nosocomial infections*, ed 4, Baltimore, 2002, Williams & Wilkins.

Woodward M: *Epidemiology: study design and data analysis*, Boca Raton, FL, 1999, Chapman and Hall/CRC.

Copyright © 2005, Association for Professionals in Infection Control and Epidemiology, Inc.

Surveillance

Kathleen Meehan Arias, M.S., C.I.C.
Arias Infection Control Consulting, LLC,
Crownsville, Maryland

ABSTRACT

Surveillance is an essential component of an effective infection prevention and control program. This chapter discusses the history, evolution, and use of surveillance programs in healthcare facilities. It outlines the steps that should be used when designing and evaluating a surveillance program, emphasizes the importance of using sound epidemiological and statistical principles, and stresses the use of surveillance data to improve the quality of healthcare. It also reviews factors that affect surveillance programs in healthcare facilities, such as the changing healthcare delivery system and emerging infectious diseases, and identifies new developments, future trends, and international issues.

KEY CONCEPTS

- Surveillance programs should be based on sound epidemiological and statistical principles.

- Surveillance methodology is evolving as the healthcare delivery system shifts outside of the traditional acute care hospital.

- A surveillance program should be designed in accordance with current recommended practices and should consist of defined elements.

- Surveillance activities should support a system that can identify risk factors for infection and other adverse advents, implement risk-reduction measures, and monitor the effectiveness of interventions.

- Surveillance plays a critical role in identifying outbreaks, emerging infectious diseases, antibiotic-resistant organisms, and bioterrorist events so that infection prevention and control measures can be instituted.

- Surveillance programs in healthcare organizations should be integrated to include infection control, performance improvement, patient safety, and public health activities.

I.   BACKGROUND

"Surveillance is a systematic method of collecting, consolidating, and analyzing data concerning the distribution and determinates of a given disease or event, followed by the dissemination of that information to those who can improve the

Copyright © 2005, Association for Professionals in Infection Control and Epidemiology, Inc.

outcomes." Surveillance is an essential component of an effective infection prevention and control program.[2,3]

In 1958, in response to nationwide outbreaks of *Staphylococcus aureus* infections in hospitals, the American Hospital Association recommended that hospitals implement a nosocomial infection surveillance program.[4] In the 1960s, the Centers for Disease Control and Prevention (CDC) recommended that hospital-based infection control programs incorporate surveillance activities, and in 1976, the Joint Commission on Accreditation of Healthcare Organizations (JCAHO) first included infection surveillance, prevention, and control standards in its requirements for hospital accreditation.[5] The Study on the Efficacy of Nosocomial Infection Control (SENIC Project) provided scientific evidence that hospitals that had strong surveillance programs coupled with strong prevention and control programs were able to improve patient outcomes by reducing nosocomial infection rates.[6] Since the publication of the SENIC Project results in 1985, much has been published regarding the use of surveillance to monitor healthcare processes and practices and healthcare-associated infections.

In the past two decades, the healthcare delivery system has shifted outside of the traditional acute care hospital, resulting in an increasing need for surveillance in other healthcare settings.[3,7] In response to this shift, infection control organizations have published recommendations for surveillance in out of hospital settings.[3,8] Infection surveillance and control programs are now required by accrediting and regulatory agencies in a variety of healthcare settings, including hospitals, long-term care, rehabilitation, ambulatory surgery, dialysis, home care, mental health, and corrections facilities (See Chapter 10). Other factors affecting surveillance programs include shorter hospital stays, the aging of the population, increased use of invasive procedures and devices, more acutely ill patient and resident populations, healthcare worker shortages, emerging infectious diseases, and the threat of bioterrorism.[7] As healthcare practices evolve, new diseases emerge, and antimicrobial resistance spreads, new surveillance methodologies are needed to meet the changing environment.

Surveillance can be used for the following purposes:

- Determine baseline and endemic rates of occurrence of a disease or event

- Detect and investigate clusters or outbreaks

- Assess the effectiveness of prevention and control measures

- Monitor the occurrence of adverse outcomes to identify potential risk factors

- Provide information that can be used by an organization to target performance improvement activities

- Measure the efficacy of interventional and performance improvement efforts

- Observe practices, such as hand hygiene and sterilizer performance monitoring, to promote compliance with recommendations and standards

- Detect and report notifiable diseases to the health department

- Identify organisms and diseases of epidemiological importance, such as antibiotic-resistant organisms and tuberculosis, to prevent their spread

- Ensure compliance with federal regulators, such as the Occupational Safety and Health Administration or the Centers for Medicare and Medicaid Services

- Ensure compliance with state regulations, such as infectious waste and occupational safety and health laws

- Ensure compliance with accrediting agency requirements, such as the Joint Commission on Accreditation of Healthcare Organizations or the Rehabilitation Accreditation Commission

- Provide information for the education of healthcare personnel

- Monitor injuries and identify risk factors for injuries in personnel

- Detect a bioterrorist event or an emerging infectious disease

- Provide data to conduct a facility risk assessment for diseases, such as legionellosis or tuberculosis.

Surveillance data has been used successfully in a variety of healthcare settings to reduce the occurrence of infections when used to identify risk factors, implement risk-reduction measures, and monitor the effectiveness of interventions.[6,9-37]

This chapter reviews the basic principles, terms, and definitions used in surveillance programs in healthcare settings. It also discusses surveillance methodologies, key elements of a surveillance program, using surveillance data for benchmarking and performance improvement, new developments, future trends, and international issues, and provides a list of supplemental resources for obtaining additional information.

II.   BASIC PRINCIPLES

Surveillance programs should be based on sound epidemiological and statistical principles. If surveillance data are properly collected and analyzed, they can provide information that can be used to improve the quality

Copyright © 2005, Association for Professionals in Infection Control and Epidemiology, Inc.

and outcomes of healthcare and to promote public health. Those who are responsible for implementing and assessing surveillance programs should be familiar with the general principles of epidemiology that are discussed in Chapter 2 and the statistical methods found in Chapters 5 and 6.

Definitions

The following are definitions of terms, as used in healthcare surveillance. Many of the definitions are adapted or taken from the Glossary (Appendix A) in "Principles of Epidemiology: An Introduction to Applied Epidemiology and Biostatistics."[38]

Attack rate: type of incidence rate used to measure the frequency of new cases of a disease or condition in a specific population during a given time period; expressed as a percentage.

Baseline: the number or value used as the basis for comparison.

Case: a person who has the disease or condition being studied.

Case definition: standardized criteria used to determine if a person has a specific disease, condition, or outcome; usually incorporates clinical, laboratory, and other diagnostic criteria.

Cluster: a group of cases that occurs closely related in time and place.

Denominator: the lower portion of a fraction used to calculate a rate or ratio.[38]

Distribution: frequency and pattern of an event in a population.

Endemic: usual presence of a disease or condition in a specific population or geographical area.

Epidemic: the occurrence of more cases of a disease than expected in a given population and place during a specified time period; synonym of outbreak.

Epidemiology: the study of the distribution and determinates of health-related states or events in specified populations, and the application of this study to the control of health problems.[38]

Incidence rate: a measure of the frequency with which an event occurs in a population over a defined time period. The numerator is the number of new cases occurring during the defined time period, and the denominator is the population at risk.

Numerator: the upper portion of a fraction used to calculate a rate or ratio. In surveillance, it is usually the number of cases of a disease or event being studied.

Population: the total number of persons in a specified place or group.

Prevalence: the number of cases or events or conditions occurring in a population.

Prevalence rate: the proportion of persons in a population who have a particular disease or condition at a specified point in time or over a specified period of time.

Proportion: a type of ratio in which the values in the numerator are included in (i.e., are a subset of) the denominator.

Rate: an expression of the frequency with which an event occurs in a defined population.[38]

Ratio: the value obtained by dividing one quantity by another.[38]

Sensitivity: the ability of a system to detect epidemics and other changes in disease occurrence.[38]

Surveillance: "The systematic, active, ongoing observation of the occurrence and distribution of disease within a population, and of the events or conditions that may increase or decrease the risk of such disease occurrence."[39]

Validity: the degree to which a measurement actually measures or detects what it is supposed to measure.[38]

Basic Statistical Measures Used for Surveillance

Common statistical measurements used in surveillance programs in the healthcare setting are measures of frequency (e.g., rates, ratios, and proportions), measures of central tendency (e.g., mean and median), measures of dispersion (e.g., standard deviation), and percentiles. Because statistical methods are discussed in detail in Chapters 5 and 6, they will only be described briefly here.

Measures of Frequency

Rates, ratios, and proportions are used to measure the occurrence and risk of an event in a specific population during a given period. These frequency measures are based on the same formula: $x/y \times 10^n$, where x (the numerator) and y (the denominator) represent the two groups being compared and 10^n represents a constant.

Rates

Rates can be used to track trends and to monitor changes in the frequency of an event in a population from one time period to another (such as the occurrence of bloodstream infections in patients in an inten-

Copyright © 2005, Association for Professionals in Infection Control and Epidemiology, Inc.

sive care unit before and after interventions implemented to reduce the risk of infection). The most commonly used rates in surveillance programs for healthcare settings are incidence, attack, incidence density and prevalence.

An incidence rate measures the occurrence of new cases or events in a specific population during a given time period. The formula for calculating an incidence rate is $x/y \times 10^n$ where x is the number of new cases or events in a population during a given time period, y is the number in the population at risk during that time period and 10^n is used to transform the result into a number that has at least one digit to the left of the decimal point. An attack rate is a type of incidence rate that is expressed as cases per 100 population, or as a percentage (i.e., where n is 2 and $10^n = 100$). An incidence density rate is another type of incidence rate in which time, such as device-days or patient-days, is incorporated into the denominator. The formula for incidence density is the number of new cases in a population during in a given time period divided by the time each person in that population is observed during that period, totaled for all persons $\times 10^n$.

Examples of incidence density rate calculations:

1. In March, there were 3 central line-associated bloodstream infections (CLA-BSI) and 491 central line-days in an ICU. The calculation for the CLA-BSI rate in the ICU in March is the # BSI in ICU patients in March/# central line days in ICU patients in March $\times 1000$ or $3/491 \times 1000 = 6.1$. In this example, $10^n = 1000$ (n=3) so that the result has one digit to the left of the decimal point. This rate is interpreted as 6.1 central line-associated bloodstream infections per 1000 central line-days in the ICU in March.

2. In June, there were 2 resident falls in a long term care (LTC) unit that had 275 resident-days. The calculation for the fall rate would be the # falls in LTC unit in June/# resident-days in LTC unit in June $\times 1000$ or $2/275 \times 1000 = 7.3$. In this example, the rate is expressed as 7.3 falls per 1000 resident-days in the LTC unit in June.

A prevalence rate measures the occurrence of existing (old and new) cases in a specific population during a given time period. The formula for prevalence rate is the # of existing cases in a population during a specific time period/# in that population during that time period $\times 10^n$.

Ratios and Proportions

A ratio is a fraction in which the values in the numerator (x) may or may not be included in the denominator (y). A ratio can be used to express a relationship between two independent groups. The device utilization ratio used in the National Nosocomial Infections Surveillance (NNIS) System is determined by dividing the number of device-days by the number of patient-days.[40] This is an example of a ratio in which the values in the numerator (device-days) are independent of the values in the denominator (patient-days).

A proportion is a ratio in which the population in the numerator is a subset of the population in the denominator. A proportion is frequently expressed as a percentage.

Examples using ratios and proportions:

In a six-month period, thirty-nine patients in a critical care unit developed ventilator-associated pneumonia—twenty-six cases are female and thirteen are male.

1. The ratio of female cases to male cases is determined using the formula $x/y \times 10^n$ in which x is 26, y is 13, and 10^n is 1 (n = 0). The ratio of females to males would be $26/13 \times 1 = 2/1$ or 2:1. Thus there are two females for every male, or twice as many females as males who developed ventilator-associated pneumonia. In this ratio, the values in the numerator (females) are not included in the denominator (males).

2. The proportion of the thirty-nine pneumonia cases who are male would be calculated using the formula $x/y \times 10^n$ in which x is 13, y is 39, and n is 0. The proportion of cases who are male would be $13/39 \times 1 = 1/3$ or 1:3. Thus one-third, or one of every three, pneumonia cases are male. This proportion can be expressed as a percentage if 10^n is 100 (or n = 2) where $13/39 \times 100 = 33\%$. In a proportion, the values in the numerator are always a subset of those in the denominator.

Measures of Central Tendency

Measures of central tendency describe the values around the middle of a set of data. Two measures of central tendency used in healthcare surveillance are the arithmetic mean and the median. The mean is the mathematical average of the values in a set of data. Although the mean is commonly used, it is important to remember that its value is affected by outliers (extremely low or high values). The median is the middle value in a ranked set of data. Because half of the measurements in the data set lie below the median and half of the measurements lie above it, the value of the median is not affected by outliers.

Copyright © 2005, Association for Professionals in Infection Control and Epidemiology, Inc.

Measures of Dispersion

Measures of dispersion measure the distribution of a set of data around its mean. Commonly used measures of dispersion in hospital epidemiology are the range, deviation, variance, and standard deviation.

The range is the difference between the smallest value and the largest value in a set of data. The deviation is the difference between an individual value in a data set and the mean (average) for the set. The variance is the deviation around the mean of a distribution. The standard deviation is a measure that reflects the distribution of values around the mean.

Percentiles

Percentiles are used to indicate the relative position of a measurement with respect to other measurements in a set of data. The median is the 50th percentile in a distribution of numbers because half of the values in the distribution are lower and half are higher than the median value. In addition to the median, commonly used percentiles for reporting surveillance data are the 10th, 25th, 75th, and 90th percentiles.

The CDC NNIS System reports percentile distributions for device-associated infection rates, device utilization ratios, surgical site infections by operative procedure, and antimicrobial usage rates among participating hospitals.[40] Hospitals that collect and analyze their data using NNIS methodology can use the NNIS data for benchmarking. An appendix in the NNIS System Reports provides instructions on how to interpret percentiles of infection rates or device utilization ratios.[40]

Additional information on how to use and calculate these statistical measures can be found in Chapter 5 of this text and in the Supplemental Resources section at the end of this chapter.

Surveillance Methodologies

Total House Surveillance

In total house surveillance, all infections are monitored in the entire population of a healthcare facility and an overall infection rate is calculated. Total house surveillance rates have been discouraged by most experts because crude overall rates are not sensitive enough to identify potential problems and therefore cannot be used to target performance improvement activities.[41-44] In addition, because overall rates are not adjusted for specific infection or injury risks, they are not appropriate for measuring trends over time, making comparisons between groups either within a facility or between facilities, or benchmarking.[43]

Targeted Surveillance

In the 1990s, the Centers for Disease Control and Prevention shifted the NNIS system away from total hospital surveillance to focus on targeted surveillance in defined populations.[45] Targeted programs focus on particular care units (such as a nursery or ICU), infections related to medical devices (such as intravascular and urinary tract catheters), invasive procedures (such as surgery), and organisms of epidemiological significance (such as methicillin-resistant *Staphylococcus aureus* [MRSA]).[16,40,41] Targeted programs usually focus on high-risk, high-volume procedures and on those healthcare-associated infections and adverse outcomes that are potentially preventable.[14,16,44]

Combination Surveillance Strategy

In practice, many infection control programs utilize a combination of targeted and modified total house surveillance. Many programs monitor targeted events that occur in a defined population and are potentially preventable while concurrently monitoring selected laboratory reports from house-wide locations. Laboratory reports can be monitored house-wide to detect the following: antibiotic-resistant organisms (such as MRSA and vancomycin-resistant enterococci [VRE]), reportable diseases, organisms of epidemiological importance, and clusters that may indicate an outbreak or breakdown of infection control practices (such as several cases of diarrhea associated with *Clostridium difficile* on a medical care unit).

Elements of a Surveillance Program: Surveillance Program Design

Much has been published about developing and evaluating surveillance programs.[8,42,46-52] Certain steps should be taken when designing a surveillance program for the healthcare setting:

Select the Surveillance Methodology

A surveillance program may measure all infections and provide an overall infection rate (i.e., total surveillance) or may be focused (targeted) on events selected by an organization.[14,41,42] Although some accrediting agencies and regulators may still require total house surveillance in certain settings, the use of an overall infection rate has been discouraged by most authorities, and overall rates are rarely used.[41-44]

Assess and Define the Population(s) to be Studied

Each organization should assess its patient, resident, and employee populations and identify those who have the greatest risk for infection or other adverse outcome.[8,42] This is done by assessing the types of persons served (e.g., newborn, pediatric, adult, geria-

Copyright © 2005, Association for Professionals in Infection Control and Epidemiology, Inc.

tric), healthcare services provided (e.g., medical, surgical, rehabilitation, long-term care, ambulatory care), surgical and other invasive procedures performed, and the conditions and diseases present in the population.

Choose the Indicators (Events) to Monitor

One of the most important steps in designing a surveillance program is the selection of appropriate health-related indicators (events) to monitor.[8,42,53] Surveillance programs should measure outcomes of healthcare, processes of healthcare, and selected events of importance to the organization.[8,42,53-60] The indicators chosen will depend on the type of healthcare setting, the population being studied, procedures performed, services provided, acuity of care, identified risk factors for infection and other adverse events, regulatory and accrediting agency requirements, available resources, the availability of the data required, public health needs, performance improvement initiatives, and organizational objectives. It is common to choose indicators that monitor high-volume, high-risk events in a specific population, especially if the information obtained can be used to guide performance improvement activities.

A surveillance program should monitor a variety of outcomes, processes, and events, and some indicators should focus on personnel.

Examples of outcome indicators that may be monitored include: healthcare-associated infections (e.g., bloodstream, urinary tract, pneumonia, surgical site, conjunctivitis, upper respiratory tract, or local IV site); infection or colonization with a specific organism (e.g., *C. difficile*, MRSA, VRE or other antibiotic-resistant organism, respiratory syncytial virus or rotavirus); decubitis ulcers; phlebitis related to peripheral intravascular therapy; pyrogenic reaction or vascular access infection in hemodialysis patients; resident or patient falls; influenza or tuberculin skin test conversions in patients, residents, or healthcare providers; and sharps injuries and blood/body fluid exposures in healthcare providers.

Examples of process indicators include: medication errors; influenza vaccination rates in personnel, residents, or patients; hepatitis B immunity rates in personnel; and personnel compliance with protocols, such as standard precautions, isolation precautions, tuberculin skin testing, hand hygiene, instrument processing, sterilization quality assurance testing, environmental cleaning, communicable disease reporting, antimicrobial prescribing and administration, and installing and maintaining barriers during construction and renovation projects.

Examples of other events of significance that may be monitored include:

the occurrence of reportable diseases and conditions; communicable and potentially communicable diseases in personnel; organisms or syndromes indicative of a bioterrorist event; results of quality assurance testing (e.g., monitoring of negative airflow in airborne infection isolation rooms, biological monitoring of sterilizers, and testing of high-level disinfectants); and the admission of a patient or resident known to be infected or colonized with an antibiotic-resistant organism.

An effort should be made to select some indicators that have validated, nationally available benchmarks that can be used for meaningful comparison, such as the NNIS system for nosocomial infections and the Vermont Oxford Network for monitoring the medical care of newborns.[40,61,62] See Chapter 9 for a detailed discussion of performance indicators.

When selecting an event and a population for study, both the number of cases (i.e., persons who have the condition) and the number in the total population at risk for that condition must be identifiable if rates are to be calculated. Rates, rather than raw numbers, must be used to accurately track trends over time. Indicators that incorporate a risk adjustment or risk stratification method should be selected, whenever possible.[8,15,40] For instance, the CDC NNIS system indicator for catheter-associated urinary tract infection (UTI) measures the development of a UTI associated with the risk of an indwelling urinary catheter in a defined population.[40] The NNIS surgical site infection component measures surgical site infection rates in patients who are risk stratified using a Risk Index based on the duration of the surgical procedure, wound classification and American Society of Anesthesiologists (ASA) score.[40,63,64]

Determine Time Period for Observation

Surveillance data for each indicator should be collected consistently and for a defined period, such as a month, quarter, or year. It is difficult to interpret rates for events that rarely occur and procedures that are infrequently performed. Therefore, if uncommon events are measured and rates are calculated, it is necessary to use an observation period that is long enough to accumulate a sufficient number of events for the measurement to be valid.

Identify Surveillance Criteria

To accurately trend surveillance data over time within a facility, or compare rates between facilities, surveillance criteria (i.e., case definitions) must be consistently used to determine the presence of a healthcare-associated infection, the occurrence of an event, or compliance with a process. If a case definition is changed, then this should be noted in the surveillance report because the number of cases identified will likely change and

Copyright © 2005, Association for Professionals in Infection Control and Epidemiology, Inc.

the rate will be affected. Criteria used should reflect generally accepted definitions of the disease or event being monitored. Criteria have been published for defining nosocomial infections in hospitals, long-term care, and home care settings.[65-68] It should be noted that criteria used to define a case for surveillance purposes may be different than criteria used for diagnosis and treatment.

Identify Data Elements to be Collected

The data elements that should be collected depend on the event being monitored and the statistical measures used to analyze the data. To use time and personnel resources efficiently, data collection should be limited only to those elements that are needed to identify a case and determine whether the case criteria is met for the condition or event being studied.

Data elements that may be collected include:

For an infectious event:

1. Case name, sex, age, unique identifier such as medical record or account number, unit or location in the facility, physician name and service, date of admission, date of onset of infection, type of infection, and date of discharge, transfer, or death

2. Information needed to determine whether the case definition is met: results of laboratory and diagnostic tests specified in the case definition, and dates performed; sites and dates cultured and organisms isolated; antibiotic susceptibility of significant isolates; and clinical signs and symptoms specific for the infection being monitored

3. Risk factors for the infection being monitored: host factors such as underlying conditions and diseases; surgical procedure and date performed, including surgeon, ASA score, wound classification, and duration of procedure; use of intravascular catheters, including date of insertion, duration of use (vascular catheter-days), catheter type and body site; use of urinary catheter, including date of insertion and duration of use (urinary catheter-days); mechanical ventilation and dates and duration of use (ventilator-days).

For a noninfectious event:

1. Case name, sex, age, unique identifier such as medical record or account number, unit or location in the facility, physician name and service, date of admission, primary diagnosis, date, time, and location of event, outcome (e.g., severity of injury), personnel involved, risk factors for the event, and date of discharge, transfer, or death.

Determine Methods for Data Analysis

Before data collection is initiated, the statistical measures that will be used to analyze the data must be determined so that the requisite data can be collected. If rates or ratios will be calculated, the values corresponding to each numerator and denominator must be defined, and the appropriate data needed to calculate each rate or ratio must be collected.

Whenever possible, data should be expressed as rates or ratios that are calculated using the same methodology as a nationally validated surveillance system. This allows a facility to compare its rates with a recognized benchmark. For instance, if ventilator-associated pneumonia (VAP) is monitored using the NNIS system criteria and methodology, both the number of VAP cases in a specified population (numerator data) and the total number of ventilator-days in that population (denominator data) must be identified to calculate VAP rates that can be benchmarked against NNIS data.[40]

Determine Methods for Data Collection and Management

Data may be collected concurrently (while a person is still under the care of the organization) or retrospectively (closed-record review after discharge). The advantages of concurrent surveillance are: data collectors may interview caregivers or observe the patient or resident if the chart does not include the information needed to fulfill the case criteria; immediate prevention and control measures, such as isolation precautions, may be instituted; clusters and outbreaks can be detected in a timely manner; and infection control personnel are available on medical care units to identify and correct potential problems and provide education to personnel, visitors, and patients or residents. The disadvantages of concurrent surveillance are the time involved in locating records on a medical care unit and incomplete medical records. The major advantage of retrospective review is that the medical record is complete and can usually be reviewed with fewer distractions. The disadvantages of retrospective surveillance is that important findings, such as the identification of an outbreak, may be delayed and missing information may not be obtainable after discharge.

Sources of surveillance data include: medical records (paper and electronic); daily reports generated by the laboratory (e.g., microbiology, immunology, and serology results); daily list of admissions, including diagnosis, from the admissions department; monthly report of patient-days and census data, by unit, provided by the finance or admissions office; nursing care plan (Kardex or computerized plan); interviews with caregivers; list of patients or residents on isolation from the care unit or computer information system; list of prescribed medications from the pharmacy; test results

Copyright © 2005, Association for Professionals in Infection Control and Epidemiology, Inc.

from the radiology department (may be available via an audio telephone reporting system or a computerized information system); incident reports; employee health reports of injuries, needlesticks, communicable diseases and exposures; procedure and activity logs from the respiratory therapy department, operating room, and medical care units; reports from others who review medical records, such as performance improvement personnel; and reports from caregivers.

Existing databases and other sources of information should be identified and utilized. Whenever possible, data should be downloaded directly into a computerized surveillance database so it can be efficiently manipulated and analyzed. Surveillance personnel can often accomplish this by working with an organization's information services department.

Personnel who are responsible for collecting and managing surveillance data must have adequate training in reviewing medical records, interpreting clinical notes, applying standardized criteria for identifying cases, using appropriate statistical and risk adjustment methods, and utilizing computer tools and technology (especially electronic records, spreadsheets and databases) to collect, store, manage, and analyze data.[2,3,8,16]

Data should be collected using a standardized data collection form (paper or electronic) that is designed to collect only those elements needed to identify a case and determine if the case criteria is met for the condition or event being studied.[8,41] To facilitate rapid data collection, the form should be designed so that data elements (such as yes/no, procedures, treatments, and risk factors) can be circled, checked, or otherwise selected. Narrative entries should be limited as much as possible. The data collection forms used in the NNIS system have been published and can be used as is or as a guide in designing a form for a specific indicator.[41] Data should be entered from a collection form into a computer spreadsheet or database so it can be sorted and analyzed. Ideally, data should be entered directly into a laptop computer or personal digital assistant (PDA) when it is collected.

Design an Interpretive Surveillance Report

A written report should be developed to provide a mechanism to interpret and disseminate surveillance data to stimulate performance improvement activities. Tables, graphs, and charts are effective tools for organizing, summarizing, and visually displaying data and should be used as applicable.[38] The format and level of detail in each report will depend on the intended audience.

A surveillance report should:

1. Define the event, population, setting, and time period studied (e.g., surgical site infections in patients undergoing coronary artery bypass graft in hospital A from January through December 2003)

2. State the criteria used for defining a case (e.g., NNIS criteria for urinary tract infection)

3. Specify the number of cases or events identified and the number in the population studied (e.g., 2 surgical site infections in 179 total hip replacement procedures performed)

4. Explain the methodology used to identify cases (e.g., case reports from personnel and review of medical records and laboratory results)

5. Identify the statistical methods and calculations used, when appropriate (e.g., fall rate on 3 North in April = # falls on 3 North in April/ # resident-days on 3 North in April × 1000 or 3/414 × 1000 = 7.2 falls per 1000 resident-days)

6. State the purpose for conducting surveillance (e.g., to reduce the rate of occurrence of an event)

7. Interpret the findings in a manner that is understandable to those who read the report

8. Describe any actions taken and recommendations made for prevention and control measures

9. Identify the author and date of the report

10. Identify the recipients of the report

Identify Recipients of the Surveillance Report

The report should be disseminated to those managers and healthcare providers in the organization who can use the findings to influence performance improvement activities.[14,16]

Develop a Written Surveillance Plan

A written surveillance plan should describe the following: the type of facility, services provided and populations served; the surveillance program purpose, goals and objectives; the indicators (i.e., events monitored) and criteria used; the reason for selecting each indicator (outcome, process, and other event); the methodology used for case identification, data collection, and analysis; the types of reports generated and to whom they are provided; and the process used to evaluate the surveillance program.

Copyright © 2005, Association for Professionals in Infection Control and Epidemiology, Inc.

Surveillance Program Evaluation

A surveillance program should periodically be evaluated to assess its usefulness and ability to meet the organization's objectives, and revisions should be made as needed. The program structure and activities should be compared with current practices and published recommendations for surveillance programs in similar settings.[2,3,8,46,49,50,69,70] The latest requirements of regulatory and accrediting agencies should be reviewed and incorporated (see Chapter 10). The resources required to manage the program, such as an adequate number of trained personnel, appropriate computer hardware and software, access to electronic mail and the Internet, provision for ongoing training, and the availability of office supplies, reference materials and related services (e.g., secretarial, information technology and laboratory support) should also be assessed and allocations made as needed.

A surveillance program should be able to support a system that can prevent the most infections and other adverse events with the resources available. Depending on the objectives of the program, a surveillance system may be considered useful if it can: detect infections, injuries, or other events in a timely manner; identify trends signaling changes in the occurrence of an event; detect outbreaks; identify risk factors associated with infection or other adverse event; provide an estimate of the magnitude of the event being monitored; assess the effectiveness of prevention and control efforts; and lead to improved practices by healthcare providers.[46]

Surveillance in Out-of-Hospital Healthcare Settings

Although the majority of literature to-date has focused on the acute care hospital, information on surveillance programs has been published for a variety of nonhospital healthcare settings: long term care,[49,50,71-85] ambulatory surgery,[86-90] outpatient hemodialysis,[91-97] physician's offices and clinics,[98-101] and home care.[69,102-111] Because surveillance methodologies evolve as the healthcare system changes, infection control personnel should review current literature and practices before evaluating or developing a surveillance program in any setting.

Using Technology

A basic requirement for those who are responsible for implementing and evaluating a surveillance program is the ability to use word processing, spreadsheet, database, and graphics programs, the Internet, and electronic mail. Data should be collected, managed, analyzed, and reported, using computers and computerized technology.[112] Specialized infection control software is available commercially, although many ICPs use basic software packages that contain word processing, spreadsheet, graphics, and database programs. Some infection control professionals use laptop computers or handheld PDAs for direct data entry.

Electronic mail (E-mail) and the Internet have become indispensable tools for infection surveillance programs. ICPs can subscribe to E-mail alert systems and Listservs, such as those from the CDC and professional organizations, such as the Association for Professionals in Infection Control and Epidemiology (APIC). These E-mail systems notify subscribers about the occurrence of disease outbreaks and emerging infectious diseases. They also provide Internet links for obtaining more information, including prevention and control measures.

A discussion of the applications of information technology in surveillance programs is found in Chapter 33.

Benchmarking

Benchmarking is the process of "comparing oneself to others performing similar activities, so as to continuously improve."[113] Although it is very appealing to compare one's rates externally with others, comparisons should be made only after ensuring that the following conditions are met:[16,43,61,114]

- Criteria for defining a case are standardized and up-to-date.

- Criteria are consistently used by all participants and all data collectors.

- The population and time period for study is well-defined.

- The surveillance methodology is standardized and consistently used by all participants over time.

- Rates and ratios are calculated using the same numerators (number of cases) and denominators (population at risk).

- The size of the population studied (denominator) is large enough to provide an accurate estimate of the true rate.

- A standardized risk adjustment method is used by all participants.

- All data collectors receive training on how to collect data and use a standardized form.

- The facility and population being compared is similar to the types of facilities and populations in an aggregate database used for external comparison (for example, data from a neonatal ICU is compared with data aggregated from other neonatal ICUs).

Copyright © 2005, Association for Professionals in Infection Control and Epidemiology, Inc.

- The aggregating organization has a mechanism for ensuring the accuracy, sensitivity, and specificity of the data submitted to it.

- The analysis and interpretation of the data provided by the benchmarking system is accurate and in a form that is understandable to the users.

- Feedback will be disseminated to those who can affect change.

- The data provided by an organization to an external aggregating system is coded for confidentiality, and the reports provided to the organization or to the public do not contain facility identifiers.

Benchmarking Systems Worldwide

Benchmarks are measures against which outcomes and processes can be compared. There are currently few external benchmarks that can be used for interfacility comparisons of healthcare-associated infections and other adverse events. Worldwide, efforts are underway to standardize infection surveillance criteria and methodology, identify methods to risk-adjust the populations studied, and develop computer technology to improve the ability to collect data and compare populations for benchmarking and performance improvement.[115-124]

In the United States, efforts have been made to establish systems for benchmarking in a variety of settings: acute care,[16,45,48,125-126] hemodialysis,[91-92] long-term care,[127] home care,[120-100] and ambulatory surgery.[131] The NNIS system for nosocomial infections surveillance in acute care hospitals is the oldest and most widely used of these.

Comparing Rates

Statistical methods should be used to compare differences between populations studied. For example, if a hospital uses NNIS methodology to collect and analyze surgical site infection data, then it can use the z-test and standardized infection ratio (SIR) to compare its risk-adjusted surgical site infection rates with the rates in the NNIS System Reports.[40,121,132] The use of z-tests and the SIR to compare rates between two defined populations is discussed in Chapter 7.

Other statistical methods that are used to compare differences between populations, such as the t-test, chi-square test, Fisher's exact test, confidence intervals, and the 2 × 2 table, are discussed in Chapter 5.

Performance Improvement, Patient Safety, and Infection Control

One of the main purposes for conducting surveillance is to provide information that can be used by an organization to target performance improvement activi-ties.[8,10,16,23] There are many published reports that demonstrate the use of surveillance data to identify potential problems and risk factors for infection, implement prevention and control measures, and document the reduction of infection rates in a variety of healthcare settings.[6,9-37,133-135] An effective infection prevention and control program will incorporate a surveillance program that enhances a healthcare organization's performance improvement activities and reduces the risk of adverse outcomes.[9,10,14] Critical elements that have been shown to be successful in reducing infection rates include: (1) voluntary participation and confidentiality; (2) standard definitions and protocols; (3) defined populations at risk (e.g., intensive care, surgical patients); (4) site-specific, risk-adjusted infection rates comparable across institutions; (5) adequate numbers of trained infection control practitioners; (6) dissemination of data to healthcare providers; and (7) a link between monitored rates and prevention efforts.[16] Further discussion of the link between infection control and performance improvement activities can be found in Chapter 8.

Since the release of the Institute of Medicine Report on patient safety and medical errors in 1999, the infection control and performance improvement communities have focused their attention on the role of infection prevention and control in patient safety.[136-139] Infection control is a critical component of patient safety.[140-143] Infection control and patient safety activities can complement and benefit each other. For example, patient safety practices, such as continuous quality improvement and root cause analysis, can augment infection prevention and control programs.[137] The use of root cause analysis has been advocated to review healthcare-associated infections that are implicated as attributable causes of death.[137,144] Conversely, traditional infection control practices that can benefit the patient safety field include the use of trained professionals and "valid definitions of infection-related adverse events, standardized methods for detecting and reporting events, confidentiality protections, appropriate rate adjustments for institutional and case-mix differences, and evidence-based intervention programs."[137]

To comply with JCAHO requirements, the surveillance program in a JCAHO-accredited organization must be able to recognize "cases of unanticipated death or major loss of function associated with a healthcare-acquired infection."[144] The relationship between patient safety and infection control is further discussed in Chapter 12.

In 2001, the CDC Division of Healthcare Quality Promotion (formerly the Hospital Infections Program) issued Seven Healthcare Safety Challenges to reduce adverse events, including infections, in a variety of

Copyright © 2005, Association for Professionals in Infection Control and Epidemiology, Inc.

healthcare settings; to eliminate occupational needlestick injuries; and to achieve 100% adherence to guidelines for immunization of healthcare personnel.[145] To meet these safety challenges, surveillance systems will be needed to determine infection rates, identify risk factors for infection and occupational injuries, measure the effectiveness of intervention measures, and evaluate immunization rates in healthcare providers.[146]

The National Healthcare Safety Network

In 2002, the Centers for Disease Control and Prevention announced that it was integrating three of its existing patient and healthcare worker surveillance systems into the National Healthcare Safety Network (NHSN). The NHSN will incorporate the:

- National Nosocomial Infections Surveillance (NNIS) System that monitors hospital-associated infections[40,45,48]

- National Surveillance System for Health Care Workers (NaSH) that monitors healthcare worker immunization and tuberculin skin-testing programs and exposures to blood and body fluids, vaccine-preventable diseases, and tuberculosis

- Dialysis Surveillance Network (DSN), which is a national voluntary surveillance system that monitors bloodstream and vascular infections in adult and pediatric patients treated in outpatient hemodialysis centers.[92,93]

The goal of the NHSN is to provide a Web-based reporting and knowledge system for patient and healthcare worker safety information, feedback of comparative data for performance improvement, and access to prevention tools and best practices (information on the National Healthcare Safety Network can be found at http://www.cdc.gov/ncidod/hip).

Detection of Healthcare-Associated Outbreaks

Only a small proportion of healthcare-associated infections are related to an outbreak.[16,50,147] In the healthcare setting, most outbreaks are suspected when routine surveillance activities detect a cluster of cases, an unusual organism, or an apparent increase in the occurrence of an organism or event; when a clinician diagnoses an unusual disease; or when a healthcare provider or laboratory worker notices a cluster of cases. In some facilities, data mining and electronic or automated surveillance programs have been used to detect potential outbreaks of infection.[148,149] The use of data mining and electronic surveillance is discussed in Chapter 33.

Surveillance for Diseases Associated with the Healthcare Environment

Surveillance of Patients and Residents

A surveillance program should monitor patients and residents in healthcare facilities for diseases that are associated with the healthcare environment. Guidelines for the surveillance of environment-associated infections, such as aspergillosis and legionellosis, have been published.[150-153]

Environmental Sampling (Culturing)

Guidelines for environmental sampling (culturing) of the environment, including air, water, and environmental surfaces, have been published by the CDC and others.[150-153] Routine or random, undirected microbiological culturing of air, water, and environmental surfaces in healthcare facilities is not recommended.[150] Culturing is indicated, however, for selected quality assurance purposes, such as biological monitoring of sterilizers using bacterial spores and cultures of water and dialysate in hemodialysis units.[90,97,150] Cultures of environmental sources may be indicated as part of an outbreak investigation if epidemiological data implicate an environmental source and results can be used to direct infection control decisions.[150] Environmental sampling should be conducted only under the guidance of a multidisciplinary team and in accordance with written protocols that define sample collection and culturing methods, how to interpret results, and what actions will be taken based on the findings.[150]

Surveillance for Public Health, Emerging Infectious Diseases, and Bioterrorism

Surveillance is the key to recognizing outbreaks and new or emerging infectious diseases so that control measures can be instituted to contain their spread. Disease surveillance in the United States is based on a passive system in which healthcare providers and laboratories report unusual or reportable conditions to a public health department. Therefore, infection control professionals and healthcare personnel play an integral role in detecting and reporting diseases of public health significance as discussed in Chapter 113.

Community outbreaks have been recognized after ICPs and other healthcare workers reported disease cases to the local health department.[154] A bioterrorist event associated with the release of anthrax spores was first detected when an astute clinician reported a case of inhalational anthrax.[155] In the past two decades, healthcare providers have been instrumental in detecting and reporting emerging infectious diseases, such as acquired immune deficiency syndrome (AIDS), hantavirus pulmonary syndrome, gastroenteritis caused by Norovirus agents, hemolytic uremic syndrome due

Copyright © 2005, Association for Professionals in Infection Control and Epidemiology, Inc.

to *Escherichia coli* O157:H7, and severe acute respiratory syndrome (SARS).[156-158] Community outbreaks, such as influenza, respiratory syncytial virus, and SARS, can affect healthcare workers, patients, and residents of healthcare institutions and can disrupt and overwhelm healthcare services.[157]

The Institute of Medicine and the Centers for Disease Control and Prevention have published recommendations for addressing the threat of emerging infectious diseases and bioterrorism that include strengthening disease surveillance systems.[156,157-160] Syndrome surveillance has been promoted to detect bioterrorist events, although its efficacy is still unknown.[161-163] Many guidelines have been published for bioterrorism response and planning, and these are discussed in Chapter 120. There is no longer any doubt about the interdependence of infection control, clinical medicine, and public health.[161] Those who are responsible for managing surveillance programs in healthcare facilities should ensure that sufficient resources are allocated for the surveillance of diseases of public health significance, including reportable conditions, emerging infectious diseases, and those associated with bioterrorism.

Surveillance for Antibiotic-Resistant Organisms

Antimicrobial resistance is increasing in both healthcare-associated and community acquired infections, and vancomycin resistance in *S. aureus* has been detected.[40,164-166] Surveillance to detect antibiotic-resistant organisms has been advocated for decades and a healthcare organization's surveillance program should monitor microbiology reports for the occurrence of resistant organisms of epidemiological importance to the facility.[167,168] The use of surveillance cultures to screen patients and residents for carriage of multidrug-resistant bacteria in nonoutbreak situations has been widely debated and there is currently no widespread consensus on this issue.[164,169,170] The Society for Healthcare Epidemiology of America recently recommended a program of active surveillance cultures and isolation precautions to control the spread of epidemiologically significant antibiotic-resistant pathogens known to be spreading in a healthcare facility.[171]

III. NEW DEVELOPMENTS

In the past decade, developments affecting surveillance programs in healthcare facilities have included:

- an ongoing shift from acute inpatient care to outpatient and long term care services[3,7,172,173]

- emphasis on the use of targeted surveillance to focus performance improvement activities[14,44]

- a decreased length of stay across the continuum of care[7]

- a focus on the use of data to demonstrate the effectiveness of an infection prevention, surveillance, and control program and the quality of healthcare[9,11-37,173]

- an emphasis on the use of benchmarking and statistical methods to compare infection rates between groups[16,91,92,114-131]

- emerging infectious diseases, such as SARS, hantavirus pulmonary syndrome, and West Nile virus[155-158]

- bioterrorism and the use of syndrome surveillance[155,162,163,174]

- the use of technology, such as the PDA, to lessen the burden of data collection[112]

- electronic and automated surveillance systems to identify cases[101,148,149,173,175-180]

- the use of surveillance to monitor noninfectious events, such as sharps injuries and compliance with hand hygiene and construction protocols[146,181]

- increased recognition of the role of the healthcare environment in the transmission of legionellosis and aspergillosis and the need for surveillance for these diseases[150-153]

- controversy over surveillance and control measures that should be used to limit the spread of antibiotic-resistant organisms[169-171]

- the use of electronic mail and the Internet to rapidly transfer information on the occurrence of outbreaks and infection prevention and control measures

IV. SUMMARY AND CONCLUSIONS

Surveillance methodology evolves in response to changes in the healthcare delivery system, the use of surveillance data, and diseases prevalent in the populations served. In the past decade healthcare delivery has continued to shift outside of the traditional acute care hospital, resulting in a growing need for surveillance in other healthcare settings. The use of surveillance data has shifted from merely measuring clinical outcomes, such as infections, to guiding performance improvement activities and demonstrating improvements in clinical outcomes. The occurrence of increasing antimicrobial resistance and outbreaks caused by emerging infectious diseases and intentionally released pathogens has highlighted the need for local, regional, national, and global surveillance systems. Those who are responsible for implementing and managing surveillance programs in healthcare facilities must ensure that their programs are based on sound epidemiological

Copyright © 2005, Association for Professionals in Infection Control and Epidemiology, Inc.

and statistical principles, designed and evaluated in accordance with current recommendations and practices, and have the resources needed to promote quality healthcare.

V.   FUTURE TRENDS/RESEARCH

Future trends that will affect surveillance programs in healthcare facilities include:

- more widespread use of post-discharge surveillance to monitor hospital-acquired infections, especially surgical site infections, that develop after discharge[178-180,182-194]

- the growth of national and global surveillance systems to detect antimicrobial resistance, bioterrorist events, naturally occurring epidemics, and emerging infectious diseases[156,158-163]

- mandatory reporting of infection rates and other adverse healthcare outcomes ("report cards")

- the use of surveillance cultures of patients and residents of healthcare institutions to detect antibiotic-resistant organisms so that infection control measures can be instituted[169-171]

- the use of electronic surveillance and information technology to identify cases and reduce the burden of collecting, managing, and analyzing data[101,112,148,149,173,175-180]

- the use of electronic mail and the Internet by more infection control professionals to rapidly transfer information on disease occurrence and infection prevention and control methods

- increased coordination of disease surveillance activities between the infection control, academic, clinical, and public health communities[196]

VI.   INTERNATIONAL PERSPECTIVES

Surveillance for Nosocomial Infections

National surveillance programs for healthcare-associated infections exist in several countries. As in the United States, infection control and infectious disease professionals in these countries are endeavoring to standardize infection surveillance criteria and methodology, develop risk-stratification methods, improve computer technology to collect, manage and analyze data, and develop benchmarking systems.[115-124]

Surveillance for Antibiotic-Resistant Organisms

Antimicrobial resistant organisms are well recognized worldwide, and many countries have surveillance programs to identify and limit their spread.[169-170,195] However, many nations do not have surveillance or control programs, and global surveillance systems are needed to rapidly detect resistant strains and institute control measures to prevent their spread.[195]

Surveillance for Outbreaks

In 2000, the World Health Organization organized the development of the Global Outbreak Alert and Response Network (see Web site at http://www.who.int/csr). This is a network of existing institutions and networks that pool resources for the rapid identification, confirmation, and response to outbreaks of international importance. The global outbreak of SARS in 2003 highlighted the need for a worldwide surveillance network. The SARS outbreak emphasized the value of the international infection control, clinical, and public health communities working together to rapidly detect cases, transfer information, and identify and implement measures to control the spread of the disease.[196]

REFERENCES AND CITATIONS

1. Lee TB, Baker-Montgomery OG: Surveillance. In *APIC text of infection control and epidemiology*, ed rev, Washington, DC, 2002, Association for Professionals in Infection Control and Epidemiology.
2. Scheckler WE, Brimhall D, Buck AS, et al: Requirements for infrastructure and essential activities of infection control and epidemiology in hospitals: a consensus panel report, *Am J Infect Control* 26:47–60, 1998. [Available at URL http://www.apic.org]
3. Friedman C, Barnette M, Buck AS, et al: Requirements for infrastructure and essential activities of infection control and epidemiology in out-of-hospital settings: a consensus panel report, *Am J Infect Control* 27:418–430, 1999. [Available at URL http://www.apic.org]
4. American Hospital Association: Prevention and control of *Staphylococcus* infections in hospitals. In U.S. Public Health Service-Communicable Disease Center and National Academy of Sciences-National Research Council: *Proceedings of the National Conference on Hospital-Acquired Staphylococcal Disease*, Atlanta, GA, 1958, Communicable Disease Center, pp 23–26.
5. Joint Commission on Accreditation of Hospitals: *Accreditation Manual for Hospitals*, Chicago, 1976, Joint Commission on Accreditation of Hospitals.
6. Haley RW, Culver DH, White JW, et al: The efficacy of surveillance and control programs in preventing nosocomial infections in U.S. hospitals, *Am J Epidemiol* 121:182–205, 1985.
7. Bernstein AB, Hing B, Moss AJ, et al: *Health care in America: trends in utilization*, Hyattsville, MD, 2003, National Center for Health Statistics. [Available at URL http://www.cdc.gov/nchs]
8. Lee TB, Baker OG, Lee JT, et al: APIC Surveillance Initiative Working Group. Recommended Practices for Surveillance, *Am J Infect Control* 26:277–288, 1998. [Available at URL http://www.apic.org]
9. Centers for Disease Control and Prevention. Monitoring hospital-acquired infections to promote patient safety—United States, 1990–1999, *MMWR* 49:149–153, 2000. [Available at URL http://www.cdc.gov/mmwr]
10. Wenzel RP, Pfaller MA: Infection control: the premier quality assessment program in United States hospitals, *Am J Med* 91(3B):27S-31S, 1991.
11. Farr B: Reasons for noncompliance with infection control guidelines, *Infect Control Hosp Epidemiol* 21:411–416, 2000.
12. Slater F: Cost-effective infection control success story: a case presentation, *Emerg Infect Dis* 7:293–294, 2001.

Copyright © 2005, Association for Professionals in Infection Control and Epidemiology, Inc.

13. Richards C, Emori TG, Peavey G, et al: Promoting quality through measurement of performance and response: prevention success stories, *Emerg Infect Dis* 7:299–301, 2001.
14. Murphy DM: From expert data collectors to interventionists: changing the focus for infection control professionals, *Am J Infect Control* 30:120–132, 2002.
15. Richardson D, Tarnow-Mordi WO, Lee SK: Risk adjustment for quality improvement, *Pediatrics* 103(1 suppl E):255–265, 1999.
16. Gaynes R, Richards C, Edwards J, et al: Feeding back surveillance data to prevent hospital-acquired infections, *Emerg Infect Dis* 7:295–298, 2001. [Available at URL http://www.cdc.gov/eid]
17. Bishop-Kurylo D: The clinical experience of continuous quality improvement in the neonatal intensive care unit, *J Perinatol Neonatal Nurs* 12:51–57, 1998.
18. Dumigan D, Kohan CA, Reed CR, et al: Utilizing National Nosocomial Infection Surveillance System data to improve urinary tract infection rates in three intensive care units, *Clin Performance Qual Improv Health Care* 6:172–178, 1998.
19. Goetz AM, Kedzuf S, Wagener M, et al: Feedback to nursing staff as an intervention to reduce catheter-associated urinary tract infections, *Am J Infect Control* 27:402–404, 1999.
20. Gaynes RP, Solomon S: Improving hospital-acquired infection rates: the CDC's experience, *J Qual Improv* 22:457–467, 1996.
21. Plsek PE: Collaborating across organizational boundaries to improve the quality of care, *Am J Infect Control* 25:85–95, 1997.
22. Centers for Disease Control and Prevention. Prevention of perinatal group B streptococcal disease: a public health perspective, *MMWR* 45(No. RR-7), 1996.
23. Gaynes RP: Surveillance of nosocomial infections: a fundamental ingredient for quality, *Infect Control Hosp Epidemiol* 18:475–478, 1997.
24. de Gentile A, Rivas N, Sinkowtiz-Cochran RL, et al: Nosocomial infections in a children's hospital in Argentina: impact of a unique infection control intervention program, *Infect Control Hosp Epidemiol* 22:762–766, 2001.
25. Lemmen SW, Zolldann D, Gastmeier P, et al: Implementing and evaluating a rotating surveillance system and infection control guidelines in 4 intensive care units, *Am J Infect Control* 29:89–93, 2001.
26. Manangan LP, Banerjee SN, Jarvis WR: Association between implementation of CDC recommendations and ventilator-associated pneumonia at selected US hospitals, *Am J Infect Control* 28:222–227, 2000.
27. Haley RW: The scientific basis for using surveillance and risk factor data to reduce nosocomial infection rates, *J Hosp Infect* 30(suppl):3–14, 1995.
28. Sohn AH, Ostrowsky BE, Sinkowitz-Cochran RL, et al: Evaluation of a successful vancomycin-resistant Enterococcus prevention intervention in a community of health care facilities, *Am J Infect Control* 29:53–57, 2001.
29. Klopf LC: Tuberculosis control in the New York State Department of Correctional Services: a case management approach, *Am J Infect Control* 26:534–538, 1998.
30. Kaye J, Ashline V, Erickson D, et al: Critical care bug team: a multidisciplinary team approach to reducing ventilator-associated pneumonia, *Am J Infect Control* 28(2):197–201, 2000.
31. Fridkin SK, Lawton R, Edwards J, et al: Monitoring antimicrobial use and resistance: comparison with a national benchmark on reducing vancomycin use and vancomycin-resistant enterococci, *Emerg Infect Dis* 8:702–707, 2002.
32. Delgado-Rodriguez M, Gomez-Ortega A, Sillero-Arenas M, et al: Efficacy of surveillance in nosocomial infection control in a surgical service, *Am J Infect Control* 29:289–294, 2001.
33. Meyer GS, Rall C: Use of evidence-based data to drive your patient safety program, *Am J Infect Control* 30:314–317, 2002.
34. Gastmeier P, Brauer H, Forster D, et al: A quality management project in 8 selected hospitals to reduce nosocomial infections: a prospective, controlled study, *Infect Control Hosp Epidemiol* 23:91–97, 2002.
35. Curran ET, Benneyan JC, Hood J: Controlling methicillin-resistant Staphylococcus aureus: a feedback approach using annotated statistical process control charts, *Infect Control Hosp Epidemiol* 23:13–18, 2002.
36. Makris AT, Morgan L, Gaber D, et al: Effect of a comprehensive infection control program on the incidence of infections in long-term care facilities, *Am J Infect Control* 28:3–7, 2002.
37. Stricof RL, DiFerdinando GT, Osten WM, et al: Tuberculosis control in New York City hospitals, *Am J Infect Control* 26:270–276, 1998.
38. Centers for Disease Control and Prevention. *Principles of epidemiology: an introduction to applied epidemiology and biostatistics*, ed 2, Atlanta, GA, 1992, U.S. Department of Health and Human Resources, Public Health Service. [Available at URL http://www.phppo.cdc.gov/PHTN]
39. Haley RW, Gaynes RP, Aber RC, et al: Surveillance of nosocomial infections. In Bennett JV, Brachman PS, editors: *Hospital infections*, ed 3, Boston, 1992, Little Brown and Company.
40. Centers for Disease Control and Prevention. National Nosocomial Infections Surveillance (NNIS) System Report, data summary from January 1992 through June 2003, issued August 2003, *Am J Infect Control* 31:481–498, 2003. [Available at URL http://www.cdc.gov/ncidod/hip/SURVEILL/SURVEILL.htm]
41. Gaynes RP, Horan TC: Surveillance of nosocomial infections. In Mayhall CG, editor: *Hospital epidemiology and infection control*, ed 2, Philadelphia, 1999, Lippincott Williams & Wilkins.
42. Pottinger JM, Herwaldt LA, Perl TM: Basics of surveillance—an overview, *Infect Control Hosp Epidemiol* 18:513–527, 1997.
43. Centers for Disease Control and Prevention. Nosocomial infection rates for interhospital comparison: limitations and possible solutions, *Infect Control and Hosp Epidemiol* 12:609–621, 1991.
44. Scheckler WE: Surveillance, foundation for the future: a historical overview and evolution of methodologies, *Am J Infect Control* 25:106–111, 1997.
45. Gaynes RP, Culver DH, Emori TG, et al: The National Nosocomial Infections Surveillance System: plans for the 1990s and beyond, *Am J Med* 91(suppl 3B):116–120, 1991.
46. Centers for Disease Control and Prevention. Updated guidelines for evaluating public health surveillance systems: recommendations from the guidelines working group, *MMWR* 50(No. RR-13), 2001. [Available at URL http://www.cdc.gov/mmwr]
47. Massanari RM, Wilkerson K, Swartzendruber S: Designing surveillance for non-infectious outcomes of medical care, *Infect Control Hosp Epidemiol* 16:419–426, 1995.
48. Emori TG, Culver DH, Horan TC, et al: National Nosocomial Infections Surveillance System (NNIS): description of surveillance methods, *Am J Infect Control* 19:19–35, 1991.
49. Smith PW: Infection surveillance in long-term care facilities, *Infect Control Hosp Epidemiol* 12:55–58, 1991.
50. Smith P, Rusnak PG: Infection prevention and control in the long-term care facility, *Infect Control Hosp Epidemiol* 18:831–849, 1997. [APIC/SHEA Position Paper available at URL http://www.apic.org]
51. Manian FA: Surveillance of surgical site infections in alternative settings: exploring the current options, *Am J Infect Control* 25:102–105, 1997.
52. Nafziger DA, Lundstrom T, Chandra S, et al: Infection control in ambulatory care, *Infect Dis Clin North Am* 11:279–296, 1997.
53. The Quality Indicator Study Group. An approach to the evaluation of quality indicators of the outcome of care in hospitalized patients, with a focus on nosocomial infection indicators, *Am J Infect Control* 23:215–222, 1995. [Available at URL http://www.shea-online.org/PositionPapers.html]
54. Crede W, Hierholzer WJ: Surveillance for quality assessment: I. Surveillance in infection control, *Infect Control Hosp Epidemiol* 10:470–474, 1989.
55. Mc Geer A, Crede W, Hierholzer WJ: Surveillance for quality assessment: II. Surveillance for noninfectious processes: back to basics, *Infect Control Hosp Epidemiol* 11:36–41, 1990.
56. Baker OG: Process surveillance: an epidemiologic challenge for all health care organizations, *Am J Infect Control* 25:96–101, 1997.
57. Baldo V, Floreani A, Dal Vecchio L, et al: Occupational risk for blood-borne viruses in healthcare workers: a 5-year surveillance program, *Infect Control Hosp Epidemiol* 23:325–327, 2002.
58. Russell ML, Ferguson CA: Using epidemiology to target staff influenza vaccination programs, *Infect Control Hosp Epidemiol* 22:525–526, 2001.
59. Pavelchak N, Cummings K, Stricof R, et al: Negative-pressure monitoring of tuberculosis isolation rooms within New York

Copyright © 2005, Association for Professionals in Infection Control and Epidemiology, Inc.

State hospitals, *Infect Control Hosp Epidemiol* 22:518–519, 2001.

60. DeFilippo VC, Bowen RW, Ingbar DH: A universal precautions monitoring system adaptable to any health care department, *Am J Infect Control* 20:159–163, 1992.
61. Emori TG, Edwards JR, Culver DH, et al: Accuracy of reporting nosocomial infections in intensive-care-unit patients to the National Nosocomial Infections Surveillance system: a pilot study, *Infect Control Hosp Epidemiol* 19:308–316, 1998.
62. Kilbride HW, Powers R, Wirtschafter DD, et al: Evaluation and development of potentially better practices to prevent neonatal nosocomial bacteremia, *Pediatrics* 111(suppl E):e504, 2003. [See also the Vermont Oxford Network at URL http://www.vtoxford.org]
63. Horan TC, Emori TG: Definitions of key terms used in the NNIS system, *Am J Infect Control* 25:112–116, 1997.
64. Culver DH, Horan TC, Gaynes RP, et al: Surgical wound infection rates by wound class, operative procedure, and patient risk index, *Am J Med* 91(suppl 3B):152S-157S, 1991.
65. Horan TC, Gaynes RP, Martone WJ, et al: CDC definitions of nosocomial surgical site infections, 1992: a modification of CDC definitions of surgical wound infections, *Infect Control Hosp Epidemiol* 13:606–608, 1992.
66. Garner JS, Jarvis WR, Emori TG, et al: CDC definitions for nosocomial infections, *Am J Infect Control* 16:128–140, 1988.
67. McGeer A, Campbell B, Emori TG, et al: Definitions of infection for surveillance in long term care facilities, *Am J Infect Control* 19:1–7, 1991.
68. APIC Home Care Membership Section: Draft definitions for surveillance of infections in home health care, *Am J Infect Control* 28:449–453, 2000.
69. Rhinehart E, Friedman MM: Surveillance of home care-associated infections. In *Infection control in home care,* Gaithersburg, MD, 1999, Aspen Publishers, pp 117–137.
70. Roy MC, Perl TM: Basics of surgical-site infection surveillance, *Infect Control and Hosp Epidemiol* 18:659–668, 1997.
71. Rosenbaum P, Pass M, Roghmann MC: Long-term care. In *APIC text of infection control and epidemiology,* Washington, DC, 2000, Association for Professionals in Infection Control and Epidemiology, pp 46–1–46–34.
72. Smith PW: Development of nursing home infection control, *Infect Control Hosp Epidemiol* 20:303–305, 1999.
73. Nicolle LE: Preventing infections in non-hospital settings: long term care, *Emerg Infect Dis* 7:205–207, 2001. [Available at URL http://www.cdc.gov]
74. Bradley SF: Long-Term Care Committee of the Society for Health Care Epidemiology of America. Prevention of influenza in long-term facilities, *Infect Control Hosp Epidemiol* 20: 629–637, 1999.
75. Centers for Disease Control and Prevention: Prevention and control of tuberculosis in facilities providing long-term care to the elderly: recommendations of the Advisory Committee for Elimination of Tuberculosis, *MMWR* 39(RR-10):7–20, 1990. [Available at URL http://www.cdc.gov/mmwr]
76. Pritchard V: Joint Commission standards for long-term care infection control: putting together the process elements, *Am J Infect Control* 27:27–34, 1999.
77. Ahlbrecht H, Shearen C, Degelau J, et al: A team approach to infection prevention and control in the nursing home setting, *Am J Infect Control* 27:64–70, 1999.
78. Stevenson KB: Regional data set of infection rates for long-term care facilities: description of a valuable benchmarking tool, *Am J Infect Control* 27:20–26, 1999.
79. Mylotte JM: Analysis of infection control surveillance data in a long-term-care facility: use of threshold settings, *Infect Control Hosp Epidemiol* 17:101–107, 1996.
80. Birnbaum D: Analysis of infection control surveillance data in a long-term-care facility: use of threshold settings [letter], *Infect Control Hosp Epidemiol* 17:348–349, 1996.
81. Beck-Sague C, Villarino E, Giuliano D, et al: Infectious diseases and death among nursing home residents: results of surveillance in 13 nursing homes, *Infect Control Hosp Epidemiol* 15: 494–496, 1994.
82. Lewis SM: The effect of surveillance definitions on nosocomial urinary tract infection rates in a rehabilitation hospital, *Infect Control Hosp Epidemiol* 16:43–48, 1995.
83. Mylotte JM, Goodnough S, Tayara A: Antibiotic-resistant organisms among long-term care facility residents on admission to an

inpatient geriatrics unit: retrospective and prospective surveillance, *Am J Infect Control* 20:139–144, 2001.
84. Golliot F, Astagneau P, Cassou B, et al: Nosocomial infections in geriatric long-term-care and rehabilitation facilities: exploration in the development of a risk index for epidemiological surveillance, *Infect Control Hosp Epidemiol* 22:746–753, 2001.
85. Nicolle LE, Garibaldi RA: Infection control in long-term care facilities, *Infect Control Hosp Epidemiol* 16:348–353, 1995.
86. Flanders E, Hinnant JR: Ambulatory surgery postoperative wound surveillance, *Am J Infect Control* 18:336–339, 1990.
87. Vilar-Compte D, Roldan R, Sandoval S, et al: Surgical site infections in ambulatory surgery: a 5-year experience, *Am J Infect Control* 29:99–103, 2001.
88. Manian FA, Meyer L: Adjunctive use of monthly physician questionnaires for surveillance of surgical site infections after hospital discharge and in ambulatory surgical patients: report of a seven-year experience, *Am J Infect Control* 25:390–394, 1997.
89. Manian FA, Meyer L: Comprehensive surveillance of surgical site infections in outpatient and inpatient surgery, *Infect Control Hosp Epidemiol* 11:515–520, 1990.
90. Association for the Advancement of Medical Instrumentation. AAMI standards and recommended practices—sterilization in health care facilities, Arlington, VA, 2001, Association for the Advancement of Medical Instrumentation. [Available at URL http://www.aami.org]
91. Stevenson KB, Adcox MJ, Mallea MC, et al: Standardized surveillance of hemodialysis vascular access infections: 18-month experience at an outpatient, multifacility hemodialysis center, *Infect Control Hosp Epidemiol* 21:200–203, 2000.
92. Tokars JI, Miller ER, Stein G: New national surveillance system for hemodialysis-associated infections: initial results, *Am J Infect Control* 30:288–295, 2002. [Available at URL http://www.cdc.gov/ncidod/hip]
93. Tokars JL: Description of a new surveillance system for bloodstream and vascular access infections in outpatient hemodialysis centers, *Semin Dial* 13:97–100, 2000.
94. Centers for Disease Control and Prevention. National Surveillance of Dialysis-Associated Diseases in the U.S., 2000. [Available at URL http://www.cdc.gov/ncidod/hip/DIALYSIS/dialysis.htm]
95. Hannah EL, Stevenson KB, Lowder CA, et al: Outbreak of hemodialysis access site infections related to malfunctioning permanent tunneled catheters: making the case for active infection surveillance, *Infect Control Hosp Epidemiol* 23:538–541, 2002.
96. Centers for Disease Control and Prevention. Recommendations for preventing transmission of infections among chronic hemodialysis patients, *MMWR* 50(RR-05):1–43, 2001. [Available at URL http://www.cdc.gov/mmwr]
97. Association for the Advancement of Medical Instrumentation. AAMI standards and recommended practices—dialysis, Arlington, VA, 2001, Association for the Advancement of Medical Instrumentation. [Available at URL http://www.aami.org]
98. Herwaldt LA, Smith SD, Carter CD: Infection control in the outpatient setting, *Infect Control Hosp Epidemiol* 19:41–74, 1998.
99. Nafzinger DA, Lundstrom T, Chandra S, et al: Infection control in ambulatory care, *Infect Dis Clin North Am* 11(2):279–296, 1997.
100. Jennings J, Thibeault M, Olmsted R, et al: Ambulatory Care. In *APIC text of infection control and epidemiology,* Washington, DC, 2000, Association for Professionals in Infection Control and Epidemiology.
101. Lazarus R, Kleinman K, Dashevsky I, et al: Use of automated ambulatory-care encounter records for detection of acute illness clusters, including potential bioterrorism events, *Emerg Infect Dis* 8:753–760, 2002. [Available at URL http://www.cdc.gov]
102. Manangan LP, Pearson ML, Tokars JI, et al: Feasibility of national surveillance of health-care-associated infections in home-care settings, *Emerg Infect Dis* 8:233–236, 2002. [Available at URL http://www.cdc.gov]
103. Rhinehart E: Infection control in home care, *Emerg Infect Dis* 7:208–211, 2001. [Available at URL http://www.cdc.gov]
104. Rosenheimer L: Establishing a surveillance system for infections in home healthcare, *Home Healthc Nurse* 13:20–26, 1995.
105. Zimay DL: Standardizing the definition and measurement of catheter-related infection in home care: a proposed outcome measurement system, *J Med Syst* 23:189–199, 1999.

Copyright © 2005, Association for Professionals in Infection Control and Epidemiology, Inc.

106. White MC, Ragland KE: Surveillance of intravenous catheter-related infections among home care clients, *Am J Infect Control* 22:213–235, 1994.

107. Rosenheimer L, Embry FC, Sanford J, et al: Infection surveillance in home care: device-related incidence rates, *Am J Infect Control* 26:359–363, 1998.

108. Goldberg P, Lange M: Development of an infection surveillance project for home healthcare, *Home Care Magazine* 1:1,4–9, 1997.

109. Rhinehart E: Developing an infection surveillance system, *Caring* 15:26–28, 31–32, 1996.

110. Smith PW, Roccaforte JS: Epidemiology and prevention of infections in home healthcare. In Mayhall CG, editor: *Hospital epidemiology and infection control,* ed 2, Philadelphia, 1999, Lippincott Williams & Wilkins, pp 1483–1488.

111. Lorenzan AN, Itkin DJ: Surveillance of infection in home care, *Am J Infect Control* 20:326–329, 1992.

112. Harr J, Olmsted RN: Applications of information technology. In *APIC text of infection control and epidemiology,* ed rev, Washington, DC, 2002, Association for Professionals in Infection Control and Epidemiology.

113. Lenz S, Myers S, Nordlund S, et al: Benchmarking: finding ways to improve, *Jt Comm J Qual Improv* 20:250–259, 1994.

114. Archibald LK, Gaynes RP: Hospital-acquired infections in the United States: the importance of interhospital comparisons, *Infect Dis Clin North Am* 11:245–255, 1997.

115. McLaws ML, Caelli M: Pilot testing standardized surveillance: hospital infection standardised surveillance (HISS), *Am J Infect Control* 28:401–405, 2000.

116. Coello R, Gastmeier R, de Boer AS: Surveillance of hospital-acquired infection in England, Germany, and The Netherlands: will international comparison of rates be possible? *Infect Control Hosp Epidemiol* 22:393–397, 2001.

117. Golliot F, Astagneau P, Cassou B, et al: Nosocomial infections in geriatric long-term-care and rehabilitation facilities: exploration in the development of a risk index for epidemiological surveillance, *Infect Control Hosp Epidemiol* 22:746–753, 2001.

118. Gulacsi L, Kiss ZT, Goldmann DA, et al: Risk-adjusted infection rates in surgery: a model for outcome measurement in hospitals developing new quality improvement programmes, *J Hosp Infect* 44:43–52, 2000.

119. Babcock HM: Surveillance for surgical-site infection: it's getting better all the time, *Infect Control Hosp Epidemiol* 24: 722–723, 2003.

120. Sands KE, Yokoe DS, Hooper DC, et al: Detection of postoperative surgical-site infections: comparison of health plan-based surveillance with hospital-based programs, *Infect Control Hosp Epidemiol* 24:741–774, 2003.

121. Monge Jodra V, Robutillo Rodela A, Martinez FM, et al: Standardized infection ratios for three general surgery procedures: a comparison between Spanish hospitals and U.S. centers participating in the National Nosocomial Infections Surveillance System, *Infect Control Hosp Epidemiol* 24:744–748, 2003.

122. Suetensi C, Savey A, Labeeuw J, et al: The ICU-HELICS programme: towards European surveillance of hospital-acquired infections in intensive care units, *Euro Surveill* 7:127–128, 2002. [Available at URL www.eurosurveillance.org]

123. McLaws ML, Taylor PC: The Hospital Infection Standardized Surveillance (HISS) programme: analysis of a two-year pilot, *J Hosp Infect* 53:259–267, 2003.

124. Vandenbroucke-Grauls C, Schultsz C: Surveillance in infection control: are we making progress? *Curr Opin Infect Dis* 15: 415–419, 2002.

125. Epps B, Edwards JR, Sohn AH, et al: Improving benchmarks for surveillance by defining types of pediatric intensive care units, *Am J Infect Control* 30:68–70, 2002.

126. Beininghen GM, Brinkous LK, Docken LA, et al: Development of a regional nosocomial infection (NI) comparative database system in small, rural hospitals (Abstract). Presented at the 27th Annual Education Conference and International Meeting of the Association for Professionals in Infection Control and Epidemiology, June 18–22, 2000, Minneapolis, MN. *Am J Infect Control* 28:282, 2000.

127. Stevenson KB: Regional data set of infection rates for long-term care facilities: description of a valuable benchmarking tool, *Am J Infect Control* 27(1):20–26, 1999. [See comment in issue 27: 1–3.]

128. Woomer N, Long CO, Anderson C, et al: Benchmarking in home health care: a collaborative approach, *Caring* 18:22–28, 1999.

129. Rosenheimer L, Embry FC, Sanford J, et al: Infection surveillance in home care: device-related incidence rates, *Am J Infect Control* 26:359–363, 1998.

130. Missouri Alliance for Home Care Infection Surveillance Project. See URL http://www.homecaremissouri.org or http://www.infectioncontrolathome.org

131. Copp NA: Benchmarking in ambulatory surgery, *AORN J* 76: 643–647, 2002.

132. Gustafson TL: Practical risk-adjusted quality control charts for infection control, *Am J Infect Control* 28:406–414, 2000.

133. Lai KK, Baker SP, Fonteccio SA: Impact of a program of intensive surveillance and interventions targeting ventilated patients in the reduction of ventilator-associated pneumonia and its cost effectiveness, *Infect Control Hosp Epidemiol* 24:859–863, 2003.

134. Alonso-Echanove J, Edwards JR, Richards MJ, et al: Effect of nurse staffing and antimicrobial-impregnated central venous catheters on the risk for bloodstream infections in intensive care units, *Infect Control Hosp Epidemiol* 24:916–925, 2003.

135. Braun BL, Kritchevsky SB, Wong ES, et al: Preventing central venous catheter-associated primary bloodstream infections: characteristics of hospitals participating in the Evaluation of Processes and Indicators in Infection Control (EPIC) study, *Infect Control Hosp Epidemiol* 24:926–935, 2003.

136. Kohn L, Corrigan J, Donaldson M, editors: *To err is human: building a safer health system,* Washington, DC, 2000, Committee on Quality of Health Care in America, Institute of Medicine. National Academy Press.

137. Gerberding JL: Hospital-onset infections: a patient safety issue, *Ann Intern Med* 137:665–670, 2002.

138. Shojania KG, Duncan BW, McDonald KM, et al: Safe but sound: patient safety meets evidence-based medicine, *JAMA* 288: 508–513, 2002.

139. Scheckler WE: Healthcare epidemiology is the paradigm for patient safety, *Infect Control Hosp Epidemiol* 23:47–51, 2002.

140. Burke JP: Patient safety: infection control—a problem for patient safety, *N Engl J Med* 348:651–656, 2003.

141. Shojania KG, Duncan BW, McDonald KM, et al. editors: *Making health care safer: a critical analysis of patient safety practices.* Evidence Report/Technology Assessment No. 43, AHRQ Publication No. 01-E058, Rockville, MD, 2001, Agency for Healthcare Research and Quality. [Available at URL www.ahrq.gov]

142. Leape LL, Berwick DM, Bates DW: What practices will most improve safety? Evidence-based medicine meets patient safety, *JAMA* 288:501–507, 2002.

143. Joint Commission on Accreditation of Healthcare Organizations. Using infection control standards to improve safety, *Jt Comm Perspect Patient Safety* 9:2, 2002.

144. Joint Commission on Accreditation of Healthcare Organizations, 2004, National Patient Safety Goals. [Published at URL http://www.jcaho.org]

145. Centers for Disease Control and Prevention. Division of Healthcare Quality Promotion Seven Healthcare Safety Challenges. [Published at URL http://www.cdc.gov/ncidod/hip]

146. Do AN, Ciesielski CA, Metler RP, et al: Occupationally acquired human immunodeficiency virus (HIV) infection: national case surveillance data during 20 years of the HIV epidemic in the United States, *Infect Control Hosp Epidemiol* 24:86–96, 2003.

147. Beck-Sague C, Jarvis WR, Martone W: Outbreak investigations, *Infect Control Hosp Epidemiol* 18:138–145, 1997.

148. Peterson LR, Brossette SE: Hunting health care-associated infections from the clinical microbiology laboratory: passive, active, and virtual surveillance, *J Clin Microbiol* 40:1–4, 2002.

149. Brossette SE, Sprague AP, Jones WT, et al: A data mining system for infection control surveillance, *Methods Inf Med* 39: 303–310, 2000.

150. Centers for Disease Control and Prevention. Guidelines for environmental infection control in health-care facilities: recommendations of the CDC and the Healthcare Infection Control Practices Advisory Committee (HICPAC), *MMWR* 52(no. RR-10):1–48, 2003. Errata: 52(42):1025–1026. [Full text version available at URL http:// www.cdc.gov/ncidod/hip]

Copyright © 2005, Association for Professionals in Infection Control and Epidemiology, Inc.

151. Freije MR: *Legionella control in health care facilities: a guide for minimizing risk,* Fallbrook CA 1996, HC Information Resources, Inc. .
152. Allegheny County Health Department. *Approaches to prevention and control of Legionella infection in Allegheny County health care facilities,* Pittsburgh, 1997, Allegheny County Health Department.
153. Maryland Department of Health and Mental Hygiene. Report of the Maryland Scientific Working Group to study Legionella in the water system in healthcare institutions, 2000. [Available at URL http://www.dhmh.state.md.us/html/legionella.htm]
154. Guerrero IC, Filippone C: A cluster of Legionnaire's disease in a community hospital—a clue to a larger epidemic, *Infect Control Hosp Epidemiol* 17:177–178, 1996.
155. Centers for Disease Control and Prevention. Update: investigation of anthrax associated with intentional exposure and interim public health guidelines, October 2001 *MMWR* 50:889–893 , 2001.
156. Lederberg J, Shope RE, Oaks SC, editors: *Emerging infections: microbial threats to health in the United States. Institute of Medicine,* Washington, DC, 1992, National Academy Press.
157. Centers for Disease Control and Prevention. Outbreak of severe acute respiratory syndrome—worldwide, 2003, *MMWR* 52:226–228, 2003.
158. Smolinski MS, Hamburg MA, Lederberg J, editors: *Microbial threats to health: emergence, detection and response,* Washington, DC, 2003, Institute of Medicine, National Academy Press.
159. Centers for Disease Control and Prevention. *Addressing emerging infectious disease threats: a prevention strategy for the United States,* Atlanta, 1994, U.S. Department of Health and Human Services, Public Health Service.
160. Centers for Disease Control and Prevention. *Preventing emerging infectious diseases: a strategy for the 21st Century* Atlanta, 1994, U.S. Department of Health and Human Services, Public Health Service.
161. Pinner RW, Rebman CA, Schuchat A, et al: Disease surveillance and the academic, clinical, and public health communities, *Emerg Infect Dis* 9:781–787, 2003.
162. Buehler JW, Berkelman RL, Hartley DM, et al: Syndrome surveillance and bioterrism-related epidemics, *Emerg Infect Dis* 9:1197–1204, 2003.
163. Henning KJ: Syndrome surveillance. In Smolinski MS, Hamburg MA, Lederberg J, editors: *Microbial threats to health: emergence, detection and response,* Washington, DC, 2003, Institute of Medicine, National Academy Press. [Available at URL http://www.nap.edu/books/030908864X/html/]
164. McGeer A: News in antimicrobial resistance: documenting the progress of pathogens, *Infect Control Hosp Epidemiol* 25:97–98, 2004.
165. Centers for Disease Control and Prevention. *Outbreaks of community-associated methicillin-resistant Staphylococcus aureus skin infections,* Los Angeles County, CA, 2002–2003.
166. Centers for Disease Control and Prevention. Staphylococcus aureus resistant to vancomycin—United States, 2002, *MMWR* 51:565–567, 2002.
167. Society for Healthcare Epidemiology of America and Infectious Diseases Society of America Joint Committee on the Prevention of Antimicrobial Resistance: guidelines for the prevention of antimicrobial resistance in hospitals, *Infect Control and Hosp Epidemiol* 18:275–291, 1997.
168. Strausbaugh LJ, Crossley KB, Nurse BA, et al: The SHEA Long-Tem Care Committee. Antimicrobial resistance in long-term care facilities, *Infect Control Hosp Epidemiol* 17:129–140, 1996.
169. Chaix C, Durand-Zaleski I, Alberti C, et al: Control of endemic methicillin-resistant Staphylococcus aureus: a cost-benefit analysis in an intensive care unit, *JAMA* 282(18):1745–1751, 1999.
170. Struelens MJ, Oliver Ronveaux O, Jans B, et al: The Groupement pour le Depistage, l'Etude et la Prevention des Infections Hospitalieres. Methicillin-resistant Staphylococcus aureus epidemiology and control in Belgian hospitals, 1991 to 1995, *Infect Control Hosp Epidemiol* 17:503–508, 1996.
171. Muto CA, Jernigan JA, Ostrowsky BE, et al: SHEA guideline for preventing nosocomial transmission of multidrug-resistant strains of Staphylococcus aureus and Enterococcus, *Infect Control*

Hosp Epidemiol 24:362–386, 2003. [Available at URL http://www.shea-online.org/pdfs/SHEA_MRSA_VRE.pdf]
172. Nguyen GT, Proctor SE, Sinkowitz-Cochran RL, et al: Status of infection surveillance and control programs in the United States, 1992–1996, *Am J Infect Control* 28:392–400, 2000.
173. Gerberding JL: Health-care quality promotion through infection prevention: beyond 2000, *Emerg Infect Dis* 7:363–366, 2001.
174. Ashford DA, Kaiser RM, Bales ME, et al: Planning against biological terrorism: lessons from outbreak investigations, *Emerg Infect Dis* 9:515–519, 2003.
175. Platt R, Yokoe DS, Sands KE: Automated methods for surveillance of surgical site infections, *Emerg Infect Dis* 7:212–216, 2001.
176. Platt R, Kleinman K, Thompson K, et al: Using automated health plan data to assess infection risk from coronary artery bypass surgery, *Emerg Infect Dis* 8:1433–1441, 2002.
177. Brossette SE, Sprague AP, Hardin JM, et al: Association rules and data mining in hospital infection control and public health surveillance, *J Am Med Inform Assoc* 5:373–381, 1998.
178. Jarvis WR: The evolving world of healthcare-associated bloodstream infection surveillance and prevention: is your system as good as you think? *Infect Control Hosp Epidemiol* 23:237–238, 2002.
179. Avato JL, Lai KK: Impact of postdischarge surveillance on surgical-site infection rates for coronary artery bypass procedures, *Infect Control Hosp Epidemiol* 23:364–367, 2002.
180. Sands K, Vineyard G, Livingston J, et al: Efficient identification of postdischarge surgical site infections using automated medical records, *J Infect Dis* 179:434–441, 1999.
181. Alvarado-Ramy F, Beltrami EM, Short LJ, et al: A comprehensive approach to percutaneous injury prevention during phlebotomy: results of a multicenter study, 1993–1995, *Infect Control Hosp Epidemiol* 24:82–85, 2003.
182. Holtz TH, Wenzel RP: Postdischarge surveillance for nosocomial wound infection: a brief review and commentary, *Am J Infect Control* 20:206–213, 1992.
183. Keeling NJ, Morgan MW: Inpatient and post-discharge wound infections in general surgery, *Ann R Coll Surg Engl* 77:245–247, 1995.
184. Sands K, Vineyard G, Platt R: Surgical site infections occurring after hospital discharge, *J Infect Dis* 173:963–970, 1996.
185. Santos KR, Bravo Neto GP, Fonseca LS, et al: Incidence surveillance of wound infection in hernia surgery during hospitalization and after discharge in a university hospital, *J Hosp Infect* 36:229–233, 1997.
186. Geffers C, Gastmeier P, Brauer H, et al: Surveillance of nosocomial infections in ICUs: is postdischarge surveillance indispensable? *Infect Control Hosp Epidemiol* 22:157–159, 2001.
187. Letrilliart L, Guiguet M, Hanslik T, et al: Postdischarge nosocomial infections in primary care, *Infect Control Hosp Epidemiol* 22:493–498, 2001.
188. Yokoe DS, Christiansen CL, Johnson R, et al: Epidemiology of and surveillance for postpartum infections, *Emerg Infect Dis* 7:837–841, 2001.
189. Thibon P, Parienti JJ, Borgey F, et al: Use of censored data to monitor surgical-site infections, *Infect Control Hosp Epidemiol* 23:368–371, 2002.
190. Noy D, Creedy D: Postdischarge surveillance of surgical site infections: a multimethod approach to data collection, *Am J Infect Control* 30(7):417–424, 2002.
191. Fanning C, Johnston BL, MacDonald S, et al: Postdischarge surgical site infection surveillance, *Can J Infect Control* 10:75–79, 1995.
192. Fields CL: Outcomes of a postdischarge surveillance system for surgical site infections at a Midwestern regional referal hospital, *Am J Infect Control* 27:158–164, 1999.
193. Couto RC, Pedrosa TM, Nogueira JM, et al: Post-discharge surveillance and infection rates in obstetric patients, *Int J Gynaecol Obstet* 61:227–231, 1998.
194. Byrne DJ, Lynce W, Napier A, et al: Wound infection rates: the importance of definition and post-discharge wound surveillance, *J Hosp Infect* 26:37–43, 1994.
195. Richet HM, Benbachir M, Brown DFJ, et al: Are there regional variations in the diagnosis, surveillance, and control of methicillin-resistant Staphylococcus aureus? *Infect Control Hosp Epidemiol* 24:334–341, 2003.
196. Heyman DL, Rodier G: Global surveillance, national surveillance, and SARS, *Emerg Infect Dis* 10:173–175, 2004.

Copyright © 2005, Association for Professionals in Infection Control and Epidemiology, Inc.

SUPPLEMENTAL RESOURCES

Arias K: Surveillance programs in healthcare facilities. APIC Infection Control Toolkit Series, Washington, DC, 2003, Association for Professionals in Infection Control and Epidemiology.

Principles of Epidemiology, 3030-G. A self-study course covering basic epidemiology principles, concepts, and procedures generally used in the surveillance and investigation of health-related events. Addresses how to calculate and interpret frequency measures (ratios, proportions and rates) and measures of central tendency, and how to use tables, graphs, and charts to organize, summarize, and display data. Information on ordering this course is available on the CDC Public Health Training Network Web site at http://www.phppo.cdc.gov/PHTN. The course (over 500 pages) can be downloaded free of charge from this site.

APIC

Bennett JV, Brachman PS, editors: *Hospital infections,* ed 4, Philadelphia, 1998, Lippincott-Raven.

Mayhall CG: *Hospital epidemiology and infection control,* ed 2, Baltimore, 1999, Lippincott Williams & Wilkins.

Wenzel RP, editor: *Prevention and control of nosocomial infections,* ed 3, Baltimore, 1997, Williams & Wilkins.

Centers for Disease Control and Prevention (CDC), http://www.cdc.gov/ncidod/hip

CDC National Center for Infectious Diseases, Infectious Disease Surveillance, http://www.cdc.gov/ncidod/osr/index.htm

Association for Professionals in Infection Control and Epidemiology, http://www.apic.org

World Health Organization, http://www.who.int

Emerging Infectious Diseases Journal (published electronically), http://www.cdc.gov/ncidod/EID/index.htm

Organizations Providing Comparative Databases for Infection Surveillance

[Note: These examples are for information only; citation does not imply endorsement by APIC]

Centers for Disease Control and Prevention Surveillance Systems, http://www.cdc.gov/ncidod/hip

Missouri Alliance for Home Care (MAHC) Infection Surveillance Project, http://www.infectioncontrolathome.org

Outpatient Parenteral Antimicrobial Therapy (OPAT) Outcomes Registry, http://www.OPAT.com

Vermont Oxford Network, http://www.vtoxford.org

Maryland Hospital Association Quality Indicator Project, http://qiproject.org

The Interactive Statistical Pages project contains web pages that perform statistical calculations: http://www.members.aol.com/johnp71/javastat.html

Links to epidemiological software and resources compiled by the Rollins School of Public Health at Emory University are available at http://www.geocities.com/ResearchTriangle/Forum/7639

The Epi Info software program—created by the Epidemiology Program Office of the CDC. Epi Info is a public domain package that provides for easy form and database construction, data entry, and analysis with epidemiological statistics, maps, and graphs: http://www.cdc.gov/epiinfo/

Steve's Attempt to Teach Statistics (STATS) available at http://www.childrens-mercy.org/stats contains much information on statistics used in health care epidemiology. The site is sponsored by Children's Mercy Hospital and Clinics.

Copyright © 2005, Association for Professionals in Infection Control and Epidemiology, Inc.

Outbreak Investigation

Patricia J. Checko, MPH, DPh
Director of Health
Bristol-Burlington Health District
Berlin, Connecticut

ABSTRACT

Outbreaks can occur in healthcare settings, communities, regions, or even on a global scale. Regardless of scope, investigation of a potential outbreak follows certain epidemiological components. Cooperation between epidemiologists, infection control professionals (ICPs), and public health experts are necessary to effectively manage outbreak situations. The ultimate goal of an outbreak investigation is to identify probable contributing factors and to stop or reduce the risk of future occurrences.

KEY CONCEPTS

- Outbreak may be suspected when healthcare-associated infections (HAIs) occur above the background rate or when an unusual microbe is recognized.

- Outbreaks may occur within the facility, in the community, or as a result of unusual new disease.

- The focus of an outbreak may be associated with specific groups of patients, locations, treatment modalities, contaminated products or devices, healthcare providers, and/or healthcare practices.

- Epidemiologic investigations of an epidemic or cluster of infections must be conducted in a standardized way that assesses the contributing factors: source(s), the pathogen(s), the host(s) and the mode of transmission.

- Ending an outbreak involves modifying one or more of these factors.

- The goals of an outbreak investigation are to identify contributing factors in order to control the outbreak and to prevent similar outbreaks in the future.

I. BACKGROUND[1-4]

The majority of healthcare-associated infections (HAIs) in a healthcare setting are endemic. However, potential outbreak may be suspected when HAIs occur above the background rate or when an unusual microbe is recognized. Outbreaks may occur within the facility (e.g., surgical site infections with same organisms) or in the community (foodborne illnesses) or even due to unusual new disease (e.g., the initial Legionnaires' disease investigation). The focus of the outbreak may be asso-

---

Copyright © 2005, Association for Professionals in Infection Control and Epidemiology, Inc.

ciated with specific groups of patients, location, treatment modalities, contaminated products or devices, particular healthcare providers and/or healthcare practices. Agents of HAIs may also be introduced into a healthcare facility by visitors, patients or personnel who have, or are harboring, an infectious disease (e.g., influenza or chickenpox).

Epidemiologic investigations of an epidemic or cluster of infections must be conducted in a standardized way. Areas that must be assessed include the source(s), the pathogen(s), the host(s) and the mode of transmission. Factors associated with these areas contribute to the development of the outbreak. Modification of one or more of these factors will end the outbreak. The goal of any outbreak investigation is to identify factors that contribute to the outbreak in order to control the outbreak and to develop and implement measures to prevent similar outbreaks in the future. This chapter will help healthcare epidemiologists and ICPs determine when a cluster of infections among patients and/or healthcare personnel should be investigated and how to conduct an investigation.

II.   OUTBREAK INVESTIGATION

Recognition of a Potential Outbreak

Surveillance is the basic tool necessary to identify endemic and epidemic HAIs (See Chapter 13, Surveillance). Endemic infections represent the usual level of a disease within a geographic area, such as a hospital or long term care facility. Sporadic (endemic) infections represent the majority of preventable nosocomial infections. This background rate may fluctuate slightly from month to month, but does not differ significantly.

Epidemic (outbreak) infections represent an excess over the expected (endemic) level of a disease within a geographic area. However, one case of an unusual disease (e.g., botulism) may constitute an epidemic. Epidemics of nosocomial infections are usually important medical problems.

While local and state health department requirements may differ, most require reporting of possible healthcare-associated outbreaks or adverse events as soon as they are suspected. State and local health departments may also be able to assist in arranging or providing epidemiologic and/or laboratory support. Any outbreak that implicates an intrinsically contaminated or defective product, such as solutions, blood or blood products, or devices, should also be reported to the Food and Drug Administration (FDA) and the Centers for Disease Control and Prevention (CDC).[3]

Conducting An Outbreak Investigation[2]

The importance and sequence of the various steps will vary, depending on the nature of the problem. It is obvious that you must complete steps 2 and 3 before attempting to formulate and test a hypothesis. However, steps often occur simultaneously, but the elements in an outbreak investigation include the following:

1. Prepare for the investigation/field work

2. Confirm that an outbreak exists

3. Establish or verify diagnosis of reported cases; identify agent

4. Search for additional cases; collect critical data; develop a line listing; collect specimens if indicated

5. Characterize the cases by person, place, and time

6. Take immediate control measures, if indicated

7. Formulate tentative hypothesis (making the best guess to explain the observations)

8. Test hypothesis (hypothesis should explain the majority of cases).

9. Plan an additional systematic study (or studies)

10. Collect specimens (e.g., culture of environment or personnel based on data)

11. Implement and evaluate control and preventive measure

12. Initiate surveillance.

13. Communicate findings; summarize investigation for requesting authority; prepare written report(s)

Sequence of Events in an Outbreak Investigation

1. Prepare for the investigation.

Get commitment and clearances from healthfacility personnel including administration and microbiology. Designate a lead investigator. Advise microbiology to save specimens and isolates for antimicrobial susceptibility testing, molecular, and non-molecular typing.[2-6] The laboratory should also be alerted to keep any subsequent isolates that may be part of the outbreak.

2. Confirm the existence of an outbreak.

Develop a case definition and use it to estimate the magnitude of the problem. The case definition may change as new information is gathered. Compare the current incidence with usual or baseline incidence.

Copyright © 2005, Association for Professionals in Infection Control and Epidemiology, Inc.

Healthcare facilities may make initial judgments based on numerator data only. Confirming the outbreak includes calculating rates. This can be done by comparing the outbreak period rate with the background rate of the same disease. If local data are not available, compare outbreak rates to the literature.

Assess the need for outside consultation and report to public health authorities if required. Institute appropriate early control measures based on the magnitude and nature of the problem. Confirm that specimens (e.g., sera) and isolates (e.g., epidemiologic markers) will be held until the investigator requests or releases them. Pseudoinfections and pseudo-outbreaks must be differentiated from a real outbreak.[7] A pseudo-outbreak may or may not be recognized at this step, but must be considered as the investigation progresses.

3. Establish or verify diagnosis of reported cases; identify agent if possible.

Develop specific criteria for the definition of a case. Initially this may be a broad definition (e.g., diarrhea in patients) that is refined as the investigation proceeds and a specific agent and diagnosis is confirmed. The final case definition may include specific laboratory components (e.g., positive blood culture with specific isolate), radiologic findings and clinical signs and symptoms. Characterize the nature of disease and signs and symptoms by reviewing patient charts. Obtain appropriate laboratory specimens to identify specific agent responsible.

4. Search for additional cases; collect critical data; develop a line listing; collect specimens if indicated.

Encourage immediate reporting of new cases by laboratory, physicians, nursing staff and others as appropriate (e.g., radiology in cases of pneumonia). Search for other cases that may have occurred retrospectively or concurrently through laboratory reports, medical records, patient charts, physicians and nursing staff, and public health data. Use a specific data collection form. Information is usually collected on a questionnaire or data abstraction form. Selected critical items may be abstracted on a line listing.

5. Characterize cases of disease by person, place and time.

Describing the outbreak by person, place and time will help to determine who is at particular risk and who should be included in further studies.

a. Time: Data regarding time are used to create an epidemic curve (see also Chapter 2, General Principles of Epidemiology). The date of onset is plotted to create the epidemic curve. The shape of the epidemic curve and line listing will provide information to facilitate identification of the mode of transmission.

   1) What is the exact period of the outbreak? (Be sure to go back to the first case or first indication of outbreak activity.)

   2) Given the diagnosis, what is the probable period of exposure?

   3) Is the outbreak common source or propagated?

b. Place: Evaluating the place of the outbreak provides clues to the population at risk and may demonstrate clustering of cases (e.g., by service, ward, operating room, etc.). This may involve the use of tables or spot maps

c. Person: Characteristics of the case patients help in defining the most likely risk factors for infection. Factors to assess include:

   1) Patient characteristics (i.e., age, sex, underlying disease)

   2) Possible exposures (i.e., surgery, nursing and medical staff, infected patients)

   3) Therapeutic modalities (i.e., invasive procedures, medications, antibiotics)

   4) Use all of the above to develop an accurate description of the population at risk.

d. Calculate rates.

6. Take immediate control measures, if indicated.

Institute control measures such as increased attention to hand hygiene, additional use of barriers (e.g., gloves and gown), or confiscating specific suspected product (e.g., patient care item). These controls may be useful, depending on the situation.

7. Formulate tentative hypothesis (making the best guess to explain the observations).

Do a "quick and dirty" evaluation of the outbreak. Record, tabulate, and review data collected from above activities to summarize common host factors and exposures. On the basis of this analysis (and literature review if necessary), develop a hypothesis (best guess) on the likely reservoir, source(s), and mode of transmission of the disease. In practice, the investigator may formulate several reasonable hypotheses, testing them simultaneously and acting on the most promising one. The hypothesis should explain the majority of cases. Frequently there will be concurrent cases not explained by the hypothesis that may be related to endemic or

Copyright © 2005, Association for Professionals in Infection Control and Epidemiology, Inc.

sporadic cases, a different disease (similar symptom-atology), or a different source or mode of transmission.

8. Test hypothesis (hypothesis should explain the majority of cases).

Many investigations do not reach this stage. The investigation may end with descriptive epidemiology (problem goes away without intervention or does not require a special study). Whether or not an investigation is carried through, the hypothesis testing phase is a function of available personnel, severity of the problem, and resource allocations. Examples of situations that should be studied include infection associated with a commercial product, infection associated with considerable morbidity and/or mortality (e.g., bacteremias) and infections associated with multiple services. For retrospective epidemiologic studies, the two types of analytic approaches are the case-control study and the cohort study. The case-control study is most frequently used in studies of HAIs.

Analyze data derived from case investigation and determine sources of transmission and risk factors associated with disease. Demonstrate significant difference of incidence or exposure in contrasted population groups. Analysis may include univariate analysis of categorical and continuous variables as well as stratified and multivariate analysis.

9 Plan an additional systematic study (or studies).

If necessary, refine hypothesis and carry out additional studies. The most important part of the investigation is the interpretation of the results. Obtaining meaningful associations between risk factors and disease depend on numerous factors.

10. Collect specimens (e.g., culture of environment or personnel based on data).[5,6]

It may be necessary to culture other patients, personnel, products, or environment if implicated as potential sources. Sample collection should be in conjunction with the laboratory to determine the appropriate type of specimen(s), collection parameters, and appropriate test(s). The laboratory may be able to perform specific comparison studies (e.g., molecular typing) or provide recommendations and coordinate with a referral laboratory.

11. Implement and evaluate control and preventive measure.

Instituting control measures may occur anywhere in the process. Identify specific preventive and control measures based on the nature of the agent and characteristics of high-risk group and sources (e.g., eliminate contaminated product, modify nursing procedures, treat implicated carriers, immunize susceptibles).

12. Initiate surveillance.

The epidemiologic study will lead to specific recommendations to stop the outbreak and prevent further transmission. The efficacy of the intervention can be measured by further surveillance to determine if cases cease to occur or return to endemic level. Use the opportunity of an outbreak to review and correct other practices related to the current situation that may contribute to an outbreak in the future.

13. Communicate findings ; summarize investigation for requesting authority; prepare written report(s).

Communication of findings may take two forms, an oral briefing for local authorities or a written report or both. A report should contain the following elements:

a. Introduction

   1) Describe circumstances leading to recognition of the problem.

   2) Background describing the setting in which the problem occurred

b. Methods (description of the studies conducted)

   1) Methods (laboratory, epidemiologic)

   2) Case definition, case-finding, and verification of diagnosis

   3) Sources of data

   4) Hypothesis testing, if any

   5) Description of type of study design; description of control group(s) and rationale for choice; statistical tests used

c. Results

   1) Facts only; no explanations

   2) May use tables, graphs, and charts

   3) Analysis of data and statistical conclusions (include p values)

d. Discussion

   1) Interpretation

   2) Description of control measures

   3) Description of other important outcomes; discoveries of new agents, reservoirs, modes of transmission; legal and economic impact, etc.

   4) Recommendations for future surveillance and control

Copyright © 2005, Association for Professionals in Infection Control and Epidemiology, Inc.

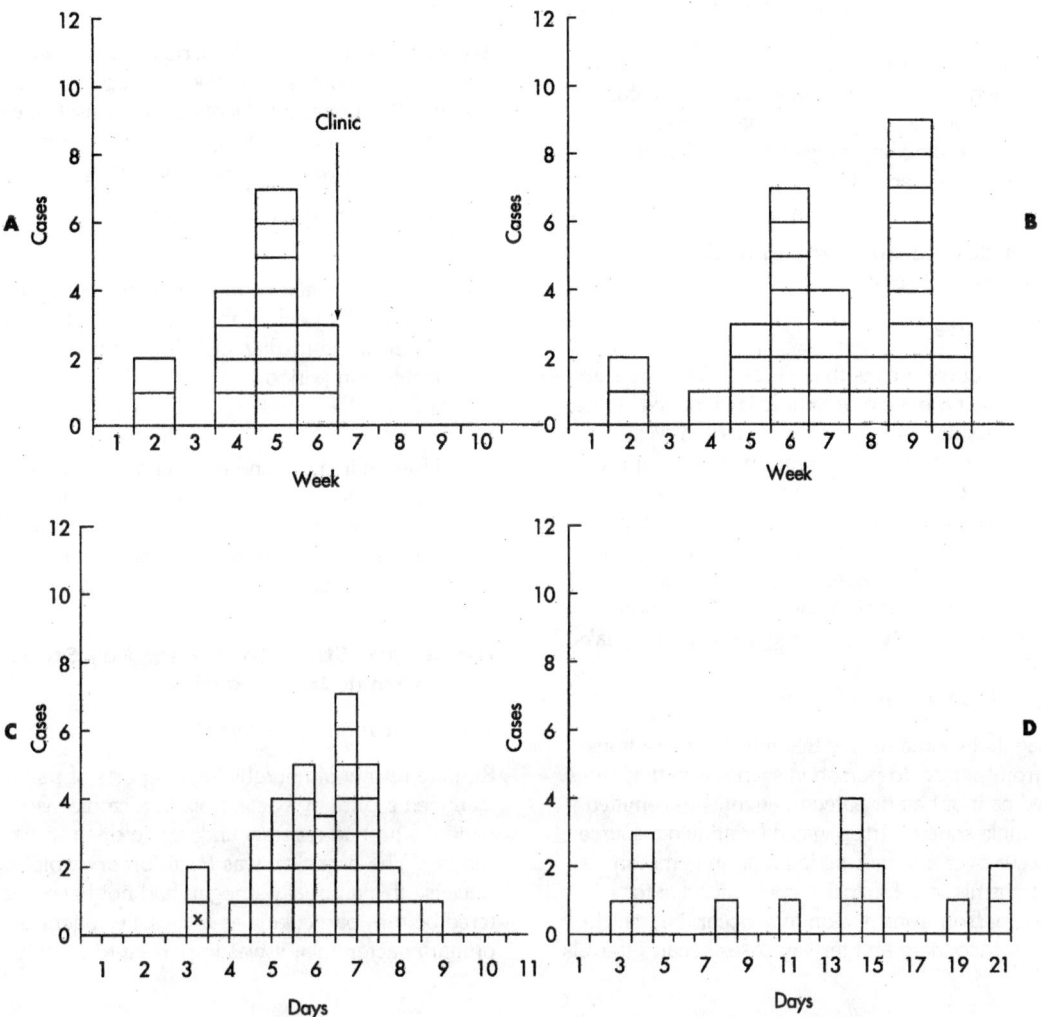

Figure 4–1 Epidemic curves; common vs. propagated source outbreak. In practice, other information gathered in the course of investigation is also used to interpret epidemic curves. **A:** Propagated source: single exposure, no secondary cases (e.g., measles). **B:** Propagated source: secondary and tertiary cases (e.g., hepatitis A). **C:** Common source: point exposure (e.g., salmonellosis following a company picnic; food handler 4 x). **D:** Common source: Intermittent exposure (e.g., bacteremia associated with contaminated blood product). NOTE: In practice, other information gathered in the course of the investigation is also used to interpret epidemic curves.

e. References

f. Disseminate to those who need to know.

The Epidemic Curve

An epidemic curve is a graph in which the cases of a disease that occurred during an epidemic period (outbreak) are plotted according to the time of onset of illness in the cases (see Figure 4–1). The shape of the curve is determined by the epidemic pattern. The epidemic curve is used to:

• Determine whether the source of infection was common, propagated (continuing), or both.

• Identify the probable time of exposure of the cases to the source(s) of infection.

• Identify the probable incubation period.

• Determine if the problem is ongoing.

Copyright © 2005, Association for Professionals in Infection Control and Epidemiology, Inc.

An epidemic curve is a histogram. Cases are plotted by date of onset of illness. Time intervals (x axis) must be based on the incubation or latency period of the disease and the length of the period over which cases are distributed. Inappropriate intervals may obscure temporal distributions [e.g., hours, days, weeks] depending on the etiologic agent and the length of time the outbreak persists.

Common Source and Propagated (Continuing) Source

Common Source

A common source means that all cases have the same origin. The same person or vehicle is identified as the primary reservoir or means of transmission. With a common source outbreak the epidemic curve approximates a normal distribution curve if there is a sufficient number of cases and if cases are limited to a short exposure with maximum incubation of a few days or less (point source). Exposure may be continuous or intermittent. Intermittent exposure to a common source produces a curve with irregularly spaced peaks.

Propagated (Continuing) Source

A propagated source means that infections are transmitted from person to person in such a way that cases identified cannot be attributed to agent(s) transmitted from a single source. Propagated (continuing) source cases occur over a longer period than in common source transmission. Explosive epidemics due to person-to-person transmission may occur (i.e., chickenpox). If secondary and tertiary cases occur, intervals between peaks usually approximate average incubation period.

To determine the probable period of exposure of cases in a common source outbreak it is necessary to know the specific disease involved, dates of onset of cases and either mean or median, or minimum and maximum, incubation period(s) for the specific disease.

Draw the epidemic curve and calculate by either – (Fig.4–2)

a. Using the mean or median incubation period: identify the peak of the epidemic or the date of onset of the median case. Count back into one incubation period

or

b. Using minimum and maximum incubation periods: start with the first case identified and count back in time the minimum incubation period; then using the last case, count back in time the maximum incubation period.

Use a Case Study to Review Key Steps in an Outbreak Investigation

1. Identification of Outbreak

Routine review of microbiologic reports of patients identified a primary bacteremia in a cardiovascular patient who had recently undergone open heart surgery. The organism was *Pseudomonas pickettii* Because this unusual pathogen had not been encountered before, particularly as a causative agent of primary bacteremia, it was important to identify a pos-

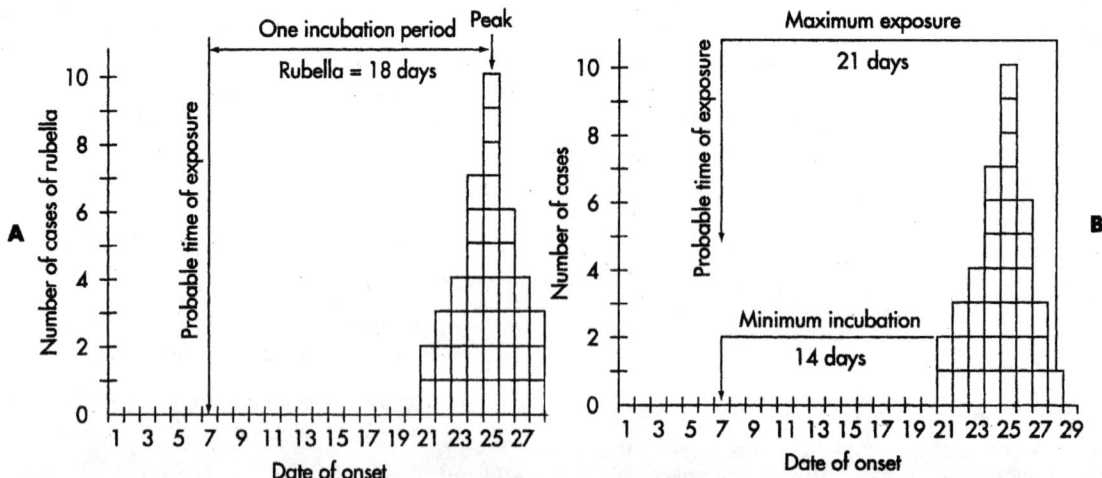

Figure 4–2 Determining the probable period of exposure in common source outbreaks using mean or median incubation period (**A**) or minimum and maximum incubation periods (**B**)

Copyright © 2005, Association for Professionals in Infection Control and Epidemiology, Inc.

sible source. A contaminated infusate or intravenous medication was the presumed source of the infection. Five days elapsed between obtaining the culture and final identification of the organism. In the interim, the patient had been transferred from the intensive care unit to a general pediatric unit. All invasive devices had been removed, and her fever had resolved. Microbiologic samples of the few remaining injectable medications were negative. The origin of this unusual organism remained obscure.

During the next two weeks, two additional surgical patients developed primary bacteremia with the same organism. Coincidentally, a prospective, unrelated study of intravenous (IV) catheter site dressings was ongoing in the institution, and most patients receiving IV therapy were enrolled. The study protocol included routine culturing of in-use IV fluids.

Ultimately, *P. pickettii* was found in the infusate of three patients who remained asymptomatic. Infection control personnel providing microbiologic support for this study recalled three previous isolates two months earlier that were positive with a nonfermentative gram-negative bacillus with similar colonial morphology.

However, the study protocol did not require full identification of all organisms if growth was minimal. The three patients were designated probable cases because isolates were no longer available for retesting. An epidemic curve was plotted. It suggested an intermittent, common source that began in January 1985 (Fig. 4–3). Multiple cases of primary bacteremia due to an unusual organism in patients undergoing clean surgical procedures were ample evidence of a nosocomial epi-

demic with the potential for a very serious outcome—death. Comprehensive investigation began immediately.

2. Data Collection

A case was defined as any surgical patient who underwent surgery between January and March 1985 and subsequently developed a primary bacteremia due to *P. pickettii* or had *P. pickettii* isolated from infusate but remained asymptomatic. Factors included in the initial line listing of implicated cases included:

a. Demographic data

- Name
- Medical record number
- Age
- Sex
- Diagnosis
- Unit
- Service
- Date of admission
- Date of surgery
- Peak and mean temperatures on the day of surgery and the first 3 days thereafter
- Date of infection onset

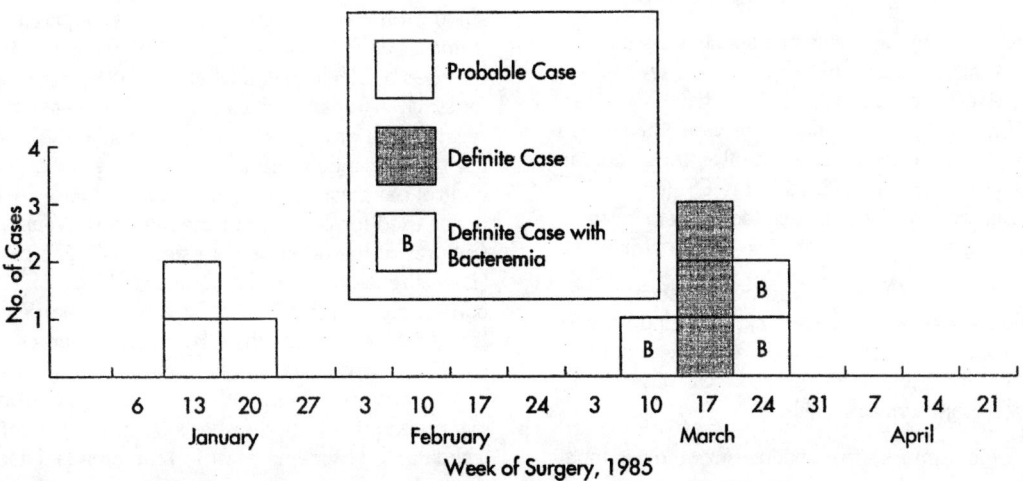

Figure 4–3 Epidemic curve for outbreak of *Pseudomonas pickettii* bacteremias and contaminated infusate traced to contaminated fentanyl.

Copyright © 2005, Association for Professionals in Infection Control and Epidemiology, Inc.

b. Risk factors

- Surgical procedure

- Operating room

- Duration of surgery

- Surgical personnel

- Anesthesia personnel

- All vascular access data

- Foley catheters

- Chest tubes

- Endotracheal tubes

- Prosthetic devices

- Steroids

- Antibiotics

- All IV medications, fluids, and blood

c. Host factors

- Renal failure

- Malignancy

- Diabetes

- Heart disease

3. Formulation of Hypothesis and Microbiologic Testing

Because none of the cases of primary bacteremia occurred before surgery, the most plausible hypothesis was that patients had received contaminated IV fluids, blood, or medication in the operating room (OR).

A selective microbiologic culture surveillance system was set up that required OR personnel to aseptically remove a small aliquot of IV fluid from each container before administration. Hopefully, this would allow identification of any low-dose, intermittent, intrinsic contamination of fluids commonly used in the OR (e.g., lactated Ringer's, dextrose in lactated Ringer's). The State Department of Health and the Centers for

Disease Control and Prevention were contacted to determine if other hospitals were experiencing nosocomial *P. pickettii* bacteremia. None were. As required in this state, the institutional outbreak was reported to the State Department of Health.

Microbiologic samples were obtained from in-use multidose medication vials on the anesthesia carts. Other drugs commonly used in operative procedures but in locked storage elsewhere in the OR were also cultured. This included medications such as hydromorphone,

morphine, meperidine, methadone, Nembutal, and fentanyl citrate. Some medications were commercially packaged in unit-dose syringes; others were predrawn from larger ampules by hospital pharmacy personnel. During the epidemic, used blood bags were returned to the blood bank and kept in refrigerated quarantine for a designated time period. To rule out the possibility of contaminated blood products, investigators retrieved and cultured the residual contents of the available bags used for implicated patients.

Other microbiologic surveillance cultures were taken from environmental sources likely to harbor *P. pickettii*, including faucets, sinks, irrigating solutions, bloodwarming baths, and distilled water. The hands of pharmacy personnel who prepared unit-dose medications were also cultured.

4. Case-Control Study

Simultaneously, a case-control study was undertaken to test the hypothesis. A case-control study can identify any factors common to the infected patients but uncommon to the noninfected patients (controls). A case control study is especially useful in hospital epidemiology because it allows one to examine events retrospectively (from the onset of recognized infection back to the event or exposure responsible for disease). Identification of significant factors may suggest an association but does not necessarily prove causality. A case-control study may also be valuable in identifying cofactors that may play a role in acquisition of disease. Nineteen control patients were selected for comparison with the nine patients meeting the case definition (six cases and three probable cases). Controls were randomly selected patients who had surgery on the same day as the cases, but whose cultures of infusion fluids initiated in the OR were negative. (The unrelated IV study protocol in progress at the time required culturing of IV fluids started in the OR. Thus this information was available.) All nine cases (100%) received IV fentanyl, whereas 9 of 19 (47%) control patients received the drug ($p < 0.007$). Although heparin was used significantly more often in the cases than in control patients, it could not explain all cases because it was used for only five of the nine cases (Table 4–1). Cultures of the heparin were sterile. All nine cases (100%) received cefazolin compared to 10 of 19 control patients (53%; $p < 0.001$). This particular drug is widely used outside the OR. However, no cases were identified in patients who had not undergone surgical procedures. Significant differences between groups were determined using Fisher's exact test for categorical data and Students t-test for continuous data.

Copyright © 2005, Association for Professionals in Infection Control and Epidemiology, Inc.

Table 4-1. Case-control analysis of risk factors for development of *P. pickettii* bacteremia or contaminated intravenous fluid.

	Cases n = 9 (%)	Controls* n = 19 (%)	p value
Age, mean	50 years	46 years	NS
Duration of surgery	4 hours	3.7 hours NS	
Type of surgery			
Cardiovascular	5 (55)	3 (16)	
General	4 (45)	16 (84)	NS
Intravenous fluids			
Lactated Ringer's	8 (89)	11 (58)	NS
Dextrose in lactated Ringer's	5 (55)	14 (74)	NS
Saline (9%)	6 (67)	4 (21)	NS
Blood products	7 (78)	4 (21)	NS
Intraoperative IV Medications			
Pentathol	4 (45)	3 (68)	NS
Lidocaine	5 (55)	5 (26)	NS
Pancuronium	5 (55)	4 (21)	NS
Heparin	5 (55)	0 (...)	<0.008†
Cefazolin	9 (100)	10 (53)	NS 0.001†
Fentanyl	9 (100)	9 (47)	<0.007†
Volume of fentanyl, mean	61.6 ml.	16.8 ml.	<0.001

* Patients randomly selected who had had surgery on the same day as case but whose cultures of IV fluid from their infusion begun in the OR were negative.
† Fisher's exact test.
n, Number of cases; NS, not significant at *p*<0.05.

5. Testing the Hypothesis

Microbiologic surveillance simultaneously revealed *P. pickettii* in IV fentanyl (in both the OR narcotic drawer and the central pharmacy) and from one distilled water tap located in the pharmacy. Because OR personnel did not have access to narcotics in the central pharmacy, it was clear that the contamination originated in pharmacy. (The case control study suggested an association, the microbiologic testing proved the hypothesis, and the hypothesis adequately explained all nine cases.)

6. Further Investigation

It was important to determine whether the fentanyl was intrinsically contaminated (during manufacturing) or extrinsically contaminated by pharmacy personnel while drawing medications into unit-dose syringes. All subsequent cultures of multiple, previously unopened vials of fentanyl tested under controlled conditions by infection control microbiologists were sterile. Query of the manufacturer revealed no knowledge of complaints by other users or an awareness of any quality control problems. Other hospitals using fentanyl from the same source were experiencing no problems. Extrinsic contamination appeared more likely.

Because fentanyl is a potent narcotic subject to illicit use, the question was raised whether the contents of syringes may have been tampered with or diluted for

purposes of diverting small portions of the drug without significantly compromising total volume or desired analgesic effect.

Additional tests using liquid chromatography compared concentrations in known sterile, pharmacy-prepared, unit-dose syringes with similarly prepared known contaminated syringes and revealed a lower drug concentration in the contaminated syringes (98.6% to 100.2% vs. 90.0% to 94.8%). This verified the suspicion that parts of fentanyl had been removed from the syringes and had been replaced with contaminated distilled water (presumably obtained from the contaminated distilled water tap in central pharmacy).

Requests to initiate urine testing of pharmacy personnel for the presence of fentanyl were denied by the hospital personnel department because of the sensitive and controversial issue of drug screening. Additional efforts to specifically identify the person responsible for drug tampering included daily, unobserved, serial culturing of stored prepared fentanyl known to be sterile. It was anticipated that this method pinpoint the period of time (within 24 hours) in which contamination occurred. One could then identify and focus on specific individuals whose usual duties required access to narcotics during that time period and, hopefully, identify a likely individual. This approach was unsuccessful. Pharmacy personnel whose duties required significant access to narcotics during the time period in which

Copyright © 2005, Association for Professionals in Infection Control and Epidemiology, Inc.

drug tampering was known to occur were questioned, but they denied involvement. Two of these individuals resigned shortly after. However, conclusive evidence that either was involved in narcotic diversion was lacking.

7. Control Measures

As soon as tampering was confirmed, pharmacy personnel made several changes to increase security. These changes ultimately became permanent control measures. No further bacteremia with *P. pickettii* have occurred.

8. Preparation of Report

The infection control unit uses a standard protocol for all epidemiologic investigations. During the investigation, several meetings were held. Appropriate departmental personnel (hospital pharmacy, administrative staff, director of personnel, hospital administration, OR administration, department of anesthesiology, and the department of security) attended.

On conclusion of the investigation, a final report detailing the above process was distributed to infection control committee members, pharmacy administration, chairman of anesthesiology, hospital administration, and the director of surgical services.

III. SUMMARY AND CONCLUSIONS

Investigation of a potential outbreak follows epidemiological principles as outlined in this chapter. Although the steps may not occur sequentially, the steps should help to guide the ICP in obtaining the goal – to identify potential cause and stop future cases. Reporting requirements for outbreaks varies and there are resources available to assist in the investigation.

IV. FUTURE TRENDS/RESEARCH

Computerized programs and reporting mechanisms are under development to provide notification and early identification of diseases. These syndromic surveillance systems are becoming available through state and regionalized public health agencies. (See also Chapter 113, Public Health, and Chapter 120, Bioterrorism and Pandemics.)

V. INTERNATIONAL PERSPECTIVES

Reporting requirements and coordination of potential outbreaks with appropriate authorities varies with geographical locale. The ICP should be familiar with these requirements as appropriate to their setting. (See also Chapter 121, International Regulatory Agencies.)

International travel has provided ample opportunities for microbes to traverse our planet in only a few hours or days. Agents may be part of the cargo (e.g., food items) or within an incubating traveler. (See also Chapter 114, Travel Health.)

REFERENCES

1. Centers for Disease Control and Prevention. *Principles of Epidemiology: An Introduction to Applied Epidemiology.* 2nd ed. Atlanta: United States Department of Health and Human Services, Public Health Service, CDC; 1992
2. Jarvis WR. Investigating endemic and epidemic nosocomial infections. In: Bennett JV, Brachman PS, eds. *Hospital Infections.* 4th ed. Boston: Little, Brown; 1998: 85–102
3. Jarvis WR. Investigation of Outbreaks. In Hospital Epidemiology and Infection Control, 3rd edition.Mayhall CG (ed). Lippincott Williams & Wilkins, Philadelphia, PA 2004: 107–122.
4. Reingold AL. Outbreak investigations – a perspective. *Emerg Infect Dis* 1998;ZS4(1):21–27.
5. Diekema DJ, Pfaller MA. Infection Control Epidemiology and Clinical Microbiology. In: Murray PR, Baron EJ, Jorgensen JH, Pfaller MA, Yolken RH (eds). Manual of Clinical Microbiology, 8th edition. ASM Press, Washington, DC 2003; 129–38.
6. Soll DR, Lockhart SR, Pujol C. Laboratory Procedures for the Epidemiological Anaylsis of Microorganisms. In: Murray PR, Baron EJ, Jorgensen JH, Pfaller MA, Yolken RH (eds). Manual of Clinical Microbiology, 8th edition. ASM Press, Washington, DC 2003; 139–161.
7. Cunha BA. Pseudoinfections and pseudo-outbreaks. In Hospital Epidemiology and Infection Control, 3rd edition. Mayhall CG (ed). Lippincott Williams & Wilkins, Philadelphia, PA 2004: 123–133.
8. Maki DG, Klein BS, McCormick RD, et al. Nosocomial *Pseudomonas pickettii* bacteremias traced to narcotic tampering: A case for selective drug screening of health care personnel. *JAMA* 1991; 265: 981–986

SUPPLEMENTAL RESOURCES

Arias K. *Quick Reference to Outbreak Investigation and Control in Health Care Facilities.* 2000. Jones & Bartlett, Sudbury, MA

Besser J, Beebe J, Swaminathan B. Investigation of Foodborne and Waterborne Disease Outbreaks In: Murray PR, Baron EJ, Jorgensen JH, Pfaller MA, Yolken RH (eds). Manual of Clinical Microbiology, 8th edition. ASM Press, Washington, DC 2003; 162–181.

CDC, Public Health Training Network: Epidemiologic case studies for download – both computer-based and classroom study at http://www.phppo.cdc.gov/phtn/casestudies/default.htm

North Carolina Center for Public Health Preparedness has outbreak investigation online courses at http://www.sph.unc.edu/nccphp/training/all_trainings/at_outbreak.htm

Outbreak investigation study group Power Point Lecture by Ebbing Lautenbach at http://www.dsf.health.state.pa.us/health/lib/health/Outbreak_Investigation. ppt

Super Course Lectures on Epidemiology and other related topics at URL http://www.pitt.edu/~super1/assist/topicsearch.htm

United States Department of Agriculture (USDA) and Food and Drug Administration (FDA) Foodborne Illness Education Information Center at URL http://peaches.nal.usda.gov/foodborne/fbindex/Outbreak.asp

University of Michigan Hospitals and Health Centers, Infection Control and Epidemiology, Outbreak Investigation Steps available at http://www.med.umich.edu/patientsafetytoolkit/infection/outbreak_steps.doc and Outbreak Investigation Checklist at http://www.med.umich.edu/patientsafetytoolkit/infection/outbreak_checklist. doc

Copyright © 2005, Association for Professionals in Infection Control and Epidemiology, Inc.

Use of Statistics

Arlene Potts, BA, MPH, CIC
Director, Infection Control Program
Robert Wood Johnson University Hospital
New Brunswick, New Jersey

Patricia J. Checko, MPH, DPh
Director of Health,
Bristol-Burlington Health District
Bristol, Connecticut

ABSTRACT

This chapter introduces basic statistical knowledge that is directly applicable to the field of infection control. While the reader is not expected to memorize formulas or know their derivation, it is important to know which formulas to use and to remember the different formulas available. The formulas presented can easily be found in most statistics books. In addition, most mathematical calculations can be performed with an inexpensive pocket calculator or in a computerized spreadsheet with a computation program. The reader who has never been exposed to statistics should not attempt to study this material without a statistics book for further reference. A calculator to complete the examples provided also is recommended.

KEY CONCEPTS

- A working knowledge of statistics is a requirement for an effective infection control professional.

- The correct statistical methods must be used if correct interpretation of the data is expected.

I. BACKGROUND

Statistical Concepts, Terminology, and Symbols

Statistics can loosely be defined as a tool:

- To aid in organizing and summarizing data

- To make inferences about data without proving anything (Statistics cannot prove either an association or causality; it can merely suggest—albeit strongly—that an association exists.)

- To communicate findings clearly and meaningfully to others.

Role of Statistics in Hospital Epidemiology

Infection control professionals (ICPs) routinely use statistical methods to prepare reports for the Infection Control Committee, identify problems or outbreaks, monitor the impact of interventions, identify areas for improvement, and monitor the progress of the improvement. These methods can be used to analyze and describe the occurrence of healthcare-associated infections within the healthcare facility. Some commonly used statistical methods are as follows:

Copyright © 2005, Association for Professionals in Infection Control and Epidemiology, Inc.

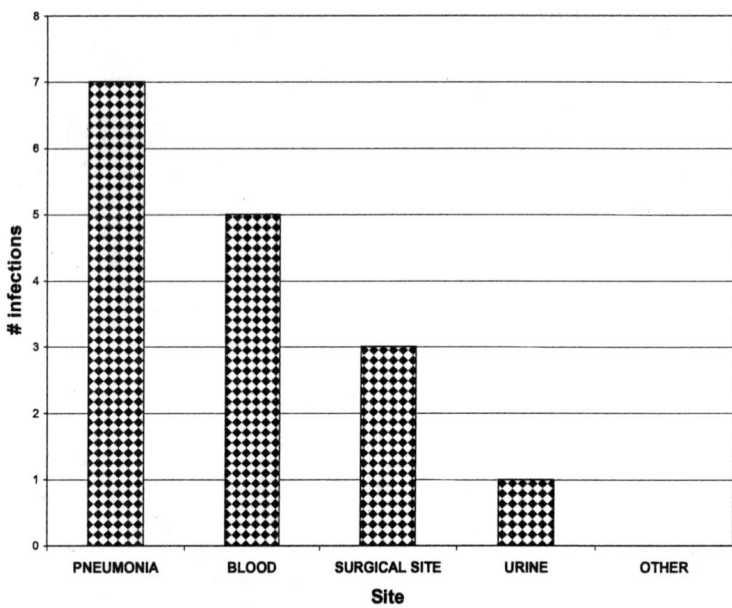

Figure 5–1 Pseudomonas aeruginosa infections by site.

- Infection rates

- Numeric summaries that describe characteristics of the population being studied (e.g., mean, average number of days of catheterization before development of a urinary tract infection)

- Frequency distributions displayed as tables, graphs, or charts (e.g., a bar graph of *Pseudomonas aeruginosa* isolates by site of infection, Figure 5–1)

II.   BASIC PRINCIPLES

The ICP is expected to be the most knowledgeable individual in the facility regarding the current literature on hospital epidemiology. Hospitals frequently decide to initiate a new policy or modify an existing one based on some publication. Some of the questions to be answered include:

- Are the findings statistically significant?

- Was the sample size large enough to demonstrate a difference if there is one?

- Are the groups being compared truly similar?

ICPs may be required to investigate an unusual cluster of cases in the facility. They will need some basic statistical skills to:

- Describe the outbreak (mean, attack rate, possibly standard deviation)

- Select control subjects who are similar to cases subjects in regard to the possible exposure

- Test hypotheses generated (χ^2 test, Fisher's Exact Test) to establish the statistical significance of an exposure (e.g., respiratory therapy) and the outcome being studied (e.g., pneumonia)

ICPs may wish to do research studies within their facilities. Designing and implementing a study requires knowledge of statistics. (Always consult with a statistician before conducting such a study to make sure that the sample size is large enough to show a difference if there is one and that the appropriate statistical tests are used.) To this end, it is imperative that the ICP has a knowledge and understanding of basic concepts of data and data analysis.

III.   USE OF STATISTICS

Definition of Data

There are two major divisions of data:

- Attribute data *counts* (e.g., the number of patients on a ventilator; the number of patients with central lines)

- Variable data *measures* (e.g., rate of ventilator-associated pneumonia, rate of line-related bloodstream infections)

Statistics

There are two types of statistics, *descriptive* and *inferential.* Descriptive statistics provides numerical information about *variables.* Inferential statistics makes an

APIC Text of Infection Control and Epidemiology

Copyright © 2005, Association for Professionals in Infection Control and Epidemiology, Inc.

assumption about a population based on a sample of the population.

Descriptive statistics include two types of data. *Discrete data* contain whole numbers and are mutually exclusive (e.g., infected or not infected, male or female, blood type). Discrete data can be *categorical* or *noncategorical*. Categorical data can count both the number of events/occurrences AND the number of nonevents/nonoccurrences (e.g., for 10 surgical site infections out of 100 surgical cases, there are 10 events (surgical site infections) and 90 nonevents (no surgical site infections). Noncategorical data can count the events/occurrences but not the nonevents/nonoccurrences (e.g., number of patient falls or number of healthcare-related infections when using 1000 patient days, ventilator days, or the like as the denominator). With noncategorical data, the number at risk can be identified but the actual number of "no infections" or "no falls" among those at risk cannot be identified.

Continuous data contain measurements of things for which there are an infinite number of possible values between the minimum and maximum value (a continuum) (e.g., serum cholesterol level; temperature, such as 98.6°F, 98.7°F, and 98.8°F; infection rates); continuous data require the process of measuring rather than counting and may contain whole numbers, decimals, or percents.

Definition of a Data Set

A data set is a group of observations whose individual values are connected in some way and are demonstrated in an *array* (a table of data that shows the observations plus the values, as in Table 5–1. In this example, patients are the observations, and the number of days signifies the values.

Definition of Variable

A variable is an observable characteristic of a phenomenon that can be measured—a quality, property, or characteristic of the person or things being studied that can be quantitatively measured or enumerated (e.g., age, sex, underlying disease, infections). The *dependent* variable is influenced or caused by another variable [e.g., ventilator-associated pneumonia (VAP), urinary tract infection]. The *independent* variable influences or causes the dependent variable (e.g., venti-

Table 5-1. Example of an *Array;* Length of Time (Days) an Indwelling Urinary Catheter Is in Place in 5 Patients

Patient	1	2	3	4	5
# days	3	10	4	6	20

Table 5-2. Example of a 2 × 2 Table with the Dependent Variable on the *x* Axis and the Independent Variable on the *y* Axis

	Pneumonia	No pneumonia	Totals (*x*)
Respiratory therapy treatments	A	B	A + B
No Respiratory therapy treatments	C	D	C + D
Totals (*y*)	A + C	B + D	A + B + C + D

lator, indwelling urinary catheter). When creating a 2 × 2 table to analyze the data, the dependent variable is always on the *x* axis (horizontal) and the independent variable is always on the *y* (vertical) axis (Table 5–2).

Scales of Measurement

Nominal Scale

The nominal scale is the simplest or crudest level of measurement. Categories are used to classify observations into mutually exclusive groups or classes. No order is implied among the classifications. These observations are known as nominal data (e.g., ill, not ill; infection sites).

Ordinal Scale

If observations are ranked so that each category is distinct and stands in some definite relationship to each of the other categories, the observations are known as ordinal data (e.g., unsatisfied, satisfied, very satisfied with socioeconomic class or staging cancer disease severity into class 1, 2, or 3, shortest to tallest).

Equal-Interval Scales

When data meet all the requirements for ordinal data and the exact distance between any 2 observations on the scale is known, they are called interval data. When the 0 point is arbitrary, the data are referred to as absolute interval data. Temperature scales (Celsius and Fahrenheit) are examples of this form of data where the 0 point is relative. Other familiar things such as blood pressure, weight, and height fall into this category.

Measurements that also have a true 0 point are sometimes referred to as ratio scale data (e.g., distance). Although certain scientists may use ratio scale measurements (e.g., Kelvin temperature scale), in the real world, most things that one would measure by equal-interval scale *do not* have a real 0 point. For practical purposes, the type of interval data does not affect the outcome of statistical procedure. Natural scientists

Copyright © 2005, Association for Professionals in Infection Control and Epidemiology, Inc.

Table 5-3. Scales of Measurements

Nominal Sex	Ordinal Rank	Interval* Weight
F	1st (minimum)	100 lbs
M	2nd	145 lbs
M	3rd	160 lbs
F	4th (maximum)	170 lbs

* Actual (pounds) weight measured in integers (exact difference between 2 observations is measurable).

(e.g., biologists, physicians) are more likely to use interval data for measurement, whereas the social scientists more frequently use nominal and ordinal scales in measuring attitudinal responses. The ICP may use both types of data (Table 5–3).

Measures of Central Tendency

Measures of central tendency describe how observations cluster around a middle value and locate only the center of a distribution measure. The methods include *mean, median,* and *mode.*

Mean

The most commonly used parameter is the arithmetic mean. Symbols used include μ for population mean and for sample mean. The formula to calculate the sample mean is

$$\bar{x} = \sum \frac{x}{n}$$

where Σ (sigma) is the symbol for "the sum of," x is the value of each observation, and n is the number of observations.

Example: You want to know the average length of stay of 7 patients (a small sample size is used for the convenience of demonstration). Create a *table* or *array* (Table 5–4). Add up all the observations and divide by the number of observations.

Table 5-4. Average Length-of-Stay of 7 Patients

Patient	# days
1	2 days
2	3 days
3	6 days
4	4 days
5	5 days
6	9 days
7	6 days

$$\bar{x} = \sum \frac{(2 + 3 + 6 + 4 + 5 + 9 + 6)}{7}$$

$$\bar{x} = \sum \frac{(35)}{7}$$

$$\bar{x} = 5$$

The mean of a data set is inaccurate if there are extreme values (outliers) in a data set.

Example:

$$\bar{x} = \sum \frac{(2 + 3 + 6 + 4 + 5 + 9 + 67)}{7}$$

$$\bar{x} = \sum \frac{(93)}{7}$$

$$\bar{x} = 13.3$$

Obviously, the value 13.3 is not reflective of the values in the data set.

Most statistical tests use the mean because it is more amenable to mathematical manipulation than the median or the mode. However, the mean is the measurement most affected by outliers (unusually high or low values), especially when the number of observations is small. As the sample size gets very large, outliers are less important.

Median

The median is the point at which 50% of the values fall below the mean and 50% of values occur above the mean. It is the midpoint of the observations. The median ignores extreme values and is better at indicating values close to an average. It is also a good measure for ordinal data or for numeric data when the distribution is skewed. The median absolute deviation is a good measure of variability and is not much affected by extreme outliers.

To calculate the median of the first data set, arrange the data in either ascending or descending order and find the middle value (i.e., for 2, 3, 4, 5, 6, 6, 9 the middle value is 5). This method assumes that there are an odd number of values. If the data set has an even number of values, arrange the set in ascending or descending order, find the middle 2 values, add them together and divide by 2.

Example:

2, 3, 4, 5, 6, 7

4 + 5 = 9

9 ÷ 2 = 4.5

The median absolute deviation is similarly computed by ranking the absolute deviations from the median and finding the median of the deviations (1.5 in this case).

Copyright © 2005, Association for Professionals in Infection Control and Epidemiology, Inc.

Mode

The mode represents the observation(s) that occur(s) most frequently in a data set and determines the height and shape of a curve. Data sets may have more than 1 mode and can be bimodal or multimodal. Small data sets may be nonmodal, (e.g., there are no repeated values). The mode is most useful for describing qualitative data; mode is used for nominal data and bimodal distributions.

Measures of Variability

Variability measures how the values are spread around the mean and includes range, deviation, standard deviation, and variance.

Range

The range provides a value that represents the difference between the highest and lowest values in a data set.

Example: Temperatures taken on patient A document the highest temperature at 103°F and a low reading of 98.6°F. The range is 4.4°F (103°F − 98.6°F). A common mistake is to say the range is 98.6°F to 103°F. That is the *raw spread* of the values. The range indicates the *extent* of the spread.

Deviation

Deviation measures the spread of each individual value from the mean of the data set and is represented by $(x - \bar{x})$, where x is the value of each observation and $\bar{x}$ represents the mean of the data set. Each individual measurement has 3 possibilities:

- Negative deviation (less than the mean)

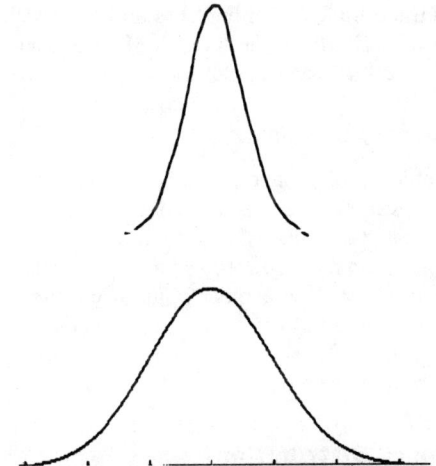

Figure 5–2 Two curves: both have the same mean but different standard deviations.

$$s = \sum \sqrt{\frac{(x - \bar{x})^2}{n-1}}$$

Figure 5–3 Formula for standard deviation (of a sample).

- Positive deviation (greater than the mean)
- No deviation (same as the mean)

The sum of the deviations must always equal 0.

Standard Deviation

Standard deviation is a measure of dispersion that reflects the variability in values around the mean. It employs the squared deviations from the mean, which therefore gives added emphasis to larger deviations. The standard deviation indicates how small the variability is (i.e., the spread) among observations. If the variability is small, all the values are close to the mean. If it is large, the values are not close to the mean (Figure 5–2).

Mathematically, standard deviation is obtained by taking all the deviations from the mean, squaring them, and then dividing their sum by the total number of observations minus 1, and, finally, taking the square root of this number. The symbol for the standard deviation of the population is σ and for the standard deviation of the sample is s. The calculation formula is the same for both.

The formula for the standard deviation of a sample is shown in Figure 5–3.

Example: To calculate the standard deviation of line days on a sample of 5 patients. (A small sample is used for the convenience of demonstration.)

- Create an array (table) (Table 5–5)
- Calculate the mean

$$\bar{x} = \sum \frac{(4 + 6 + 4 + 7 + 3)}{5}$$

Table 5-5. An Array of Line Days of 5 Patients

Patient	# line days
1	4 days
2	6 days
3	4 days
4	7 days
5	3 days

Copyright © 2005, Association for Professionals in Infection Control and Epidemiology, Inc.

Table 5-6. Patient Value Mean Deviation

	x $\bar{x}$	$(x - \bar{x})$
1	3	4.8 −1.8
2	4 4.8	−0.8
3	4 4.8	−0.8
4	6 4.8	+1.2
5	7 4.8	+2.2
	$\Sigma (x - x) = 0$	

- Calculate the deviations and sum up the total (must always add up to "0") (Table 5–6)

- Square each deviation and sum up the total (Table 5–7)

- Divide the total of the deviations squared by the number of observations minus 1. Calculate the square root.

The significance of the standard deviation is that with normal (bell-shaped) distributions, the following (Empirical rule for the normal curve) rules apply:

- The interval from 1 standard deviation below the mean to 1 standard deviation above the mean contains approximately 68% of the measurements.

- The interval from 2 standard deviations below the mean to 2 standard deviations above the mean contains approximately 95% of the measurements.

- The interval from 3 standard deviations below the mean to 3 standard deviations above the mean contains approximately 99.7% (or approximately all) of the measurements (Figure 5–4).

Variance

Variance is the square of the standard deviation of the measurements. The variance is a useful indicator of variability; however, standard deviation is more commonly used. Standard deviation has the same units as the original data.

Table 5-7.

Pt	x $\bar{x}$	$(x - \bar{x})$	$(x - \bar{x})^2$
1	3 4.8	−1.8	3.24
2	4 4.8	−0.8	0.64
3	4 4.8	−0.8	0.64
4	6 4.8	+1.2	1.44
5	7 4.8	+2.2	4.84
	$\Sigma (x - \bar{x})^2 = 10.8$		

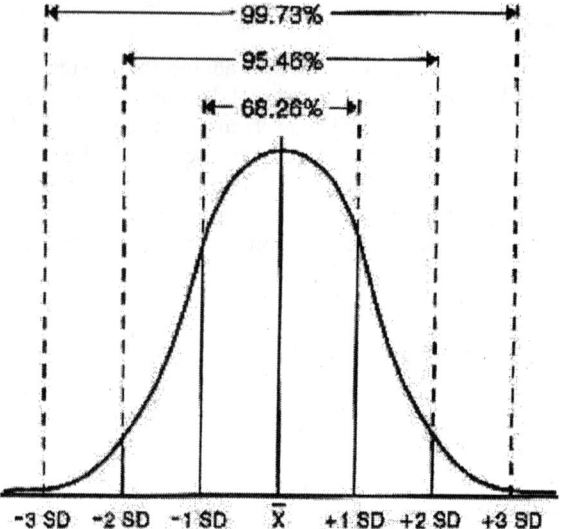

Figure 5–4 The normal distribution.

Example: Square the standard deviation of the previous example to obtain the variance (e.g., $1.64^2 = 2.7$). The variance of a population is represented by the symbol σ^2 and the sample population, s^2.

The mean and the standard deviation or the variance are necessary to use many of the formulas involved in hypothesis testing, (e.g., z test, t test).

Standard Error of the Mean

The standard error of the mean (SEM) is the standard deviation adjusted for by the sample $SEM = \sigma/\sqrt{N}$ size and is often the better measure for comparative purposes.

95% Confidence Interval

The 95% confidence interval (CI) of a mean can be calculated using the value of the SEM and t, thus 95%CI = $\bar{x} - (t \times SEM)$ to $\bar{x} + (t \times SEM)$. The value of t is close to 2 for large sample sizes.

Coefficient of Variation

The coefficient of variation (CV) is a unitless measure of relative variability and is useful for comparison of populations. It is defined as the ratio of the standard deviation to the mean, expressed as a percentage. The coefficient of variation is meaningful only if the variable is measured on a ratio scale. Because this measure is an index, the CV remains unchanged if all sample values are multiplied by a constant.

Frequency Distribution

If the distribution (spread) of the values is even on both sides of the mean (both halves are equal), it is a

APIC Text of Infection Control and Epidemiology

Copyright © 2005, Association for Professionals in Infection Control and Epidemiology, Inc.

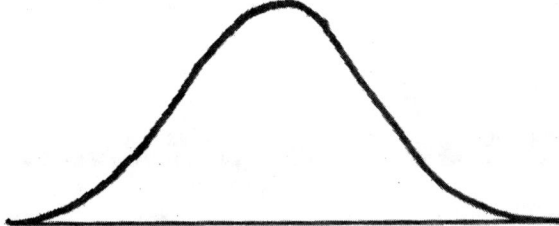

Figure 5-5 Mean = median = mode

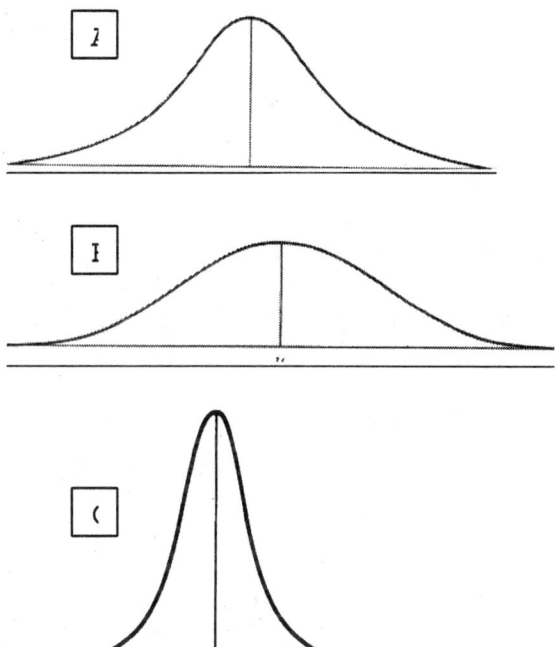

Figure 5-7 Kurtosis refers to how flat or peaked a curve is.

normal distribution. The curve is bell shaped (Gaussian distribution) and symmetrical. The mean, median, and mode are all equal (Figure 5–5). The normal distribution is the situation in which the population of things or persons clusters around a central point and then trails off symmetrically in both directions with fewer and fewer large and small individuals at the upper and lower ends, respectively. Normal distribution reflects data that are influenced by many small and unrelated random effects. As a sample size increases in number, the effects of the random influences are diminished and the data get closer to a normal distribution.

The distribution (spread) also can be asymmetrical (skewed). The skew indicates the direction that extreme values fall from the mean. The skew can be positive or negative. If the mean is greater than the median, it is a positive skew. If the mean is less than the median, it has a negative skew. References to a left or right skew refer to the direction of the tail of the curve. The shape and height of the curve are determined by the spread of the values from the mean and the mode (Figure 5–6). When the data are highly skewed, the median more accurately reflects where the bulk of data fall than does the mean. Most computer packages calculate skewness. A value of 0 means there is no skew. A positive number indicates skew to the right, and a negative number indicates skew to the left.

Two terms are used to describe the shape of a frequency distribution: *skewness* and *kurtosis*. Kurtosis refers to how flat or peaked a curve is. The 3 curves in Figure 5–7 are all symmetric but differ in kurtosis.

- **Curve A** is a typical bell-shaped curve or normal distribution (mesokurtic).

- **Curve B,** the more peaked curve, is leptokurtic.

- **Curve C**, the flatter curve, is platykurtic.

Statistical packages calculate kurtosis. A value of 0 indicates mesokurtosis, positive numbers indicate leptokurtosis, and negative numbers indicate platykurtosis.

Quantiles and Percentiles

Quantiles or Quantifiable Groupings

Quantiles, or quantifiable groupings, are useful for a detailed study of a variable's distribution.

Quartiles group the values in ascending order such that 25% of the observations are in the first grouping, 25% in the second, and so forth. Deciles are groupings of 10% blocks of the observations, and percentiles are 1% groupings.

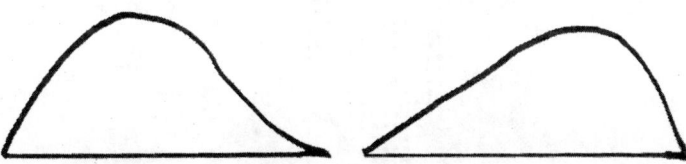

Figure 5-6 Negative skew (left); positive skew (right).

Copyright © 2005, Association for Professionals in Infection Control and Epidemiology, Inc.

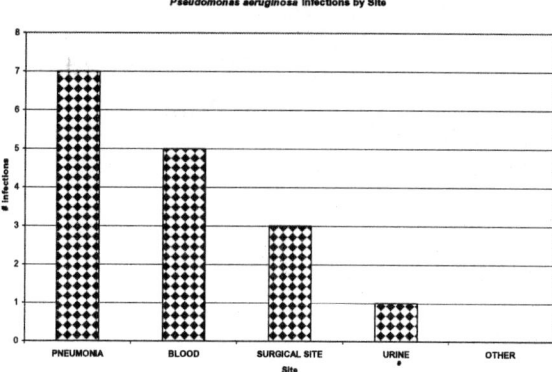

Figure 5-8 Bar chart.

Percentiles

Percentiles are often used in the context of the *p*th percentile, with the value having *p*% of the measurements below it and (100 – *p*)% above it. Percentile is used to designate the number in a frequency position below which a certain number of scores will fall. (If 50 people took a test and you scored better than 40 others, you would be in the 80th percentile or in the top 20% of the group.) The median is a specialized case of a quantile, defined as the 50th percentile.

Percentage

Percentage is the relative frequency of occurrence of some event to a total (e.g., an attack rate is a percentage, number of infections divided by the number at risk in the same time interval multiplied by 100).

Pictorial Statistics

Pictorial statistics present the numerical data that have been collected in graphs or charts, creating a picture of the data. The ICP must know the type of data being presented to select the appropriate graphic display.

Table 5-8. Ogive.

Ages of residents residing at the Golden Home of the Aged (small data set)

98 99 100 99 101 101 100 98 101 100 101 100 99 102 103 102 102 102 100

Age	Frequency of Each Value (Age)							
98	2	99	3	100	5	4	3	103	1

Length of Stay (Days) of 20 Patients (Larger Data Set) (Frequency Intervals)

Days	Frequency					
1–9	10	10–19	5	20–29	3	30–39	2

With discrete data, the most frequently used graphic displays are bar charts and pie charts.

- Bar charts compare the size and magnitude of the differences. The bars are unconnected, depicting data that are mutually exclusive. Bar charts display qualifying (names) and quantifying (numbers) data (Figure 5-8).

- Pie charts have an advantage over bar charts of depicting what portion of the total each item represents. Each portion (slice) of the pie must add up to the total of the whole (pie). If the slices are displayed as percents, the totals must add up to 100% (Figure 5-9).

Ogive (line chart), frequency polygon, or histogram are the most appropriate selections for continuous data.

An ogive is a cumulative line graph that plots data points over time. Frequency polygons and histograms show how many events occur in each category. The method involves grouping data into frequency intervals and is used to condense large data sets into manageable numbers. With large data sets, more intervals are used to avoid misrepresentation of the distribution of the data. With smaller data sets, fewer intervals are needed. Once again, it must be stressed that the

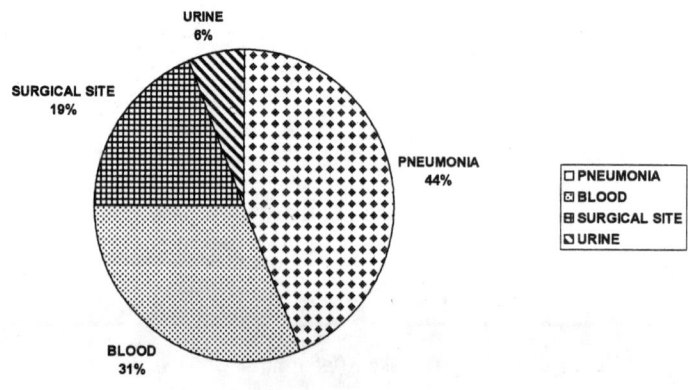

Figure 5-9 Pie chart.

Copyright © 2005, Association for Professionals in Infection Control and Epidemiology, Inc.

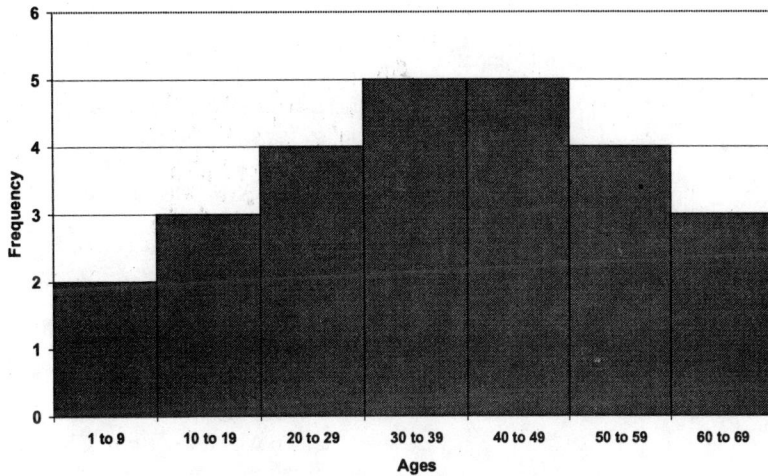

Figure 5-10 Frequency histogram.

example in Table 5-8 contains a small samples for the convenience of demonstration.

Both frequency polygons and histograms place the data point over the center point of the data range. With a frequency histogram, the bars are connected and placed so that the center of the bar is placed over the midpoint of the intervals. (Figures 5–10 and 5–11).

Inferential Statistics

Inferential statistics makes an assumption about a population based on a small sample size and is used to show an association between cause and effect, (e.g., development of pneumonia and being on a ventilator). There are calculations to show the strength of the association between the cause and effect but cause can NEVER be statistically proven. There are only methods

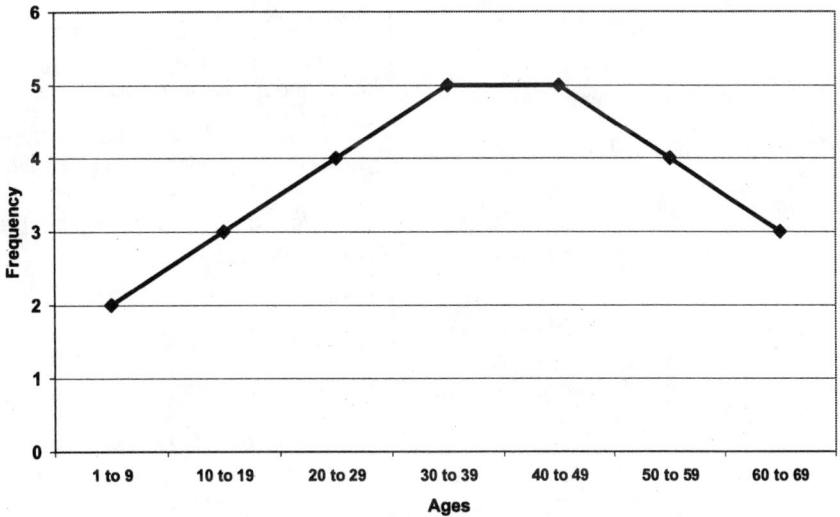

Figure 5-11 Frequency polygon.

Copyright © 2005, Association for Professionals in Infection Control and Epidemiology, Inc.

to validate the strength of the association. Inferential statistics are part of our everyday life and are used in election polls, medical testing, environmental monitoring, and manufacturing quality control. Inferential statistics relies on probability (laws of chance). The history of probability dates back to early Egypt where it was developed to increase the odds of winning in a game of chance (gambling). The first written document on probability dates back to the Roman Emperor, Claudius (circa 60 BC) who wrote on how to win in a game of dice.

Common Statistical Terms

Comparing Population and Sample

Population

Population is the set of all observations of interest to the investigator (the universe). These may be individuals, procedures, or any type of measurement. The population (sometimes called parent population) is the total from which the sample is selected (e.g., all hospitalized patients, all burn patients).

Sample

The sample is a group of observations selected from a population and chosen to represent the population whole.

Basic Principles of Sampling

The purpose of sampling is to obtain observations (measurements) that are representative of the population of interest, using a portion of that population (i.e., a sample). Two major principles underlie all sample designs:

- To control bias in the selection procedure

- To achieve the maximum precision in measurement

Sources of Bias in Sample Selection

The following are potential sources of bias in sample selection:

- Use of a nonrandom method (i.e., the selection is consciously or unconsciously influenced by human choice, such as a telephone survey would exclude those without a telephone)

- The sampling frame (population record), which serves as the basis for selection, does not cover the population adequately, completely, or accurately

- Some sections of the population are impossible to find or refuse to cooperate

Impact of Bias or Lack of Precision in Sample Selection on a Study

Bias causes systematic, noncompensating errors. These errors cannot be eliminated or reduced by an increase in sample size (e.g., *Literary Digest* presidential survey of 1936 picked the sample from telephone directories; it was biased because the poor were unlikely to have telephones).

Comparison of Types of Samples

Random Sample A random sample is a sample in which each person (patient) in the population has an equal chance of being selected (probability sample).

Nonrandom Sample A nonrandom sample is a sample in which the study subjects are not selected according to a random selection scheme (nonprobability sample).

Evaluation of the Use of Random and Nonrandom Approaches

Random Sample Advantages A random sample:

- Minimizes influences of bias on sample selection

- Tests statistical significance assuming random sampling of the population

- Is more generalizable to the target population

Random Sample Disadvantages Disadvantages of random samples are that they:

- Are more costly

- Are more time-consuming

- May require the use of mechanical or other devices (i.e., random number table)

- Does not ensure that sample is representative of the population, especially with small samples

Nonrandom Sample Advantages Nonrandom samples are:

- Less costly

- Administratively easy

- Less time-consuming

Nonrandom Sample Disadvantages Disadvantages of nonrandom samples are that they:

- May fail to secure a representative sample

Copyright © 2005, Association for Professionals in Infection Control and Epidemiology, Inc.

- Have questionable generalizability of conclusions

- Have possible bias because selection is nonrandom

Importance of Sample Size in Statistical Inference

Generally, the larger the sample, the stronger the inference. Variability is inversely proportional to the square root of sample size; therefore, as the size of the sample increases, variability decreases. The larger the sample, the less likely that the observed difference is due to chance alone; small samples are more subject to error.

Definition of Power and Its Relationship to Sample Size

The power of a test is its ability to detect a specified difference (e.g., the probability of rejecting the null hypothesis when it is false). The greater the specified differences to be detected are, the more powerful a sample will be in its ability to reject a false null hypothesis.

Because statistical testing for significant differences is based on the number of outcomes, a researcher must always determine how much of a difference might be expected (the power of the test) to calculate the power of the test and to determine a sample size appropriate for the study. The smaller the difference expected, the less the power of any given sample size has to detect a true difference.

Determination of sample size involves simultaneous consideration of risk factor frequency, disease frequency, and desired degree of sensitivity. A study to detect a slight difference or slight increase in disease risk with great precision will require more individuals than for less precise detection of large differences.

Sampling Distribution

All inferential statistics assume some type of sampling distribution (normal or skewed) against which the observed data from sampling are compared. Statistical inference based on the normal distribution, sometimes referred to as the bell-shaped curve, is the type most frequently encountered in the literature. In the day-to-day surveillance and data collection conducted by ICPs, the sample sizes (number of infections) are usually small and a normal distribution cannot be assumed. The test for each type of data, normal distribution and distribution unknown, will be reviewed in this chapter.

Hypothesis Testing

A common use of statistics is hypothesis testing. Hypothesis testing uses the distribution of a known area in the normal curve. It estimates the likelihood (probability) that a result did not occur by chance. First, a research or alternate hypothesis is formulated. The hypothesis states the expectation to be tested (e.g., Doctor A has a higher surgical site infection rate than Doctor B). Then a statement that is opposite to the research or alternate hypothesis is developed (e.g., Doctor A has a lower infection rate than Doctor B). The latter is called the null hypothesis (H_o). The H_o is always stated to be rejected. The research or alternate hypothesis (H_a) is the desired result. Only 2 outcomes are possible with hypothesis testing: the null hypothesis is accepted or rejected.

To test a hypothesis, the cut-off value must be selected in advance. Do you want to be 95% certain that your result did not occur by chance (selecting to 2 standard deviations)? This would tell you that there is still a 5% chance that your results did occur by chance. This number is called the critical or tabled value because it is looked up in a table. If the null hypothesis can be rejected, that is taken as evidence in favor of the alternate hypothesis. Because a test is rarely conclusive, one cannot state that the alternate hypothesis has been "proved," only that the theory has been supported.

Directional hypothesis specifies the expected relationship between variables. It can be 1 or 2 tailed.

One-tailed example: Direction is specified in advance. Concern is with only 1 direction from the mean.

> Research hypothesis: Doctor A has a higher surgical site infection rate than Doctor B.
>
> H_o: Dr. A infection rate $<$ Dr. B
>
> H_a: Dr. A infection rate $>$ Dr. B

When the intent is to test whether the true population mean is significantly greater than the value hypothesized under the null hypothesis, then the rejection region is 1-tailed in the upper tail or right-hand side. When the intent is to test whether the true population mean is smaller than the value hypothesized by the H_o, then the rejection region is in the lower tail or left-hand side. Whenever the direction is predicted, 1-tailed tests are preferable to 2-tailed tests.

Two-tailed example: Direction is not specified. Concern is with difference in both directions, regardless of the direction.

> Research hypothesis: The surgical site infection rate for Doctor A is not the same as the infection rate of Doctor B
>
> H_o: Dr. A infection rate $=$ Dr. B
>
> H_a: Dr. A infection rate $\neq$ Dr. B

Copyright © 2005, Association for Professionals in Infection Control and Epidemiology, Inc.

When interest is to determine if the true mean is either greater than or less than, that is, in any way different from, the value hypothesized under Ho, then the rejection region consists of 2 tails.

The rejection region for a 1-tailed test is determined by placing the entire alpha level in 1 tail to find the cutoff point calculated for a test statistic value in the appropriate statistical table.

The decision to select a 1-tailed or 2-tailed test is not purely statistical.

There are risks associated with hypothesis testing:

• A Type I error (α) means rejecting the null hypothesis when it is true and attributing significance when there is none. The probability of committing a type I error is referred to as the *significance level*. The α level is always stated.

• A Type II error (β) means accepting the null hypothesis when it is false or not attributing significance when it exists.

The following shows ways to reduce the risk of errors:

• Type I (α) error can be reduced by decreasing the length of the "rejection" area. Keeping the α level very small (e.g., 0.05, 0.01) will decrease the risk of committing a Type I error.

• Type II (β) error can be reduced by increasing the sampling size. Recall that as the sample size increases, the data get closer to a normal distribution. With infection control data, sample size cannot be controlled (e.g., number of infections, number of line days). It may not be obvious when an β error has been has been met.

Types I and II errors are inversely related. Once the sample size is fixed, decreasing the risk of committing a Type I error increases the risk of committing a Type II error. Therefore, it is impossible to control for both types of errors simultaneously.

Inferential Statistics

Inferential statistics are divided into 2 types: parametric and nonparametric.

Parametric

Parametric statistics assume a normal distribution of the parent or sample population. Most parametric techniques require measurements on a continuous-interval scale. There are many statistical tests in each category, but the 2 examples that have application for infection control are the *z* test and Student's *t* test. The for-

mulas can be found in any statistics book and will not be detailed in this text.

The *z* test is the most appropriate to test that the means of 2 samples are not different (2-tailed hypothesis). An example of its use is to compare the mean of infection rates against the National Nosocomial Infections Surveillance (NNIS) mean or another benchmark mean. It requires a normal distribution and a sample size of 30 or more.

An English statistician, W.S. Gossett, working in Dublin for the Guinness brewery and writing under the pseudonym "Student," developed the *t* test named for him for quality control in brewing. Student's *t* test also works best with a normal distribution, but it can be used when the sample size is less than 30. It can be used with continuous data (e.g., infection rates) and can be 1 or 2 tailed. There are 2 types of *t* test:

• Independent sample: experiment versus a control

• Paired sample: 2 measures from the same sample (e.g., before and after)

While the formulas for the *z* test and *t* test are not detailed in this chapter, degrees of freedom (df) must be mentioned if calculations are to be performed manually. The degree of freedom is a parameter used to help select the critical value in some probability distributions. It is necessary to know the df to select the correct critical value from the table. The formula to calculate degrees of freedom can be found in any statistics book.

Nonparametric

Nonparametric data makes no assumption about the distribution of the population values and can be used with discrete data (e.g., infection, no infection), nominal and ordinal data, and interval data. The main advantage of nonparametric methods is that the assumptions of normality are not required.

One nonparametric statistical technique to test an association is called the Chi square (χ^2) test. The χ^2 test can analyze 2 or more groups and measures the observed (the interest of study) against the expected (baseline, benchmark, or historical data).

The formula for χ^2 is as follows: (Figure 5–12)

• Chi-square distributions are positive numbers and are skewed to the right.

$$(a,b) = \sqrt{\bar{x} \pm z \times s/n}$$

Figure 5–12 Formula for χ^2.

Copyright © 2005, Association for Professionals in Infection Control and Epidemiology, Inc.

Table 5-9. 2 × 2 Table

	VAP	No VAP	Total
Current	A	B	A + B
Baseline	C	D	C + D
Total	A + C	B + D	A + B + C + D

Table 5-11.

	VAP	No VAP	Total
Current	15	45	60
Baseline	8	95	103
Total			

- A χ^2 test can be used to compare any number of proportions.

The χ^2 test is appropriate when comparing infection rates of Doctor A versus Doctor B as mentioned in the section addressing hypothesis testing. It also can be used to support a theory that the infection rate calculated during the current month is higher than the baseline (previous months).

Example: There is a sense the current month's VAP rate is higher than the rates of prior months. The immediate past month had 15 patients who developed VAP out of 60 patients who were on ventilators. Data from the previous 12 months documented 8 patients with VAP of 103 on ventilators. The null hypothesis is stated to be rejected: The current VAP rate is lower than the baseline. Ho: Current rate is less than baseline rate. The alternate (desired outcome) hypothesis is stated as "the current VAP rate is higher than the baseline." Ha: Current rate is greater than baseline rate (1-tailed). A 95% level of significance level is selected [a 5% (1 of 20) risk of being wrong, rejecting the null hypothesis when it is true].

- Create a 2 × 2 table (Table 5–9).

- Enter the known values into the cells in the row titled "current" (15 into cell A under VAP, 60 under the "total" heading), in the row titled "baseline" (8 into cell C under VAP and 103 under the "total" heading) (Table 5–10).

- Calculate the values for cells B and D by subtracting the value in cells A and C from the row totals (Table 5–11).

- Total up the 2 columns (A + C and B + D).

- Total up the 2 rows (A + B and C + D).

- Total up all row and columns (A + B + C + D) (Table 5–12)

- Calculate the degrees of freedom. The formula for calculating degrees of freedom for a χ^2 test is as follows: Cn – 1 × Rn – 1 (Cn represents the number of columns and Rn, the number of rows. In a 2 × 2 table (2 rows and 2 columns) the formula would be 2 – 1 × 2 – 1 = 1 df

- Plug in the values using the formula for χ^2 listed previously:

$$\chi^2 = (1) \left[(15 \times 95) - (45 \times 81) - \frac{163}{2} \right]^2$$
$$\times \frac{163}{60} \times 103 \times 23 \times 140$$

- When calculations are done manually or using a calculator, the appropriate table must be used to verify the result (i.e., χ^2 Critical Values Table for χ^2). The value in the appropriate table is called the *critical value* (Table 5–13).

- Find df of "1" in the column on the left side of the table. Go across the row to the right until you find a value closest to your calculated result. The calculated (computed) result is 7.92. The calculated value is between 7.88 and 9.14 in the table. The *p* values above 7.88 and 9.14 are 0.005 and 0.0025 respectively. For a 95% probability that the result did not occur by chance, a *p* value of .05 needed to be met. The calculated result exceeds that minimum requirement so the Ho can be rejected with a 95% probability that the result did not occur by chance.

The Fisher's exact test is used in place of the χ^2 when the sample size number is less than 20 or any 1 cell in the table is less than 5 (Table 5–14).

Table 5-10.

	VAP	No VAP	Total
Current	15		60
Baseline	8		103
Total			

Table 5-12.

	VAP	No VAP	Total
Current	15	45	60
Baseline	8	95	103
Total	23	140	163

Copyright © 2005, Association for Professionals in Infection Control and Epidemiology, Inc.

Table 5-13. χ^2 Critical Values Table

χ^2 Critical Values Table										
df	.25	.20	.15	.10	.05	*p* .025	.02	.01	.005	.0025	.001
1	1.32	1.64	2.07	2.71	3.84	5.02	5.41	6.63	7.88	9.14	10.83
2	2.77	3.22	3.79	4.61	5.99	7.38	7.82	9.21	10.60	11.98	13.82
3	4.11	4.64	5.32	6.25	7.81	9.35	9.84	11.34	12.84	14.32	16.27

Definition of Test Statistic

A test statistic is a numeric measure computed from a set of sample measurements that quantifies the magnitude of discrepancy between the hypothesized population parameter and the statistic computed from the sample. It can be converted to a probability value (i.e., level of significance) using special tables. Different test statistics (e.g., χ^2, *t* test) use different statistical tables for interpretation of significance. A *p* value is not the probability that an observed result is due to chance alone. Instead, it is the probability, given that the null hypothesis is true, of collecting a random sample of the same size from the same population that yields a test statistic at least as extreme as the 1 calculated from the sample.

Definition of Level of Significance

The level of significance is the probability value arbitrarily chosen by the researcher as the desired level of probability at which one may feel secure in rejecting the null hypothesis. When using sample data, it is not possible to be absolutely certain that the hypothesis being accepted is true. Therefore, a probability that the finding is due to chance is stated. This probability of rejecting a null hypothesis when it is true is the level of significance or α level. Most researchers use .05 (5%) or .01 (1%) values for α to minimize the chances of incorrectly rejecting the null hypothesis. This specified level states a sufficiently small likelihood that the given observation could occur by chance variation alone (e.g., .05 or a 1-in-20 chance). The researcher finds the appropriate rejection region for a test statistic at a given α level and rejects the null hypothesis for those values of the test statistic that lie beyond the specified value. Simply stated, α level is the level of risk. It is the level of risk a researcher is willing to take of being wrong.

Confidence Intervals (CI)

A sample mean is an *estimate* of the population mean (μ). It is a point estimate that may include some error. To compensate for this margin of error, a calculation is performed to identify a range of possible values the population mean might take. This range is known as the confidence interval (CI).

To calculate a CI, the data must have a normal distribution. The researcher determines what level of confidence to select. The common selection is 90% (e.g., you want to be 90% certain the outcome did not occur by chance).The formula for calculating a CI of a sample is as following:

The result will give a plus and minus (a, b) value because 1 value will be less than the sample mean and the other, greater than the mean (a range is being calculated).

The *z* score is a unit of measurement and is commonly used for standardized observations that tell us how many standard deviations the original observations falls from the mean and in which direction. The value for the *z* score is found by going to an Areas of the Standard Normal Curve table.

Example: You are participating in a program to monitor obesity among the male senior students from a local high school. The enrollment number of male seniors is 320. You take a sample of 100 seniors and weigh them. You calculate a mean of 177 lbs and a standard deviation of 28 lbs. You want to be 90% certain that the sample mean is a true reflection of the mean of all senior male students. You are aware that the mean from the sample is a point estimate and you want to increase the accuracy of your result by calculating a possible range of weights.

- Calculate the *z* score: For a 90% confidence that the result did not occur by chance, the first step is to divide .90 by 2 = 0.4505 (remember, you are looking for a plus and minus value. If you select 95%, you divide 95 divide by 2 and go to the table

Table 5-14. Fisher's Exact Test

	VAP	No VAP	Total
Current	2(<5)	5	7
Baseline	6	6	2
Total	8	11	19 (<20)

APIC Text of Infection Control and Epidemiology

Copyright © 2005, Association for Professionals in Infection Control and Epidemiology, Inc.

Table 5-15. Areas of the Standard Normal Curve z μ to z

0.00 .0000	0.25 .0987	0.50 .1915	0.75 .2734	1.00 .3413	1.25 .3844	1.50 .4332
0.01 .0040	0.26 .1026	0.51 .1950	0.76 .2764	1.01 .3438	1.26 .3962	1.51 .4345
0.02 .0080	0.27 .1064	0.52 .1985	0.77 .2794	1.02 .3461	1.27 .3980	1.52 .4357
0.03 .0120	0.28 .1103	0.53 .2019	0.78 .2823	1.03 .3485	1.28 .3997	1.53 .4370
0.04 .0160	0.29 .1141	0.54 .2054	0.79 .2852	1.04 .3508	1.29 .4015	1.54 .4382
0.05 .0199	0.30 .1179	0.55 .2088	0.80 .2881	1.05 .3531	1.30 .4032	1.55 .4394
0.06 .0239	0.31 .1217	0.56 .2123	0.81 .2910	1.06 .3554	1.31 .4049	1.56 .4406
0.07 .0278	0.32 .1255	0.57 .2157	0.82 .2939	1.07 .3577	1.32 .4066	1.57 .4418
0.08 .0319	0.33 .1293	0.58 .2190	0.83 .2967	1.08 .3599	1.33 .4082	1.58 .4429
0.09 .0359	0.34 .1331	0.59 .2221	0.84 .2996	1.09 .3621	1.34 .4099	1.59 .4441
0.10 .0398	0.35 .1368	0.60 .2257	0.85 .3023	1.10 .3643	1.35 .4116	1.60 .4452
0.11 .0438	0.36 .1406	0.61 .2291	0.86 .3051	1.11 .3665	1.36 .4131	1.61 .4463
0.12 .0478	0.37 .1443	0.62 .2324	0.87 .3078	1.12 .3686	1.37 .4147	1.62 .4474
0.13 .0517	0.38 .1480	0.63 .2357	0.88 .3106	1.13 .3708	1.38 .4162	1.63 .4484
0.14 .0557	0.39 .1517	0.64 .2389	0.89 .3133	1.14 .3729	1.39 .4177	1.64 .4495
0.15 .0596	0.40 .1554	0.65 .2422	0.90 .3159	1.15 .3749	1.40 .4192	1.65 ??.4505
0.16 .0636	0.41 .1591	0.66 .2454	0.91 .3186	1.16 .3770	1.41 .4207	1.66 .4515
0.17 .0675	0.42 .1628	0.67 .2486	0.92 .3212	1.17 .3790	1.42 .4222	1.67 .4525
0.18 .0714	0.43 .1664	0.68 .2517	0.93 .3238	1.18 .3810	1.43 .4236	1.68 .4535
0.19 .0753	0.44 .1700	0.69 .2549	0.94 .3264	1.19 .3830	1.44 .4251	1.69 .4545
0.20 .0793	0.45 .1736	0.70 .2380	0.95 .3289	1.20 .3849	1.45 .4265	1.70 .4564
0.21 .0832	0.46 .1772	0.71 .2611	0.96 .3315	1.21 .3869	1.46 .4279	1.71 .4564
0.22 .0871	0.47 .1808	0.72 .2642	0.97 .3340	1.22 .3888	1.47 .4292	1.72 .4573
0.23 .0910	0.48 .1844	0.73 .2673	0.98 .3365	1.23 .3907	1.48 .4306	1.73 .4582
0.24 .0948	0.49 .1879	0.74 .2704	0.99 .3389	1.24 .3925	1.49 .4319	1.74 .4591
0.25 .0987	0.50 .1915	0.75 .2734	1.00 .3413	1.25 .3944	1.50 .4332	1.75 .4599

and look for the z score that corresponds to 0.4750). Going to the table (Table 5–15), look for 0.4505, and you find that the z score is 1.65.

- Plug the numbers into the formula: (Figures 5–13 and 5–14).

- CI = 177 ± 4.6 lbs

$$\chi^2 = \frac{(df)[(ad-bc)-(\frac{-n}{2})^2(n)}{(a+b)(c+d)(a+c)(b+d)}$$

Figure 5–13 Formula for confidence interval.

$$(a,b) = \sqrt{177 \pm 165 \times 28/n}$$

—CI = 177 ± 4.6 lbs

Figure 5–14 Confidence interval calculations.

- Interpretation: We can be 90% certain the mean weight of all senior male students is between 172 lbs and 182 lbs.

Definition of Rejection Region

The rejection region of a test of hypothesis specifies which values of the test statistic are "sufficiently large" to warrant rejection of the null hypothesis. The size of the rejection region depends on the level of significance for the test (Figure 5–15).

Drawing Conclusions From Statistical Tests

Statistical Significance

The question is "Is chance or sampling variation a likely explanation for the difference between a sample statistic and the corresponding null hypothesis population value?" If the answer is yes, it means that the difference is likely to occur by chance alone, and this sample result is compatible with the null hypothesis,

Copyright © 2005, Association for Professionals in Infection Control and Epidemiology, Inc.

Two tests at the same probability level (96%)

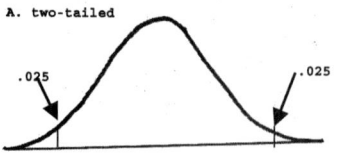

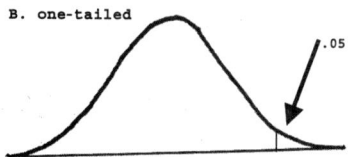

Figure 5-15 Area of rejection under the curve.

and therefore is **not statistically significant.** If the answer is no, it means that the observed difference is not likely to occur by chance variation and the sample result is not compatible with the null hypothesis, and therefore is **statistically significant.**

- Statistically significant: Reject the null hypothesis because there is sufficient evidence to support that sampling variation or chance is unlikely explanation for difference between Ho and sample values. This does not prove that the null hypothesis is true.

- Not statistically significant: Do not reject null hypothesis. There is not sufficient evidence that sampling variation is likely explanation for difference between Ho and sample values.

Remember that the null hypothesis of a statistical test refers to the parameter(s) of the population(s) of interest. The test statistic that is to be calculated from sample data has a distribution, called the sampling distribution. To understand this distribution, consider a population of numbers from which you take all possible samples of a particular size n. From each of these samples, you can calculate a test statistic to test some null hypothesis (perhaps that the mean of the population is 0). These test statistics will not all be equal; they will have a distribution (perhaps a t distribution). Thus, it may be possible to calculate the probability of collecting a sample where the value of the test statistic is greater than (or less than) or equal to some specified value. The p value will be the probability of observing a sample in which the test statistic is greater than or equal to the test statistic for the sample which you actually did observe. For a 1-tailed test, this probability is equal to the area under 1 tail of the distribution; for a 2-tailed test it is the area under both tails.

- If the p value is small, you can conclude that the null hypothesis of your test is probably not true.

- If the p value is large, you do not have sufficient evidence to reject the null hypothesis.

The p value is commonly compared to α, the specified significance level of the test. If $\alpha = .05$, then a p value less than .05 would cause you to reject the null hypothesis, whereas a p value greater than .05 would cause you to fail to reject the null hypotheses.

Steps in Performing a Statistical Test

- Collect the data to be analyzed.

- Organize the data set.

- Developed the assumptions required (e.g., normal distribution).

- State the null hypothesis (Ho).

- State the significance level (usually 0.05 or 0.01).

- Determine if 1-tailed or 2-tailed test is appropriate.

- Select the rejection region (critical ratio).

- Calculate the appropriate test statistic and its p value.

- Accept or reject the null hypothesis. Use caution: One should use the p value as an indication of the strength of evidence against the Ho.

Calculation and Use of Frequency Measures, Rates, and Ratios Used in Epidemiology

Appropriate Use of Rates

A rate measures the probability of occurrence (i.e., frequency) in a population of some particular event such as cases of disease or deaths. Epidemiologists use rates to summarize the experience of a population over time. A rate provides a means of comparing the occurrence of an event in 1 population to similar populations by adjusting for differences in population sizes. To avoid inaccurate conclusions from focusing solely on numerators, choice of the appropriate denominator is 1 of the most important aspects when measuring disease/event frequency.

Basic Formula for All Types of Rates

Rate = numerator/denominator × constant

$$\frac{x}{y} \times k$$

where

x = the numerator, which equals the number of times the event (e.g., infections) has occurred during a specified time interval.

APIC Text of Infection Control and Epidemiology

Copyright © 2005, Association for Professionals in Infection Control and Epidemiology, Inc.

y = the denominator, which equals a population (e.g., number of patients at risk) from which those experiencing the event were derived during the *same* time interval.

k = A constant used to transform the result of division into a uniform quantity so that it can be compared with other, similar quantities. A whole number (fractions are inconvenient) such as 100, 1000, 10,000, or 100,000 is usually used (selection of k is usually made so that the smallest rate calculated has at least 1 digit to the left of the decimal point) or is determined by accepted practice (the magnitude of numerator compared with denominator).

There are 3 important aspects of the formula:

- Persons in the denominator must reflect the same population from which the numerator was taken.

- Counts in the numerator and denominator should cover the same time period.

- At least in theory, the persons in the denominator should have been at risk of the event or occurrence.

The following discussion shows how to calculate commonly used rates.

Incidence Rate

An incidence rate is a measure of the frequency with which an event occurs in a population over a specified period of time. Incidence indicates the risk of disease in a population over a period of time. The incidence rate equals the number of new cases of a disease for a specified time period divided by the population at risk for same time period multiplied by a constant.

Example: During 1994, 840 patients in Hospital A developed urinary tract infections (UTIs). The hospital had 45,628 total discharges for the year. What is the annual incidence of UTIs per 1000 discharges?

The incident rate = $840/45{,}628 \times 1000 = 18.4/1000$ discharges.

Prevalence (or Point Prevalence) Rate

A prevalence rate is the proportion of persons in a population with a particular disease or attribute at a specific point in time (point prevalence) or over a specified time period (period prevalence). Prevalence depends on the duration of disease. The prevalence rate equals the number of existing cases of disease from a specified interval or point in time divided by the population at risk for same time period multiplied by a constant.

Example: On a specified day, the ICP identifies 16 patients with healthcare-associated UTIs. On the day of the study the hospital census is 403. What is the prevalence of UTIs per 1000 patients?

Prevalence rate = $16/403 \times 1000 = 39.7/1000$ patients

There are 2 approaches to determining the numerator for prevalence surveys. Both approaches are acceptable provided the composition of the rates is clearly defined. In both cases, the denominator would be number of charts reviewed, number of patients examined, or the like.

- Only active cases of healthcare-associated infection are included in the numerator, that is, all cases from a point in time up to a second point in time are included (e.g., for a 10-day period). This method reduces the prevalence rate and more nearly reflects incidence.

- All healthcare-associated infections up to a certain point in time are included, whether they are active or inactive, that is, all infections on the day(s) of the study are counted, regardless of their date of onset. This method produces a higher prevalence rate because it counts all cases, regardless of state of infection.

Attack Rate

An attack rate is a special form of incidence rate. In fact, it is not truly a rate, but a proportion. It is the proportion of persons at risk who become infected over an entire period of exposure or a measure of the risk or probability of becoming a case. It is usually expressed as a percentage and is used almost exclusively for epidemics or outbreaks of disease where a specific population is exposed to a disease for a limited period of time. In hospital epidemiology, attack rates are also used to describe the probability of acquiring a healthcare-associated infection during hospitalization. An attack rate has no specification of time in the denominator. The attack rate equals the number of new cases of disease (for a specified time period) divided by the population at risk for same time period multiplied by 100. Attack rate is the same as incidence rate, except that attack rates are always expressed as cases per 100 populations or as a percentage.

Example: During a 34-month period, there were 158 admissions to the burn–trauma unit of a hospital, with 52 of the patients subsequently contracting an infection with *Staphylococcus aureus*. Of the 158 total admissions to the burn–trauma unit, 129 were admitted with burns. The remainders were trauma cases. Of the 52 patients with *S. aureus* infections, 49 had burns. Of the 129 burn patients, 81 had burns that covered less than 20% of the body; 48 had burns that covered more than 20% of the body. Of the 49 infections in burn patients, 16 were inpatients with

Copyright © 2005, Association for Professionals in Infection Control and Epidemiology, Inc.

burns that covered less than 20% of the body; 33 were inpatients with burns that covered more than 20% of their body. The following rates can be calculated:

- Overall attack rate = 52/158 × 100 = 32.9%

- Burn patient attack rate = 49/129 × 100 =38%

- Trauma patient attack rate = 3/29 × 100 = 10.3%

- Attack rate for burn patients with less than 20% burns = 16/81 ×100 =19.8%

- Attack rate for burn patients with greater than 20% burns =33/48 × 100 = 68.8%

Incidence Density

Incidence density is a type of incidence rate that incorporates time into the denominator. Each person in a group is observed from a fixed beginning time to an established end point. End points include onset of disease, death, loss to follow-up, and end of study. In this case, the numerator is still the number of new cases, but the denominator is different. The denominator is the sum of the time each person was observed during the study, which is totaled for all persons. Another perspective might be the number of persons at risk multiplied by the time for which each remains at risk (e.g., person-time units). Incidence density equals the number of cases (during observation period) divided by the time each person was observed (totaled for all persons) multiplied by 10.

Incidence density is usually used in cohort studies of diseases with long incubation or latency periods, such as chronic diseases and occupationally acquired diseases, or when people are not followed up for the same length of time. The estimated incidence density for a disease is also called the estimated hazard for developing a disease, person-time rate, or force of morbidity/mortality. Like all quantities meeting the formal definition of a rate, the incidence density is expressed as a change per unit of time.

A closely related concept is that of the risk or probability of developing a disease over a given time period. The cumulative incidence rate is used to express this probability. It is not a true rate, but a measure of average risk. It is the proportion (i.e., probability) of a fixed population that becomes diseased in a stated period of time.

Mortality Rate

A mortality rate is the measure of the frequency of death in a defined population during a specified time (usually a year). The crude mortality rate measures the proportion of the population dying each year from all causes. The cause-specific mortality rate measures mortality from a specified cause for a population.

mortality rate

$$\frac{x}{y} \times k$$

where

x = The number of people in a defined population during a specified interval of time who (1) die of any cause (crude rate) or (2) die of a specified cause (cause-specific rate)

y = Estimated population at midyear (i.e., July); crude rates use 1000 or 100,000

k = Is usually an assigned value of 1000 when calculating crude rates: 100,000 is used for cause-specific rates

Example: In a city of 250,000 population, 2106 persons died during the year; 12 persons died from bacterial meningitis. What is the crude mortality rate per 1000? What is the cause-specific rate per 100,000?

- Crude mortality rate = 2106/250,000 × 1000 = 8.42 deaths/1000 population

- Cause-specific mortality rate = 12/250,000 × 100,000 = 4.8/100,000 population

Purpose of Adjusting Rates

In the example of the burn unit, it is clear that certain patient characteristics increase the risk of infection (e.g., extensive burns). If only overall attack rates were examined, these differences would not be apparent. However, when the data are stratified (i.e., group data by specific subsets), it becomes clear that there are differences within groups. This type of adjustment for the purposes of comparison removes the effect of differences in composition of groups. This is why site-specific rates are calculated.

Epidemiology texts often refer to age adjustment comparing morbidity or mortality for each specific age group. A more sophisticated form of adjustment uses a "standard population" to compare rates from 2 different sources (e.g., cities and hospitals). A standard population is an arbitrary distribution of a characteristic (e.g., age) used as a common standard for 2 groups when comparing their rates. Because the composition of the population of 2 hospitals may be very different (e.g., average age, underlying disease, socioeconomic status), it is impossible to compare infection rates unless a standard population of some type is used. Adjusted rates permit unbiased comparison of groups. Comparison of crude rates in 2 populations may be misleading when there is a variable (i.e., factor) related to the event you are interested in measuring and the

Copyright © 2005, Association for Professionals in Infection Control and Epidemiology, Inc.

variable is distributed differently for the 2 populations. The classic example of adjustment is age adjustment for crude death rates. Age is a variable obviously related to mortality. If the age distribution of 2 populations is very different, the 1 with the larger proportion of older persons often has a higher crude death rate. To remove the effect of age, statistical methods are used to adjust rates. Age-adjusted mortality rates for comparison of 2 or more populations are calculated by multiplying age-specific death rates for each age group by the population in the same age group in a standard population. The 1940, 1970, or 2000 US populations are usually used for this type of direct rate adjustment.

Stratification is another method of adjustment that is important when measures of association may vary over strata. It is an important analytic tool for controlling the effect of confounding variables and describing variables that are effect modifiers.

Controversies Associated With Calculation, Use, and Comparison of Incidence Rates in Hospital Epidemiology

The numerator and denominator used to calculate infection rates do not have the same dimension. In fact, the incidence rate is actually an infection ratio that is treated as if it were a rate.

• Numerator equals infections

• Denominator equals patients

The numerator and denominator are not drawn from the same population at risk. Discharges do not necessarily reflect the actual month patients are admitted. The infection proportion is the number of patients with 1 or more infections divided by the number of persons at risk during the same time period. About 18% of persons with healthcare-associated infections have more than 1 infection. Therefore, the infection ratio is about 1.27 times larger than the infection proportion. It is easier to get the data for the infection ratio. The ratio is commonly used as the infection rate in hospital epidemiology.

$$\frac{\text{Number of infections acquired in month A}}{\text{Number of patients discharged in month A}} = \text{Incidence rate}$$

This equation does not take into account the influence of time in the denominator. Incidence rates must take into consideration not only the population at risk but also the time (at risk) contributed by each individual during the study period. To calculate incidence densities, a measure of risk of healthcare-associated infection corrected for time and some estimate of length of hospital stay per admission or discharge would be required. As currently calculated (i.e., infection rates per 100 discharges or attack rates), comparisons

cannot be made between hospitals because of the unknown effect of duration on the equation.

Definitions of rates and proportions are not always followed strictly, nor is the difference between prevalence and incidence always recognized. In the literature, these rates, which are not directly comparable, have sometimes been used interchangeably or lumped together as "infection rates." Rates from different populations are frequently compared without appropriate concern for comparability. No standard adjustment methods are widely used that allow for comparison of different populations. (For example, although your facility is a community hospital, it is not appropriate to assume that your rates should be the same as those reported by community hospitals in the NNIS system. The 2 groups have differences that do not permit unbiased comparison.)

Denominators should reflect the appropriate population at risk as much as possible. Only patients who are truly at risk should be included in the denominator, but practical difficulties determine the use of less precise denominators such as admissions or discharges to a specific service during a specified time. Recently the Centers for Disease Control and Prevention initiated inclusion of device-days (i.e., ventilator-days or central line–days) as part of the data collected in intensive care units for NNIS system. Device-days have been incorporated in the denominator of rates used for interhospital comparison. Using central venous catheter–days as the denominator takes into account the utilization rate of central lines by various hospitals and adjusts rates for a variable that may affect the outcome of interest.

Various measures of association are used in epidemiology to quantify the magnitude of the effect of risk factors on disease risk. Epidemiological studies are performed not only to identify risk factors related to disease but also to quantify the magnitude of risk associated with them. The measures of association used most frequently in epidemiology are those based on incidence rates and on the risk of developing disease.

Measures of Association Used to Assess Risk of Disease

Incidence Rate

Please see the earlier section on rates.

Relative Risk (Risk Ratio)

Relative risk (RR) is a measure of the strength of association used in prospective and experimental studies. It is the probability of developing a disease if the risk factor is present divided by the probability of developing disease if the risk factor is not present. It is sometimes called the risk ratio or the ratio of the 2 incidence

Copyright © 2005, Association for Professionals in Infection Control and Epidemiology, Inc.

Table 5-16.

	PNE	No PNE	Total
Vent			
No vent			
Total			

Table 5-18.

	PNE	No PNE	Total
Vent	10	5	15
No vent	5	20	25
Total	15	25	40

rates. It estimates how much more likely disease is to occur in exposed groups compared with the unexposed. Relative risk:

- Is used for cohort studies [a group of individuals who share a common experience (e.g. central lines)]

- Is prospective, starts at point 0 and continues into the future (e.g. begins before the event occurs)

- Asks the question: What is risk of developing disease if exposed to the risk factor?

Example: At time of admission, 40 patients are followed through to discharge and monitored for the development of pneumonia. Of the 40 patients, 15 developed pneumonia during their stay. Of the 15 who developed pneumonia, 10 had mechanical ventilation prior to the development of pneumonia. A total of 15 patients the 40 received mechanical ventilation.

- Create a table (Table 5–16).

- Enter the known values into the appropriate cells (Table 5–17).

- Calculate and enter the unknown values (Table 5–18).

- Calculate a relative risk using the formula

$$RR = \frac{\left(\dfrac{A}{R1}\right)}{\left(\dfrac{C}{R2}\right)}$$

$$RR = \frac{\left(\dfrac{10}{15}\right)}{\left(\dfrac{5}{25}\right)}$$

- RR = 3.3.

- Interpretation: The relative risk of developing pneumonia if exposed to mechanical ventilation is 3.3 to 1 (3.3:1). Those exposed to mechanical ventilation were 3.3 times more likely to develop pneumonia than those who were not exposed to mechanical ventilation.

As a general rule:

- If RR = 1 is no significance

- If RR >1 is positive association

- If RR < 1 is a negative association (protective)

Odds Ratio

The odds ratio (OR) is another measure of association that is closely related to relative risk. It is the probability of having a particular risk factor if a condition or disease is present divided by the probability of having the risk factor if the disease or condition is not present. It is used for all types of studies with nominal data but is used mostly for retrospective and cross-sectional studies. The odds ratio is sometimes called the cross-product ratio or relative odds.

Odds ratio:

- Is used with case control studies [Begin with subjects who already have event (disease) and compare to those who do not have event (disease).]

- Is retrospective (disease already present)

- Looks at prevalence so it is not appropriate to use with chronic diseases

- Asks the question, If disease is present, what is the likelihood of having been exposed to the risk factor?

Example: During a 1 month period, 15 patients developed pneumonia in a 30-bed ventilator-dependent intensive care unit. During the same month, the other

Table 5-17.

	PNE	No PNE	Total
Vent	10		15
No vent			
Total	15		40

Table 5-19.

	PNE	No PNE	Total
TF	11	2	
No TF			
Total	15	15	30

APIC Text of Infection Control and Epidemiology

Copyright © 2005, Association for Professionals in Infection Control and Epidemiology, Inc.

15 patients in the unit did not develop pneumonia. All 30 patients were exposed to mechanical ventilation. Chart review for commonalities revealed that 11 of the 15 with pneumonia had tube feedings, while only 2 of the 15 without pneumonia did.

- Create a table and enter known values into the appropriate cells (Table 5–19).

- Calculate and enter the unknown values (Table 5–20).

- Calculate the odds ratio using the formula:

$$OR = \frac{(a \times d)}{(c \times b)}$$

$$OR = \frac{(11 \times 13)}{(4 \times 2)}$$

- OR = 17.9.

- Interpretation: ratio of odds of having tube feedings if pneumonia is present to the odds of having tube feedings if pneumonia is not present is 17.9 to 1 (17.9:1). The odds of having tube feedings if a patient had pneumonia is 17.9 times greater than among the patients who did not have pneumonia.

Testing for Validity

The most common statistics used to describe diagnostic tests or presence of disease are sensitivity and specificity. Understanding the following definitions will help to understand the methodology.

- **Prevalence** is the probability of disease in the entire population at any point in time (i.e., 2% of the US population has diabetes mellitus).

- **Incidence** is the probability that a patient without disease develops disease during an interval.

- **Sensitivity** is the probability of a positive test among patients with disease.

- **Specificity** is the probability of a negative test among patients without disease.

In the 1800s, Reverend Thomas Bayes tried to answer the question, "What is the probability of disease given a negative or positive test for the disease?" He developed an equation to answer that question (Bayes' Equation):

Table 5-21.

	Disease	No disease
Positive test	TP	FP
Negative test	FN	TN

$$\text{Posttest odds} = \text{pretest odds} \times \left(\frac{\text{Sensitivity}}{1 - \text{Specificity}} \right)$$

where the pretest odds is the prevalence, thus:

- Probability of disease given a positive test = (prevalence × sensitivity) divided by (prevalence × sensitivity) plus [(1 − prevalence) × (1 − specificity)]

- Rule of thumb: Sensitivity test is when a negative rules out disease; specificity test is when a positive rules in disease

- A 2 × 2 table is used (Table 5–21): TP = true positive, FP = false positive, TN = true negative, FN = false negative

  − Sensitivity = TP/(TP + FN)

Specificity = TN/(TN + FP)

Where TP = true positive, FP = false positive, TN = true negative, FN = false negative

Example: A pharmaceutical company "Drugs R Us" is researching a test to identify SARS. The company screened 238 people who were admitted to a hospital with a diagnosis of "rule out" SARS (Table 5–22).

Using the formulas mentioned previously:

Sensitivity = 18/(18 + 23) = 44%

Specificity = 3/(215 + 3) = 99%

Interpretation: Positive predictive value = TP/(TP + FP); that it, patients with a positive test were most likely have the disease (18 out of 21 or 86%).

Bivariate Relationships

Correlation

Correlation is used to calculate the direction and magnitude of a relationship between 2 variables. Correlation calculates a value, r, which measures the degree of the

Table 5-20.

	PNE	No PNE	Total
TF	11	2	13
No TF	4	13	12
Total	15	15	30

Table 5-22.

	SARS	No SARS
Positive test	18	3
Negative test	23	215

Copyright © 2005, Association for Professionals in Infection Control and Epidemiology, Inc.

Table 5-23. Correlation Between Number of Hours Studied and the Exam Score

Student	Hours Studied	Score
1	2	68
2	6	69
3	8	70
4	10	72
5	12	76
6	13	77
7	17	82
8	24	84
9	30	88
10	40	92
$r =$	0.97	

relationship. The calculated values can range between +1 and −1. The closer r is to ±1, the stronger the relationship. A positive correlation exists when as 1 variable increases so does the other (e.g., the longer a foley is in place, the greater the risk of developing a urinary tract infection). A negative correlation occurs when as 1 variable increases; the other decreases (e.g., increased handwashing results in fewer infections). As r approaches 0, the less the association between 2 variables, (with a value of zero there is no correlation).

With correlation, both variables are free to vary; the researcher does not control either one. The graphic display would use a scatter gram.

Example: Ten ICPs study for the certification exam. Each is asked how many hours they studied. After taking the exams, the scores are correlated to the hours studied (Table 5–23; Figure 5–16).

Interpretation: There is a positive correlation between the hours studied and the exam score.

Regression

Regression assesses the influence of 1 or more variables on another. Correlation measures association; regressions measures influence. Correlation describes how a response (dependent variable) changes as the influence (independent variable) changes. If there is only 1 independent variable, the relationship is expressed in a straight line (linear regression). Only 1 variable is free to vary, the other is controlled by the researcher (e.g., new drug treatment). It is an inferential procedure, meaning you can draw conclusions about a population based on a sample. A straight line can be represented by the following equation: $y = a + bx$, where y is the variable on the vertical axis, x is the variable on the horizontal axis, a is the y value where the line crosses the vertical axis (intercept), and b is the amount of change in y (slope).

Lurking Variables

Correlation and regression show only association and do not prove causation. Both correlation and regression have limits on predictions called "lurking variables." It is a variable that has an important effect on the result but is not among the variables being studied. A lurking variable can suggest a false relationship between variables or it can hide a relationship that exits.

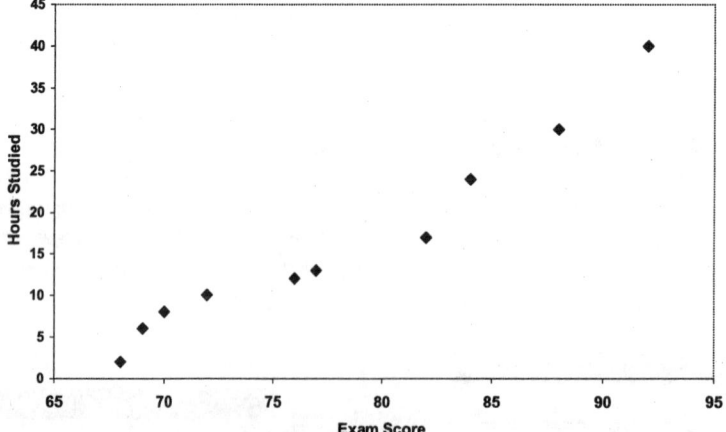

Correlation Between Hours Studied and Exam Score

Figure 5–16   Scatter gram.

APIC Text of Infection Control and Epidemiology

Copyright © 2005, Association for Professionals in Infection Control and Epidemiology, Inc.

Example: A group of college students enrolled in a geriatric course wanted to study depression in the elderly. To capture a constant population, they decided to work with residents of a nearby long-term care facility. Their project focused on providing books with positive plots to the residents. On the first visit, the students administered a psychological test designed to measure depression. Every Wednesday for the next 3 months, they provided a new book assignment and the visits ended with group discussions on the stories read. At the end of the study period, the same test for depression was administered and a statistically significant improvement was noted. This result did not surprise the facility's administrators because they said that the overall improvement in mood was noticed in better appetites, more interaction among the residents, and fewer physical complaints. The students concluded that reading books helped alleviate depression. What factors not included in the study could have resulted in the outcome? Could it have been the actual visits by the students? Very possible, as the administrators noted a return to the mood levels prior to the study once the visits stopped. This occurred even though an extensive library was provided for the residents.

Table 5-24. Commonly Used Symbols and Abbreviations

μ	population mean (mu)
$\bar{x}$	sample mean
σ	population standard deviation (lower case sigma)
s	sample standard deviation
σ^2	population variance
s^2	sample variance
Σ	upper case sigma meaning "take the sum of"; indicates that a group of numbers are to be summed
N, n	Sample size (number of items/observations in a sample)
χ^2	chi square
P, p	probability of an event (observation) occurring
df	degrees of freedom
H_o	null hypothesis
H_a	alternate (research) hypothesis
$<$	less than
$>$	greater than
$\neq$	not equal to
$\pm$	plus and minus
α	(alpha) – significance level: probability of rejecting a null hypothesis when it is true (Type I Error)
β	(beta) probability of accepting a null hypothesis when it is false (Type II Error)
$1 - \beta$	power of a test: the ability of the test to detect a specified difference

IV. SUMMARY AND CONCLUSIONS

This chapter is an introduction to the discipline of statistics. For those whose interest has been stimulated to read further, many of the references listed in the references are excellent resources for the ICP. Statistics provide the ICP with the ability to present credible data that can be transformed into information; information that will be used by the facility to improve outcomes and quality of care. Data is power, and the keeper of the data has the power to effect change. Please see Table 5–24 for a list of commonly used symbols and abbreviations used in this chapter.

REFERENCES AND CITATIONS

1. Knapp RC: *Basic statistics for nurses,* New York, NY, 1978, John Wiley & Sons.
2. Colton T: *Statistics in medicine,* Boston, Mass, 1974, Little, Brown.
3. Rosner B: *Fundamentals of biostatistics,* ed 3, Belmont, Calif, 1990, Duxbury.
4. Stahl S, Hennes J: Reading and understanding applied statistics, ed 2, St Louis, Mo, 1980, Mosby.
5. Mattson DE: Statistics: difficult concepts, understandable explanations, St Louis, Mo, 1981, Mosby.
6. Dawson-Saunders B, Trapp RG: *Basic and clinical biostatistics,* ed 2, Norwalk, Conn, 1994, Appleton & Lange.
7. Norman GR, Streiner DL: *Biostatistics: the bare essentials,* St Louis, Mo, 1994, Mosby.
8. Centers for Disease Control and Prevention: *Principles of epidemiology,* ed 2, Atlanta, Ga,1992, US Department of Health and Human Services, Public Health Service, CDC.
9. MacMahon B, Pugh TF: *Epidemiology: principles and methods,* Boston, Mass, 1970, Little, Brown.
10. Haley R, Gaynes RP, Aber RC, et al: Surveillance of nosocomial infections. In Bennett JV, Brachman PS, editors: *Hospital infections,* ed 3, Boston, Mass, 1992, Little, Brown, pp 79–108.
11. Fleiss JL, editor: *Statistical methods for rates and proportions,* ed 2, New York, NY, 1981, John Wiley & Sons.
12. Freeman J., McGowan JE Jr: Methodologic issues in hospital epidemiology. I. Rates, case-finding and interpretation, Rev Infect Dis 3:658–667, 1981.
13. Rhame FS, Sudderth WD: Incidence and prevalence as used in the analysis of the occurrences of nosocomial infections, *Am J Epidemiol* 113:1–11, 1981.
14. Townsend TR: New aspects of case-control studies and clinical trials. In Wenzel RP, editor: *Prevention and control of nosocomial infections,* Baltimore, Md, 1987, Williams & Wilkins, pp 578–590.
15. Mausner JS, Kramer KS: *Mausner and Bahn epidemiology: an introductory text,* Philadelphia, Pa, 1985, WB Saunders.
16. Victora CG: What's the denominator? *Lancet* 342:97–99, 1993.
17. Friedman GD: Primer of epidemiology, ed 4, New York, NY, 1994, McGraw-Hill.
18. Kelsey JL, Thompson WD, Evans AS: *Methods in observational epidemiology,* Boston, 1986, Little, Brown.
19. Rothman KJ: *Modern epidemiology,* Boston, Mass, 1986, Little, Brown.
20. Haley RWet, Hooton TM, Culver DH, et al: Nosocomial infections in U.S. hospitals, 1975–76: estimated nationwide frequency by selected characteristics of patients, *Am J Med* 70:947, 1981.
21. Freeman J, McGowan JE Jr: Methodologic issues in hospital epidemiology. II. Time and accuracy in estimation, *Rev Infect Dis* 3: 668–677, 1981.
22. Martin SM, Plikaytis, BD, Bean NH: Statistical considerations for analysis of nosocomial data. In Bennett JV, Brachman PS, editors: *Hospital infections,* ed 3, Boston, Mass, 1992, Little, Brown, pp 135–157.
23. Schlesselman JJ: *Case-control studies: design, conduct, analysis,* New York, NY, 1986, Oxford.

Copyright © 2005, Association for Professionals in Infection Control and Epidemiology, Inc.

24. Lilienfeld DE, Stolley PD: *Foundations of epidemiology,* ed 3, New York, NY, 1994, Oxford.
25. Riegelman RK: *Studying a study and testing a test,* Boston, Mass, 1981, Little, Brown.
26. Ingelfinger JA, Mosteller F, Thibodeau LA, et al: *Biostatistics in clinical medicine,* ed 2, New York, NY, 1987, Macmillan.
27. Harrigton HJ, Hoffherr GD, Reid RP: *Statistical Analysis Simplified,* New York, NY, 1998, McGraw-Hill.
28. Zolman JF: *Biostatistics: Experimental Design and Statistical Inference,* New York, NY, 1993, Oxford Press.
29. Ott, L: *An Introduction to Statistical Methods and data Analysis,* Boston, Mass, 1977, Duxbury Press.

Copyright © 2005, Association for Professionals in Infection Control and Epidemiology, Inc.

Statistical Process Control

Arlene Potts, BA, MPH, CIC
Director, Infection Control Program
Robert Wood Johnson University Hospital
New Brunswick, New Jersey

ABSTRACT

Traditional methods of quality control (QC) in U.S. manufacturing were based on "inspection" of the product(s) at the end of the production process. This type of QC may be compared with quality assurance (QA) in healthcare. In traditional QA, adverse patient outcomes, such as healthcare-associated infection, may be monitored concurrently but are usually reported after discharge. Frequently, a month or more intervenes between the event(s) and reporting. Like traditional QC in industry, this strategy does not allow for examination and monitoring of the process of care while it is being provided. Therefore, hospital quality improvement programs, including infection control, must develop methods to monitor both process and outcome. Measurement of process should be concurrent.

KEY CONCEPTS

- Statistical process control is an essential component of QC and performance improvement.

- The principles of statistical process control are used to monitor both the process and the outcome in a systematic manner.

- Using the elements of statistical process control enables the infection control professional (ICP) to construct charts and graphs that visually represent data.

- Analysis of the data can assist the ICP in determining special cause or common cause variations important to an epidemiologic investigation.

I.   BACKGROUND

Walter Shewhart is the individual primarily credited with the development of statistical process control (SPC). In 1924, Dr Shewhart, a research physicist with Bell Laboratories, used rudimentary statistical methods to develop the control chart.[1]

Joseph Juran and W Edwards Deming, two individuals now well known in the quality movement, were protégés of Shewhart. In 1947, Dr. Deming traveled to Japan to contribute to the post-World War II recovery efforts by assisting Japanese industry. Deming brought SPC to the Japanese and taught them to incorporate the SPC methods into the quality management programs within the manufacturing industries. Deming developed his theories for total quality

Copyright © 2005, Association for Professionals in Infection Control and Epidemiology, Inc.

management in Japan during the years after the war. The results of this effort and the success of Japanese industry are now legendary. One of Deming's Japanese students was Professor Kaoru Ishikawa.[1,2]

The methods and tools of Shewhart, Juran, Deming, and Ishikawa formed a nucleus for continuous quality improvement (CQI). These methods were not considered for serious application in the United States until the 1980s, when Deming and his methods were featured in an NBC television special. Since then, application of total quality management has become a common means for success and improved quality in U.S. industry. The concept of CQI, applying the tools and methods as described by Deming and his colleagues, was introduced into healthcare in the National Demonstration Project in 1987.[3]

The Joint Commission on Accreditation of Healthcare Organizations (JCAHO) revised its approach to the accreditation process beginning in 1989 through the Agenda for Change. This revised approach requires implementation and application of CQI methods, including SPC, by healthcare organizations for performance measurement and improvement.[4]

II. BASIC PRINCIPLES

- SPC may be applied to monitor outcomes (rates and frequency of healthcare-associated infection) or to monitor the process of care.

- The occurrence of healthcare-associated infection is usually the result of random variation in the process of care that is attributable to regular or ordinary causes.

- In general, efforts to decrease variation lead to improved quality and decreased costs.

- Run charts are useful for identifying variations and trends, and SPC charts can help identify special causes for variation.

- ICPs who have a firm understanding of SPC can establish a quality and performance monitoring process to quickly identify variations in practice or outcomes, determine if and when interventions are necessary to address those variations, and measure the impact of such interventions.

III. STATISTICAL PROCESS CONTROL

SPC in Infection Control

SPC was developed in industry to concurrently monitor the production process. Its main objective is to ensure that the process is performed consistently within predetermined parameters, thereby ensuring that the final product (or outcome) does not include defects (e.g., 0 defects).

For example, SPC is applied to the manufacturing of parts for a motorcycle engine by measuring specified dimensions of all the parts (or a sample of the parts) as they are manufactured. Parts must be within the specifications of the design to ensure that the engine will run properly once the parts are assembled. If a part is defective (e.g., wrong diameter), it is replaced before the entire motor is assembled and adversely affected by the bad part. This concurrent approach to process control provides greater potential benefit for saving time and money by identifying a defect before the final product is assembled.

SPC is a method of ensuring and improving quality based on sound statistical principles and methods. It focuses on process (as the term implies) and is based on the principle of random variation. SPC is a tool that ICPs can use to measure and improve healthcare quality; it has the advantages of objectivity and a sound statistical foundation.

A healthcare-associated infection is an adverse outcome that may occur as a result of an error (defect) in the process of care. Although some risk factors for healthcare-associated infections cannot be controlled (e.g., host factors), many of those relating to the process of care can be controlled (e.g., patient care practices).

For example, perioperative antibiotics are used to reduce the risk of surgical site infection. Research has determined that the optimal time to administer the first dose is within 2 hours before surgery. In a study by Classen et al.,[5] the authors examined the process of administration and found that prophylactic antibiotics were not administered within the optimal period in 40% of the elective surgical cases included in the study. Reducing the variation in administration of preoperative antibiotics through process improvement was projected to result in a significant decrease in the rate of the adverse outcome, surgical site infection.

SPC provides for the monitoring and evaluation of processes and outcomes and facilitates the determination of common cause (expected) variation versus special cause variation based on statistical probability.

SPC may be applied in infection control programs to monitor outcomes (rates and frequency of healthcare-associated infection) or to monitor the process of care. Process improvement efforts such as those reported by Classen et al.[5] may contribute to an overall reduction in the risks of endemic healthcare-associated infection, which may in turn lead to a reduction in incidence.

Copyright © 2005, Association for Professionals in Infection Control and Epidemiology, Inc.

Process Variation

Variation in process is a key concept in quality improvement and SPC. In general, efforts to decrease variation lead to improved quality and decreased costs.

As a quality management tool, SPC focuses on monitoring processes and outcomes to minimize or decrease variation. SPC was developed using the basic principles of normal distribution and random variation. A German mathematician, Carl Gauss, first described the concept of normal distribution within a sample population. He also developed the calculation for standard deviation (SD) in the study of random variation within the normal distribution.

Quality theory teaches us that variation can have two sources: common cause and special cause.

Common Cause Variation

All processes have variation. Variation is part of the design of the process and is attributable to regular or ordinary causes. A good demonstration of common cause variation is to compare 10 signatures from the same person. Close examination of each signature will show differences in size and shape of some letters.

Common cause variation results in a stable process because the variation is predictable. It is the normal or expected variation within a population or sample and is commonly known as "noise." This type of variation explains why infection rates in a facility have some variability from month to month. An example of common cause is the endemic levels of urinary tract infections that are influenced by age, sex, instrumentation, duration or frequency of instrumentation, and infection at another site.

Special Cause Variation

Special cause variation occurs when an event or process is affected or influenced by an event or cause outside the process system. It results in an unstable process because it is not predictable. This type of variation can be positive or negative (i.e., a decrease or an increase in infections). An example of a special cause event would be a cluster or outbreak of surgical site infections attributed to a breakdown in instrument processing. The source of special cause variation should be identified and eliminated.

Based on Gaussian theory of normal distribution and SD, common cause variation results in a distribution that lies within 3 SDs above and below the mean. This includes 99.73% of all probable events. Therefore special cause variation should occur in less than 0.27% of events sampled. The occurrence of endemic healthcare-associated infection is usually the result of random variation based on common cause.

Analyzing Variation

Two methods are available to measure and plot variation. Run charts are useful in identifying trends, and SPC charts identify special cause. Run charts—

- plot the movement of observation (infections and the like over a given period of time).

- can be used with any type of data (e.g., discrete, continuous, nominal).

- compute no statistical calculations.

- use the median of the data set.

- Need at least 16 data points for reliability

- use the 7,7,1 rule:
  - 7 data points above the median
  - 7 data points in row going up or down (may cross the median)
  - 1 large spike (Figure 6–1)

The following is an example of the construction of a run chart: On May 30, you receive a call from the microbiology laboratory stating that there are six cultures positive for *Serratia* isolated from sputum specimens in the surgical intensive care unit. To determine whether this is a true increase, you ask the microbiology laboratory to produce a retrospective printout of all positive cultures from that unit dating back to January of the previous year. You put the data into a table in a spreadsheet (Table 6–1). The next step is to calculate the median of the data set; it is 3.4. Construct a line graph using the data points and the median (Figure 6–2).

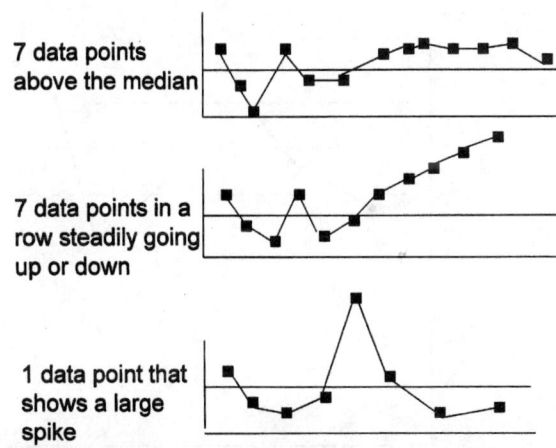

7 data points above the median

7 data points in a row steadily going up or down

1 data point that shows a large spike

Figure 6–1 The 7, 7, 1 Rule.

Copyright © 2005, Association for Professionals in Infection Control and Epidemiology, Inc.

Table 6-1. Spreadsheet

Month	No. Isolates	No. Patient Days	Rate/1000 Patient Days	Median
Jan	1	307	3.3	3.4
Feb	2	247	8.1	3.4
Mar	0	266	0.0	3.4
Apr	1	258	3.9	3.4
May	0	273	0.0	3.4
Jun	0	265	0.0	3.4
Jul	2	229	8.7	3.4
Aug	1	218	4.6	3.4
Sep	0	208	0.0	3.4
Oct	2	267	7.5	3.4
Nov	1	278	3.6	3.4
Dec	3	264	11.4	3.4
Jan	1	304	3.3	3.4
Feb	2	270	7.4	3.4
Mar	1	305	3.3	3.4
Apr	1	298	3.4	3.4
May	1	336	3.0	3.4
Jun	0	359	0.0	3.4
Jul	6	375	16.0	3.4
Median			3.4	3.4

SPC charts—

- are more sensitive than run charts.

- use statistical calculations [mean ($\overline{X}$) and sigma (σ)].

- use σ (the standard error measurement that quantifies the precision with which the sample mean estimates the population mean; measures the reliability of estimates).

Elements of a SPC Chart

- The data are plotted in time sequences.

- Calculations provide an upper and lower control limits (σ) and a mean ($\overline{X}$).

- Special cause is identified by dividing the chart into zones (Figure 6–3).

Selecting a SPC Chart

The types of data and frequency of events determine type of control chart. There are two types of data: discrete and continuous. Discrete data may be categorical (the events and the nonevents can be counted) or noncategorical (the events can be counted, but the nonevents cannot). Events that occur frequently usually follow a normal distribution; those that occur infrequently may not (e.g., Poisson distribution). Type of

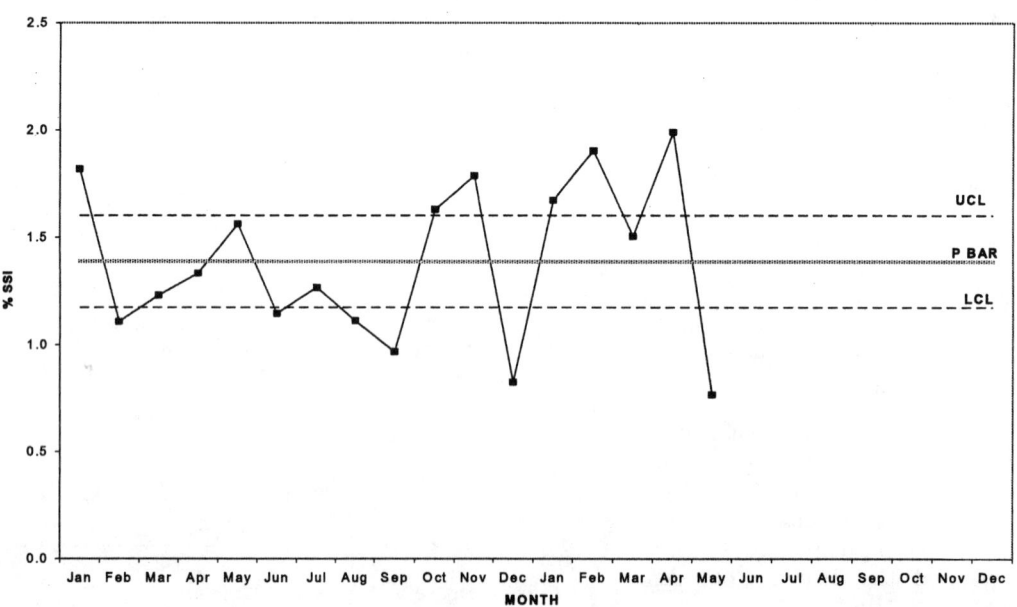

SURGICAL SITE INFECTIONS AMONG PATIENTS UNDERGOING CORNARY ARTERY BYPASS SUGERY
JANUARY 1, 2002 - MAY 31, 2003

Figure 6–2 Run chart.

APIC Text of Infection Control and Epidemiology

Copyright © 2005, Association for Professionals in Infection Control and Epidemiology, Inc.

Figure 6-3 Creation of "zones" in a control chart.

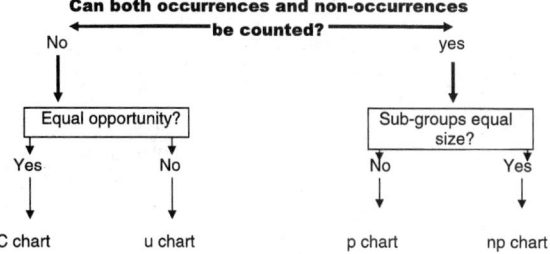

Figure 6-5 Discrete data.

data, frequency of the event being monitored, and stability of the denominator (sample) are used to determine which type of control chart is applicable to the situation being studied (Figures 6–4, 6–5; Table 6–2)

Types of SPC Charts

- $\bar{X}$ and R chart (mean and range): These types of charts might be used to measure increased complaints from the emergency department about turnaround times for laboratory reports. Collect three complete blood counts (CBCs)/day for 23 consecutive weekdays (sample size of 3 CBCs is less than 10).

- $\bar{X}$ and s chart (mean and sample standard deviation): These charts are the same as $\bar{X}$ and R but collect 15 CBC/day for 23 consecutive weekdays (sample size of 15 CBCs is greater than 10).

- XmR (Individuals chart): An XmR chart shows daily blood pressure readings on 1 individual patient for 1 month.

- c chart: If a facility wants to reduce the number of patient falls, it might implement a new program followed by 24 months of data collection. Stable census, for example, long-term care with consistent occupancy rates.

- u chart: If a facility wants to reduce the number of patient falls, it might implement a new program followed by 24 months of data collection. Census fluctuates, for example, acute care hospital.

- p chart: A facility wants to use a control chart to plot surgical site infections. In this case, it knows the number of events (infections) and number of nonevents (cases without infections). Because the number of cases is not the same each month, this facility can use a p chart.

- np chart: This chart can be used to follow 10 type and cross-match orders each week (sample size stable) and monitor for appropriate checks and patient identification procedures.

The chart most commonly recommended for tracking healthcare-associated infections with noncategorical data (the events can be counted but the nonevents cannot) is the u chart.[8] However, there is new debate on that issue and the alternative may be a XmR chart.[9] Until more studies are conducted to verify this finding, a u chart remains the accepted choice.

When creating control charts using continuous data, the number of "subgroups" also needs to be deter-

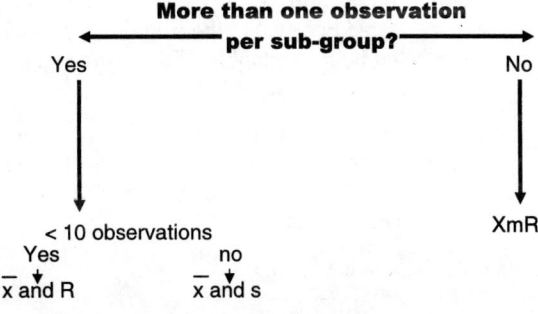

Figure 6-4 Continuous data.

Table 6-2. Selection of a Control Chart Based on the Data

Chart		
p Chart	Discrete	Proportion of defects (e.g., surgical site infections – healthcare-associated infections if using number of admissions or discharges as the denominator)
np Chart	Discrete	Number of defects when sample is stable (e.g., from a sample of 100 stat lab orders each week, how many are not done in the prescribed time?)
c Chart	Discrete	Infrequent event in a sample size (e.g., number of CNS infections)
u Chart	Discrete	Infrequent event; sample size is variable (healthcare-associated infections using patient days as the denominator – Rate of ventilator-associated pneumonia when using number of ventilator days as the denominator).

Copyright © 2005, Association for Professionals in Infection Control and Epidemiology, Inc.

mined. A subgroup represents a sample of data selected from continuous measurements of a process. For example,

- Obtaining one CBC per day for 30 days on the same patient for 30 days is one subgroup (*1 patient*)

- Collecting one CBC per day for 30 days on 10 patients is more than one subgroup (*10 patients*)

General Steps in Constructing a Control Chart[1]

1. Collect and enter data into a spreadsheet for analysis.

2. Historical data may be used if it meets the definition selected or developed for the current study or project. If not, a definition must be developed, and data must be collected prospectively.

3. After a sufficient sample is available, depending on the control chart selected, calculate the parameters required to construct the control chart.

Construction of Specific Types of Control Charts

Construction of u Chart

Let's say you have been monitoring ventilator-associated pneumonia (VAP) for the past 15 months (Table 6-3).

Table 6-3. Spreadsheet

Month	No. VAP	No. vent days
Jan	1	307
Feb	2	247
Mar	0	266
Apr	1	258
May	0	273
Jun	0	265
Jul	2	229
Aug	1	218
Sep	0	208
Oct	2	267
Nov	1	278
Dec	5	264
Jan	1	304
Feb	2	270
Mar	1	305
Apr	1	298

- Calculate the (rate) of defects by subgroup (e.g., monthly) by dividing a number of VAP by the number of ventilator days (within the same time period) and multiplying by a constant (k). For a rate, multiply by 1000.

- Calculate the $\bar{u}$ mean of all the subgroups (months) by dividing the total number of infections in the data set by the total number of patient days (within the same time period).

- Calculate $\sigma = \dfrac{\sqrt{\bar{u}}}{\bar{\bar{X}}}$

- Calculate the upper and lower control limits: the upper control limits are $\bar{u} + 3\sigma$ $\bar{u} + 2\sigma$ $\bar{u} + 1\sigma$. Lower control limits are $\bar{u} - 1\sigma$ $\bar{u} - 2\sigma$ $\bar{u} - 3\sigma$.

- To create the chart, select the columns containing the VAP rate, $\bar{u}$, and all 6 upper and lower control limits, and create a line chart. Customize the chart to represent zones of control limits, $\bar{u}$ bar, and infection rates and add titles (Figure 6–6).

- It is suggested that you create a chart with months included beyond the study periods. This will eliminate the need to construct a new chart each month (Table 6–4). Note. As each new month's data are added to the spreadsheet, remember to add the new cell numbers (column and row) to the "number of infections" and "number of procedures." This will recalculate the $\bar{u}$ bar (average) and make the necessary adjustments to the data.

Construction of a p Chart

Let's say, for example, for the past 16 months, you have been collecting data on sternal wound infections among patients undergoing coronary artery bypass surgery.

- Collect the data on both numerators (defects/infections) and denominators (sample size/number of procedures).

- Calculate the rate of defects (surgical site infections) by subgroup (e.g., monthly) by dividing the number of surgical site infections in the data set by the number of procedures (within the same time period) and multiplying by a constant (k). For a percentage, multiply by 100.

- Calculate the $\bar{p}$ mean rate of all subgroups (months) by dividing the total number of infections by the total number of procedures and multiplying by 100 (if calculated as a percentage).

- Subtract the $\bar{p}$ value from 1.

- Calculate $\sigma = \sqrt{\dfrac{\bar{p}(1 - \bar{p})}{n}}$. If $1 - \bar{p}$ has a negative value, the absolute value must be used. Use the

APIC Text of Infection Control and Epidemiology

Copyright © 2005, Association for Professionals in Infection Control and Epidemiology, Inc.

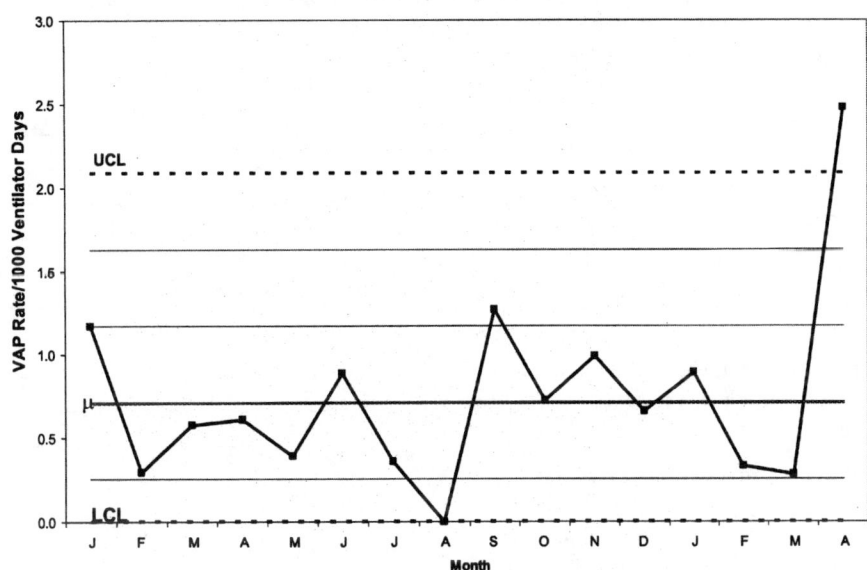

Figure 6-6 Ventilator-associated pneumonia control chart (U chart).

Table 6-4. Ventilator-Associated Pneumonia Data

Month	No. VAP	No. vent days	VAP rate/1000 vent days	ū	σ	3	2	1	1	2	3
Jan	1	307	3.3	4.7	3.3	14.47	11.2	8.0	1.4	0	0
Feb	2	247	8.1	4.7	5.7	14.47	11.2	8.0	1.4	0	0
Mar	0	266	0.0	4.7	0.0	14.47	11.2	8.0	1.4	0	0
Apr	1	258	3.9	4.7	3.9	14.47	11.2	8.0	1.4	0	0
May	0	273	0.0	4.7	0.0	14.47	11.2	8.0	1.4	0	0
Jun	0	265	0.0	4.7	0.0	14.47	11.2	8.0	1.4	0	0
Jul	2	229	8.7	4.7	6.2	14.47	11.2	8.0	1.4	0	0
Aug	1	218	4.6	4.7	4.6	14.47	11.2	8.0	1.4	0	0
Sep	0	208	0.0	4.7	0.0	14.47	11.2	8.0	1.4	0	0
Oct	2	267	7.5	4.7	5.3	14.47	11.2	8.0	1.4	0	0
Nov	1	278	3.6	4.7	3.6	14.47	11.2	8.0	1.4	0	0
Dec	5	264	18.9	4.7	8.5	14.47	11.2	8.0	1.4	0	0
Jan	1	304	3.3	4.7	3.3	14.47	11.2	8.0	1.4	0	0
Feb	2	270	7.4	4.7	5.2	14.47	11.2	8.0	1.4	0	0
Mar	1	305	3.3	4.7	3.3	14.47	11.2	8.0	1.4	0	0
Apr	1	298	3.4	4.7	3.4	14.47	11.2	8.0	1.4	0	0
May				4.7		14.47	11.2	8.0	1.4	0	0
Jun				4.7		14.47	11.2	8.0	1.4	0	0
Jul				4.7		14.47	11.2	8.0	1.4	0	0
Aug				4.7		14.47	11.2	8.0	1.4	0	0
Sep				4.7		14.47	11.2	8.0	1.4	0	0
Oct				4.7		14.47	11.2	8.0	1.4	0	0
Nov				4.7		14.47	11.2	8.0	1.4	0	0
Dec				4.7		14.47	11.2	8.0	1.4	0	0

Copyright © 2005, Association for Professionals in Infection Control and Epidemiology, Inc.

```
=SQRT(#CASES*(ABSOLUTE( 1-P BAR)/ P BAR *100))
=SQRT (10881*(ABS(-0.4)/1.4*100))
```

Figure 6–7 Converting a negative value into an "absolute" value.

spreadsheet's functionality to convert a negative to an "absolute" (Figure 6–7).

- Calculate the control limits: $p \pm 3 \times \sigma$ (Table 6–5).

- To create the chart, select the columns that contain the infection rate, p, and upper and lower control limits and create a line chart. Customize the chart to represent zones of control limits, $\bar{p}$, and infection rates and add titles.

- It is suggested that you create a chart with months included beyond the study periods. This will eliminate the need to construct a new chart each month (Figure 6–8). Note. As each new month's data are added to the spreadsheet, remember to add the new cell numbers (column and row) to the "number of

Table 6-6. Spreadsheet

	#inf	#cases
Jan	12	660
Feb	7	632
Mar	8	651
Apr	8	601
May	11	704
Jun	8	699
Jul	8	632
Aug	7	630
Sep	6	621
Oct	11	675
Nov	11	616
Dec	5	605
Jan	11	658
Feb	11	578
Mar	10	664
Apr	12	603
May	5	652

infections" and "number of procedures." Table 6–6). This will recalculate the p bar (average) and make the necessary adjustments to the data.

Interpretation of Control Charts to Identify Special Cause

Not only data points are examined to determine whether they are within the UCL and LCL; trends in data are considered as well. Process is defined as "out of control" if 1 of the following occurs:

- One data point is above the UCL or below the LCL

- Two of three consecutive points are in zone A or beyond (>2 SDs but <3 SDs) on oneside of the mean

- Four of five consecutive points are in zone B (>1 SD but <2 SDs) on one side of the mean

- Seven consecutive points are in zone C or beyond on side of the mean

- Six or more points are in a row steadily increasing or decreasing (if you have 20 or fewer data points) and seven or more points if you have 21 or more data points

- Fourteen consecutive points alternate up or down (forming a saw tooth pattern)

- Fifteen consecutive points are in zone C (1 SD) above or below the mean

Table 6-5. P Chart

	No. inf	No. cases	No. inf	$\bar{p}$	UCL	LCL
Jan	12	660	1.8	1.4	1.6	1.2
Feb	7	632	1.1	1.4	1.6	1.2
Mar	8	651	1.2	1.4	1.6	1.2
Apr	8	601	1.3	1.4	1.6	1.2
May	11	704	1.6	1.4	1.6	1.2
Jun	8	699	1.1	1.4	1.6	1.2
Jul	8	632	1.3	1.4	1.6	1.2
Aug	7	630	1.1	1.4	1.6	1.2
Sep	6	621	1.0	1.4	1.6	1.2
Oct	11	675	1.6	1.4	1.6	1.2
Nov	11	616	1.8	1.4	1.6	1.2
Dec	5	605	0.8	1.4	1.6	1.2
Jan	11	658	1.7	1.4	1.6	1.2
Feb	11	578	1.9	1.4	1.6	1.2
Mar	10	664	1.5	1.4	1.6	1.2
Apr	12	603	2.0	1.4	1.6	1.2
May	5	652	0.8	1.4	1.6	1.2
Jun				1.4	1.6	1.2
Jul				1.4	1.6	1.2
Aug				1.4	1.6	1.2
Sep				1.4	1.6	1.2
Oct				1.4	1.6	1.2
Nov				1.4	1.6	1.2
Dec				1.4	1.6	1.2

APIC Text of Infection Control and Epidemiology

Copyright © 2005, Association for Professionals in Infection Control and Epidemiology, Inc.

SURGICAL SITE INFECTIONS AMONG PATIENTS UNDERGOING CORNARY ARTERY BYPASS SUGERY
JANUARY 1, 2002–MAY 31, 2003

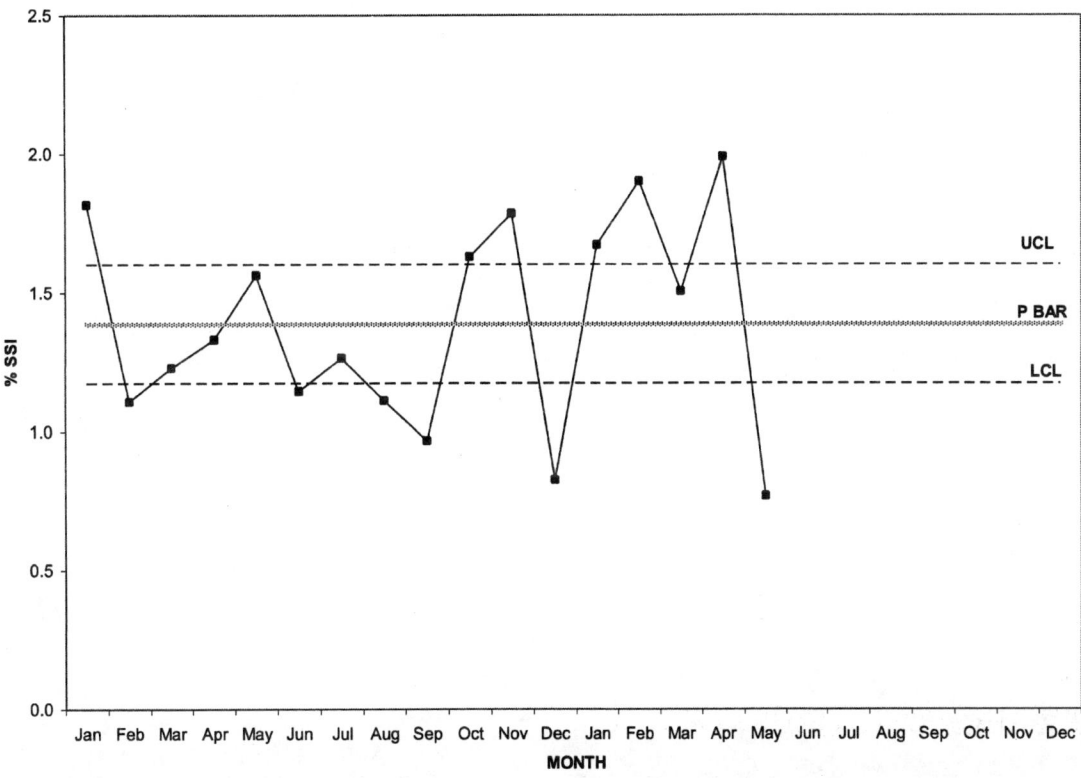

Figure 6–8 Surgical site infection control chart (P chart).

Some healthcare providers have expressed concern that 3 SDs as a "threshold" for action may not be sufficiently sensitive in a clinical situation. When employing SPC in infection control, users should consider the specific circumstances and may select a more conservative "threshold" (e.g., 2 SDs). However, users should also consider that experts in SPC would warn that interference with a system using too narrow a threshold is consider "tampering" and overcontrol of a system.

IV. SUMMARY AND CONCLUSIONS

The need to ensure that decisions are made using the best information available requires that the ICP have a firm understanding of the basics involved in statistical process control. This means the ability to establish a quality and performance monitoring process that enables the users to quickly identify variations in practice or outcomes and determine if and when interventions need to be made as well as the impact of those interventions.

REFERENCES AND CITATIONS

1. Sloan D: *How to lower health care costs by improving health care quality,* Milwaukee, Wis, 1994, American Society for Quality Control, Quality Press.
2. Ishikawa K: *Guide to quality control,* Tokyo, 1971, Asian Productivity Organization.
3. Berwick D, Godffey AB, Roessner J: *Curing healthcare,* San Francisco, 1990, Jossey-Bass.
4. Joint Commission on Accreditation of Healthcare Organizations: *Framework for improving performance,* Oakbrook Terrace, Ill, 1994, JCAHO.
5. Classen DC, Evans RS, Pestotnik SL, et al: The timing of prophylactic administration of antibiotics and the risk of surgical-wound infection, *N Engl J Med* 326(5):281–286, 1992.
6. Berger RW, Hart TH: *Statistical process control: a guide for implementation,* New York, 1986, Marcel Dekker, ASQC Press.
7. Brown SC, Coombs W: Use of statistics in continuous quality improvement (CQI) initiatives. Course presented at Saline Community Hospital, Saline, Mich, 1993.
8. Sellick JA: The use of statisical process control chart in hospital epidemiology, *Infect Control Hosp Epidemiol* 14(11):649—656, 1993.
9. Garner JS, Jarvis WR, Emori TG, et al: CDC definitions for nosocomial infections, *Am J Infect Control* 16(3):128—140, 1988.
8. Carey RG, Lloyd RC: *Measuring quality improvement in healthcare: a guide to statistical process control applications,* New York, 1995, Quality Resources.
9. Gustafson TL: Practical risk-adjusted quality control charts for infection control, *Am J Infect Control* 28(6):406—414, 2000.

Copyright © 2005, Association for Professionals in Infection Control and Epidemiology, Inc.

Developing and Comparing Infection Rates

Jonathan R. Edwards, MS
Healthcare Outcomes Branch
Division of Healthcare Quality Promotion
Centers for Disease Control and Prevention
Atlanta, Georgia

Teresa C. Horan, MPH, CIC
NNIS Coordinator
Chief, Performance Measurement Section
Healthcare Outcomes Branch
Division of Healthcare Quality Promotion
Centers for Disease Control and Prevention
Atlanta, Georgia

ABSTRACT

Infection control and epidemiology professionals make external and internal comparisons of risk-stratified and risk-adjusted infection rates and ratios. Simple Z-tests can be used to give approximate *p*-values and to determine whether significant differences exist. The ability of infection control professionals to make such comparisons enhances the usefulness of surveillance data and better enables them to focus prevention and control activities to enhance patient safety and improve outcomes.

KEY CONCEPTS

- Comparing surgical site infection (SSI) rates requires that they be appropriately stratified and/or adjusted by risk.

- Risk-stratified and/or risk-adjusted SSI rates account for differences in the distribution of the important risk factors.

- Z-tests can be used to compare risk-stratified and risk-adjusted SSI rates between a hospital and a standard population, a surgeon and a standard population, and one surgeon and another.

- The National Nosocomial Infections Surveillance (NNIS) System is currently the only source of risk-stratified and risk-adjusted nosocomial infection rates in the United States.

I.   BACKGROUND

"How do our facility's surgical site infection (SSI) rates compare with those of others? How have they changed over time?" These are important questions that we must be able to answer with the surveillance data we collect. However, such answers require that the SSI rates we calculate be appropriately stratified and/or adjusted by risk. Such risk-stratified/risk-adjusted rates are those that account for the differences in the distribution of the important risk factors associated with the event's occurrence. Only when we have gathered the necessary data and calculated risk-stratified/risk-adjusted SSI rates can we make interhospital (external) and intrahospital (internal) comparisons.[1,2] This chapter provides examples of the use of Z-tests to compare risk-stratified/risk-adjusted SSI rates between a hospital and a standard population, a surgeon and a standard population, and one surgeon

Copyright © 2005, Association for Professionals in Infection Control and Epidemiology, Inc.

and another. The standard population data used in these examples are those reported from hospitals that participate in the NNIS System. (The data in the examples in this section are unpublished and are for training purposes only. Refer to the latest CDC publication for current NNIS data.) NNIS is currently the only source of risk-stratified/risk-adjusted nosocomial infection rates in the United States. The NNIS surveillance methods, definitions, and rates have been reported elsewhere.[1-7]

II.   METHODS FOR DEVELOPING AND COMPARING INFECTION RATES

The Null Hypothesis

When comparing SSI rates, the hypothesis being tested is that the rates are not different from each other. This is called the null hypothesis. Z-tests can be used to test this null hypothesis and will yield Z statistics. For nosocomial infection rates, we are usually interested in the direction of a difference in the rates (i.e., higher or lower), so we conventionally use one-tailed p-values to quantify the significance of any difference detected. After the Z statistic has been calculated, the p-value can be obtained from a table of the normal probability distribution, which can be found in any basic statistics textbook.

Stratification and Standardization

Stratification and/or standardization methods may need to be used to adjust for differences in patients' risks of acquiring a nosocomial SSI, to account for small numbers of operations performed, or to control for differences in the distributions of operations in the comparison and standard populations. Stratification is the grouping together of patients at similar risk for an event (e.g., acquiring a nosocomial SSI). The examples of risk-stratified rates used in this chapter show SSI data that have been stratified by operative procedure and risk index (i.e., procedure-risk category rates). The standardization method we most often use in nosocomial infection surveillance is indirect standardization. Indirect standardization is a means of risk adjustment in which the raw rate of an event is divided by the average risk of the occurrence of the event. In Examples 2 and 3 we use indirect standardization to calculate the standardized infection ratio (SIR). As shown there, the SIR is calculated by dividing the SSI rate of a surgeon by the SSI rate of a standard population or, equivalently, by dividing the observed number of SSIs by the expected number of SSIs. The rate of the standard population represents the average risk of the occurrence of SSIs.

Sample Size Considerations

When comparing infection rates, it must be recognized that the size of the denominators are a critical factor in determining the appropriateness of the Z-test and the ability of the test to detect any differences that may exist. The Z-test may be inappropriate if the denominators are too small. Formula 1 requires large denominators (at least 20). The Z-test formulas for comparing SIRs used in Examples 2 and 3 can be used only when the expected number of SSIs is at least 1. Therefore, as a general rule of thumb, do not compare procedure-risk category SSI rates when the number of operations in the denominator of either rate is less than 20. Also, do not use the SIR to perform comparisons when the denominator of the SIR (the expected number of SSIs) is less than 1. If comparison is necessary when denominators are small, other statistical tests must be used (e.g., Fisher's Exact test or a Poisson test).

Formula for Z-test that is used for comparing two procedure-risk category SSI rates

$$Z = \frac{r - R}{\sqrt{P(100 - P)\left(\frac{1}{n} + \frac{1}{N}\right)}}$$
Formula 1

where

r = SSI rate (expressed as a percent, i.e., number of SSIs per 100 operations)

n = number of operations in SSI rate (i.e., the denominator)

R = SSI rate of a standard population (expressed as a percent; i.e., number of SSIs per 100 operations)

N = number of operations in the SSI rate of the standard population (i.e., the denominator)

P = pooled rate, obtained from the two rates being compared by using Formula 2 below:

$$P = \frac{i + I}{n + N} \times 100$$
Formula 2

where

i = number of SSIs detected (i.e., the numerator of the SSI rate)

I = number of SSIs in the standard population (i.e., the numerator of the SSI rate of the standard population).

Formulas 1 and 2 are used in Example 1, which compares procedure-risk category SSI rates for certain operative procedures for Hospital A to corresponding aggregated NNIS rates (i.e., the standard population's rates).

Copyright © 2005, Association for Professionals in Infection Control and Epidemiology, Inc.

Z-Test and the Standard Normal Curve

Z statistics are normally distributed (i.e., if we plotted the Z statistics from many different comparisons along a horizontal and vertical axis, their distribution would be more or less a bell-shaped curve). To determine the probability of the occurrence of an event from this type of curve, the area under the curve must be defined as 1 or 100%. Such a curve is called a standard normal curve, or Z-curve, and has a mean of 0 and standard deviation of 1 (Fig. 7–1).[8] When we use a Z-test for comparing SSI rates, the area under the curve to the right of the Z statistic (if it is positive) or to the left (if it is negative) represents the probability of obtaining a difference in rates as large as that observed, or larger if the null hypothesis is true (one-tailed Z-test). If that probability is 5% or lower, we generally reject the null hypothesis and state that the rates we are comparing are significantly different (p \H 0.05). The value of the Z statistic where this 5% probability occurs is Z = 1.645 or Z = -1.645, or approximately Z = ±1.6 (see Fig. 7–1).

Interpretation of Z > 1.6

When Z > 1.6, the SSI rate is significantly *higher* than that of the standard population. This may mean that there is an infection control problem that needs further investigation.

Interpretation of Z < -1.6

When Z < -1.6, the SSI rate is significantly *lower* than that of the standard population. If case-finding has been adequate, there is evidence that rate is better than that of the standard population.

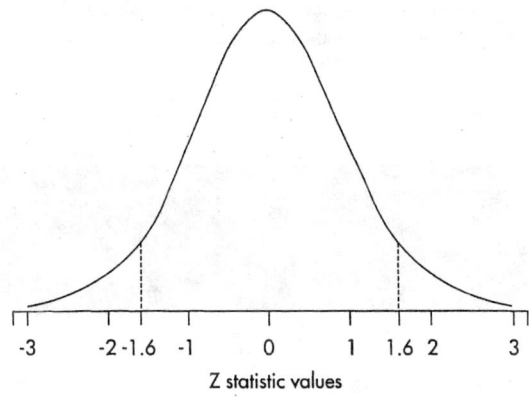

Figure 7–1 Standard normal curve with mean of 0 and standard deviation of 1. The critical values -1.6 and 1.6 correspond to a **p** value of 0.05.

Interpretation of Z Between -1.6 and 1.6

When Z is between -1.6 and 1.6, the SSI rate is *not* significantly different from that of the standard population. Depending on the rates that were compared and the denominator of these rates, there still could be an infection control problem. Example 3 illustrates this concept.

Examples of Risk-Stratified Rate Comparisons Using a Z-test

Example 1: Comparing Procedure-Risk Category Rates and Testing for a Significant Difference

Suppose we want to compare hospital A's procedure-risk category SSI rates to that of a standard population (i.e., an external comparison). Using the data in Table 7–1, we'll compare Hospital A's risk category SSI rates for coronary artery bypass graft (CABG) and cardiac surgery (CARD) to the corresponding NNIS rates. For each procedure-risk category, we can use Formula 1 of the Z-test to compare the rates and obtain a Z statistic.

Example 1a: CABG   Formula 1

$$Z = \frac{r - R}{\sqrt{P(100 - P)\left(\frac{1}{n} + \frac{1}{N}\right)}}$$

$$= \frac{5 - 6.34}{\sqrt{6.33(100 - 6.33)\left(\frac{1}{20} + \frac{1}{2475}\right)}} = -0.22$$

r = 5

n = 20

R = 6.34

N = 2475

P = 6.33 (obtained using Formula 2 below):

$$P = \frac{i + I}{n + N} \times 100 = \frac{1 + 157}{20 + 2475} \times 100 = 6.33$$

Since Z is between -1.6 and 1.6, the risk category SSI rate for Hospital A for CABG is *not significantly different* from the NNIS rate. From a table of normal probability distribution, we can find the *p* value that corresponds with the value of the Z statistic. In this example, p = 0.41.

Example 1b: CARD   Formula 1

$$P = \frac{i + I}{n + N} \times 100 = \frac{1 + 157}{20 + 2475} \times 100 = 6.33$$

Copyright © 2005, Association for Professionals in Infection Control and Epidemiology, Inc.

Table 7-1. Data for Example 1

Risk index category	Operative procedure	NNIS* No. of SSIs (I)	No. of operations (N)	Rate (%) (R)	No. of SSIs (i)	Hospital A No. of operations (n)	Rate (%) (r)
2,3	CABG	157	2475	6.34	1	20	5.00
2	CARD	21	362	5.80	8	59	13.56

* Unpublished data; for training purposes only. Refer to latest CDC publication for current NNIS data.
CABG, coronary artery bypass graft; *CARD*, cardiac surgery; NNIS, National Nosocomial Infections Surveillance; SSI, Surgical site infection

$r = 13.56$

$n = 59$

$R = 5.8$

$N = 362$

$P = 6.89$ (obtained using Formula 2):

$$P = \frac{8+21}{59+362} \times 100 = 6.89 \qquad \text{Formula 2}$$

Because $Z > 1.6$, the risk category SSI rate for Hospital A for CARD is *significantly higher* ($p = 0.01$) than the NNIS rate and warrants further investigation.

Note 1: Using Z-test Formula 1, external and internal comparisons of risk-adjusted ratios obtained from nosocomial infection surveillance can be made. For example, you can make an external comparison of Intensive Care Unit (ICU)-specific device utilization ratios to NNIS ratios (e.g., ventilator use in the surgical ICU to NNIS) or an internal comparison of such ICU ratios from one time period to another (e.g., last year's ventilator use compared to that of this year for the surgical ICU).

Note 2: A Fisher's exact test can be performed easily by using EpiInfo 6 software. First select Programs, then select EPITABLE calculator, then select Probability, then Fisher's Exact Test. Enter the observed frequencies into the cells of the 2x2 table as follows:

Observed	No. w/ SSI	No. w/o SSI	No. of Operations
Hospital	i	n – i	n
NNIS	I	N – I	N

Press the Enter key to calculate. The one- and two-tailed *p*-values will be displayed; report the one-tailed value.

Example 2: Calculating a Standardized Infection Ratio by Pooling Data Across Procedure-Specific Risk Categories and Testing for a Significant Difference

In this example, we want to make an external comparison of a surgeon's SSI experience following a specific operative procedure to that of a standard population. Using the data in Table 7–2, we'll compare Dr. X's cholecystectomy (CHOL) SSI experience to that of NNIS.

As we did in Example 1, a comparison of Dr. X's SSI rates with those of NNIS can be performed for risk index categories 0 and 1 (e.g., for risk category 0, Dr. X's rate of 5% can be compared with the NNIS rate of 1.1%). We cannot use Formula 1 to compare the 2,3 risk category because Dr. X only performed 10 cholecystectomies. Therefore, we might want to compare his summary experience across all risk categories. However, we cannot compare Dr. X's summary

Table 7-2. Data for Example 2

Risk index category	NNIS* Observed number of SSIs	Number of operations (N)	Operations (%)	Rate** (R)	Dr. X Observed number of SSIs	Number of operations (n)	Operations (%)	Rate** (r)
0	41	3770	54	1.1	1	20	40	5.0
1	51	2546	36	2.0	2	20	40	10.0
2,3	37	682	10	5.4	3	10	20	30.0
Total	129	6998	100	1.9	6	50	100	12.0

* Unpublished data; for training purposes only. Refer to latest CDC publication for current NNIS data.
** Per 100 operations.
NNIS, National Nosocomial Infections Surveillance; SSI, Surgical site infection.

APIC Text of Infection Control and Epidemiology

Copyright © 2005, Association for Professionals in Infection Control and Epidemiology, Inc.

CHOL SSI rate (12%) with that of NNIS (1.9%) because of the difference between the distribution of Dr. X's operations among the risk categories (40%, 40%, and 20%) and the distribution of those of NNIS (54%, 36%, and 10%). Note that 20% of Dr. X's operations were in risk index category 2,3 versus only 10% of those of NNIS. Thus, intuitively, we would expect the surgeon's summary rate to be higher than that of NNIS. To validly make a comparison using a single summary measure of Dr. X's SSI experience, we must control for the difference in distribution of the operations between the two groups. One method is to calculate the SIR using steps 1 and 2 that follow.

The SIR is an example of indirect standardization, in which the observed rate ("raw rate") is divided by the expected rate ("average risk of the occurrence of the event"). Or, equivalently, the observed number of SSIs is divided by the expected number of SSIs. The expected rate or expected number of SSIs is the number that would be expected if the surgeon's experience had been the same as that of the standard population. In step 1, using Formula 3, we calculate the expected number of SSIs (E) by using risk category–specific rates from the standard population (R) and the number of operations (n) in each risk category performed by a surgeon, a surgical subspecialty service, or a hospital. In step 2, using Formula 4, we divide the observed number of SSIs (O) by the expected number of SSIs (E) to get the SIR. To test for a significant difference, we use a Z-test to compare the surgeon's SIR to the nominal value of 1 (i.e., where O = E in the standard population).

Step 1: Use Formula 3 to calculate the expected number of SSIs for Dr. X.

$$E = \Sigma\,(R \times n)\,/\,100 \qquad \text{Formula 3}$$

In this example, to calculate the expected number of SSIs for Dr. X (E_x), multiply the NNIS risk category–specific CHOL SSI rate (R) times the number of Dr. X's operations in that risk category (n) and sum across all risk categories.

$$E_x = \frac{[(1.1 \times 20) + (2.0 \times 20) + (5.4 \times 10)]}{100} = 1.16$$

Step 2: Use Formula 4 to calculate the SIR for Dr. X.

$$SIR = \frac{\text{Observed number of SSIs}}{\text{Expected number of SSIs}} = \frac{O_x}{E_x} \qquad \text{Formula 4}$$

$O_x = 6$

$E_x = 1.16$

$$SIR \text{ for Dr. X} = SIR_x = \frac{6}{1.16} = 5.2$$

The interpretation of this value of the SIR is that Dr. X had 5.2 times as many SSIs as predicted by the rates

of the standard population (NNIS). It represents a 420% increase over the nominal value of 1. Note, however, that Dr. X performed a total of only 50 cholecystectomies. We must ascertain that this result was not due to chance. To do this, we must perform another Z-test and calculate a *p*-value. In Step 3, we answer the question "Is Dr. X's SIR significantly higher than 1?."

Step 3: Use Z-test Formula 5 to compare the SIR of Dr. X against 1.

$$Z = 2(\sqrt{SIR_x} - 1)(\sqrt{E_x}) \qquad \text{Formula 5}$$

Comparing the SIR of Dr. X against 1 using Formula 5 is equivalent to comparing the observed number of SSIs of Dr. X (O_x) against the expected number of SSIs of Dr. X (E_x) using Formula 6. Either formula can be used.

$$Z = 2(\sqrt{O_x} - \sqrt{E_x}) \qquad \text{Formula 6}$$

Use of both formulas is shown, where $SIR_x = 5.2$, $O_x = 6$, and $E_x = 1.16$:

$$Z = 2(\sqrt{SIR_x} - 1)(\sqrt{E_x}) \qquad \text{Formula 5}$$
$$Z = 2(\sqrt{5.2} - 1)(\sqrt{1.16}) = 2.76$$

$$Z = 2(\sqrt{O_x} - \sqrt{E_x}) \qquad \text{Formula 6}$$
$$Z = 2(\sqrt{6} - \sqrt{1.16}) = 2.76$$

Because $Z > 1.6$, Dr. X's SIR for CHOL is *significantly higher* ($p = 0.003$) than 1 and warrants further investigation.

Note: The numerator of an SIR, the observed number of SSIs, has an approximate Poisson distribution. When the denominator of the SIR, the expected number of SSIs, is 1 or more, the Z-test of Formulas 5 or 6 and the Z-test of Formula 7 in the next example can be used as good approximations to more accurate statistical tests.[9] However, if the expected number of SSIs is less than 1, the approximation is poor, and misleading results could be obtained.

A Poisson test can be performed easily by using EpiInfo 6 software. First select Programs, then select EPITABLE calculator, then select Probability, then Poisson. Enter the value of O for the "observed number of events" and the value of E for the "expected number of events." The *p*-value is displayed as the "probability that the number of events found is" $\geq O$ (when $O > E$) or $\geq O$ (when $O < E$).

Copyright © 2005, Association for Professionals in Infection Control and Epidemiology, Inc.

Table 7-3. Data for Example 3

	Operation-risk index category	Observed no. of SSIs (0)	No. of operations (n)	Rate" (r)	NNIS rate*" (R)	Expected no. of SSIs (E)
Dr. X	FUS: 0	0	239	0	0.75	1.79
	FUS: 1,2	2	106	1.9	2.62	2.78
	FX: 0,1	3	38	7.9	1.45	0.55
	FX: 2,3	1	5	20.0	3.61	0.18
Total		$0_x = 6$	388	1.5	–	$E_x = 5.30$
Dr. Y	PROS: 0	2	56	3.6	1.11	0.62
	PROS: 1	1	19	5.3	2.32	0.44
	PROS: 2,3	0	2	0	5.43	0.11
	FX: 0,1	2	26	7.7	1.45	0.38
	FX: 2,3	1	15	6.7	3.61	0.54
						$E_y = 2.09$
Total		$0_Y = 6$	118	5.1	–	

* Unpublished data; for training purposes only. Refer to latest CDC publication for current NNIS data.
" Per 100 operations.
FUS, spinal fusion/lamineclomy; *FX*, open reduction of fracture; *PROS*, Joint prosthesis.

Example 3: Calculating Two SIRs (e.g., the SIRs of Two Surgeons) and Testing for a Significant Difference

We might want to make an internal comparison of the SSI experience of two surgeons, even when they did not do the same exact procedures. In this example, we'll use the data in Table 7–3 to compare the experience of the two orthopedic surgeons. Both of them performed open reduction of fracture procedures, but Dr. X also did spinal fusions and laminectomies, whereas Dr. Y did joint prosthesis procedures. Six SSIs occurred among each of the surgeon's patients, but Dr. Y's rate was 5.1% versus Dr. X's rate of 1.5%. We would like to determine whether this difference in SSI experience is statistically significant. Just as in Example 2, we need to calculate the SIR for each surgeon and then compare the SIRs to each other.

Step 1: Use Formula 3 to calculate the expected number of SSIs for each surgeon (E_X, E_Y).

$$E = S (R \times n)/100 \quad \text{Formula 3}$$

$$E_x = \frac{[(0.75 \times 239) + (2.62 \times 106) + (1.45 \times 38) + (3.61 \times 5)]}{100}$$

$$= \frac{179 + 278 + 55 + 18}{100} = 5.30$$

$$E_y = \frac{[(1.11 \times 56) + (2.32 \times 19) + (5.43 \times 2) + (1.45 \times 26) + (3.61 \times 15)]}{100}$$

$$= \frac{62 + 44 + 11 + 38 + 54}{100} = 2.09$$

Step 2: Use Formula 4 to calculate the SIR for each surgeon (SIR_x, SIR_y).

$$SIR = \frac{\text{Observed number of SSIs}}{\text{Expected number of SSIs}} = \frac{0}{E} \quad \text{Formula 4}$$

$$SIR_x = \frac{6}{5.30} = 1.13$$

$$SIR_y = \frac{6}{2.09} = 2.87$$

Step 3: Use the Z-test in Formula 7 or a binomial test to compare the SIRs.

$$Z = \frac{2(\sqrt{SIR_y} - \sqrt{SIR_x})}{\sqrt{\frac{1}{E_y} + \frac{1}{E_y}}} \quad \text{Formula 7}$$

$SIR_x = 1.13$
$SIR_y = 2.87$
$E_x = 5.30$
$E_y = 2.09$

$$Z = \frac{2(\sqrt{2.87} - \sqrt{1.13})}{\sqrt{\frac{1}{2.09} + \frac{1}{5.30}}} = 1.54$$

Because Z is very close to 1.6, the *p*-value is 0.06. This borderline *p*-value suggests, and another look at the data in Table 7–3 and the SIRs for each surgeon reinforces, that we might still suspect that Dr. Y could have a problem. His SIR is 187% higher than the nominal value of 1, and he had six SSIs when he should have had only about two, if his experience had been like that of the standard population. At this point, it is appropriate to perform an external comparison using Formula 5. In other words, we'll compare Dr.

APIC Text of Infection Control and Epidemiology

Copyright © 2005, Association for Professionals in Infection Control and Epidemiology, Inc.

Y's SIR to that of the standard population (i.e., the nominal value of 1).

$$Z = 2(\sqrt{SIR_y} - 1)(\sqrt{E_y})$$ Formula 5

$SIR_y = 2.87$

$E_y = 2.09$

$$Z = 2(\sqrt{2.87} - 1)(\sqrt{2.09}) = 2.02$$

Now we can see that Dr. Y's SIR is *significantly higher* than 1 ($p = 0.02$) and supports our position to further investigate.

Note: An exact *p*-value can be obtained by performing a binomial test using the EpiInfo 6 software. First select Programs, then select EPITABLE calculator, then select Probability, then Binomial. Enter O_Y for the "numerator," $O_X + O_Y$ for the "total observations," and

$$\frac{E_y}{E_x + E_y} \times 100$$

for the "expected percentage." The p-value is then displayed as the "Probability that the # of cases" (i.e., "events") $\geq O_Y$.

III. SUMMARY AND CONCLUSIONS

At times, we want to know how our nosocomial infection experience compares to that of others or how it has changed over time within our institution. Such external and internal comparisons may be done only when risk-stratified and/or risk-adjusted rates are available. Simple Z-tests can be used to give approximate *p*-values and determine whether significant differences exist. Example 1 used Z-test Formula 1 to illustrate how to perform an external comparison of risk-stratified SSI rates. It was noted that this formula of the Z-test also can be used to compare risk-adjusted ratios, such as ICU-specific device utilization ratios.

Sometimes we want or need to compare the summary experience of one or more surgeons. However, such a comparison can be difficult because a small number of procedures were performed in some or all of the procedure-risk categories, because the distribution of the patients in the procedure-risk categories is not the same in the two groups being compared, or because the procedures themselves are not identical. The first two problems were apparent in Example 2, and all three were evident in Example 3. To validly compare the summary experience of the surgeons in each of these examples, we used indirect standardization and calculated SIRs. Then we tested for a significant difference by using either Z-test Formula 5 or 6 for the external comparison to a standard population in

Example 2, and by using Formula 7 for the internal comparison of the two surgeons in Example 3.

It was noted that these formulations of the Z-test could only be used when the expected number of SSIs was 1 or more. It was also noted that exact *p*-values could be obtained by using a Fisher's exact test (Example 1), a Poisson test (Example 2), or a binomial test (Example 3).

The ability of the infection control epidemiology professional to make external and internal comparisons of risk-stratified/risk-adjusted infection rates and ratios can greatly enhance the usefulness of surveillance data. Full use of the data will help focus prevention and control efforts, as well as enhance the quality, of patient care in the hospital.

IV. FUTURE TRENDS/RESEARCH

As the patient safety agenda continues to gain momentum, increased attention is being placed on reduction of negative patient outcomes. Public reporting of results, including SSI, and tying performance to payment will continue to provide motivation to both the healthcare facilities as well as the individual clinician. Providing credible feedback using well-designed processes will enhance both the acceptance of results as well as compliance with improvement initiatives.

V. INTERNATIONAL PERSPECTIVES

Although NNIS is currently the only source of risk-stratified/risk-adjusted nosocomial infection rates in the United States, other countries have developed and are developing similar processes. Recognizing the ties that exist between countries, sharing of information and continued use of well-designed processes will promote appropriate comparisons and heighten the success opportunities.

REFERENCES

1. Centers for Disease Control and Prevention. Nosocomial infection rates for interhospital comparison: limitations and possible solutions. *Infect Control Hosp Epidemiol* 12:609–621, 1991.
2. Culver DH, Horan TC, Gaynes RP, et al. Surgical wound infection rates by wound class, operative procedure, and patient risk index. *Am J Med* 91(Suppl 3B):152S–157S, 1991.
3. Emori TG, Culver DH, Horan TC, et al. National nosocomial infections surveillance system (NNIS): description of surveillance methods. *Am J Infect Control* 19:19–35, 1991.
4. Gaynes R, Culver DH, Banerjee S, et al. Meaningful interhospital comparisons of infection rates in intensive care units. *Am J Infect Control* 21:43–44, 1993.
5. Garner JS, Jarvis WR, Emori TG, et al. CDC definitions for nosocomial infections, 1988. *Am J Infect Control* 16:128–140, 1988.
6. Horan TC, Gaynes RP, Martone WJ, et al. CDC definitions of nosocomial surgical site infections, 1992: a modification of CDC definitions of surgical wound infections. *Infect Control Hosp Epidemiol* 13:606–608, 1992.

Copyright © 2005, Association for Professionals in Infection Control and Epidemiology, Inc.

7. Gaynes RP, Horan TC. Surveillance of nosocomial infections. In Mayhall CG, ed. *Hospital Epidemiology and Infection Control.* Baltimore, MD: Williams & Wilkins, 1996:1017–1031, Appendix A-1–Appendix C-1.
8. Rimm AA, Hartz AJ, Kalbfleisch JH, et al. *Basic Biostatistics in Medicine and Epidemiology,* Norwalk, CT: Appleton-Century-Crofts, 1980.
9. Centers for Disease Control and Prevention: NNIS IDEAS user's guide. Unpublished, 1994:121.

SUPPLEMENTAL RESOURCES

Gaynes RP, Culver DH, Horan TC, et al. Surgical site infection (SSI) rates in the United States, 1992–98: the NNIS basic SSI risk index. *Clin Infect Dis* 2001.

http://www.cdc.gov/ncidod/hip/surveill/NNIS.htm

Copyright © 2005, Association for Professionals in Infection Control and Epidemiology, Inc.

Quality Concepts

Marlyn T. Conti, RN, BSN, CPHQ
Quality Consultant, Intermountain Health Care
Salt Lake City, Utah

Dallin Poulsen, MBA./HSA
Data Manager, Statistician, Intermountain
Health Care
Salt Lake City, Utah

ABSTRACT

There are many approaches to quality improvement, some of which have been around for a long time and others of which are newly emerging. A new infection control professional (ICP) may be confused by all the approaches to quality improvement in the literature. The authors will describe how continuous quality improvement (CQI), total quality management (TQM), performance improvement (PI) and quality management (QM) concepts can all be linked using a simple model of planning, measurement, and improvement (PMI) to achieve the desired outcomes for an infection control program. The concepts that are key to defining quality capitalize on many of the attributes of organizational development, the scientific process, the discipline of epidemiology, and the methodology of statistical process control. An integrated multidisciplinary approach—use of teams, tools, and methodologies—such as described in this chapter can help ICPs find the best fit for their program that will ensure good patient outcomes.

KEY CONCEPTS

- Quality

- Planning

- Deming's 14 Key Concepts

- Focus on customers, mission, vision, values

- Focus on improvement

- Measurement

- Understanding variation

- Improvement teams

- Methods and tools

- Processes

I.   BACKGROUND

Since the end of World War II, the work of W. Edwards Deming, his disciples, and his 14 Key Concepts regarding quality have greatly influenced U.S. industries and, more recently, healthcare.[1, 2,3] The planning, measurement, and improvement (PMI) model incorporates many of these models and recommended approaches. The planning concepts, which follow Deming's advice, focus on meeting

Copyright © 2005, Association for Professionals in Infection Control and Epidemiology, Inc.

customers' needs and expectations; on implementing the mission, vision, and values identified by the business; and on achieving measurable outcomes. Planning activities might follow existing models, such as the Shewhart cycle (PDCA), Hoshin planning,[4] General Electric's PICOS, Six Sigma, or the Baldrige approach, and may include planning tools and/or outcome and benchmark data. Cyclical strategic planning activities and a regular evaluation of the plan's effectiveness can focus an organization's efforts to improve quality, both qualitatively and quantitatively.

Measurement requires a good understanding of variation and measurement methodologies to improve processes. Examples of measurement tools include check sheets, run charts, histograms, Pareto charts, and statistical process control charts. The relationship between variation and cost is referred to as *quality waste*.

Improvement, a key methodology, promotes the use of multidisciplinary teams to deploy changes and improvements. A quality-focused culture values the knowledge and skills of its frontline workers. The continuous process of improvement entails a variety of methods and tools, including documentation of the process steps. Finally, in infection control there are examples of departmental or programmatic improvements and of larger-scale healthcare initiatives related to improving outcomes.

II.   BASIC PRINCIPLES

Definitions of Quality

Quality can be defined in many ways by different organizations and industries. Below are some examples. The authors recommend that the ICP choose a definition and approach for the program that has meaning in his or her specific practice setting and stick with it. Quality is:

- Defined by its attributes: effectiveness, efficiency, optimality, acceptability, legitimacy, and equity

- The interrelationships between structure, process, and outcome

- 3. hassle elimination

- The result of planning, measuring (monitoring), and improving (team efforts); improvements in quality are achieved by understanding processes and variation

- The relationship between the use of quality, the scientific approach, and team work[5] (Fig. 8–1)

- Conformance to specifications

- Meeting or exceeding customer expectations 100% of the time

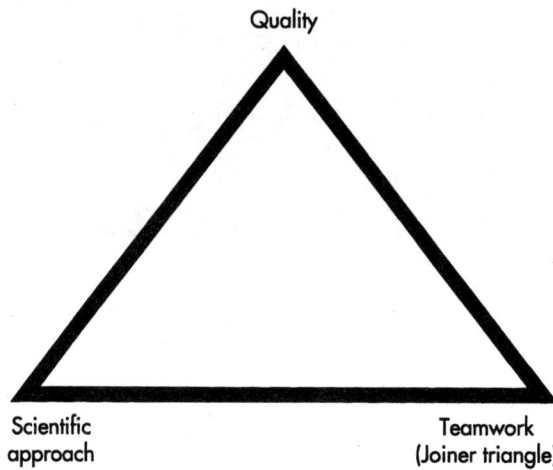

Figure 8–1   Excellent quality depends on scientific methodology and multidisciplinary team effort.

- The degree to which health services for individuals and populations increase the likelihood of desired health outcomes and are consistent with current professional knowledge (Joint Commission on Accreditation of Healthcare Organizations, JCAHO)

An infection control (IC) program whose primary role is surveillance (inspection), rather than "improving outcomes" (reducing healthcare-acquired infection), in general will be attempting to eliminate problems rather than focusing on process improvement. This approach is often perceived as the traditional "sort and shoot" mentality or Tayloristic Management model.[3] Some outcomes focus activities in this type of program might be:

- Surveillance for adverse outcomes or infections rather than conformance to practice standards

- Identifying root causes

- Returning to previously established baseline rates of infection

- Reporting individual physician rates of infection with the hope of identifying and correcting practice patterns associated with undesirable rates

- Maintaining an acceptable average rate of infection

An IC program that is instead focused on improving outcomes/quality, rather than inspection, will attempt to study processes and discover a higher level of performance rather than seeking a return to baseline or a previous level of quality. This program will, in general, attempt to eliminate problems by planning and defining expectations, goals, and desired outcomes; by measuring and collecting performance information; and by changing defective processes. For example, ICPs learn about the process of prescribing and admin-

Copyright © 2005, Association for Professionals in Infection Control and Epidemiology, Inc.

istering antibiotics used prior to surgery, discover a new standard regarding timing and appropriate antibiotic for surgical site, implement the new standard, and substantially reduce postoperative wound infections. (See JCAHO and CMS Patient Safety recommendations.)

III. QUALITY CONCEPTS

CONCEPTS: Deming's 14 Key Concepts Regarding Quality

W. Edward Deming established 14 Key Concepts that can help organizations improve quality and reduce costs. These principles are also referred to as *continuous quality improvement*, *industrial quality control*, or *total quality management*. Incorporation of the 14 concepts into an organization or IC program can provide a structure and foundation for good continuous improvement.[1] The 14 Key Concepts are: (1) create constancy of purpose; (2) do things right the first time; (3) cease dependence on mass inspection; (4) constantly and forever improve the system; (5) remove barriers to pride of workmanship; (6) drive out fear; (7) break down barriers between departments; (8) eliminate slogans, exhortations, and targets; (9) eliminate work standards, quotas, and numerical goals; (10) institute modern methods of leadership; (11) institute training on the job; (12) create a learning environment; (13) do not award business based on price alone; and, finally, (14) everyone must work to accomplish the transformation. Listed below are each of the concepts with a brief and description and some IC examples:

1. Create constancy of purpose.

All IC programs should have clear mission, vision, and goals that are linked to and aligned with those of their organizations. Those documents should be widely shared and understood by all levels of the organization. One possible mission statement is:

> To provide expertise and resources leadership, departments, and medical staff to support the achievement of organizational goals and reduce the risk for infections. This is accomplished through the application of quality improvement initiatives, including data management, process improvement, benchmarking, and team facilitation.

An example goal for a surgical program might be: "to prevent postoperative wound infections." Subsequently, healthcare providers should work together to align improvement, prevention, and educational strategies. A facility might also choose to make compliance with recommended surgical prophylactic antibiotic use and timing one of its corporate-wide patient safety goals and quality process measures.

2. Do things right the first time.

ICPs should teach and monitor compliance with approved and proven patient care practices. For example, ICPs might develop protocols for personnel to use for insertion of indwelling urinary catheters to follow and thereby eliminate variation in practice. By providing the necessary knowledge, skills, and abilities to staff and by monitoring compliance, an ICP can reduce the risk for catheter-associated infections. Other examples might be to use the correct preoperative hand scrub procedure and disinfectant or to properly insert intravenous catheters. Although these practices must continue at some relevant level, efforts to improve key processes and "doing it right the first time" must be a primary focus.

3. Cease dependence on mass inspection.

Mass inspection breeds mistrust and a feeling of being controlled from above. In healthcare, surveillance, reviews, and audits feel like "mass inspection" and tend to focus attention on the few unfortunate events rather than on improving usual practices and the delivery of care. The ICP could move to intermittently inspecting or sampling to allow time for process improvement. One way to approach this is through the use of a simple Pareto analysis of infections data from your institution. The Pareto principle, or 80/20 rule, will lead you to focus on the areas where the most benefit will be derived. Vilfredo Pareto was an Italian economist during the mid-1800s. He discovered that 80% of the land was owned by 20% of the population. He found this percentage to hold true in many areas, including his garden. He observed that 80% of his peas came from 20% of his seeds.[7]

4. Constantly and forever improve the system.

An IC program values research and improvement and works to ensure that resources are in the organization's budget. ICPs should keep abreast of the latest publications, guidelines, and community standards. The expectation that one can launch an improvement project and reach perfection in a short time has led many ICPs to become frustrated. The assumption should be that there is always room for improvement and other, better ways to do what we are doing.

5. Remove barriers to pride of workmanship.

The ICP should work to ensure that staff members involved in any process improvement are rewarded and allowed to celebrate their achievements. Team efforts, successes, and failures should be recognized and rewarded by management and peers in formal and informal ways. Give credit where credit is due. Build and support ownership at the frontline, patient care interface. For example, providing staff members with the time and resources necessary to publish their expe-

Copyright © 2005, Association for Professionals in Infection Control and Epidemiology, Inc.

riences contributes to pride of work. This can be done by holding storyboard fairs, publishing newsletters, displaying poster boards, awarding prizes, and so forth.

6. Drive out fear.

It is important for the ICP to involve frontline healthcare professionals in the collection of data and assist them in the study design and analysis. This level of participation supports accountability and ownership, thereby reducing fear. It gets the ICP out of the inspector or "cop" role. Another way to drive out fear might be to celebrate failure as a lesson learned, not a mistake to be covered up. The ICP might participate in an in-depth analysis or root cause analysis to prevent the process failure from re-occurring.

7. Break down barriers between departments.

When ICPs facilitate the design and implementation of an improvement project, they can encourage multidisciplinary and intradepartmental involvement. Working across department lines on a common process with a focus on the patient or on good outcomes goes a long way to break down barriers between departments. The same can be said for collaboration across organizations, such as among the hospital, suppliers, home health agencies, and long-term-care facilities.

8. Eliminate slogans, exhortations, and targets.

Slogans such as "drown a germ," do little to improve knowledge or change behavior. Signs and posters become invisible after a while if they are not supported by active involvement in process improvement. Satisfaction with an overall 5% rate of healthcare-acquired infection is acceptance of an arbitrary target or threshold. Rates should be shared and understood at all levels of the organization, and improvements should be ongoing.

9. Eliminate work standards, quotas, and numerical goals.

Work schedules that specify the exact number of hours to be spent on a given task, say data collection, limit people's desire to improve performance, say by finding better ways to collect data. Focusing on work quotas limits the ICP's ability to meet and exceed expectations or find a higher level of performance. Additionally, work standards are often arbitrary and may not be indicative of the best performance. If teams are allowed to set their own best performance or outcome standards, they often achieve a higher threshold than management would expect.

10. Institute modern methods of leadership.

The ICP's job description should include broad areas of responsibility, such as coach, teacher, and developer. They should participate, train, and plan with hospital

staff rather than supervise, manage, monitor, or oversee.

11. Institute training on the job.

The expectation is that management supports and provides educational opportunities as part of staff members' daily work and annual performance expectations. If staff members and ICPs are not continually improving their knowledge, skills, and abilities, they will lose ground. ICPs can take advantage of local, relevant in-service programs, journals and publications, conferences, and training in new knowledge, practices, and technologies. ICPs can, in turn, share this new knowledge with other healthcare professionals. Teaching at a nursing school may create a relationship that ensures a more competent labor force in the future.

12. Create a learning environment.

ICPs can promote self-improvement and retraining by acknowledging that all learning opportunities are valuable. When the ICP gains computer skills, attends a conference, acquires new clinical skills, or re-certifies, she or he demonstrates and provides an example of the value of learning. Learning and new skills should be part of the ICP's job expectations and evaluation process. Each team and project should be examined for lessons to be learned. We learn by doing and evaluating.

13. Do not award business based on price alone.

Developing criteria other than price (quality, satisfaction, ease of use) with a medical supply company may ensure an optimal product or service. Study after study proves that high quality will cost less in the long run. It is also recommended by the U.S. Centers for Disease Control and Prevention (CDC) and JCAHO that ICPs participate on their facility purchasing committees to help ensure the use of safe, high-quality equipment and supplies.

14. Everyone must work to accomplish the transformation.

Knowledge in the methods of data collection, measurement, and statistical analysis must be shared and owned by the entire team to create broad accountability. It takes the participation of all employees at all levels and across all departments to move the organization forward and build a quality culture.

PLANNING: Focus on Customers, Mission, Vision, Values, and Measurable Outcomes

In this section, we will describe several tools, concepts, and approaches to planning that ICPs can incorporate into their programs. According to Deming et al.,[8] strategic planning and goal setting should be based on a

Copyright © 2005, Association for Professionals in Infection Control and Epidemiology, Inc.

clear understanding of mission and vision but also the customers' needs, wants, and expectations.

A customer is anyone with an expectation about delivery and content of IC services. A quality-based IC program should be focused on its customers and should include a process for regularly assessing and evaluating how the program meets the need of the identified customers.

Customers can be loosely defined as internal or external customers. Internal customers are individuals within the organization who have expectations about IC services. ICPs' internal customers are physicians, nurses, administrators, departmental supervisors, ancillary, and support staff. Defining the staff's role and increasing ICPs' awareness of their customers' needs is an ever-evolving process. Each healthcare worker must understand his or her role in infection prevention and control, integrate it into daily activities, and articulate this role to others.

External customers are individuals or groups outside of the immediate organization who have expectations of IC services. ICPs' external customers include patients, patients' family and significant others, visitors, regulatory agencies (Center for Medicare and Medicaid Services [CMS], JCAHO, Occupational Safety and Health Administration [OSHA]), the community, other ICPs, and the public.

Customers' expectations are often based on personal values and cannot be mandated, although they can be understood and possibly changed through education. ICPs' external customers may value low cost, excellent care, their own health, comfort, and information, whereas ICPs' internal customers may value availability, accuracy, quick turnaround times, and responsiveness.

ICPs should find methods to measure their customers' expectations in many different ways: satisfaction surveys, complaint lines, suggestion boxes, and focus group interviews. Internal customers may want reports of surveillance activities, a review of IC policies, orientation sessions, updates on current practice, and information about risk. What is important here is that the ICP assesses customer satisfaction regularly and that goals and activities be readjusted as needed.

A clear, concise mission statement is key to providing a foundation for an IC program and the facility quality program. A mission statement answers the question: "What are we trying to accomplish?" The answer should be expressed as specific expectations regarding the scope and work of the service, committee, or team, to create constancy of purpose. The mission statement should reflect the program's purpose for existing and should be developed by the whole committee, not just the ICP. For example, "Our program

exists to prevent infections in hospital patients through proactive surveillance, prevention, and education of staff."

A vision statement provides a picture of the IC service you want in the future, based on the needs of the customers or community served and on relevant changes in the healthcare environment. Here are a few sample vision statements: "The highest quality and the best cost." "High quality, patient focused care." "Quality is Job 1" (Ford Motor Company). Your vision statement should be simple, clear, and easily remembered, and it should become part of daily work processes.

A values statement demonstrates the ICP's understanding of the moral values of patients, families, and providers; the social values implicit in social and scientific policy; and the professional values implicit in standards of care and practice. Values are culturally determined and cannot be mandated. They provide rules to guide actions on a day-to-day basis. Examples of a values statement include: "Customers are always right." "Accuracy first.." "Team work, mutual respect, accountability, clinical excellence." "Trust."

The Malcolm Baldrige National Quality Award Program approach to excellence in healthcare is another framework that can be adapted to a specific facility or IC program. This approach is adapted from National Institute of Standards and Technology framework and includes seven core values and concepts:

1. leadership;

2. strategic planning;

3. focus on patients, other customers, and markets;

4. information and analysis;

5. staff focus;

6. process management, and

7. organization performance results.[8]

All of the concepts and approaches discussed in this chapter can fit into this model as well.

PLANNING: Activities that Assist a Focus on Improvement

It is important to remember that planning is a cyclical activity. An organization or program doesn't do planning just once. It needs to occur at least annually as part of the ICP's annual evaluation. Examples include the Shewhart/Deming Cycle of Plan, Do, Check, Act (PDCA)[2] (Fig. 8–2).

1. Plan

Specify what the IC program wants to accomplish over time and how to get there. Activities that occur in the

---

Copyright © 2005, Association for Professionals in Infection Control and Epidemiology, Inc.

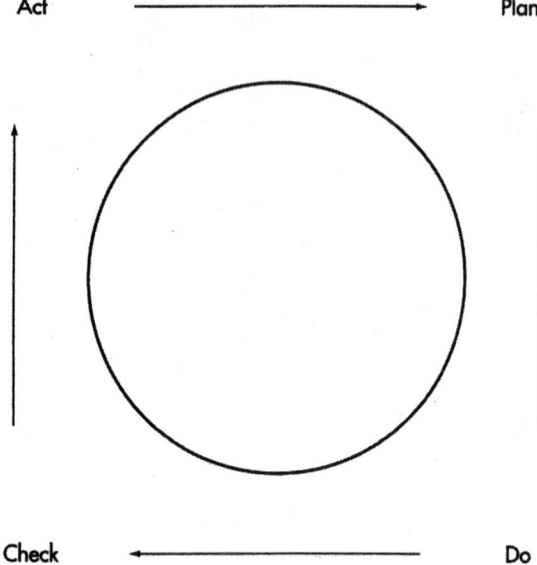

Figure 8–2 The Shewhart/Deming cycle describes a systematic approach for improvement.

planning stage include development of a mission statement, vision statement, and/or goals. Tools used in planning might include an interrelationship diagram, cause-and-effect diagram, affinity digraph, or a tree diagram.

2. Do

The IC program performs or implements its action plan to further the goals. Activities that occur in this stage include implementation of process improvement, a new policy, or education.

3. Check (Study)

The IC program compares the goals with what was actually achieved. During this phase, measuring infection rates occur.

4. Act

The IC program makes continuous changes to more closely achieve the goals. This is when changes become permanent by building them into the processes and monitoring activities.

When the PDCS cycle is complete, it should start all over with planning. The cycle should be repeated as often as necessary until the right solution is found. Tom Nolan and The Institute for Healthcare Improvement (IHI) advocate a series of quick process cycles in their approach termed *rapid cycle improvement*.[9,10]

Planning should include benchmarks or desired outcomes, which are not to be confused with arbitrary thresholds. It is extremely important to be clear about how one will measure success so the team or committee know when they have arrived. For example, implementing a new OSHA tuberculosis prevention program might seek the idealistic outcome of compliance with policy and *no* new hospital-acquired tuberculosis cases or employee PPD conversions. Many benchmarks can be derived from the National Nosocomial Infections Study (NNIS) published in August 2001.[11]

Planning often involves use of both qualitative and quantitative data. Planning requires descriptive information that assists program implementation, process analysis, and outcomes understanding. It is important to include the customers, both internal and external, in the planning processes. Qualitative data may be obtained from in-depth, open-ended interviews, direct observation, and written documents, such as questionnaires, diaries, and records. Quantitative data can be obtained from a surveillance program, facility case mix databases, and medical records.

Planning requires knowledge of basic quality improvement tools and processes to support improvement. The ICP must have knowledge of systems and of the interactions and interrelationships between related processes. Proposed improvement activities should complement each other. System design starts with a focus on outcomes and asks: "How do we design systems that achieve the desired outcome?" Planners must decide whether processes are needed and what value they add to the IC program's mission. Goldmann[12] reports that hospital leaders at one institution were provided with strategic goals to significantly impact antimicrobial resistance. A multidisciplinary group used published evidence and a consensus process to develop goals related to process and outcome measures, antimicrobial use optimization, detection, reporting, and prevention of transmission of antimicrobial-resistant organisms.

Planning also requires knowledge of the program's scope, the system of delivery, and types of services. Scope is often defined as the type of services delivered in a specific setting by specially trained staff. It includes volumes, major diagnoses or patient populations served, service site(s), hours of operation, and types of staff members who provide each service. A good understanding of that scope of service and how the system works provides a good foundation. A system is comprised of input, processes, and output (Fig. 8–3). Use of the system tool with the IC program committee can be very helpful. The ICP can have the committee review all of their "inputs, process/system steps and outputs" as part of the annual program evaluation or in conjunction with strategic planning.

Copyright © 2005, Association for Professionals in Infection Control and Epidemiology, Inc.

A System

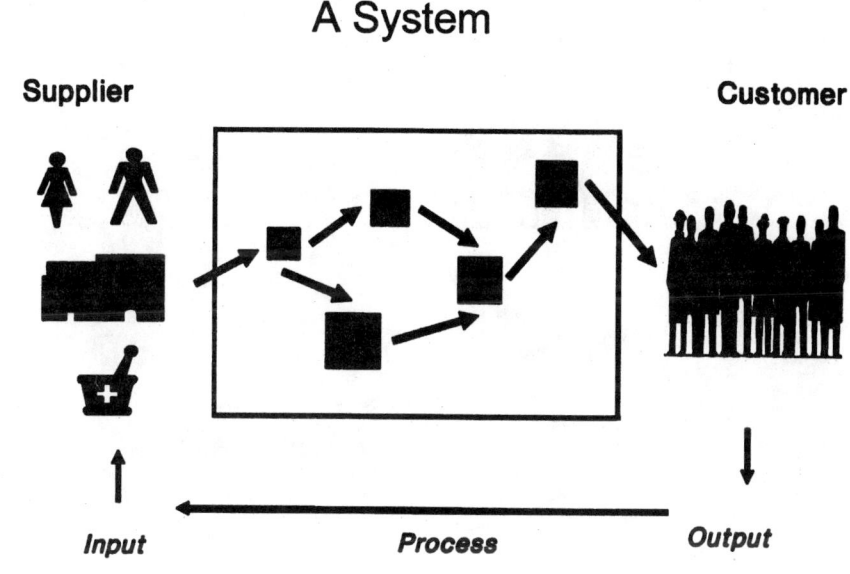

Supplier

Customer

Input   *Process*   *Output*

©.LDSH 1990

Figure 8–3   A system consists of processes that convert input (supplies) into output (customer outcomes).

MEASUREMENT: Understanding Variation

Statistical process control (SPC) is also called *continuous quality improvement, total quality management, total quality control* or *industrial quality control.* SPC assumes that the limits of randomization in any task or process can be charted with control limits established. Processes that are within statistical control limits are considered to be under control. Processes that exceed their control limits are considered out of statistical control, and adjustments in the process may be needed. SPC may also signal a special cause variance and need a focus study.[19,20]

Variation is described as the difference in process steps and outputs. Consistent and predictable processes—processes without variation—are easier to improve than erratic processes. One of the first steps in the Joiner triangle, using the scientific approach, requires that one eliminate variation in a process before manipulating the process to improve quality. This means that the process being worked on has been stabilized, and random variation has been minimized.

There are two types of variation: special-cause and common-cause. Special-cause variation is also referred to as *attributable, assignable* or as *first order change.* Special-cause variation is either not part of the system (or process) all of the time or does not affect everyone; it arises out of specific circumstances. To reduce special-cause variation, look for different conditions or procedures that lead to differences in results.[21] For example, one might develop a cause-

and-effect diagram using analysis of people, methods, machines, materials, operating conditions, and measurement tools (Fig. 8–4). Removing special-cause variation results in a return to the average or expected performance level of the system achieved some time in the past. The impact is usually felt in the present or near future. For example, an ICP seeks to standardize across surgeons, eliminate variation in timing or in the antiseptic agents used to prepare the operative site. As another example, the ICP introduces a new procedure that fundamentally alters the preparation process, admitting practices, and the incidence of post-procedural infection.

Common-cause variation is also called *random variation* or *second order change.* Common-cause variation is inherently part of the system (or process) over time and affects everyone working and all outcomes. To reduce common-cause variation, the process or system must be fundamentally changed, designed, or redesigned. Reducing common-cause variation improves the system beyond historical levels. The impact is felt far into the future. Reducing common-cause variation usually results in improvement of several measures of the system simultaneously. For example, a high prevalence of group B streptococcal carriage in the community may result in a higher incidence of neonatal infection. If there is indeed a higher prevalence in the community, this common cause cannot be easily eliminated or reduced. But the ICP could implement screening and prevention processes.

Quality Concepts

Copyright © 2005, Association for Professionals in Infection Control and Epidemiology, Inc.

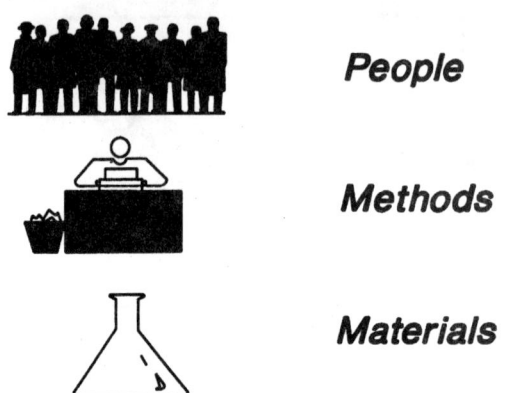

Sources of Variation

People

Methods

Materials

from NDP 1989

Figure 8–4   Varation in systems is usually related to three sources: people, methods, and materials.

There are tools and methods to control and reduce variation of a process. Understanding variation requires knowledge of data—the results from the recording of observations or from making measurements, both qualitative and quantitative. For example, an investigation of consistently high rates of intravenous site infection may lead to identification of poor site preparation and management, which was, unfortunately, a consistent and predictable process variation.

Data collection is important to process improvement. Ask the right question. Collect the data and facts to answer the question. Determine what type of data is needed. Determine where the data can be found. Decide who can provide the data. Check the accuracy of the data, and use methods that reduce the risk of error. Organize and present the data in a manner that answers the question.

A check sheet, or tally, is a basic tool that helps answer how often a specific event occurs. To develop a check sheet, decide which specific event will be observed and recorded. Establish the time to begin and end data collection, and visually display the patterns and trends.

Run charts are epidemiological tools that are frequently used to identify how process specifications change over time (e.g., the number of healthcare-acquired infections occurring within a hospital over a given period of time). They allow for the mean or average to be determined as well as showing changes in the mean/average. They can also demonstrate special-cause varia-

tion when there is a steady pattern of observation points falling above and below the mean/average line in an equal pattern.

Control charts identify variation that is normal or common for the process and variation that is not. The upper and lower control limits are calculated using standard deviation (Fig. 8–5).

Clinical practice guidelines are tools, such as algorithms and consensus statements, to reduce variation in practice to control behavior, contain spending, and improve care and outcomes. Strategies to develop, disseminate, and implement guidelines are often based on social influences that affect healthcare practitioner behavior. For example, standardization of diagnosis of pneumonia along with timely administration of the appropriate antibiotic reduces morbidity and mortality.

The relationship between variation and cost is referred to as "quality waste," or the "cost of poor quality" and is the cost of fixing a failure, such as new construction hazards. It reflects the cost of complex processes, re-work loops, and missing steps. Quality waste results in low productivity and increased costs and includes the cost of efforts to prevent, detect, and react to quality problems. JCAHO requires that Construction Risk Assessments be done prior to each significant remodel or new construction in an effort to prevent quality waste. Hospital-acquired infections can also be an example of quality waste, if an infection occurs and policies and procedures were not followed.

APIC Text of Infection Control and Epidemiology

Copyright © 2005, Association for Professionals in Infection Control and Epidemiology, Inc.

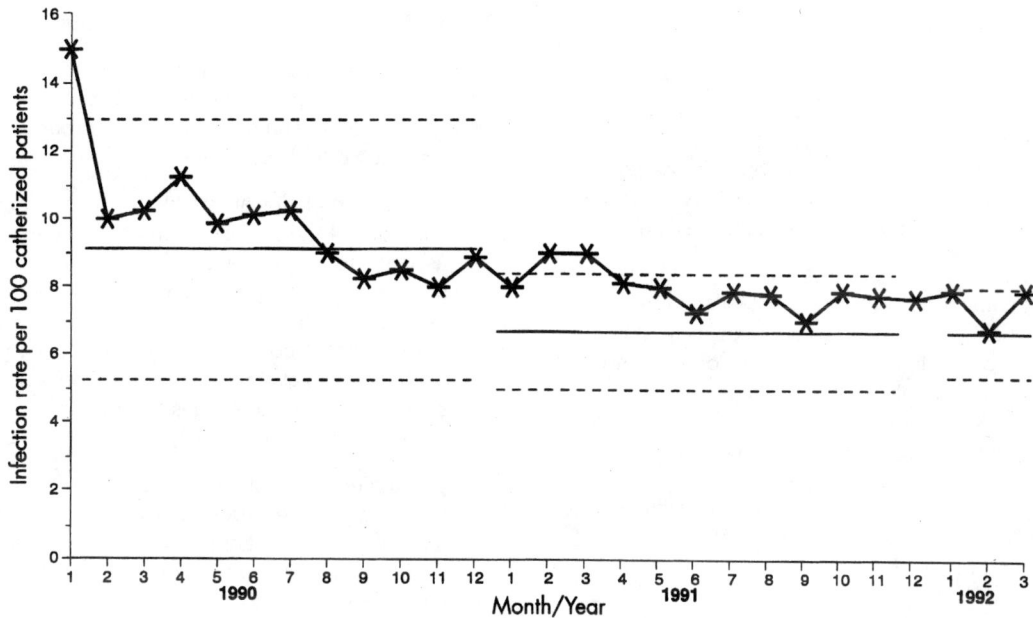

Figure 8-5 This control chart identifies special-cause variation (January 1990) and narrowing of control limits as the process was improved.

Stabilizing a process by focusing on variation involves detecting and eliminating special-cause variation. Only common-cause variation should exist in a stable process. Variation within the upper and lower control limits is common variation, and the process is considered to be in statistical control. The chief use of a control chart is to detect assignable or special-cause variation. Control limits will narrow over time as the process improves. If they do not narrow, the process may not be stable and the team needs to pursue process improvement. The logical order is to stabilize the process before implementing change. In the scientific process this must be done before testing hypotheses.

IMPROVEMENT: Teams

Multidisciplinary teams are a valuable tool in deploying a quality-focused culture or process. Successful teams increase problem solving and efficiency, raise morale *and* productivity, use integrative rather than imposed solutions, increase acceptance of the solution, and tap the potential in people and their fundamental knowledge of the process. They also align with mission, vision, and values of the organization and identify customers and expectations. Below are some guidance for working with teams, but "The Team Handbook"[5] includes more information and facilitator assistance.

Teams may experience failure for many reasons. Some teams may lack commitment or full attendance by team members. They may have a leader who believes

that she or he is the only one right. They may be unclear about the goal or mission or confused about their team's role. Meetings may be unproductive or the team as a whole may not have been given ample credit, reward, or recognition. Teams may accomplish their work but find their suggested changes are not implemented by upper management. An evaluation of a failed team can determine causes and can be a valuable learning experience.

Ground rules, or operational rules, are the IC program's guiding rules of operation or policies and should be agreed upon by team members. Team or committee ground rules should address attendance, participation, meeting places and times, assignments, completion dates or time frames, and clear role definitions for all team members.

A guidance team for an IC program may be an established entity such as an infection control committee, which approves, launches, and oversees the project team. It may rest with the committee to pick the process or project to be improved and to provide a clear mission statement and desired outcomes. The committee may be involved in the formation of the actual project team and will certainly assist in mobilizing resources as needed. Using an existing body as the guidance team may help remove institutional barriers and speed implementation of the changes recommended.

Copyright © 2005, Association for Professionals in Infection Control and Epidemiology, Inc.

A project team or committee is composed of people who do the work. The team leader retains the management responsibility, has expertise in the process under study, and liaises with the guidance team. The facilitator is a technical advisor, teacher, and expert on the team process, although not necessarily on the process under review or study. Team members have the fundamental knowledge of the process under study and are usually frontline employees.

Team or committee conflict is inevitable and natural. It is usually due to differences in behavior, beliefs, and values that cause differences in style. Conflict is *not* necessarily a result of people being right or wrong; rather it can arise when people have strengths in different areas or when individuals defend a value position rather than concentrating on objective facts. Conflict can be productive and foster creativity, but the team facilitator must be able to negotiate, arbitrate, counsel, and resolve conflict.

IMPROVEMENT: Methods and Tools

Use of multiple tools or techniques will help the team focus effort on purpose, uncover problems, sort confusing information and data, and make progress. Some commonly used tools include:

Brainstorming helps an existing or newly organized team define the project or process they are assigned to improve and enhance their problem solving potential by identifying a large number of ideas from which to choose. It can also generate theories about possible causes of identified problems and help clarify ideas so that *everyone* understands intent. It encourages creative and innovative thinking.

Affinity diagrams gather large amounts of language data and creatively group these data based on lines of natural relationships. Data are usually collected from brainstorming or customer surveys (Fig. 8–6).

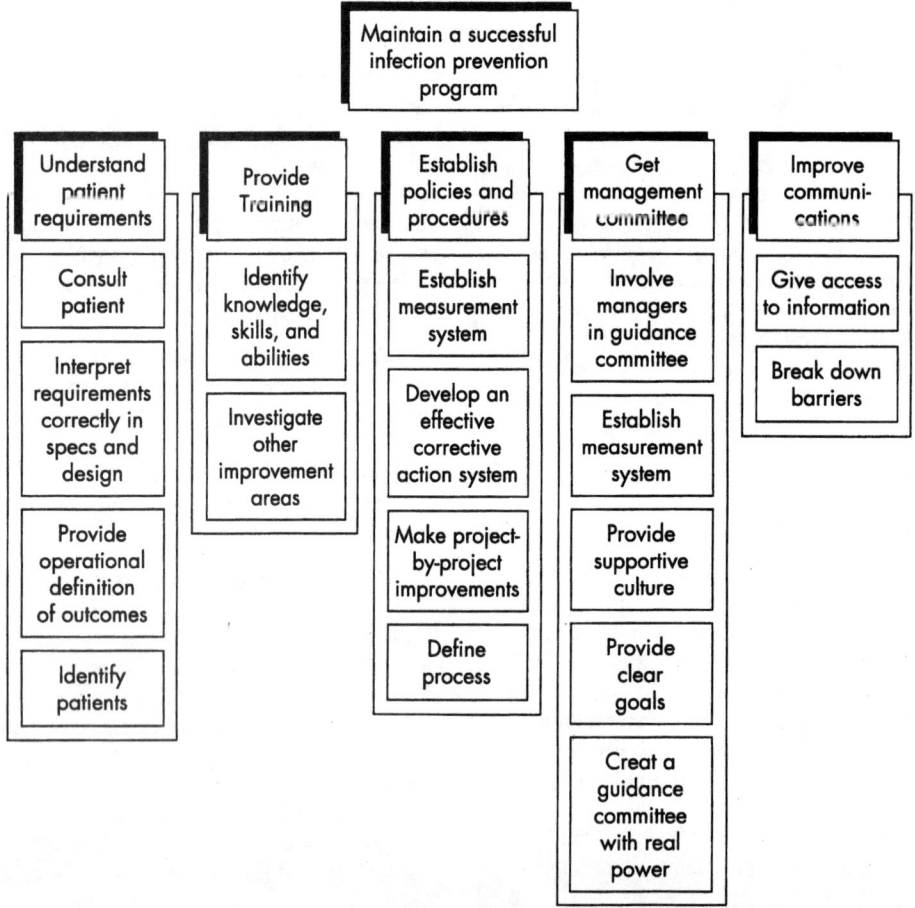

Figure 8–6   An affinity diagram organizes large amounts of qualitative data into natural groupings.

Copyright © 2005, Association for Professionals in Infection Control and Epidemiology, Inc.

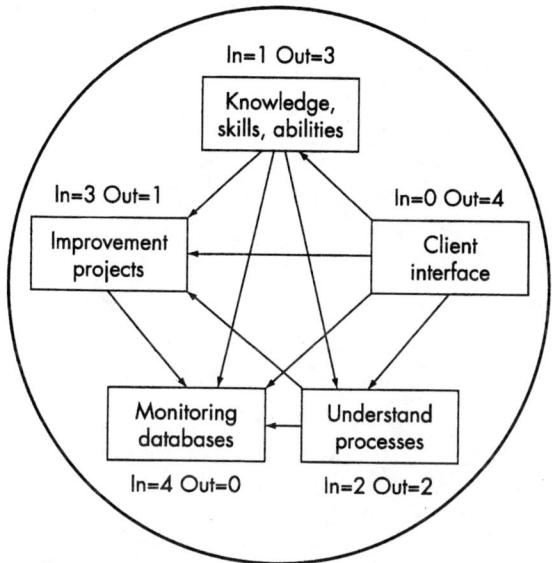

Figure 8-7 This simple variation of an inter-relationship diagraph helps to identify root cause and to priortize an action plan.

Interrelationship digraphs take complex, multivariable problems and graphically display all of the interrelated factors. They may also suggest cause-and-effect relationships, thereby providing focus for the team or project (Fig. 8–7).

Tree diagrams map in detail the full range of paths and tasks that must be accomplished to achieve a primary goal and related subgoals. This is the "meat and flesh" of your strategic plan (Fig. 8–8).

Cause-and-effect or *fishbone diagrams* (Fig. 8–9) identify a specific problem, find the root cause of the problem by backtracking through all the steps until the source is found, represent the relationship between possible causes of specific problems and effects or outcomes, and practically document and organize complex interactions that occur when dealing with *many* causes. The effect or outcome (whether desired or undesired) is on the right side of the chart, and the possible causes are on the left. The main lines branching off the large arrow represent major categories of causes: manpower, methods, machines, materials, people, policies, procedures, plant, environment, and equipment.

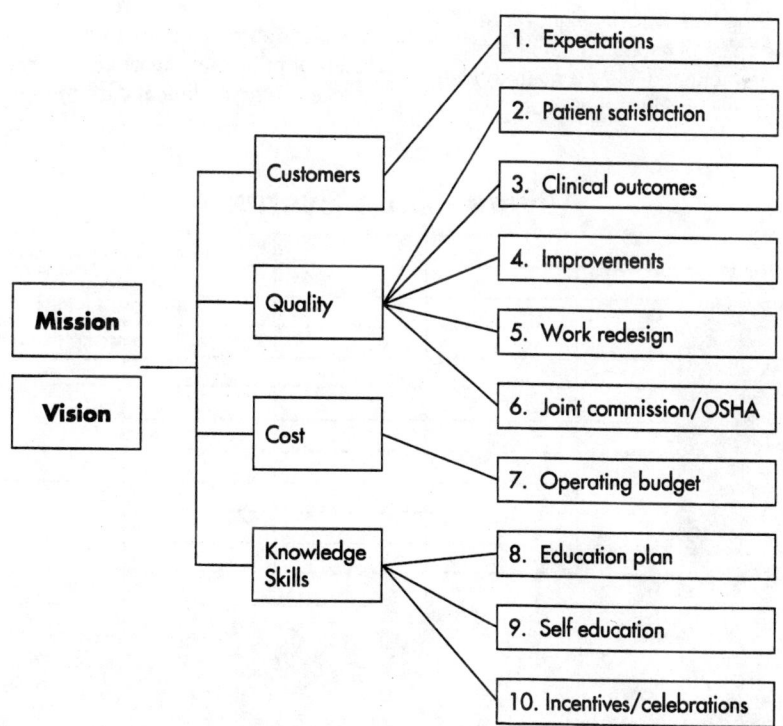

Figure 8-8 The tree diagram adds increasing detail as the team moves from major goals to specific objectives and tactics.

Copyright © 2005, Association for Professionals in Infection Control and Epidemiology, Inc.

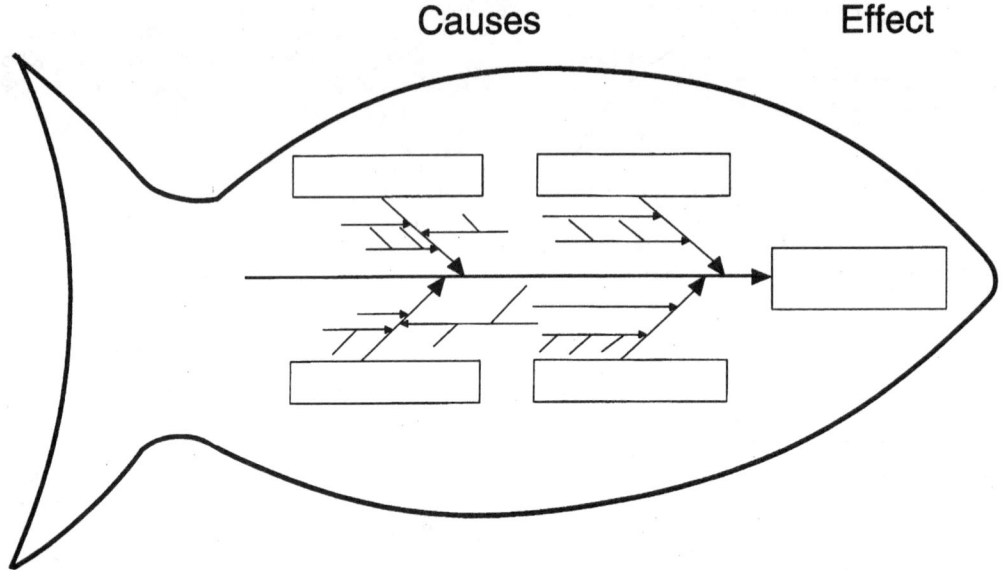

Causes   Effect

Figure 8-9 A fishbone diagram begins with a desired or undesired effect and provides a tool to group causes.

Pareto charts (Fig. 8–10) are a series of vertical bars arranged, sorted, in descending order of height from left to right with a cumulative percent line on the second Y-axis. They can be used to categorize data using bars whose height represents the discrete value of each compared against the unit of measurement and allow a team to identify where its effort will produce the greatest value.

IMPROVEMENT: Documenting Process Steps

As discussed previously, we know that a process consists of inputs and a series of activities that produce an output. In healthcare, process often refers to what healthcare providers do to diagnose and treat patients. Clinical processes are often referred to as *clinical process maps, clinical care models,* and *critical*

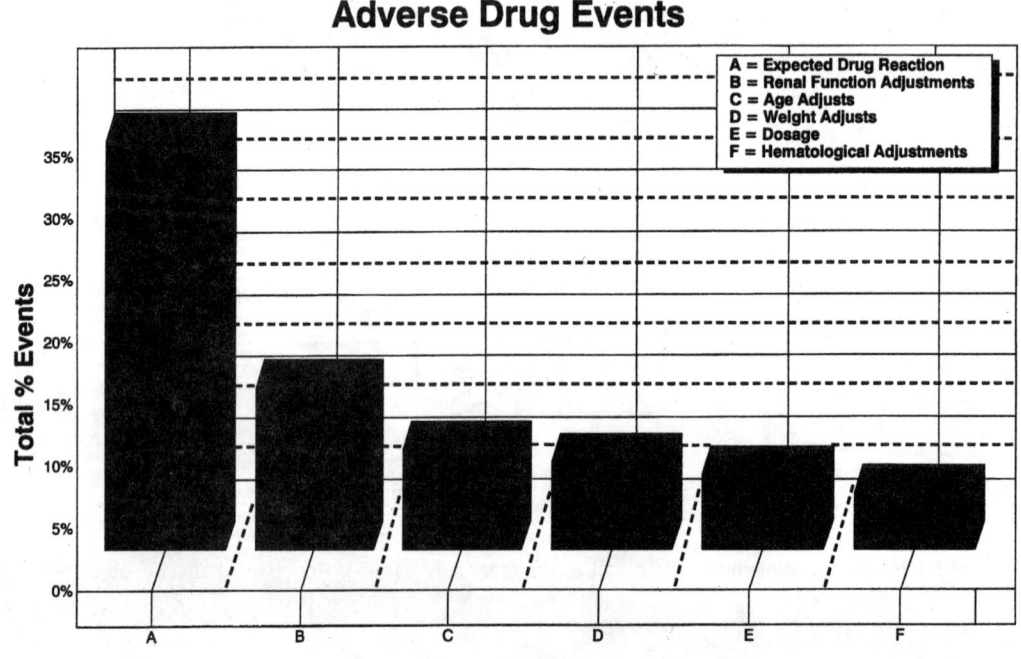

Adverse Drug Events

A = Expected Drug Reaction
B = Renal Function Adjustments
C = Age Adjusts
D = Weight Adjusts
E = Dosage
F = Hematological Adjustments

Figure 8-10 Sample Pareto Chart.

APIC Text of Infection Control and Epidemiology

Copyright © 2005, Association for Professionals in Infection Control and Epidemiology, Inc.

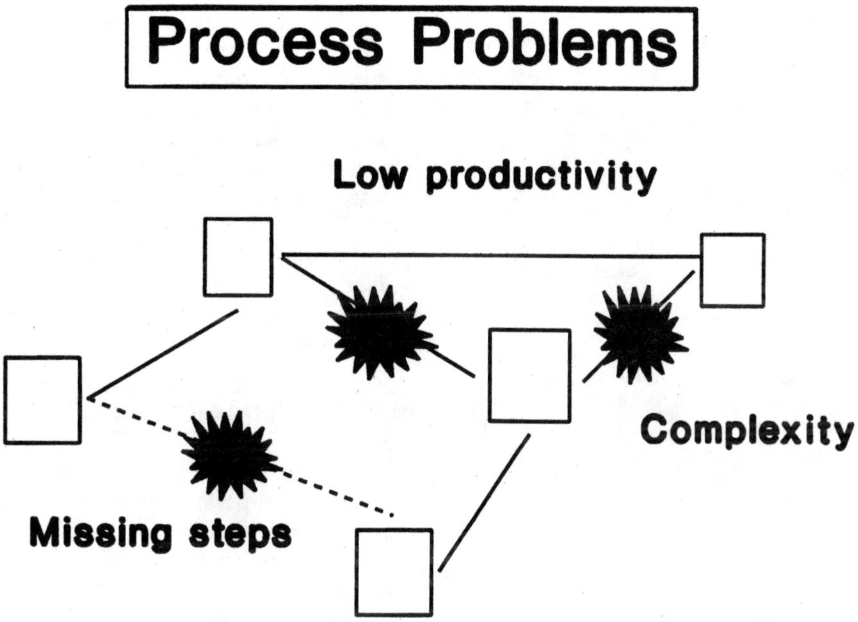

Process Problems

Low productivity

Complexity

Missing steps

Figure 8-11 Typical process problems are low productivity, missing steps, and complexity.

paths. Surveillance, education, and policy development are examples of IC processes. Most processes cross departments or services and require multidisciplinary teams to study and improve them.

If quality is conformance to specifications, then nonconformance or variation is "nonquality." Complexity and missing steps, or low productivity, are common problems with processes. An example of complexity is that patients are repeatedly required to provide the same demographic data at multiple services points in the same care process. An example of a missing step might be the frequent absence of proper handwashing after patient contact (Fig. 8–11).

Every process is a series of steps, all interconnected and usually hierarchical in nature. Process steps that causally determine whether the output will meet quality expectations should be specified and measured. To understand a process, document it, by writing down the steps in a sequential format. During documentation, special cause variation is frequently identified and may lead to immediate improvement. Constructing a process flowchart can help delineate the process steps and assist with measuring the variation or process specifications.

The steps in process flowchart construction are identified in Figure 8–12. They include:

- Identify a process to improve

- Define the boundaries of the process (start small)

- Create by a team with firsthand knowledge of the process (include customers when appropriate)

- Describe and displaying the steps of a process

- Discover weak areas or problems in the process that have the potential for improvement

- Compare with another flowchart depicting the ideal process

- Use flowchart symbols: terminal, activity, decision, flow lines, and connectors

Quality improvement processes should start with an explicit, measurable, statement regarding an important attribute of an output as well as explicit specifications that will form the basis for an objective measurement system that can then be used to measure process improvement. The aim is to eliminate variation from every step so that only random noise (common-cause variation) is present when measured.

IMPROVEMENT: Infection Control Examples

As described by Nicotra,[13] a multidisciplinary team in an acute care facility targeted ventilator-associated healthcare-acquired infections that were higher than the national standard. The team focused on closed suction systems, policies, and procedures for cleaning ventilators, and staff education. Their efforts resulted in a reduction of the ventilator-associated healthcare-acquired pneumonia infection rate to 8.3 per 1,000

Copyright © 2005, Association for Professionals in Infection Control and Epidemiology, Inc.

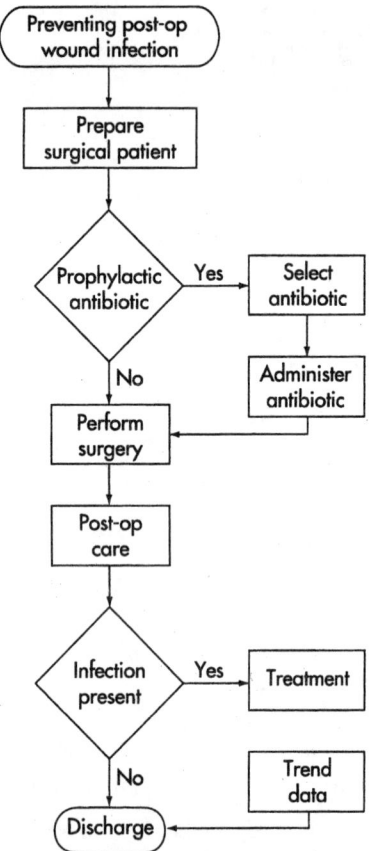

Figure 8-12 In a process flow chart, ovals are terminal symbols, boxes represent activities, triangles are decisions, and lines indicate flow of information.

ventilator days and a cost savings of more than $580,000.

In an intensive care unit, a multidisciplinary group used quality improvement techniques to significantly reduce their endemic ventilator-associated lower respiratory tract infection rate, also improving protocol compliance and management of ventilated patients and reducing management cost.[16]

Another team described the use of CQI to achieve proper isolation of patients with suspected tuberculosis. These projects used multidisciplinary teams, process flowcharting, self-administered knowledge testing, and monitoring and measurement of outcomes. As a result, the time spent in isolation to rule out tuberculosis was decreased, exposures were decreased, and associated costs were reduced.[15]

At one large healthcare company, an improvement initiative focused on improving the timing of preoperative antibiotics. After experiencing success at one large facility, the company launched a team at the corporate level that involved a good cross-section of facilities and

disciplines to implement an education and tracking system in all 21 of the company's hospitals. Through education, use of the Medical Letter guidelines on prophylaxis, and implementation of a data collection system, the initiative achieved a significant decrease in incisional wound infections, from 0.54% to 0.34%. Deep wound infections decreased from 0.41% to 0.30%, and organ space dropped from 0.50% to 0.27%. The company concluded that systematic reporting, consistent education of staff, and regular feedback of each sites data resulted in significant improvement.[17]

IV.   SUMMARY AND CONCLUSIONS

In summary, this chapter presents a framework for ICPs that incorporates the many and varied approaches to quality into a simple model of planning, measuring, and improving—starting with Deming and moving on to current initiatives, such as the national patient safety goals and the Baldrige Excellence in Health Care Award process. Planning is cyclical and ongoing and should be focused on the customers, internal and external. Measuring is the only way to determine know where you have been and where you are now. Measurement is an integral part of any infection control program, but measuring for its own sake can be wasteful. Focusing measures on important and high-risk processes is more beneficial. The use of planning and measuring in a continuous improvement model can lead to improvement, the third component of the framework. ICPs can select among the many approaches and tools explored in this chapter to determine a "best fit" for their programs within their organization's quality improvement structure. Good quality is indeed a continuously improving process.

V.   FUTURE TRENDS

Infection control programs are increasingly expected to link process to improved outcomes. The degree to which outcomes can be directly linked to processes of care continues to be challenging. To understand process and outcome measures, we need definitive evidence of links, stronger relationships between technology assessment and quality assessment, reliable and valid outcome measures, and continued development of health status measures, benchmarking or industry comparative data, setting and measuring thresholds, and satisfaction measures.

ICPs will also be expected to use quality improvement methodology as well as epidemiological approaches and quantitative methods to analyze diseases in populations, whether iatrogenic or noniatrogenic, to determine causal factors, and to evaluate the efficacy of

Copyright © 2005, Association for Professionals in Infection Control and Epidemiology, Inc.

interventions. Adverse outcomes, including infections, are associated with

diagnostic studies, surgical procedures, administration of medications and anesthesia, and nursing care. Huskins et al.[16] adapted the continuous quality improvement methodology in a demonstration project for hospitals in low- and middle-income countries to reduce the incidence of surgical-site infections. Again, their approach was to stabilize or standardize the process steps, implement best practice, and measure the outcomes.

ICPs will be expected to be familiar with advances in technology that improve the quality of healthcare delivered, leading to improved outcomes for patients. New medical technologies diagnose and treat but are often associated with an increase in complications and adverse outcomes. Objective provider-specific data (evidence-based medicine) can assist decision making and maximize benefits and minimize risks. For example, latex Foley catheters are associated with a higher incidence of urinary tract infection than silicone catheters.

Healthcare institutions may also meet an increasing expectation that their quality outcomes measures are made known to their customers. How and when to make data on hospital quality available to the public is an issue being addressed by federal and state governments, business and purchaser coalitions, and hospital programs. Although private groups, such as the Joint Commission on the Accreditation of Healthcare Organization (JCAHO) and the National Committee on Quality Assurance (NCQA), can establish quality measures and offer accreditation, the government can require hospital data collection and disclosure. The Healthcare Financing Administration (HCFA) and CMS, for example, have released hospital or nursing home data to the public, including on public Web sites (e.g., *http://www.cms.hhs.gov/quality/nhqi/*). Other quality indicators, such as readmissions within 30 days of discharge and unplanned returns to the operating room, have been proposed as outcomes that reflect quality of care. Challenges that must be addressed when considering outcomes disclosure include adjusting for severity of illness so that accurate benchmarking between facilities is possible. It is clear that we can measure outcomes, but their link to specific diagnoses and processes is not as clear. The risk management approach currently in use is based on tort law and screening with quality indicators to discover cases, assuming that quality of care contributes directly to the indicator occurrences. Labor-intensive peer review provides retrospective analysis of problems and focuses attention on damage control.

Current outcome assessments focus on the measurement, monitoring, and feedback of outcomes. Projects usually address a particular condition or procedure.

Data are often severity adjusted or stratified, and algorithms or process flowcharts are employed. Monitoring, or the repeated measurement of indicators, permits causal inferences about care processes and resources used to achieve patient outcomes, particularly reducing symptoms and improving health status. Health status assessment tools measure functional or health status outcomes related to physical condition, emotional condition, and pain. The technology is maturing and tools (for example, the John Ware SF-36, a functional status assessment comprised of thirty-six questions) are now brief, valid, reliable, easy to administer and score, and suitable for use in clinical practice.[18]

ORYX/Core measures, implemented by JCAHO, are mandatory reporting of outcome measures and measures specific to disease processes. Participating facilities are required to collect data on acute myocardial infarcts, heart failure, community-acquired pneumonia, and other proposed categories. They are quantitative measures of processes or outcomes of care associated with the delivery of clinical services. Using control charts, hospital performance will be compared and benchmarked against its national peers (see *http://www.jcaho.org/pms/index.htm*).

Community-oriented outcome measures are also being increasingly applied. Recent partnerships between healthcare systems and public health programs, such as those sponsored by the National Patient Safety Foundation and the Harvard/Pilgrim Projects, are promoting measures such as employee turnover, substance abuse rates, immunization rates, homicide and accident rates, use of screening and preventive measures, and occurrence of diseases.

The Centers for Disease Control and Prevention (CDC) has become engaged in promoting use of proven prevention guidelines. It has identified a set of health status indicators to monitor and evaluate progress toward the *Healthy People 2000 Objectives* and to encourage states and local communities to adopt them (see *http://www.cdc.gov/nchs/otheract.htm*).

HEDIS (Health Plan Employer Data and Information Set) measures quantitative indicators of performance that are used by the NCQA to evaluate and accredit health maintenance organizations. Examples of these measures include childhood immunization rates and mammography screening rates. Eventually, NCQA will share these data with consumers and purchasers (see *http://www.ncqa.org/Communications/News/sohc2003.htm*).

REFERENCES

1. Mann N: *The keys to excellence: the story of the Deming philosophy*, Los Angeles, 1989, Prestwick.
2. Juran J: *Juran on leadership for quality*, New York, 1989, Collier Macmillan.

Copyright © 2005, Association for Professionals in Infection Control and Epidemiology, Inc.

3. Walton M: *The Deming management method*, New York, 1986, Putman.
4. King B: *Hoshin planning: the developmental approach*, 1989, Bob King, GOAL/QPC.
5. Scholtes P: *The team handbook*, ed 3, Madison, WI, 2003, Oriel Incorporated.
6. Gilleum T: Deming's 14 points and hospital quality: responding to the consumer's demand for the best value health care, *J Nurs Qual Assur* 2:70–78, 1988.
7. Burr JT: *SPC: Tools for operators*, Milwaukee, 1989, Quality Press.
8. National Institute of Standards and Technology Administration. The Malcolm Baldrige National Quality Award. Gaithersburg, MD, 1993, NISTA.
9. Langley GJ, et al: *The improvement guide: a practical approach to enhancing organization performance,* San Francisco, 1996, Jossey-Bass.
10. Carver P: *Reducing delays and waiting times throughout the healthcare system*, Boston, 1996, Institute for Healthcare Improvement.
11. National Nosocomial Infections Surveillance (NNIS) System Report, *Am J Infect Control* 29(6):404–421, 2001.
12. Goldmann DA, et al: Strategies to prevent and control the emergence and spread of antimicrobial-resistant microorganisms in hospitals: a challenge to hospital leadership, *J Am Med Assoc* 275:234–240, 1996.
13. Nicotra D, Ulrich C: Process Improvement Plan for the reduction of nosocomial pneumonia in patients on ventilators, *J Nurs Care Qual* 10:18–23, 1996.
14. Joiner GA, Salisbury D, Bollin GE: Utilizing quality assurance as a tool for reducing the risk of nosocomial ventilator-associated pneumonia, *Am J Med Qual* 11:100–103, 1996.
15. Cook JD, Lewis L, Thomassen KA: The use of continuous quality improvement to achieve proper isolation of patients with suspected tuberculosis, *Am J Infect Control* 23:323–328, 1995.
16. Huskins WC, Soule BM, et al: Hospital infection prevention and control: a model for improving the quality of hospital care in low- and middle-income countries, *Infect Control Hosp Epidemiol* 19:125–135, 1998.
17. Larsen RA, et al: Improved peri-operative antibiotic use and reduced surgical wound infections through use of computer decision analysis, *Infect Control Hosp Epidemiol* 10:316–320, 1989.
18. Ware JE Jr: SF-36 health survey update, *Spine* 25(24):3130–3139, .
19. Batalden PB, Stoltz PK: A framework for the continual improvement of health care: building and applying professional and improvement knowledge to test changes in daily work, *Jt Comm J Qual Improv* 19:424–452, 1993.
20. Batalden PB, et al: Linking outcomes measurement to continual improvement, *Jt Comm J Qual Improv* 20:167–180, 1994.
21. Cleveland WS: *The elements of graphing data*, Monterey, CA, 1985, Wadsworth Advanced Books and Software.

SUPPLEMENTAL RESOURCES

Block P: *Flawless consulting: a guide to getting your expertise used,* San Diego, 1981, Pfeiffer & Co.

Brassard M: *The memory jogger: a pocket guide of tools for continuous improvement,* Metheun, MA, 1988, GOAL/QPC.

Brassard M: *The memory jogger plus,*. Metheun, MA, 1989, GOAL/QPC.

Crosby PB: *Quality is free,* New York, 1979, Penguin Books.

Desatnick R: *Long live the king,* 1989, Quality Progress, pp 24–26.

Donabedian A: Defining and measuring quality in health care. In Wenzel RP, editor: *Assessing quality health care: perspectives for clinicians,* Baltimore, 1992, Williams & Wilkins,

Friedman C, et al: Use of the total quality process in an infection control program: a surprising customer–needs assessment, *Am J Infect Control* 21:155–159, 1993.

James B: *Quality management for health care delivery*, Chicago, 1990, American Hospital Association.

Institute of Medicine: *Crossing the quality chasm: a new health system for the 21st Century*, Washington, DC, 2001, National Academy Press.

Kohn LT, et al: *To err is human: building a safer health system*, Washington, DC, 1999, Institute of Medicine, National Academy Press.

Kume H: *Statistical methods for quality improvement*, Tokyo, 1989, The Association for Overseas Technical Scholarship.

Lawton R: Creating a customer-centered culture for service quality, *Qual Prog* 34–36, 1989.

Markson LE, Nash DB: Overview: public accountability of hospitals regarding quality, *Jt Comm J Qual Improv* 20:359–363, 1994.

Massanari RM: Quality improvement: controlling the risk of adverse events. In Wenzel RP, editor: *Assessing quality health care: perspectives for clinicians,* Baltimore, 1992, Williams & Wilkins, .

Nelson EC, Berwick DM: The measurement of health status in clinical practice, *Med Care* 27:S77–S89, 1989.

Ozeki K, Asaka T: *Handbook of quality tools: the Japanese approach,* Cambridge, MA, 1990, Productivity Press.

Scherkenbach W: *The Deming route to quality and productivity,* Milwaukee, 1990, Quality Press.

Thompson D, et al: The strategic use of outcome information. *Jt Comm J Qual Improv* 26(10):576–586, 2000.

Townsend PL: *Commit to quality,* New York, 1990, John Wiley & Sons.

Wenzel RP, editor: *Assessing quality health care: perspectives for clinicians,* Baltimore, 1992, Williams & Wilkins.

Zenger JH, et al: *Leading teams: mastering the new role,* Homewood, IL, 1994, Zenger Miller.

Web Sites of Interest

Centers for Disease Control (CDC) Division of Healthcare Quality Promotion, *http://www.cdc.gov/ncidod/hip/Guide/guide.htm*

CDC Healthy People 2000 plus other initiatives, *http://www.cdc.gov/nchs/otheract.htm*

CMS Hospital Quality Initiative, *http://www.cms.hhs.gov/quality/hospital/*

CMS Nursing Home Compare, *http://www.cms.hhs.gov/quality/nhqi/*

Institute for Healthcare Improvement (IHI), *http://www.ihi.org/*

International Organization for Standardization (ISO), *http://www.iso.ch/iso/en/aboutiso/introduction/index.html*

JCAHO ORYX Core measures, *http://www.jcaho.org/pms/index.htm*

Juran Institute, *http://www.juran.com*

National Association for Healthcare Quality, *http://www.nahq.org/*

APIC Text of Infection Control and Epidemiology

Copyright © 2005, Association for Professionals in Infection Control and Epidemiology, Inc.

National Committee for Quality Assurance (NCQA), *http://www.ncqa.org/index.asp*

The American Health Quality Association, *http://www.ahqa.org/pub/inside/158_670_2426.cfm*

Six Sigma: Quality tools and templates, *http://www.isixsigma.com/*

Copyright © 2005, Association for Professionals in Infection Control and Epidemiology, Inc.

Performance Indicators

Marlyn T. Conti, RN, BSN, CPHQ
Quality Consultant
Intermountain Health Care
Salt Lake City, Utah

ABSTRACT

Much work has been accomplished nationwide on the development and use of quality indicators (QIs) in the past few years. The Joint Commission for Accreditation of Health Care Organizations (JCAHO) launched its ORYX outcome measures in 1997. The Centers for Medicare and Medicaid Services (CMS) launched national comparative measures for long-term care in 2002, home care in 2003, and in 2004, hospital reporting with the launch of the National Voluntary Hospital Reporting Initiative. The Institute of Medicine published its reports on quality, *To Err is Human* [1] in 1999 and *Crossing the Quality Chasm* [2] in 2001. Our quality world has come to be much more definitive with regard to the use of indicators. This chapter will review many of the systems and processes available for measuring quality and will provide a framework for evaluation, development, and use of effective indicators.

KEY CONCEPTS

- Quality indicators are events or steps in a process that lead to high quality or are evidence that high quality exists in the care process under investigation.

- Outcome measures are the result of a care process or delivery system.

- Process measures are indicators of interim process steps.

I.   BACKGROUND

As the healthcare industry makes progress in the quest for quality, issues of cost, access, and outcomes continue to be the primary elements of discussion. The debate about cost and quality, while of interest and concern to both providers and purchasers of healthcare, needs to be balanced with the use of good indicators to identify improvement in quality for patients.

This chapter outlines some epidemiological principles, suggested standards, and precautions for the design and use of quality indicators (QIs), as well as a reasonable approach for infection control professionals (ICPs) to follow in the quest for quality improvement indicators to prevent wasted effort and expenditure of healthcare dollars. Some approaches, although well intended, carry the risk of generating misleading information. "The potential for subsequently flawed decision making can only compound an already complex situation."[3]

Copyright © 2005, Association for Professionals in Infection Control and Epidemiology, Inc.

Much of this chapter draws on the work of the QI Study Group findings published in 1994 and 1995.[3,4] The QI Study Group was created by the governing boards of the Society for Healthcare Epidemiology of America (SHEA), the Association for Professionals in Infection Control and Epidemiology (APIC), and the Surgical Infection Society. The QI Study Group conducted a literature review, interviewed experts in the field, and focused on how best to evaluate QIs, with an emphasis on nosocomial infection. QIs used in epidemiology, nosocomial infection control, infection prevention, and quality-of-care improvement were evaluated. This report reviewed pertinent issues and, where possible, provided specific advice on how to evaluate QIs and QI systems. The objective was to enable the reader to be able to discuss, develop, and evaluate QIs, and to better collect, aggregate, analyze, and use quality data.

The 1995 Quality Indicator Project final report, published in *Infection Control and Hospital Epidemiology* in 1995, expanded and refined the interim report[4] and represented a multiauthor collaboration by doctors and nurses currently performing epidemiological research, providing direct patient care, or managing clinical epidemiology and quality improvement programs. The consensus views and advice evolved with the final goal of distinguishing areas of clear understanding from areas of uncertainty.

Other groups that may be interested in the concepts outlined herein include decision makers and senior managers in acute care institutions who have been, and continue to be, solicited or required to participate in QI projects. This chapter should facilitate a more knowledgeable participation in mandatory QI programs, such as that implemented by the Joint Commission for Accreditation of Health Care Organizations (JCAHO) and the Centers for Medicare and Medicaid Services (CMS).

Providers and users of quality data must be fully knowledgeable of sound epidemiological principles that apply to use and development of QIs. They also must be aware of the many perils and missteps that may result if these principles are ignored or not fully employed in the design, collection, aggregation, and analysis of data related to QIs. (See Table 9–1.)

A final audience for this chapter may be purchasers (health plans, insurers, and businesses) and receivers (patients and families) of healthcare. They too may have remained unsatisfied in the quest to define quality healthcare. This information may provide them with new insights into future methods to measure quality of care.

Table 9-1. Important concepts in QI development

- Selection of outcome or process
- Definitions: numerator and denominator
- Feasibility
- Reliability
- Accuracy and completeness
- Timeliness
- Training (consistency, cost, personell)
- Comparability and use (internal or external)
- Quality improvement strategies

Current Status of Utilization of QIs

In October 1994, the Quality Indicator Project conducted a survey of statewide indicator systems with the SHEA state liaisons in the 48 states where at least one liaison was present. Responses were received from representatives in 28 states. It is remarkable that only about 58% (28 of 48) of the states responded and 46% (13 of 28) of those were participating in a QI system. Liaisons from the following 15 states indicated that no formal statewide QI system was planned or in use at that time: Alabama, Arizona, Arkansas, Colorado, Florida, Kentucky, Maine, Mississippi, Nebraska, North Carolina, Oregon, Tennessee, Texas, Vermont, and Washington. Liaisons from another 13 states indicated that some type of statewide QI system was being promoted. The following states however, did indicate participation in statewide indicators: California, Connecticut, Georgia, Indiana, Maryland, Massachusetts, New Hampshire, New York, North Dakota, Ohio, Rhode Island, West Virginia, and Wisconsin.[3,4] In personal communication, some of the original task force members, (Gross, Weinstein and Scheckler) reported that the work of this group has been continued in their various professional organizations [i.e., SHEA, Centers for Disease Control and Prevention (CDC), JCAHO, and APIC].

The speed of the development of QIs and their implementation has accelerated since publication of the Quality Indicator Project. Three organizations have been involved extensively in the development of QIs for use in acute care hospitals: the Maryland Hospital Association Quality Indicator Project (MHAQIP), JCAHO, and CMS. More specific to ICPs are the CDCs National Nosocomial Infection Surveillance (NNIS) study measures, which are discussed in more detail later.

The Maryland project began in 1985 as a small voluntary project involving seven hospitals. "It was designed to provide tools to hospital trustees, management, and medical staff leadership to improve hospital performance." The MHAQIP had approximately 950 hospi-

Copyright © 2005, Association for Professionals in Infection Control and Epidemiology, Inc.

tals participating in the QI project as of late 1994. As of 2004, there are 835 Acute Care hospitals, 250 Psychiatric, 88 Long Term Care and 22 Home Care facilities/agencies according to information on its Web site.Each hospital receives a summary of its own information along with a comparison of that information to the overall database. Participation is coordinated through state hospital associations and other hospital networks. Participating hospitals collect and provide their data through their sponsoring organization. Aggregate data are produced and provided to participants for their internal use. MHAQIP makes it clear that it is not conducting clinical research or outcome studies.[5] The MHAQIP includes several nosocomial infection indicators. It currently has indicators for acute, psychiatric, long-term, and home care. MHAQIP is also a qualified vendor for the JCAHO ORYX measures.

JCAHO began the development of its Indicator Measurement System as part of the "Agenda for Change" in 1989. Initial indicators were common outcome measures such as mortality, surgical site infection rates, and adverse drug reactions. With pilot projects completed, the ORYX reporting system began in 1997. All accredited hospitals were required to select a data intermediary (vendor) and begin submitting at least four measures on a quarterly basis. These data are intended for comparison with other facilities, performance improvement, and the accreditation of hospitals. Beginning in January 2003, JCAHO instituted the next level of measures: CORE. CORE are designed around diagnostic groups such as acute myocardial infarct, community-acquired pneumonia, and heart failure.[6] Of interest to ICPs would be the pneumonia measures; patients who receive their first does of antibiotics within 4 hours after arrival at the hospital, patients older than 65 years who are screened for pneumococcal vaccine status, and patients who are administered vaccine prior to discharge. These are good examples of process indicators.

Under a new federal law, CMS provides an incentive to hospitals to submit quality performance data on 10 required quality measures to receive the full annual payment update (See Table 9–2). Since October 2003, CMS has reported data on a set of 10 hospital quality measures submitted voluntarily by hospitals on at the CMS Web site. Hospitals that do not participate in "Reporting Hospital Quality Data for Annual Payment Update" will receive a reduction of 0.4% in the annual payment update. To receive the full annual payment update, hospitals must register with a vendor and on their QualityNet Exchange. Data must be submitted beginning July 2004 for cases discharged after January 1, 2004.[7]

Table 9-2. CMS Voluntary Quality Measures[7]

CMS 10 measures in 3 disease areas are as follows:

- Heart attack (acute myocardial infarction)
  - Was aspirin given to the patient when upon arrival at the hospital?
  - Was aspirin prescribed when the patient was discharged?
  - Was a beta-blocker given to the patient upon arrival at the hospital?
  - Was a beta-blocker prescribed when the patient was discharged?
  - Was an ACE Inhibitor given for the patient with heart failure?
- Heart failure
  - Did the patient get an assessment of his or her heart function?
  - Was an ACE Inhibitor given to the patient?
- Pneumonia
  - Was an antibiotic given to the patient in a timely way?
  - Had a patient received a pneumococcal vaccination?
  - Was the patient's oxygen level assessed?

The NNIS system of CDC was "established in 1970 when selected hospitals in the United States began reporting their nosocomial infection surveillance data for aggregation into a national database."[9] Because nosocomial infections are considered to be valid QI measures by most health care practitioners, the ICP should be very familiar with the most recent NNIS publications. NNIS currently monitors (1) site-specific nosocomial infection rates in patients at risk in intensive care units (e.g., ventilator-associated pneumonias) and (2) surgical site infection rates, stratified by a risk index that is tailored to the population of patients undergoing a specific surgical procedure. The current NNIS methodology is a useful benchmark against which nosocomial infection QIs from other sponsors can be compared.[8,9]

Important Concepts in Evaluating QIs

Use of Outcome or Process Indicators

Quality measures are usually believed to be related to processes or outcomes. In the pursuit of quality, most organizations include an analysis of a variety of events or complications that occur during or after care. Some of these events may not be related directly to an outcome per se [e.g., percentage of residents who have/had a catheter inserted and left in the bladder (CMS Nursing Home measure) or the frequency of central line dressing changes]. Those events that are not directly related to an outcome are considered process measures. Many organizations further divide outcomes into 3 types of outcome indicators; cost, quality, and satisfaction. Cost is an outcome indicator that reflects efficiency and is believed to be helpful in understanding the balance between cost and benefit. Satisfaction indicators, a subset of outcomes, are an assessment of how well the primary customer, the patient, was satisfied by his or her care. The use of nos-

Copyright © 2005, Association for Professionals in Infection Control and Epidemiology, Inc.

ocomial infections as QIs are at the top of the indicator list and are generally better accepted due to their longer history of use and comfort with definitions and data collection methodologies.

Process indicators do not measure a patient outcome but rather a step in the care process. They can be useful to evaluate quality if they can be linked to an outcome measure (e.g., urinary tract infection, wound infection, or bacteremia). Process indicators may be worthwhile if the outcome to be measured is rare in occurrence. Intravascular device associated bacteremias are associated with aseptic insertion, dressing changes, line changes, and the like. Process measures are also helpful in evaluating the effectiveness of an educational effort as a measure of behavior (e.g., compliance with dressing change or handwashing policy). Many process measures can be taken directly from the CDC's Infection Prevention guidelines. Its category 1 and 2 recommendations lend themselves well to this type of monitoring.

For instance, the category 1A recommendation for administration of a pre-operative antibiotic appropriate to the type of surgery prior to surgical site incision.[10(p267)]

Selection of QIs

The question of what makes an indicator an accurate measure of quality is difficult to answer without a universally accepted definition. In the absence of a definition, there can be an active evaluation of various indicators and a finding of best fit or best business strategy. "Perhaps the best approach would be to ask the question: As the indicator's performance improves (e.g., decrease in the occurrence of adverse events such as nosocomial infections), do patient outcomes improve as well?"[4(p310)] The answer to this question can only be found through analysis and trial of the chosen indicators. The NNIS study[11] noted that those hospitals participating in NNIS had more improvement in nosocomial rates over time than did their counterparts who were not participating. It also found that NNIS participants had more ICP hours per patient bed, a process measure, and more active involvement by their ICPs in clinical operations, teams, and planning.

Indicator rates may change because of changes unrelated to changes in quality, such as a change in the case mix or in the system of case finding.[4] As changes in demographics, the baby boomer population, and local economics occur, the case-mix and severity of illness for patient populations may change. However an organization chooses to define quality and no matter which QIs it selects, it is important that the decision is made, supported, and funded by the highest levels. Several data collection systems that most facili-

ties are already participating in (JCAHO ORYX/CORE measures, CMS, and NNIS) have been discussed already. Many states also have mandatory reporting. These state indicators should be collected, analyzed, and used for board reports, clinical programs, and department- and practitioner-level quality improvement. Gray reports in his book, *Evidence-Based Healthcare*, that "Every decision will have to be based on a systematic appraisal of the best evidence available."[12]

Definition of an Indicator, Numerator, and Denominator

The numerator can be defined as the event being tracked (e.g., a patient fall, wound infection, intravenous dressing change). The selection of specific nosocomial infections as QIs should focus on those QIs that have clear-cut definitions, are supported by prior studies, and can be applied readily in most hospitals. They also should be considered clinically important in a given patient population. In addition, they may need to be amenable to risk stratification.[12-14] "No indicator can be perfectly appropriate for every institution or for every patient population. It is also important to avoid overly broad indicators, such as all nosocomial infections."[4(p311)] Some important indicators such as pneumonia may be difficult to measure accurately. Nosocomial pneumonia is a cause of significant hospital morbidity, yet the clinical case definition of nosocomial pneumonia is neither sensitive nor specific; conversely, nosocomial urinary tract infections are easily defined and detected[15] but are infrequently important factors in patient morbidity or mortality. Table 9–3 compares several factors that are important when selecting specific nosocomial infections as indicator events.[4]

The denominator is the patient population at risk of experiencing the event defined in the numerator. The selection of denominators for the indicator events (and definition of a time period, i.e., with in

Table 9-3. Factors Important in selecting numerators[a]

- Clear case definition
- Ease of specimen collection
- Ease of Surveillance; laboratory, clinical, relative frequency
- Importance of the event: morbidity and mortality
- Potential of interventions to reduce rates
- Ease of stratification; exposure risk factors, severity of illness
- Denominator by device days
- Availability; ease of data collection and/or detection

[a] Adapted from An approach to the evaluation of Quality Indicators of the Outcome of Care in Hospitalized Infection Indicators. The quality Indicator Study Group, *Infect Control Hosp Epidemiol* 16:308–316, 1995.[4]

Copyright © 2005, Association for Professionals in Infection Control and Epidemiology, Inc.

30 days) allows the development of indicator rates (numerator/denominator rate). Two important decisions in developing or selecting a denominator are how specific to be and how to stratify patients by their risk factors.[4]

The specificity should include the decision to use patient discharge, patient-days, or device-days. The denominator chosen needs to be applicable, easy to collect, and timely. Examples of indicator events are hospital discharges, hospital admissions, patient-days for hospital or unit, exposure days to a certain device, prescriptions, or doses of medications.

Because rates may be tracked over time and compared among units, services, and institutions, it may be important to stratify the data by separating it into homogeneous subgroups. Usually, the more specific the stratification, the more meaningful the comparison. For example, surgical site infection rates can be divided into groupings, or strata, that account for differences in infection risk.

> Stratifying on a composite risk score that considers general physical status (for example, the American Society of Anesthesiologists preoperative classification score), wound contamination classification, and/or the length of the procedure may produce more meaningful comparisons than lumping all wound infection numerators together or stratifying on wound class alone. [4,13,14]

Feasibility and Ease of Data Collection

The size of the list of QIs must be manageable for a hospital's resources.

> For broad application, QI data elements must be amenable to accurate and consistent collection. Benefits gained or lost by adding or deleting specific elements must be weighed carefully. The evaluation of benefit should reflect the likelihood that the additional information will assist in clinical decision making and, ultimately, in improved outcomes. Limited resources ordinarily would be directed toward issues (1) for which documentation exists that correlates data collection and reporting with improved outcomes,[15] (2) having the greatest theoretic potential for improvement, or (3) having the most grave consequences.[4(p 313)]

Human resources, staffing needs, data collection, and analysis of personnel hours should also be considered. The development of guidelines for staff allocation is a critical research item for any QI system. Researchers have the tendency to say, "While we are in the patient chart, let's collect this . . . ." This thinking can rapidly add complexity and significant cost to the data collection process. Questions that should be asked include the following: Who already has these data? Who already has a need to review this record? What database do we have that could give us a framework to build on? Frequently after asking these questions, researchers, ICPs, or quality staff may find that they can piggyback to an existing data collection process or data set.

Reliability of Data Collection

To be useful, QIs must be able to be collected in a reliable and reproducible method. "Reliability may be defined as the degree to which the QI correctly identifies the targeted event. Reproducibility evaluates whether the findings can be repeated consistently when applied to new populations, to different institutions, or by different individuals." [4(p 313)] Collection methods should have a high degree of inter-rater reliability, which means two raters (surveillance staff) reviewing the same set of information could consistently classify the QIs in the same way. Any new data collection method should be tested. A recommended process includes a data collection template, tested on a sample of charts (10 to 30 is reasonable), then application of the methodology. It is important to build in regular reevaluation intervals to allow the tool or method to be revised to support accurate data collection. Another process might be to build in regular reaudits by impartial auditors or collectors. An ICP group might bring charts to a central meeting and pass the charts around the room to ICPs from another facility for review to determine if the same data could be abstracted.

Definitions and data collection procedures need to be agreed on and put in writing. Those written documents should include enough detail to support consistent methods, whether for 1 or numerous data collectors.[4,7] In the IHCexperience discussed previously, it has a system whereby the definitions of numerators, denominators, and data collection methodologies are not only in writing but also available on the Web site in documents that can be searched, shared, and reproduced.[16] This system supports consistent training and strict adherence to criteria. Regular data audits to ensure validity are required by JCAHO and CMS for their measurement systems and should be a part of any QI system.

The limitations of small sample sizes also should be considered. While the data collected may be accurate, analyses and subsequent conclusions may be limited by small numbers in the studied population. Organizations with small populations are limited, and few guidelines exist regarding how to address the evaluation of QIs in such settings.[4] Some studies propose using process measures that have documented association with specific high-quality outcomes. Since the outcome is so uncommon, monitoring of process measures that have

Copyright © 2005, Association for Professionals in Infection Control and Epidemiology, Inc.

been documented to prevent the untoward outcome would be more appropriate. The CDC guideline for prevention of infectionsis an excellent source of process measures that can be used. Examples are observation of handwashing, frequency of central line dressing changes, and administration of the preoperative prophylactic antibiotic. Even with large numbers, sometimes the use of risk stratification methods can result in small numbers in some risk strata, thus limiting comparisons and use of the data.

Accuracy and Completeness of Data Collection

Equally important to reliability and accuracy of the collected data is the completeness of data collection. Every system should have explicit written descriptions of data collection methods that minimize ad hoc, off-the-cuff decisions. Surveillance intensity must be consistent if data are to be compared over time or among institutions. Some additional questions that you will need to consider are related to frequency, reliability, staff involved, and data sources. Are you collecting prevalence data or incidence data? Are you collecting data using the same staff members or are multiple staff members involved? Are data collected the same way when the facility has suboptimal staffing or uncovered absences of the data collection personnel? Treating data collection as a low-priority activity may result in retrospective chart reviews when concurrent data collection is the preferred method. Inadequate computer, programmer, and data input staff resources and incomplete chart information or availability also may affect the completeness and accuracy. In addition, data gleaned from computer data bases can be significantly affected by new coding staff and a different level of education or experience.

Methods should be in place to verify the completeness of ongoing monitoring.

> These would be linked to reliability determination procedures and should be formalized and performed routinely. If healthcare systems, consortia, or other bodies aggregate data from multiple institutions, these data quality monitors are mandatory, and commitment to them should be part of the initial enrollment prerequisites. Without validation of completeness and accuracy of data, comparisons by aggregating systems probably are meaningless and, potentially, very misleading. [4]

"Measures should also be incorporated to verify the accuracy of data gleaned from automated databases."[4(p 312)] By using of an overreading process for a sample of records, input by other staff, appropriate error checks in the software, and by methods to determine data integrity routinely. These methods for database validation also need to be in writing and agreed upon. Case vignettes have been used to evaluate the accuracy of use of standard definitions of nosocomial infections.[17]

Timeliness of Data Collection and Reports

Data are most useful when the time between data collection and reporting is short. In terms of intrahospital use, rapid analysis of data is key to the ability to identify opportunities for improvement. Generation of timely internal reports is important to the function of supplying data useful by clinicians. The concept of "report cards" has gained popularity because leadership decides which measures need to be collected in "real time" and presented daily, weekly, or monthly. IHCs philosophy, Brent James, MD, is that "you manage what you measure."[16] Also important is the ability of the individual organization to generate its own analyses from data collected for the indicator system; this may require that centrally distributed software have ad hoc reporting capabilities or, at the least, generate data files of a known and standard format. The rapid reporting of data to an aggregating agency can assist in ensuring completeness of the overall database.

Training

"Implementation of a QI system should include not only formal training of those who will be collecting, analyzing, and communicating data, but also appropriate training of the management, leadership, trustees and medical staff." [4(p 312)] This supports an environment that will promote the implementation and use of the monitoring system. When senior managers are not aware of the implications of the QI system, including the resources required for its implementation and the appropriate use of data for comparative analyses, barriers to successful implementation and interpretation are likely to be encountered.

Ideally, training data collection personnel should include the opportunity to practice data abstraction, chart review, data entry, and the like, as well as to provide feedback on performance.[17,18] Training can be a critical aspect of ensuring the reliability and reproducibility of future data. Methods of appropriate training include formal courses with practice workshops to self-instructional methods, such as computer-assisted instruction,[18] to mentoring. The involvement of experts from the related field (e.g., for infection control indicators, experts in infection control and infectious diseases, as well as epidemiologists and other process experts) is key to the success of training is. [4]

Copyright © 2005, Association for Professionals in Infection Control and Epidemiology, Inc.

Comparability of Populations

Severity and Case-Mix Realities

When assessing a healthcare process or outcome indicator, adjustment for case-mix and severity is important.[19] Comparison of the performance of healthcare practitioners or institutions may be misleading without appropriate adjustment. The comparability among institutions of indicator results that have been severity adjusted cannot be assumed. Severity of illness indicators must be used with proper statistical methodology, or very misleading results can occur, as a group from Pennsylvania demonstrated.[20] Data comparison can be aided by including the severity or case-mix detail so that the receiving entity can test the data abstraction. It also enables the receiving entity to analyze its own data in a like manner. For example, if you chose to compare surgical site infection rates for the total number of hip patients, you would want the patients' age, co-morbidity, complications, antibiotic timing, and wound classification to more fairly compare patient populations.

The level to begin the comparison is also critical. If the level is too coarse, or "macro," the heterogeneity in the case-mix may be too great for meaningful comparison. If the level is too refined or "micro," the number of cases available for comparison is likely to be small, compromising the statistical power of the comparison.

> Within the diagnosis related group (DRG) system, a gradient of homogeneity exists. The progression from the least to the most homogeneous is as follows: MDC (Major Diagnostic Category), (DRG) Diagnosis Related Group, ICD-9-CM (*International Classification of Diseases, 9th Revision, Clinical Modification*) severity system score.[20] Since the advent and use of the APR-DRG classification system that enables a Severity of Illness (SOI) and Risk of Mortality (ROM) score helps classify patients into similar groups that the regular DRG and ICD-9 system do not allow.[4]

Comparison at the DRG level usually is a common starting place for analysis in an attempt to yield meaningful numbers, but the reliability of comparison at this level may not be great if the case-mix and severity vary significantly among the institutions being compared. As an example, consider mortality from pneumonia at 2 hospitals. Analysis could begin with all patients in DRG 89 [simple pneumonia and pleurisy: age >17 years with complications or comorbidity (C)] Cs and DRG 90 (simple pneumonia and pleurisy: age >17 years without CCs. The problem is that DRGs 89 and 90 include at least 15 different diagnostic codes, such as ICD-9-CM 481 (pneumococcal pneumonia), 482.9 (unspecified bacterial pneumonia), and 487.0 (influenza with pneumonia). One community hospital may have a preponderance of pneumococcal pneumonia patients (with low severity of illness scores) in the DRG, whereas the other hospital may have a large organ transplant service and many patients with unspecified bacterial pneumonia (and high severity of illness scores).

Available systems for assessing severity have different forms and uses.[19] Some systems are intended for almost all diseases, such as APACHE II or III or Medis-Groups.[20,21] Others are procedure specific, such as the NNIS risk index for surgical site infections.[10]

Internal Tracking Versus External Comparisons

Once an indicator has been determined to be appropriate for comparing healthcare practitioners within an institution, the decision as whether it is inappropriate for comparing results at two or more institutions needs to be made. Gray's book *Evidenced-Base Healthcare* gives excellent guidelines on how to benchmark, develop, and use outcomes.[12] An indicator always should be validated before any new use, particularly for comparisons with external sites. The data collection concepts discussed here would be important to reassess as data are compared across facilities. Are the data collected using the same methodologies, the same level of training, database, and chart reviews? Are the data collected concurrently or retrospectively? Local peer review organizations (PROs) can often help in this area. For example, CMS is currently conducting a feasibility study for hospital QIs in rural facilities. It has developed audit tools, methodologies, and definitions. CMS has completed initial training of data collectors and is in the process of validating those chart reviews. Each facility abstracts a small number of charts, then submits the data collected and a copy of the chart to HealthInsight, the Utah PRO, and StratisHealth the Minnesota PRO. The next step is to audit those records to determine whether an independent reviewer can glean the same data from those charts. Once this process is complete, each hospital will then re-collect their data and resubmit to HealthInsight.[22]

Before using a reported indicator rate as a benchmark, it is critical to know whether the setting and data collection techniques are comparable. For example, was surveillance at the benchmarking institution comparable to the other institutions? Are the definitions of disease and risk comparable? Given that true benchmarking requires knowing who is "best in class" for a given outcome or process, you need to be able to determine who the "best" is so they can be used as a resource to improve care. Most comparative databases do not identify the reporting institutions so that true benchmarking is not possible. Usually results at an organization simply are compared with the range of results reported by similar institutions. Large severity-adjusted databases

Copyright © 2005, Association for Professionals in Infection Control and Epidemiology, Inc.

have been gathered by commercial healthcare organizations.[20,23-26]

Appropriate statistical testing should be part of both internal and external comparison exercises. This is critical especially when comparative data are used in the process of credentialing and privileging individual practitioners or in institutional accreditation. Further, accurate analysis of data can ensure that resources are directed toward clinically important issues.[4]

Sharing Methods and Data in the Medical Literature

In the United States, many organizations have supported the development of guideline and indicator outcome activities. Differing methodologies and nomenclatures have been employed. Some have been specifically for or related to infection control. To avoid duplication and to increase effectiveness and the timely implementation of the use of indicators and guidelines, it is important to share methodologies, analyses, and results across a wide population of users.

The Institute of Medicine of the National Academy of Science published a monograph in 1990 reviewing the development and use of clinical practice guidelines.[2] This report listed desirable attributes of guidelines and the medical review criteria used in their development. These qualities may be considered as equally important features of indicators. They include validity, reproducibility, clinical applicability, flexibility, clarity, sensitivity, specificity, feasibility, and documentation of the methods used in development and of the evidence used for assumptions. The Institute of Medicine further published, *To Err is Human* in 1999 and *Crossing the Quality Chasm* in 2001, which built on the previous recommendations.[1,2] These subsequent reports give specific recommendations as to how healthcare as a business and healthcare organizations can begin to build the structural and strategic bridges to better quality.[27]

Many authors recommend the development of indicators by using a consistent process that allows good benchmarking, identification of best practice, team involvement, and iterative process improvement. Steps might include the following: (1) an in-depth review of the literature regarding the topic or diagnostic group you have decided to focus on, (2) presentation of the findings of the review to a panel of experts or clinical team, (3) development of a consensus, (4) pilot testing, (5) data analysis and aggregation, and (6) next steps or process changes.[1,2,5,12,16,27]

Once completed, indicators must be piloted or field tested. Pilot testing may be through retrospective cohort studies, but subsequent field testing (the so-called alpha and beta testing) should be accomplished under actual practice conditions with the intended data collectors, not research personnel. Results of these analyses should be shared with the expert development group, and corrections should be made to improve efficacy and efficiency. Many indicators and guidelines do not perform well outside the artificial development environment and fail at this point. Indicators surviving these tests are ready for release.

Successfully developed indicators must be disseminated widely to the appropriate users. One method of ensuring another level of quality review and broad dissemination to the practicing field is the presentation of indicators in peer-reviewed scientific journals respected by the targeted users.

Relation to Quality Improvement

Accurate indicator data that include nosocomial infections can be useful and supportive of quality improvement efforts within an organization. In the CQI/TQM paradigm, clinical decisions are based on data that are gathered and analyzed over time using appropriate statistical tools and feedback to clinicians. CQI efforts can address both endemic levels of disease (as common-cause variation), as well as epidemic levels of disease (as special cause variation). Good epidemiology is as important for use of data internally as it is for external comparisons.[4(p 314)]

Indicator systems can measure outcomes, such as infections; in addition, related processes also are of interest in the CQI world. Multidisciplinary teams can address the multivariate nature of the risk of infections in an effort to improve both processes and their associated outcomes.[1,2]

As institutions aggregate surveillance data on nosocomial infection rates to use for interhospital comparisons, debate among hospital epidemiologists, infection control professionals, and quality staff continues as to which indicators best reflect true quality.[12] At the time of the publication of the QI study group findings, participation in a multihospital surveillance system was not as common as it is now. For example, those facilities that hold JCAHO accreditation status are now required to select indicators and collect and submit their data per JCAHO requirements. CMS recently launched its Nursing Home Compare Web site (http://www.medicare.gov) to provide consumers with rates on many indicators that reflect the overall quality of nursing homes and skilled care centers in their communities. CMS is also beginning data collection for the National Voluntary Hospital Reporting Initiative.

The decision to participate is no longer optional. The decision as to which indicators should be used for your organization's patient population should be discussed

Copyright © 2005, Association for Professionals in Infection Control and Epidemiology, Inc.

at all levels—from senior management to front-line caregivers. There must be a link between the collection of such data and your organization's continuous improvement strategy support clinical teams use of data to improve the quality of healthcare. "One of the main reasons total quality management has failed to transform health care as it has other industries, is the lack of investment in outcome measurement."[16] In Thompson's 2000 report in the Journal on Quality Improvement, he reported on a case study at Intermountain Health Care (IHC) in Salt Lake City. In 1997, IHC made a strategic decision to implement clinical quality teams around its key clinical process areas, such as cardiovascular, women and newborn services, and primary care services. Guidance teams with administrative, nursing, and medical staff participation chose indicators of process and outcome for high-volume and high-risk diagnostic groups and developed systems for reporting of those indicators widely. IHC instituted processes for regular, timely reports that can be aggregated across the corporation and each of its 21 hospitals or detailed to an individual practitioner level. These reports are published in hard copy and are available electronically on the IHC intranet. Further, Thompson stated that, "Health care executives will not willingly invest in outcomes until they believe that the outcomes have business value."[16(p 585)]

II.   SUMMARY AND CONCLUSION

This chapter has endeavored to identify many QIs and systems in use, to present concepts and guidelines for development of indicators, and to share methods for use in healthcare. Existing indicator systems are in a constant state of flux and development so that producing a listing comparing current systems would be difficult, if not impossible. The NNIS system, however, is well developed, as noted in the bibliography, and can provide excellent guidance to ICPs. QI "report cards" for evaluation of outpatient, home health, long-term, and managed care systems are recently deployed and could provide good examples for ICPs wanting to refine and enhance their system of monitoring. ICPs' use of the epidemiological approach provides a sound framework for participation in organizational quality improvement programs and strategies.

REFERENCES

1. Kohn LT, Corrigan JM, and Donaldson MS, editors: *To Err Human: Building a Safer Health System,* Washington, DC, 1999, Institute of Medicine, National Academy Press.
2. IOM: *Crossing the Quality Chasm,* Washington, DC, 2001, Institute of Medicine, National Academy Press.
3. Scheckler WE: Interim report of the quality indicator study group, *Am J Infect Control* 23:215–222, 1995.
4. An approach to the evaluation of quality indicators of the outcome of care in hospitalized infection indicators. The Quality Indicator Study Group, *Infect Control Hosp Epidemiol* 16: 308–316, 1995.
5. Vibbert S, Strickland D, Migdail K, et al: Major projects–Maryland quality indicator project. In Vibbert S, et al., editors: The 1995 *medical outcomes and guidelines sourcebook*: A progress report and resource guide on medical outcomes research and practice guidelines: Developments, data, and documentation, New York, 1994, Faulkner & Gray, pp 29–31.
6. Joint Commission for Accreditation of Healthcare Organizations: Specifications manual for national implementation of hospital core measures, _Chicago, 2003, JCAHO.
7. CMS Announces Guidelines for Reporting Hospital Quality Data, *Medicare News.* January 28, 2004.
8. Emori TG, Culver CH, Horan TC, et al: National Nosocomial Infections Surveillance (NNIS) system: Description of surveillance methodology, *Am J Infect Control* 19:19—35, 1990.
9. Solomon S, Horan T, et al: National Nosocomial Infections Surveillance (NNIS) System repot, data summary from January 1992 through June 2003, *Am J Infect Control* 8;ZS481–498, 2003.
10. Mangram JA, Horan TC, Pearson ML, Silver LC, Jarvis WR: Guideline for Prevention of Surgical Site Infections, 1999. Hospital Infection Control Practices Advisory Committee, *Infect Control Hosp Epidemiol* 4:247–278, 1999.
11. Richards, C, Emori, TG, Edwards J, Fridkin S, Tolson J, Gaynes R: Characteristics of hospitals and infection control professionals participating in the National Nosocomial Infections Surveillance System, *Am J Infect Control* 29:400–403, 2001.
12. Gray, JAM: *Evidence-based healthcare.* Churchill Livingstone, 1997, NewYork.
13. New classification of physical status, *Anesthesiology* 24:111, 1963.
14. Owens WD, Felts JA, Spitznagel EL Jr: ASA physical status classification: A study of consistency of ratings, *Anesthesiology* 49: 239—243, 1978.
14. Culver DH, Horan TC, Gaynes RP, et al: Surgical wound infection rates by wound class, operation, and risk index in U.S. hospitals, 1986—1990, *Am J Med* 91(suppl 3B):152S-157S, 1991.
15. Garner JS, Jarvis WR, Emori TG, Horan TC, Hughes JM: CDC definitions for nosocomial infections, *Am J Infect Control* 16: 128–40, 1988.
16. Thompson DI, Sirio C, Holt P: The strategic use of outcome information, *Jt Comm J Qual Improv* 26:576–586, 2000.
17. Larson E, Horan T, Cooper B, Kotilainen HR, Landry S, Terry B: Study of the definition of nosocomial infections (SDNI), *Am J Infect Control* 19:259—267, 1991.
18. Lancaster D, Willis MA: Computer-assisted instruction (CAI): A time-saving, individualized teaching methodology, *Am J Infect Control* 22:179—181, 1994
19. Gross PA: Use of severity of illness indices. In Mayhall G, editor: *Hospital epidemiology and infection control,* Baltimore, 1995,Williams & Wilkins. 20. Localio AR, Hamory BH, Sharp TJ, et al: Comparing hospital mortality in adult patients with pneumonia: A case study of statistical methods in a managed care program, *Ann Intern Med* 122:125—132, 1995.
21. Iezzoni LI, Hotchkin EK, Ash AS, Schwartz M, Mackiernan Y: MedisGroups databases: The impact of data collection guidelines on predicting in-hospital mortality, *Med Care* 31:277—283, 1993.
21. Rural Health Network Development Technical Assistance Program, Office of Rural Health Policy (ORHP). http://networkassist.ruralhealth.hrsa.gov
23. HCIA-Sachs Institute: *The guide to hospital performance,* Baltimore, 1993, HCIA.
24. Fine MJ, Singer DE, Hanusa BH, Lave JR, Kapoor WN: Validation of a pneumonia prognostic index using the MedisGroups comparative hospital database, *Am J Med* 94:153—159, 1993.
25. *Acuity index method database,* San Mateo, Calif, 1993, lameter.
26. Berwick DM: The clinical process and the quality process, *Qual Manag Health Care* 1:1–8, 1992.
27. O'Leary DS: The measurement mandate: Report card day is coming, *Jt Comm J Qual Improv* 19:487—491, 1993.

Copyright © 2005, Association for Professionals in Infection Control and Epidemiology, Inc.

SUPPLEMENTAL RESOURCES

Quality Indicator Project: http://www.qiproject.org

CDC Guidelines & Recommendations Prevention of Healthcare-Associated Infections: http://www.cdc.gov/ncidod/hip/Guide/guide.htm

The Official U.S. Government Site for People with Medicare: http://www.medicare.gov/default.asp

Centers for Medicare and Medicaid Services Web site: www.cms.hhs.gov

Copyright © 2005, Association for Professionals in Infection Control and Epidemiology, Inc.

10

REVISED 2004

Accrediting and Regulatory Agencies

Judene Bartley, MS, MPH, CIC
Vice President, Epidemiology Consulting
Services, Inc.
Beverly Hills, Michigan

ABSTRACT

This chapter presents administrative issues for infection prevention and control programs (IPCPs) and addresses historical and current pressures affecting accrediting and regulatory agencies at all levels affecting IPCPs. A brief description of the agencies, their relationships to each other, and their impact on the IPCP is provided, including a table with contact and Web site information for retrieval of more information.

KEY CONCEPTS

- The Agency for Healthcare Research and Quality (AHRQ) was charged with developing a plan to reduce adverse patient outcomes and improve the safety of healthcare workers and patients.

- The focus on medical safety continues to develop in healthcare organizations across the United States and includes all aspects of IPCP.

- Accrediting agencies, such as JCAHO, encourage organizations to place more emphasis on IPCP.

- There has been increasing collaboration among federal agencies and new partnerships among the federal agencies and private and professional organizations to develop performance measures and improve consumers' ability to compare healthcare delivery.

- To function effectively, infection control professionals (ICPs) require a basic knowledge of the key agencies.

- Most agencies with impact on infection control programs emanate from the executive branch, primarily within the Department of Health and Human Services (DHHS) and its major divisions of the Public Health Service (PHS): Centers for Disease Control and Prevention (CDC), National Institute for Occupational Safety and Health (NIOSH), Food and Drug Administration (FDA), Health Resources and Service Administration (HRSA), National Institutes of Health (NIH), Agency for Toxic Substances and Disease Registry (ATSDR), Agency for Healthcare Research and Quality (AHRQ), and a separate department, the Centers for Medicare and Medicaid Services (CMS) , formerly known as the Health Care Financing Administration (HCFA).

Copyright © 2005, Association for Professionals in Infection Control and Epidemiology, Inc.

I. BACKGROUND

Extraordinary change occurring in the healthcare field has had a profound effect on current infection prevention and control programs. In the past, regulatory changes have driven related policy development of infection prevention and control programs (IPCPs) (see Chapter 1: Infection Control and Prevention Program). Competitive forces have provided such impact that even voluntary accrediting agencies have effected program changes in all care sites, for example, acute care, extended care, pre- and post-hospital care, homecare, and ambulatory care clinics. Examples of historical changes affecting IPCPs throughout the 1990s and the present include:

- Joint Commission on Accreditation of Healthcare Organizations (JCAHO) standards published first in 1976 required hospitals seeking accreditation to have infection control programs.

- Development of the prospective payment system, a fixed payment hospital reimbursement system, motivated hospitals to prevent costly infections.

- SENIC: Publication of the results of the ten-year (1974–1983) Study on the Efficacy of Nosocomial Infection Control (SENIC) established the efficacy of hospital infection control programs.[1]

- The evolution of the AIDS epidemic challenged healthcare to meet the medical needs of a growing number of very ill patients and to address occupational concerns and educational needs of all healthcare workers.

- Managed care systems and prospective payment system for long-term care continued throughout the 1990s, exerting pressure on resizing systems. This includes redesign of infection control programs for systems well beyond the borders of acute-care setting.

- Threats from emerging pathogens and bioterrorism had a major impact on IPCPs beginning in late 2001. The era was initiated with the dramatic event of *Bacillus anthracis* transmission through the U.S. Postal system, continuing with current planning responses to potential biological agents, such as smallpox. IPCPs played a major role in developing strategies for *Vaccinia* vaccination programs as part of the smallpox response plan. These major events along with responding to new and emerging pathogens, such as Severe Acute Respiratory Syndrome (SARS), added a major shift in priorities for programs already concerned with potential threats of an overdue influenza pandemic.

II. BASIC PRINCIPLES

The impact of the Institute of Medicine's (IOM) reports beginning in 1999 has had a dramatic affect in healthcare, focusing on the importance of the healthcare environment's effect on patient outcomes.[2] The Agency for Healthcare Research and Quality (AHRQ) was charged with developing a plan to reduce adverse outcomes and improve the safety of workers and patients. This focus on medical safety continues to develop in healthcare organizations across the United States and includes all aspects of IPCP. Given this emphasis on patient safety, accrediting agencies, such as JCAHO, encourage organizations to place increasing focus on IPCP as evident in the most recent infection control (IC) standards revision. One very visible result has been increasing collaboration among federal agencies as well as increasing partnerships between the federal agencies and the private sector. These changes have a profound impact on IPCP. For example, federal agencies concerned with quality and/ or performance standards and guidelines (e.g., Centers for Medicare and Medicaid [CMS], Agency for Healthcare Research and Quality (AHRQ), Centers for Disease Control and Prevention [CDC]) are partnering with private and professional organizations, such as the American Hospital Association (AHA) and the National Quality Forum (NQF). The goal of the collaborative effort is development of similar performance measures in each care setting, improving the consumer's ability to compare healthcare delivery in similar care sites. One such initiative is the public reporting on several quality measures in hospitals, nursing homes and home care, all of which include infection-related complications. These efforts grow continuously, and to function effectively, infection control professionals (ICPs) require a basic knowledge of the key agencies and an understanding of their relationship to each other and to their specific program.

III. ACCREDITING AND REGULATORY AGENCIES

Against this backdrop, the federal and state agencies remain a powerful influence, and their relationships within the government structure are described briefly. A summary table (Table 10–1) accompanies the following explanatory remarks, provides a quick reference guide for easy access, and includes the current address for online resources (URL) available at the time of publication.

Government Agencies and Activities

Governmental agencies can be placed organizationally in terms of their relationship to the three branches of the United States government. That is, agencies fit as

Copyright © 2005, Association for Professionals in Infection Control and Epidemiology, Inc.

Table 10-1. Regulatory Compliance: Accreditation, Regulatory and Professional Agencies, National and State Agencies with Impact on Infection Control and Epidemiology Programs

Major Dept. or Agency	Specific Agency	Programs or AHJ*	Phone, Fax, or Online Resource	Regulatory or Voluntary	Key Rules/Impact	Comment
Executive Branch PHS Health & Human Services: Public Health Services	Centers for Disease Control & Prevention **CDC**	National Center for Infectious Diseases **NCID**	http://www.cdc.gov	Not regulatory but often perceived as regulatory in the sense of setting a "community standard"	Multiple guidelines; travel medicine; emerging pathogens program; antibiotic usage	Publishes guidelines; major impact on acute care and multiple care delivery settings
PHS	CDC	Hospital Infections Program DHQP	www.cdc.gov/ncidod diseases/hip/hip.htm	Not regulatory; as above	NNIS/NHSN: surveillance program; antibiotic usage	Source of national comparative data for NIR rates and data
PHS	CDC				Dialysis; occupational exposure to HIV; disinfection and antiseptics	Guidelines and support for practice areas
PHS	CDC	Hospital infection control program advisory committee **HICPAC**	http://access.gpo.gov/su_doc/index.html (To access guidelines published in the federal register)	Not regulatory; as above	Advises CDC on patient care guidelines	Also published in journals (isolation, VRE, pneumonia, IV; HCW, environmental infection control guidelines)
PHS	CDC	Advisory Committee on Immunization practices **ACIP**	www.cdc.gov/nip	Not regulatory; as above	Sets guidelines for immunization practices	"Gold Standard" for vaccination recommendations
Executive Branch PHS Health & Human Services: Public Health Services	CDC	Agency for Toxic Substances and Disease Registry **ATSDR**	www.cdc.gov/publications/atsdr	Not regulatory; guidance for communities; hospitals Haz substances; EP planning	Issues related to medical waste & definitions; safety planning for hazardous materials	Agency defined medical waste: 1990 Report to congress
PHS	CDC	Public Health Emergency Preparedness and Response	www.bt.cdc.gov	Not regulatory; as above	Provides guidance education, training biological, chemical agents, national pharmaceutical stockpile	This is a coordinating function involving many divisions, e.g., immunization
PHS	Food & Drug Administration **FDA**	Safe Medical Device Act **SMDA** Safe Blood Supply (both FDA and CDC) Food safety for all but meat, poultry, & eggs	www.fda.gov	Regulatory; Enforces SMDA (germicides as antiseptics; medical devices); medical device systems; food contamination (**HAACP**- See USDA)	Interaction with safety enforcement and recalls; needle device safety, per health department; OSHA	Major focus on needles; surgical implants; latex issues; sterile gloves; medical devices, including reuse of single use devices (SUD)
PHS	Health Resources and Services Administration **HRSA**	Health Delivery Services	www.hrsa.gov	Regulatory; National Practitioner data bank; Organ procurement transplant/funding aspects	Licensure; privileges meet conditions for funding (Ryan White funding)	Report of adverse actions; may include infection-related events

(Continued)

Table 10-1. Continued

Major Dept. or Agency	Specific Agency	Programs or AHJ*	Phone, Fax, or Online Resource	Regulatory or Voluntary	Key Rules/Impact	Comment
PHS	Agency for Healthcare Research and Quality **AHRQ**	AHRQ Guidelines	www.ahrq.gov	Not regulatory; guidelines may heavily impact reimbursement; adopted by CMS	AHRQ guidelines include protocols and pathways; affects Medicare programs	Multiple guidelines related to IC, e.g., pressure sores; UTI, HIV/AIDS; Quality measures
PHS	National Institutes of Health **NIH** National Library of Medicine **NLM**	Improve health of nation 14 research institutes	www.nih.gov/ www.nih.nlm.gov	Not regulatory; Major research in all areas; transfusion safety impacts regulations	NIAID Allergy & Infectious Disease; Natl. heart lung blood institute; National Library of Medicine	Impact on national health goals; Agenda: emerging pathogens program
PHS	Center for Medicare and Medicaid **CMS** (Separate branch)	Oversight for Medicare/Medicaid Participation: Conditions	www.cms.gov (Access for Medicare databases for LTC, homecare)	Regulatory; hospital certificate; quality screens; (Mortality IC & QA Standards); CLIA	Enforces "Safe & Sanitary" facility by Infection Control; CLIA for labs and offices.	CMS Rules; QA finalized January 10, 2003
Executive Branch EPA Environmental Protection Agency	Independent agency **EPA**	Regulated Medical Waste **RCRA** Antimicrobial pesticides	http://www.epa.gov/oppad001/chemregindex.htm Antimicrobial hotline: 1 (703) 308-0127 (9–5 M-F)	Regulatory; disinfectant/cleaner versus FDA & antiseptics; medical devices; Pesticides FIFRA	Med. waste regs. & incinerators chemical cleaner disinfectant; hotline for antimicrobial pesticides	Major impact on programs for waste disposal; claims for chemical cleaners disinfectant; and label checks
Executive Branch DOL Department of Labor	Occupational Health & Safety **DOL-OSHA**	General Safety & Health Standards	www.osha.gov	Regulatory; bloodborne pathogens; environmental chemical germicides	Enforces universal precautions; HBV vaccination offer; BBP exposure follow-up	Enforced by federal OSHA or by states with state-plan OSHA agency
Executive Branch DOL Department of Labor	**OSHA**			Regulatory; May enforce under the general duty clause	Enforces CDC TB guideline with a CPL based on general duty clause.	Enforced in states by state plan OSHA agencies; 20 states have own plan
Executive Branch DOT Department of Transportation	Independent agency **DOT**	Research & Special Programs **RSPA**	www.dot.gov	Regulatory; Regulates hazardous and medical waste crossing state lines.	Regulates infectious substances; impact on state regulations for medical waste	Enforcer for regulated medical waste crossing state lines
Executive Branch USDA Department of Agriculture	Independent agency **USDA**	Food Safety Inspection Service **FSIS**	www.usda.fsis.gov	Regulatory; Food inspections for commercial food providers	Recall of food products; enforcement	Healthcare facility cafeterias inspected if serving the public; may use local health dept.
Legislative Branch **Congress** Congressional information agencies	**Congress – GAO** Expenditures; Government Accounting Office	Provides Congress with information on public spending **GAO**	www.gao.gov	Not regulatory; Informational	Reports, e.g., one evaluating VA versus non-VA Infection Control programs.	Resources about and for infection control, e.g., cost benefit of safer sharps devices
Legislative Branch **Congress** Congressional information agencies	**Congress OTA** Office of Technology Assessment *Closed in 1997*	Analytical arm for legislative policy makers **OTA**	*No current office*	Not regulatory; informational; APIC and other groups provided input to OTA	OTA: 1991 HIV in Workplace TB white paper	Resources for Infection Control in the past; information located from other government agencies

Category / Name	Description	Notes	URL	Status	Role / Enforcement	Core indicators / Comments
Voluntary Accreditation **JCAHO** Commission on Accreditation of Health Care Org.	Nongovernmental accreditation; **JCAHO**; NCQA equivalent for HMO systems	Outgrowth of AHA,ACS, AMA;ADA, ACP Oryx: 1998–99	www.jcaho.org	Voluntary; Gives deemed status for Medicare/Medicaid in lieu of CMS agent	Accredit for reimbursement; IC indicators; Sentinel event policy; enforces other's regulations	Core indicators include catheter-related BSI, UTI and ventilator-related pneumonia
Voluntary Accreditation **NCQA** National Committee on Quality Assurance	Nongovernmental accreditation **Other:** HMO **NCQA:** Accredits HMO and outpatient settings	Collaboration as of 1998 with JCAHO, AMAP for quality council & measurement	www.ncqa.org	Voluntary; provides for reimbursement agreements for private and possibly government funding	Accredit for reimbursement; HEDIS provides major measurement set used for HMO reimbursement	Indicators, such as immunization rates; infection control input critical
Voluntary Accreditation **Laboratory CAP COLA**	College of American Pathologists **CAP** Commission on Office Lab Accreditation **COLA**	Certifies Laboratories; JCAHO recognizes as 'deemed status'	www.cap.org www.cola.org	Voluntary; Standards set for Lab Tests	JCAHO or CAP or COLA required for 3rd party payer reimbursement to meet CLIA standards	Requirement for meeting basic of laboratory safety and infection control: UP; asepsis; medical waste
State Department(s) of public or community health	Disease Control; Laboratory Services	Infectious disease control services of some type	URL is state specific	Regulatory; CCD and reporting AIDS/HIV, HIV;MRSA VRE Guidelines	TB Testing; DNA typing; HIV reporting	Communicable disease reporting; immunization issues; state guidelines
States Agencies charged with health care facility enforcement	Enforcement of COP with Medicare/Medicaid; OBRA & ECF; Construction codes; Office of fire safety; Enforce CLIA	Licensing bureau	URL is state specific	Regulatory; Ventilation Codes; Authority for clinical & physical plant surveys	Enforces CMS CoP; State codes enforced (Role for JCAHO & deemed status)	CMS CON Facility review construction; state codes based on 96/97 AIA GD; enforces CLIA
State Agencies charged with enforcement of MW Incinerators	Medical Waste Program	State Plan Environmental quality of some type	URL is state specific	Regulatory; Medical Waste Hazardous/chem waste & incinerators	Incinerators & medical waste are controversial issue over dioxins	Major impact on medical waste program; safety programs
State- Plan-State Occupational Safety, Health Act	OSHA Occupational Health; Radiation Health	State Plan Occupational Safety & Health	URL is state specific	Regulatory; BBPR enforcement; TB enforcement	Major enforcer of CDC guidelines BBP and TB involving HCW	Enforces negative air pressure for TB control; RMW Occ injury for HCW
State- Plan- State Labor Department &/or Occ. Safety, Health Act	General Safety Labor: General Safety Program	State Plan Labor division	URL is state specific	Regulatory; Safety Programs; Workman Compensation; Levies fines	Labor inspections wall-to-wall surveys every 3–5 years involves IC.	Includes barrier-free hallways, trip hazards, etc.; impacts on isolation; traffic
Local Local Health Dept.	Jurisdiction may be separate from state health depts	Communicable Disease agency	URL is state specific links	Regulatory; communicable disease reporting and follow-up	Laboratory & infection control interaction	Reporting of CD according to local rules and regulations
Local Fire Marshall; Water jurisdiction	Departments of public health or city	Food, Water, Waste	URL is state-specific links	Regulatory; inspections for food safety, water department for effluent, etc.	IC and interaction with dietary, facility services, environmental services, etc.	Concerned with hazardous/chemical spills; mercury formaldehyde, etc., into waste water

* AHJ, authority having jurisdiction.

extensions of the legislative, executive, and judicial branches of governmental structures.[3] The accompanying table highlights the fact that most agencies with impact on infection control programs emanate from the *executive branch*, primarily within the Department of Health and Human Services (DHHS) and its major divisions of the Public Health Service (PHS): Centers for Disease Control and Prevention (CDC), National Institute for Occupational Safety and Health (NIOSH), Food and Drug Administration (FDA), Health Resources and Service Administration (HRSA), National Institutes of Health (NIH), the Agency for Toxic Substances and Disease Registry (ATSDR), the Agency for Healthcare Research and Quality (AHRQ), and a separate department, the Centers for Medicare and Medicaid Services (CMS) , formerly known as the Health Care Financing Administration (HCFA). Other independent, key agencies of the executive branch include the Department of Labor's (DOL) Occupational Safety and Health Administration (OSHA), the Environmental Protection Agency (EPA), the U.S. Department of Agriculture (USDA) and the Department of Transportation (DOT).

The *legislative branch* has two agencies important to Congress for communication; these include the Government Accounting Office (GAO) and the Office of Technology Assessment (OTA). However, the OTA office has been closed, and other resources provide the services.

Public Health Service

Centers for Disease Control and Prevention

CDC is responsible for providing leadership and direction in prevention and control of diseases and preventable conditions, and for responding to public health emergencies. CDC responded to a national anthrax mail scare and continues to provide critical direction and leadership for all aspects of programs involving bioterrorism and related agents, including massive smallpox vaccination programs. The Emerging Pathogens program has developed important initiatives in recent years and ranges from new pathogens to new levels of antimicrobial resistance, for example, vancomycin-resistant *Staphylococcus aureus* or VRSA. CDC provided major leadership with the World Health Organization (WHO) in responding to the SARS epidemic, identifying a new variant of corona virus with enormous public health implications around the world. As noted in the table, CDC publishes a number of guidelines that are applied to appropriate settings. Although many consider their recommendations "standard setting," they are not regulatory in nature nor are they enforced as regulatory standards.

The Division of Healthcare Quality Promotion, formerly the Hospital Infections Program

CDC's DHQP is one of ten divisions within the National Center for Infectious Diseases and is composed of three main branches: Epidemiology and Laboratory, Prevention, and Evaluation and Healthcare Outcomes. DHQP (1) conducts research, surveillance, investigations, laboratory and field studies of healthcare-associated infections as well as research on methods of preventing and controlling infections; (2) collects and processes clinical and environmental specimens; (3) rapidly diagnoses disease and identifies unusual sources of infection; (4) evaluates medical devices as sources of infection; and (5) analyzes and reports antimicrobial resistance.

- Dialysis: DHQP has primary responsibility for prevention of dialysis-associated disease, including guidance for equipment disinfection and other means of prevention of disease transmission. The Dialysis Surveillance Network (DSN), a voluntary national surveillance system monitoring bloodstream and vascular infections in adults and pediatrics was initiated by CDC in 1999.

- Disinfection and sterilization: DHQP develops disinfection and sterilization procedures and recommends broad strategies for proper use of sterilants, disinfectants, and antiseptics to prevent the transmission of infection in the healthcare environment. This includes both environmental and medical device issues.

- National surveillance of nosocomial infections and National Healthcare Safety Network: National surveillance of nosocomial infections begun in 1970, is conducted through DHQP's National Nosocomial Infections Surveillance System (NNIS) to estimate the magnitude and nature of nosocomial infections and to provide hospitals with comparative data to evaluate prevention and control efforts. DHQP is incorporating NNIS into a Web-based knowledge system identified as the National Healthcare Safety Network (NHSN). NHSN is a system for accumulating, exchanging, and integrating relevant information and resources to protect patients and promote healthcare safety. NHSN will eventually include the elements of NNIS, NaSH (National Surveillance System for Healthcare Workers) and DSN, forming an integrated data repository at CDC.

- Bloodborne pathogens: DHQP conducts studies on the nature, frequency, and risk factors for transmission of bloodborne pathogens in healthcare and develops guidelines to reduce these risks.

Copyright © 2005, Association for Professionals in Infection Control and Epidemiology, Inc.

Healthcare Infection Control Practices Advisory Committee (formerly Hospital Infection Control Practices Advisory Committee)

HICPAC was established in 1991 to provide guidance to CDC and develop guidelines on specific infection control practices in healthcare. Guidelines are published cooperatively in professional journals, including the *American Journal of Infection Control*. Drafts are usually published for comment in the Federal Register. The guidelines are used as major resources for policy development and modified for facility-specific needs; they are not regulatory in nature.

The Advisory Committee on Immunization Practices

ACIP was established in 1974 to provide guidance to CDC on the most appropriate application of antigens and related agents, for example, vaccines, antisera, and immunoglobulins, as well as to recommend specific immunization practices and strategies to improve national immunization efforts. Recommendations are published and updated in the *Morbidity and Mortality Weekly Report* (*MMWR*) as well as in periodic *MMWR Recommendations* and/or *Summaries*. The 1997 *Immunization of Health-Care Workers* guideline (*MMWR* 46 RR18) for healthcare workers was a joint initiative between ACIP and HICPAC.

The National Institute for Occupational Safety and Health

NIOSH was established by the 1970 Occupational Safety and Health Act. This agency conducts research on occupational hazards, provides technical assistance and recommendations to the Occupational Safety and Health Administration (OSHA), and participates in the training of occupational safety and health experts. However, its charge is based on a premise of determining "zero" risk of exposure, without being compelled to determine the cost/benefit of required interventions. Enforcement agencies like OSHA may accept or reject recommendations from NIOSH.

The Agency for Toxic Substances and Disease Registry

ATSDR is responsible for providing leadership and direction to programs and activities designed to protect both the public and workers from exposures to hazardous substances. Safety committees are familiar with its expertise and leadership in developing emergency preparedness programs. A notable activity of ATSDR involved medical waste and resulted in the 1990 report to Congress: "The Public Health Effects of Medical Waste." The agency concluded that the general public is not likely to be adversely affected by medical waste generated in the traditional healthcare setting.

The Food and Drug Administration

The FDA develops, implements, monitors, and enforces standards for the safety, effectiveness, and labeling of all drugs and biologics, including food, blood and blood products, medical and radiological devices, antimicrobial products, and chemical germicides used in conjunction with medical devices. Some confusion among the agencies with overlapping jurisdictions (FDA, EPA, and OSHA) for chemicals was addressed through memoranda of understanding related to enforcement concerns. Historically, the Environmental Protection Agency (EPA) was the organization in the federal government that registered new chemical sterilants. There were approximately forty formulations approved in the United States. Following the agreement between the EPA and FDA that sterilants and high-level disinfectants that were intended for use on medical devices would be the responsibility of the FDA, the FDA required all such products to be cleared by the 510 (k) process. As a result, there are fewer formulations on the market. FDA enforces final regulations governing reuse of single-use devices (SUDs).

- Blood safety: The FDA is responsible for the safety of the nation's blood supply. The FDA has specific standards for collection, testing, and distribution of blood as well as disposal of contaminated or untested blood. These standards apply to all facilities that have blood-banking operations and are being comprehensively revised.

- Chemical germicides: The FDA regulates chemical germicides that are formulated as antiseptics, preservatives, or drugs to be used on or in the human body, or as preparations to be used to inhibit microorganisms on the skin. Based on data voluntarily provided by the manufacturer, chemical germicides are divided into three categories: category I: safe and effective; category II: not safe or efficacious; and category III: insufficient data to categorize. Chemical germicides, when used in conjunction with specific medical devices, may also require FDA approval.

- Medical Device Act (1974) and Safe Medical Device Act (SMDA) of 1990: The Medical Device Act of 1974 required the classification of medical devices according to their potential to cause harm. The SMDA of 1990 expanded FDA's authority in this area by improving incident reporting, removing defective or dangerous devices in a timely manner, and ensuring that only safe and effective devices enter the marketplace.

The Health Resources Service Administration

HRSA provides leadership and support efforts to integrate health-service delivery programs with the public and private financing programs.

Copyright © 2005, Association for Professionals in Infection Control and Epidemiology, Inc.

- National Practitioner Data Base: The NPDB, created as part of the Health Care Quality Improvement Act of 1986, collects and disseminates information concerning adverse actions affecting physicians, dentists, and other healthcare professionals. Hospitals are required to report to the data bank adverse disciplinary actions against practitioners, query the bank every three years, and query again at the time of medical staff appointment.

- Organ Procurement: HRSA administers grant-supported programs such as operation of the Organ Procurement and Transplantation Network.

Agency for Healthcare Research and Quality

AHRQ is an agency developed by Congress to define the appropriateness or necessity of medical care. It was formerly known as the Agency for Healthcare Policy and Research and was reauthorized in 1999 by the Healthcare Research and Quality Act. Its mission is to assess and enhance the quality of medical care through outcomes research and development of clinical-practice guidelines. The role of this office has taken on a new dynamic with the 1999 publication of the Institute of Medicine's "First Do No Harm."[2] AHRQ was given the charge to coordinate all federal quality improvement efforts, provide health services research oversight, and lead this effort through the Quality Interagency Coordination Task Force (QuIC).

National Institutes of Health

NIH with its fourteen specialized institutes is responsible for improving the health of the nation. NIH is the world's largest biomedical research organization and maintains the National Library of Medicine, the world's largest center of medical literature.

Other Federal Agencies

Center for Medicare and Medicaid Services (formerly, Health Care Financing Administration)

CMS was established by DHHS in 1977 and is responsible for oversight and reimbursement monitoring of Medicare and Medicaid programs. Its regional offices maintain close working relationships with state health departments for enforcement activity.

- Infection Control Standards and Medicare/Medicaid: CMS maintains independent standards for infection control in hospitals, long-term care and home care facilities/agencies, and enforces compliance with these as conditions for certification and participation in Medicare and Medicaid Programs (COP).
  - Long-term care: Nursing homes were required in 1998 to transmit data electronically to CMS on each patient in a set of assessments termed

Minimum Data Set or MDS. This covers all aspects of patient care, including infections.
  - Home Care: CMS published a notice in the Federal Register (June 18, 1999) announcing the effective date for the mandatory use, collection, encoding, and transmission of the Outcome and Assessment Information Set (OASIS) to fulfill conditions of participation in Medicare and Medicaid for home health agencies as part of their quality assurance and improvement demonstration requirements. As recently as June 2002, CMS was making continued effort to reduce Medicare's paperwork requirements so that more attention can be focused on providing quality care to patients.
  - Acute Care: The most recent update affecting infection control was published in the Federal Register in December 1997. On January 24, 2003, CMS published the Final rule for Quality Assessment and Performance Improvement (FR 2003; Vol. 68(16): 3435–3455). New emphasis is being placed on performance standards and outcome measurements (e.g., healthcare-associated infection rates).

- Construction: Construction codes and standards for physical plant/environmental standards were revised with a new requirement for infection control input. The consensus Guideline is revised every few years, for example, 2001 *Guidelines for Design and Construction of Hospital and Health Care Facilities*, published jointly by the American Institute of Architects, Academy of Architecture for Health/Facilities Guideline Institute, with assistance from the Department of Health and Human Services.[4] Hospital construction and costs are directly related to the charge of CMS's mission. Although CMS does not adopt the Guidelines as regulations per se, the agency does concur with the recommendations. Each state may adopt the guidelines as a whole or may adapt it as a basis for their own state codes. CMS then enforces construction codes or the Guidelines through health department surveyors as agents of CMS for Conditions of Participation (COP) in Medical and Medicaid. (Refer to Chapters 108 and 106.) The 2001 Guidelines have expanded requirements for a documented "infection control risk assessment" or ICRA, including many issues beyond the determination of needed number of airborne infection isolation (AII) rooms.

- Deemed status and state exemptions: Healthcare facilities accredited by JCAHO, a voluntary agency, are deemed to be in compliance with CMS requirements and are exempted from routine federal or state inspections. CMS follows and validates approximately five percent of accredited hospitals following a facility survey. State health department surveyors

Copyright © 2005, Association for Professionals in Infection Control and Epidemiology, Inc.

enforce CMS Conditions for Participation (COP) in Medicare/Medicaid in facilities that have foregone voluntary accreditation, whether JCAHO or American Osteopathic Accreditation (AOA).

- Medicare Quality Improvement Organizations, formerly known as State Peer Review Organizations: Quality improvement organizations (QIO) operate under contract with CMS to ensure that medical services provided to Medicare patients in hospitals and certain outpatient settings are medically necessary and appropriate and meet recognized standards of care. Their approach has been moving from individual performance to that of trending and outcome measurements in line with CMS requirements. These organizations are key for collaborative efforts in developing and publishing public performance measures.

- Clinical Laboratory Improvement Act: In 1988, Congress passed legislation (CLIA 88,42 CFR 493) to amend the Clinical Laboratory Improvement Act (CLIA) of 1956. In 1992, CMS issued final regulations to implement the statutory authority granted by CLIA. Those regulations, which became effective in July 1, 1992, extend the scope of CLIA to all laboratory testing, including physician office labs and clinics, and mandate specific personnel, proficiency testing quality control, patient tests, management, and computer systems. There is still no umbrella organization to coordinate the standardization of accreditation standards of all entities awarding CLIA certificates. States typically enforce CLIA through CMS Licensing and Certification divisions of state health departments.

Environmental Protection Agency

The EPA is an independent agency responsible for regulation and registration of chemical germicides formulated as sterilants and disinfectants used on devices or environmental surfaces as part of the Federal Insecticide Fungicide and Rodenticide Act (FIFRA).

- EPA and FDA germicide responsibilities: The EPA and FDA have entered an interagency agreement to jointly test all registered sterilants, those products seeking registration, and those products (sterilants and hospital-type disinfectants) making unsubstantiated claims about controlling tuberculosis. Information regarding products and their approval status is routinely available from EPA's Hotline, both by fax and on the Internet.

- Resource Conservation and Recovery Act (RCRA): Through the RCRA of 1976, the EPA was designated the authority for developing regulation for management of solid waste, including regulated medical waste.

- Incinerators and medical waste: The EPA has been directed to develop and publish regulations on medical waste incinerators regarding emissions control and ash disposal as part of recent revisions of the Clean Air Act.

Occupational Safety and Health Administration

OSHA is a division of the U.S. Department of Labor. Its programs are administered under the jurisdiction of federal Occupational Safety and Health Act and through approved state plans.

- General Duty Clause: Basic to OSHA's activity is the general duty clause of the 1970 Occupational Safety and Health Act requiring that an employer is responsible for providing a workplace free of occupational hazards. Specific standards are developed according to identified hazards, and compliance documents (CPL) are developed to interpret the standard. Publication of the bloodborne pathogens rule in 1991 was the first to address specifically infection-related activity. In the event that a newly identified hazard does not have an existing standard (e.g., tuberculosis), OSHA develops an emergency CPL to interpret and enforce compliance under the General Duty clause. The documents can be requested from the agency; OSHA is not required to publish a CPL for external distribution. Although a TB standard had been proposed in 1997, OSHA withdrew the proposal on May 27, 2003, because it did not meet the criteria to justify promulgation of a standard. Nevertheless, there are standards addressing respiratory protection programs?one for *Mycobacterium tuberculosis* (CFR 1910.139) and the general standard that applies to all other respirators (CFR 1910.134).

- Compliance inspection: OSHA conducts inspections of healthcare facilities on a predetermined schedule, in response to a serious hazard or as a result of an employee complaint. Recently, the agency has developed a targeted approach, focusing on injuries of high frequency and seriousness in specific industries. More than twenty states are state-plan states in which implementation of the OSH Act may be under the jurisdiction of different agencies within a state. Nevertheless, standards and compliance with those standards developed within states must be at least as effective as federal OSHA. Many states adopt the specific federal standard by reference.

- Occupational illness/injury logs: OSHA issues regulations to protect workers from occupational illness and injury. Recent standards have addressed hazard communications (chemical exposure), bloodborne pathogens, and possibly in the future, ergonomics. OSHA's Record keeping rule was revised January

Copyright © 2005, Association for Professionals in Infection Control and Epidemiology, Inc.

19, 2001, and includes provisions for recording injuries involving contaminated needlestick and sharps.

United States Department of Agriculture (USDA); Food Safety Inspection System (FSIS)

The USDA has responded to increasing problems of food contamination and consumer demand for safer food products following outbreaks of pathogens, for example, *Escherichia coli* 0157:H7, Hepatitis A, and antimicrobial resistant microorganisms. Specific program initiatives are collected and managed under the program of Hazard Analysis Critical Control Points (HACCP). More information is available from FSIS through its online resources. (See Chapters 58 and 99.)

Department of Transportation; Research and Special Programs Administration

While the DOT has broad responsibility for ensuring safe transport of goods, the RSPA has important linkages to regulated medical waste (RMW) and its transport across state lines. Although definitions and management of RMW disposal are under the jurisdiction of the EPA, as discussed earlier, DOT raised major concerns in waste management industries when it proposed regulations using performance-oriented packaging standards for RMW. The DOT promulgated its final regulation in 1996 using criteria-based definitions, and its final packaging and labeling requirements remain consistent with the OSHA bloodborne pathogens standard. The regulation allows an exemption for laboratory cultures and stocks by subjecting them to stringent packaging requirements. Another exemption of importance to ICPs is that related to transport of laundry and medical devices as long as procedures conform to OSHA bloodborne pathogens regulations. In the *Federal Register* of September 1998 (63; 1700), the RSPA published proposed further revisions to its packaging standards, that is, Hazardous Materials: Revisions to standards for infectious substances and genetically modified microorganisms (49 *CFR* Parts 171, 172, 183, and 178). The proposal considers revising the standards, including RMW, to adopt defining criteria, hazard communication, and packaging requirements for Division 6.2 materials consistent with international standards. The revision was also to revise broad exceptions for diagnostic specimens and biological products and improve safety and ease in understanding the regulations. Input was solicited in an electronic public meeting in September, and the final outcome was published for enforcement in February 2003. The major impact is actually on the waste hauling companies, with new requirements focusing on packaging. Healthcare requirements involve requirements for education of staff managing waste.

Congressional Information Agencies

Office of Technology Assessment and current status

The OTA provided legislative policy makers with independent and timely reports about the potential effects of technological applications. Recent reports included "Issues in Medical Waste Management" and "HIV in the Health Care Workplace." Reports were distributed through the Government Printing Office, but the office has since closed and its function incorporated in other government offices.

Government Accounting Office

The GAO, an agency of the legislative branch, is responsible for providing Congress with information on expenditures and financial management issues at the request of Congress. One report evaluated infection control programs in the Department of Veteran Affairs (VA) and a sample of non-VA hospitals. A recent GAO report (GAO-01–60R) *Cost and Benefit of Needlestick Prevention* estimated the cost-effectiveness of sharps with safety features. Others assessed the government's bioterrorism preparedness and smallpox vaccination programs. Published reports are available through the U.S. General Accounting Office, PO Box 6015, Gaithersburg, MD 20877. Others can be identified and ordered through online resources.

Voluntary Accreditation Agencies

A number of accreditation agencies have considerable effect on healthcare organizations, and the resulting certification has implications for both marketing and reimbursement of funding, if deemed status is at stake.

Joint Commission on Accreditation of Healthcare Organizations (JCAHO)

The JCAHO was established in 1915 as a hospital standard-setting program of the American College of Surgeons. Currently, the American College of Physicians (ACP), the American Medical Association (AMA), the American Hospital Association (AHA), the American College of Surgeons (ACS), and the American Dental Association (ADA) govern the JCAHO. The American Osteopathic Association (AOA) provides a similar accreditation to osteopathic hospitals, with similar standards.

- Accredited organizations and JCAHO initiatives: A variety of healthcare organizations (e.g., ambulatory care clinics, long-term care, home-care) are accredited by JCAHO. Standards and scoring guidelines are published annually, and a three-year accreditation is awarded to hospitals found to be in compliance. Major changes in the accreditation

APIC Text of Infection Control and Epidemiology

Copyright © 2005, Association for Professionals in Infection Control and Epidemiology, Inc.

process began in 2003 under the initiative termed "Shared Visions-New Pathways." By 2004 organizations will be doing their own Periodic Performance Review midway in their review cycle, followed by the actual survey. Unannounced surveys will be routine by 2006. The new process required major streamlining of standards to ensure each element is scorable. During this process the Infection Control Standards were revised with major input from infection control experts. Healthcare-associated infection (HAI) received increased attention from JCAHO when it announced that reduction of HAI would be added as the latest National Patient Safety Goal (NPSG) for 2004. Compliance is to rely heavily on implementation of CDC's Hand Hygiene guidelines.

- Indicator Measurement System (IMS): As part of its "agenda for change" during the 1990s, the JCAHO began a long-term project to develop quantitative indicators measuring certain aspects of quality patient care. These indicators were to have been built into the JCAHO's IMS, which was national and voluntary. However, after massive testing of the system, the IMS indicators were changed considerably and developed into another initiative known as "ORYX."

- ORYX and Core measures: During 2003, the ORYX initiative (not an acronym but a term coined by the JCAHO for this project) began a replacement into sets of measurements termed "Core measures." This latest set of indicators is aligned with CMS initiatives overseen by state QIOs, as well as with AHQR measures and others proposed by organizations in the private sector. The intent is alignment of mandatory and voluntary quality measures and standardized definitions. Indicators important to infection control (catheter-related bloodstream, catheter-related urinary tract and ventilator-associated pneumonia infections) are included.

Laboratory Inspection and Certification

The College of American Pathologists (CAP) conducts voluntary inspections and certifications of laboratories. In addition, CAP performs quality-control studies using research to improve laboratory performance. These are done every two years, with laboratories carrying out self-surveys in the odd year. Successful surveys may provide "deemed status " for laboratories also accredited by the Joint Commission. However, JCAHO surveys continue to review broad laboratory performance improvement measures in which the laboratory interacts with the rest of its affiliated healthcare organization, beyond basic CAP quality control measures. The Commission on Office Laboratory Accreditation (COLA) is another laboratory accrediting agency affecting offices and clinics and is also recognized by

JCAHO. JCAHO has recently entered into another collaborative accreditation effort with CAP and the American Proficient Institute (API) termed the Lab Advantage™, emphasizing a quality improvement approach.

Other Accrediting Organizations

Other well-known organizations accredit specific entities, such as health maintenance organizations, clinics and offices, for example, National Committee on Quality Assurance (NCQA) and the American Medical Accreditation Programs (AMAP). Along with JCAHO, NCQA and AMAP are the preeminent healthcare accrediting organizations. NCQA is recognized as one the top organizations providing voluntary accreditation for managed care organizations, that is, Health Maintenance Organizations or HMOs. HMOs primarily measure outcomes in an ambulatory care setting. NCQA has developed a summary of measures known as Health Plan Employer Data and Information Set (HEDIS), which is increasingly used as an outcomes report. HEDIS includes important preventive measures of health, for example, immunization rates. JCAHO, NCQA, and AMAP have developed a Performance Measurement Coordinating Council or PMCC to ensure efficiency and consistency in their activities within these various organizations. Infection related surveillance outcomes should be considered in each of these initiatives. The Commission on Accreditation of Rehabilitation Facilities (CARF) provides voluntary accreditation to facilities meeting their standards for quality in the United States, Canada, and Europe.[www.carf.org and list as additional resource]

State and Local Agencies

State Agencies

States have multiple departments that parallel functions of the federal agencies outlined above, that is, jurisdictions related to health, education, welfare, environment, agriculture, and so forth. The organizational structures vary by name and grouping of functions or programs; linkage to federal programs occurs frequently through funding or regulatory requirements. For example, federal OSHA administers occupational health and safety programs in many states, but at least twenty states have independent OSH programs. State-plan state programs must provide enforcement that is at least as effective as that of OSHA. ICPs should identify the agencies that establish laws, rules, and regulations for healthcare facilities as well as for professional licensure, certificate of need, and environmental regulations, such as medical waste or management of pesticides. Designated state agency surveyors act as agents of CMS to enforce the COP for Medicare and Medicaid within states and are linked to federal agencies through

Copyright © 2005, Association for Professionals in Infection Control and Epidemiology, Inc.

regional offices. These affect healthcare service delivery processes and design standards for healthcare facilities as discussed earlier. Interaction with state and local agencies has become increasingly important for bioterrorism program planning as well.

Local Jurisdiction

ICPs also need to familiarize themselves with public health and education laws regulated by specific state and local health departments. Regulations for reportable communicable diseases vary from state to state regarding what and how reporting takes place. The regulations include reporting of laboratory based infectious agents and clinical diseases and may also define processes for reporting outbreaks and related interventions. State regulated healthcare construction codes may be influenced or modified by local authorities having jurisdiction over issues such as water quality, levels of discharged contaminants, and local fire marshal regulations. (See Table 10–1.)

Clinical Practice Guidelines

Efforts to contain costs have heightened consumer desire for information about healthcare quality and value. Purchasers of healthcare demand information about providers and the care delivered compared to accepted clinical practice guidelines and standards.

American College of Physicians and Practice Guidelines

The American College of Physicians defines *practice guidelines* as a means of providing knowledge derived from a scientific analysis of the practice of medicine, in a useful format to physicians, patients, and others, about the best use of healthcare resources. As part of the information management and quality improvement, healthcare facilities integrate practice guidelines into their professional credentialing activities. The JCAHO is developing new standards requiring hospitals to consider their use when measuring patient care management.

Other Professional Resources and Guidelines

By the mid-1990s, more than sixty professional organizations developed well beyond 1,500 practice guidelines raising concern about focus, resources, and scientific validation.[3] The Performance Measurement Coordination Council may be a start in grappling with consistency and efficiency. However, consumer demand and purchaser pressure for accountability related to healthcare costs led to increased frequency of public reporting of outcome measurements. Data began being published by facility and physician name in many areas of the United States by the late 1990s.

These measurement "report cards" may ultimately lead to improved efforts of validation and better resource utilization. As noted earlier, the American Hospital Association, in collaboration with other organizations, such as JCAHO and HHS, announced an initiative identifying a set of common indicators that would ultimately be published as a "report card" in all hospitals, similar to CMS efforts in nursing homes and home care.

Professional and Trade Organizations

Numerous professional and trade associations have influenced hospital infection prevention and control programs with the development of guidelines and standards on various aspects of infection control practice. Although these groups are voluntary, they often become the standard of practice for governmental and accreditation bodies. Several organizations have also published journals dedicated to hospital epidemiology and infection control practice to provide a forum for exchange of scientific and professional information. The Association for Professionals in Infection Control and Epidemiology (APIC) provides published guidelines and resources as well as online resources to inquire and/or research existing standards and practices. The Certification Board in Infection Control (CBIC) offers professional certification in infection control. APIC's governmental and legislative affairs staff assist members in developing collaboration and coalition building with many of professional groups with similar interests and alliances.

IV. SUMMARY AND CONCLUSIONS

Effective IPCPs function through a variety of multidisciplinary activities within all healthcare delivery settings. Organizations rely on ICPs to understand the related accrediting and regulatory requirements and to recommend policy and actions based on current standards and guidelines. Continuous changes require ICPs to maintain currency in the regulatory milieu in to maintain an effective and credible program, regardless of the care setting.

REFERENCES

1. Haley RW, Culver DH, White JW, et al: The efficacy of infection surveillance and control program in preventing nosocomial infections in U.S. hospitals, *Am J Epidemiol* 121:182–205, 1985.
2. Kohn LT, Corrigan JM, Donaldson MS, editors: *To err is human: building a safer health system,* Washington, DC, 1999, Institute of Medicine National Academy Press, pp 1–223.
3. McDonald LL, Pugliese G: Regulatory, accreditation, and professional agencies influencing infection control programs. In Wenzel RP, editor: *Prevention and control of nosocomial infections,* ed 3, Baltimore, 1997, Williams & Wilkins, pp 58–69.
4. 2001 Guidelines for design and construction of hospital and healthcare facilities, Washington, DC, 2001, AIA Press.

Copyright © 2005, Association for Professionals in Infection Control and Epidemiology, Inc.

Education and Training

Harriette A. Carr, RN, MSN, CIC
Infection Control Specialist
C.R. Bard, Inc.
Carmichael, California

Patricia L. Hinson, CIC
Corporate Compliance Specialist
Carolinas Healthcare System
Salisbury, North Carolina

ABSTRACT

Learning is a way to transform knowledge, insights, and skills into behavior. Adult learners are unique. They seek out learning experiences to satisfy a personally perceived need based on past experiences. The more success adult learners have, the more likely they are to willingly seek out learning experiences. Healthcare's growing complexity and rapid change require that theories of learning be incorporated into a trans-cultural educational experience, which addresses issues of literacy, cultural diversity, multiple-skilled workers, and technological advances. Those who plan and implement educational activities in healthcare should be familiar with the more accepted learning theories for adults. They should assess the educational needs of the learner population, the institution, and the community as they relate to infection control. They should provide an appropriate climate for learning, demonstrating creativity and flexibility and using a team concept to accomplish mandatory training.

KEY CONCEPTS

- The most basic goal of healthcare education and training is to improve job skills and competencies.

- Adult learning is a response to current situations and tends to be problem-centered.

- Adults have strong reasons for learning, and learning retention increases when immediate application follows instructions

- Workplace education is business driven and tied to administrative and financial goals, productivity, and the need to benchmark against the best professional practices.

- Educational needs represent deficiencies in knowledge, skills, or attitude that can be identified by Needs Assessments or performance improvement studies.

- The educator controls the learning experience with a well-defined plan using goals, objectives, and appropriate teaching methods. Goals are statements that communicate the intent of the curriculum and provide a direction for planning the education session. Expectations are clearly defined in terms of time and available resources.

- Management should be included in educational Needs Assessment, and training should be linked to a facility's organizational vision, mission, and values.

Copyright © 2005, Association for Professionals in Infection Control and Epidemiology, Inc.

I. BACKGROUND

Learning is a way to change knowledge, insights, and skills into behavior. It uses consistency and reasonable explanations to link new knowledge to the familiar. Learning is a voluntary, active, goal-directed process that requires personal commitment to the process. The participant may experience self-doubt, conflict, and resistance. Behavioral change is facilitated in a climate of trust and interaction with others.[18]

Learning reflects the human need or drive to solve problems, acquire new skills, initiate improvement, explore new ideas, and satisfy curiosity; it is a lifelong process. Not all learning takes place in the same way. Bloom's Taxonomy[47] of learning identified three domains of educational activities: cognitive, affective, psychomotor. Cognitive learning involves the development of intellectual abilities such as recall, application, and analytical levels of knowledge. Affective learning embraces new attitudes, values, beliefs, and ways of feeling. Increased self-esteem and the desire to learn occur in a caring, respectful relationship. Finally, psychomotor learning involves the performance of new skills or new ways of performing.[18]

Learning also happens in distinct stages:

- Awareness—learner perceives a need to think, feel, or act differently.

- Information or data gathering—curiosity is increased as the learner seeks to understand and explore the learning need.

- Intellectual insight—learner weighs advantages and disadvantages of the alternatives and conducts mental "trial or practice runs" (cognitive learning).

- Emotional insight—learner practices the new behavior in real situations; this is usually a time of conflict in trying to get the change to "feel right" (affective learning).

- Behavioral change—new knowledge becomes a part of learner's way of thinking, feeling, and behaving.[18]

II. BASIC PRINCIPLES

Major Goals in Teaching

The most basic goal of healthcare education and training is to improve job skills and competencies. A greater emphasis is being placed on learner "gap analysis" to distinguish performance issues from other needs. Healthcare's growing complexity and rapid change, however, demands more. The issues of literacy, cultural diversity, multiple-skilled workers, and technological advances are addressed through education. Outcomes should include increased competence

in identifying problems, critical thinking, managing existing situations, and coping effectively with stress.[47]

An increasingly diverse workforce has driven the need for education to increase tolerance for diversity. Cultural diversity and a mixed workforce are regarded as organizational strengths. People who do not think alike help to create a competitive advantage when problem-solving. Similarly, providing opportunities for workers to network with other personnel and share their expertise within the organization will expand learner creative abilities. This interaction can be effective in stimulating learning and is invaluable to the learning process.

Learning Theories that Explain Learner Motivation

Those planning and implementing educational activities in healthcare should be familiar with some of the more accepted learning theories. Adult-learning theories differ from those of children; therefore, the theory most appropriate to the group of learners must be selected. Approximately fifty distinct theories of learning have been published.

- The Psychoanalytic school asserts that behavior or learning is motivated by inner forces or urges.

- The Behaviorism school focuses on objectively observed behaviors that lead to the development of new behaviors. Pavlov's dog experiments are an example of this style of learning.[33]

- The Humanistic school uses a holistic approach to teaching. The learner is recognized as being capable of growth and self-direction.

- The Constructivism thinking movement emphasizes how learners think, connect ideas, and make judgments. It uses mind-mapping or thinking maps as tools to "unlock and expand learning." Mind mapping was designed primarily to help the student take notes in a manner that would maximize his or her ability to relate and remember facts and concepts.[8,21]

- The Andragogy Theory of Knowles was developed specifically to address the art and science of helping adults to learn. This theory emphasizes that adults expect to take responsibility for their learning.
  - Adults tend to be self-directed.
  - Adults have a rich reservoir of experience to draw upon.
  - Adults readiness to learn is affected by their need to know or do something.
  - Adults are generally motivated to learn due to internal or intrinsic factors as opposed to external or extrinsic forces.[1]

APIC Text of Infection Control and Epidemiology

Copyright © 2005, Association for Professionals in Infection Control and Epidemiology, Inc.

The Adult Learner

Adult learners can generally be characterized as having a readiness to learn, although patterns of interest tend to change with normal shifting of focus during life transitions. This is predictable and growth producing. Old interests provide continuity and stability, whereas new interests provide excitement and discovery. Engaging in change can be anxiety producing. Learning is often motivated by job needs, such as the need for new skills or the desire for promotion and increased salary.[48]

Adults generally prefer practical rather than academic knowledge. They tend to learn what they can use. Adults usually concentrate on areas of personal experience to improve on what is already known and enjoyed.

Adults see themselves as producers and as able to manage their own lives. They need to be perceived by others as self-directed and expect to be treated with respect. Many regard aging as an altered state of being but not a lesser state.

Adults have a great volume and variety of life experience upon which to draw in solving problems. Life experiences influence judgment both positively and negatively. They attach greater value to personal experience. The educator can capitalize on this experience when introducing new material. In some cases, adults may assume the educator role or lead group discussions. In general, adults are not hesitant to speak out or walk out, if learning needs are not being met. They will provide honest feedback if encouraged to do so.

In general, adult learning is a response to current situations and tends to be problem-centered. Adults have strong reasons for learning, and learning retention increases when immediate application follows instructions.[1]

Roadblocks to Learning

Educators must also be aware of and plan to confront common roadblocks to the learning process. For example, what people know is not always predictive of how they will behave. We cannot assume workers will perform better because they attend classes and acquire new knowledge. Providing experienced educators and a well-designed curriculum initiates the learning process only and does not ensure the application of learning on the job.

The passive learner response must also be challenged. It is important for the educator to recognize during training that what happens at the front of the classroom has little effect on what participants will implement in the work setting. Adult learners can become bored rapidly. A mix of activities and presentation methods will hold their interest longer in the topic.[49]

To increase learning retention and motivate the learner to change practice behaviors, the educator should assume a facilitator role, limit monologues or lectures, and opt for more interactive classroom approaches. A "rule of thumb" for the active/passive ration is a minimum of 60/40.[2]

Adult learners require a safe learning environment. Providing a low-risk, nonintimidating learning environment can also facilitate class interaction. Adults learn when they believe that they need to learn something new. Convincing the adult learner to participate in a classroom activity can be difficult as they are often worried about being embarrassed, acknowledging what they "don't know," and feel at risk in stating an opinion or taking a position. If the facilitator critiques the learner in the class, identifying all the mistakes that were made, the learner will be less likely to try to use the new skill in the work setting.

Learners must overcome a fear of failure as they process new information and learn new skills. The facilitator must recognize that participants will only try to use the skills they successfully performed in class. Adult learners need transfer of learning activities before and after the training event, if the training is to impact their on-the-job behaviors. A more effective approach would be to allow learners to evaluate themselves, identify areas needing improvement, and plan for further education. The facilitator encourages the learner to leave his or her comfort zone and persist in skill development in spite of the fear of failure, awkwardness of the situation, or negative feedback from friends or superiors.

In planning the course, it is important to focus on measurable outcomes. The facilitator builds into the course design a method to assess learning retention and transference of learning to the workplace. If students are unable to meet the performance objectives or unable to implement the knowledge acquired in the classroom, then it is the instruction that has failed and not the student.[35]

Educators should avoid a "one-size-fits-all" teaching approach. Workplace education is business driven and tied to administrative and financial goals, productivity, and the need to benchmark against the best professional practices. Healthcare providers require teaching methods that address their unique value systems, learning preferences, and job requirements. Just-in-time competency training in infection control practices should be available in various instructional formats to measure and improve worker performance.

Copyright © 2005, Association for Professionals in Infection Control and Epidemiology, Inc.

III. EDUCATIONAL PROGRAM DEVELOPMENT

Educational needs represent deficiencies in knowledge, skills, or attitude that can be identified by Needs Assessments or performance improvement studies. Assessing educational needs of the learner population, the institution, and the community, as it relates to infection control, is the first step in effective program planning.[18]

Fortunately, the infection control learning needs of the healthcare workers, the institution and the community at large are interrelated. Healthcare worker participants need to know principles of infection control and/or prevention and current policies and procedures that govern infection control practice in their assigned areas of work. Facility administrators need to know how to develop institutional guidelines, policies, and procedures in accordance with accrediting and regulating groups. The citizenry or community populations need to know the factors that influence the development and spread of infectious disease.

Assessing Educational Needs

Performing a Needs Assessment[29] will enable the educator to measure the gaps between what is and what ought to be to focus educational activities. It is directed at the level of policy and programs not the individual learner. Properly done it can be used to assess the success of the educational activity.

Adult learners prefer learning experiences that make sense, are related to their needs, and enhance self-responsibility. Studying target-learner populations assists the educator in developing educational programs that are relevant and reasonable. A systematic Needs Assessment will determine the interests of the group, readiness to learn, professional experience, and the cognitive differences in clinical reasoning.[18]

Methods that the infection control professional (ICP) can use to determine educational needs of the leaner population include:

- Learner self-assessment. The learner develops a self-achievement model and compares the present situation to the standard.

- Focus group discussion. Learning needs are assessed in small groups with members assisting each other to clarify needs.

- Interest-finder surveys. These are data-gathering tools, such as checklists or questionnaires. Findings are reported to the surveyed population (e.g., healthcare worker satisfaction with protective barriers used to prevent exposure to blood and body fluids).

- Test development. Tests can be used as diagnostic tools to identify areas of learning deficiencies. Tests may also be seen as threatening or intimidating.

- Personal interviews. The educator consults with random or selected individuals to determine learning needs.

- Job analysis and performance reviews. These methods provide specific, precise information about work and performance. Job analysis is time-consuming and difficult to do; seek assistance from one trained in job analysis techniques. Discussions of on-the-job expectations with supervisors can be used to identify learning needs.

- Observational studies. Direct observation of personnel working can be performed by quality management analysts or ICPs (e.g., handwashing study in critical care units).

- Review of incident reports, occupational injury and illness reports, and performance improvement studies. Reviews may indicate specific learning needs of healthcare providers.[18]

Goals and Objectives

The educator controls the learning experience with a well-defined plan using goals, objectives, and appropriate teaching methods. Goals are statements that communicate the intent of the curriculum and provide a direction for planning the education session. Expectations are clearly defined in terms of time and available resources.

Once the purpose of the program is established, the educator determines the specific actions the learner will perform because of instruction. These actions are known as *instructional objectives*. Properly written instructional objectives describe the expected behavior of the learner in measurable terms. The objective includes conditions (restrictions or limitations) under which learning will occur. The level of expected learner performance in terms of speed, accuracy, and the quality or acceptable deviation from the designated standard will be indicated[19] (Fig. 11–1) .

Recognizing that there are different levels of cognitive skills, one objective should be written for each level of skill attainment. However, depending upon the results of the Needs Assessment not all levels of cognitive skills will need to be included in each educational program.

Copyright © 2005, Association for Professionals in Infection Control and Epidemiology, Inc.

Basic Rules for Writing Objectives

1. **The objective must be specific.** Use clear, precise language to identify the end goal of learning; describe what the learner is expected to achieve. When the emphasis is on performance, the learner may not achieve insight, wisdom, or understanding.

2. **The objective must be measurable.** Use action verbs to describe what the learner is expected to do; select verbs that are open to little interpretation, such as *calculate* or *evaluate,* instead of *believe, know,* or *understand.* It is difficult to measure learners' level of knowledge or understanding.

3. **The objective must be achievable.** Choose verbs that accurately indicate the expected level of reasoning, skills, and psychomotor performance (acting and doing).

4. **The objective must be relevant to the material presented.** Recognize that behavioral changes are defined in terms of knowledge, skills, or attitude; use appropriate verbs to convey the desired learning.

5. **The objective must have a separate outcome.** Outcomes may take time to become evident and may be demonstrated over time.

Figure 11–1 Basic rules for writing objectives

TX>Cognitive levels include:

- Recall—objectives that measure learner recognition of specific information. The objective requires the learner to list, name, define, or repeat. At this level, the learner performs by rote.

- Comprehension—objectives that require the learner to understand the meaning, interpretation, translation, or interpolation of a problem. This objective requires the learner to comprehend, explain, generalize, predict, or paraphrase.

- Application—objectives that require the learner to comprehend and manipulate data or concepts. The objective requires the learner to interpret, demonstrate, illustrate, or employ.

- Analysis—objectives at a higher cognitive level. The objective requires the learner to contrast, criticize, differentiate, or solve.

- Synthesis—objectives that build a structure from a pattern of diverse elements. Key words for this objective would include *categorize, compile, devise, explain, plan, rewrite* or *summarize.*

- Evaluation—objectives that require the learner to make judgments. Key terms for this objective would include *appraise, compare and contrast, defend, describe, evaluate* or *justify.*[6]

There is no one correct method or style for writing educational objectives. To provide criteria of accepted competency, objectives must be measurable. The objectives clue the learner to the content of a test or evaluation.

Each objective will include the task/behavior the learner must perform, the conditions under which this task/behavior will be performed, and the standard of how well it will be performed. One action verb is used for each task/behavior anticipated. Actiona verbs such as discuss, describe, demonstrate, solve, identify, measure, compare, contrast, evaluate, or prepare should be used when writing educational objectives.

Improving learning transfer to workplace practices must be a high priority in the planning phase. Educators must link the previous knowledge and experience of participants to what is being taught, using workplace situations to illustrate major points. The program content must be relevant, practical, and "doable" and should include practice sessions as a part of class activities. ICPs should plan for reinforcement of knowledge in the work setting and ensure support from key leaders and supervisors.[9]

Management Support

Winning management support for training can be crucial for a program's success. Management should be included in educational Needs Assessment, and training should be linked to a facility's organizational vision, mission, and values. When seeking management support for an educational plan, the ICP should include justification of need, costs, level of involvement for each level of management, and the type of evaluation planned.

Copyright © 2005, Association for Professionals in Infection Control and Epidemiology, Inc.

Managers should be encouraged to partner with ICPs to both team-teach and provide pre-class goals and post-class follow-up in terms of evaluation and plans to reinforce learning. When an educational activity has been completed, publicize its success in a newsletter and provide reports of educational successes in department managers meetings. Have a written statement for the recording secretary to ensure inclusion in the meeting minutes.[32]

Fiscal Responsibility

A critical part of planning educational programs involves budgeting skills. If this is not the forte of the educator, consideration should be given to the assignment of this responsibility to one who is adept in resolving fiscal management problems. Direct costs to consider in planning an educational program include speaker honoraria and expenses, cost of a facility and refreshments for participants, preparation of teaching materials (e.g., copying expenses), promotional costs, secretarial/clerical assistance, unplanned expenses, and the general loss of revenue experienced by employees or employers while the learner is away from work. Indirect costs will include the salary expenses for the learners and replacement costs of learner in the work area. In an institution wide program, different costs will be incurred for each department involved in the training program.

Basic Principles of Effective Teaching

The educator must provide an appropriate climate for learning and controls the educational session with a well-defined teaching plan. The plan includes creating an environment that learners want to be in. This principle establishes a foundation for all that follows. Adults are more self-directed and independent in learning experiences; they learn what they want to learn and what is useful to them.

The learning space should be private and congenial, with comfortable seating, room temperature, and illumination. The room should be properly arranged for learning transactions and should maximize physical and sensory potential. Adjust the room temperature to a comfortable level; this item will invariably receive comment in the program evaluation, which underscores the fact that adults have less tolerance for increased heat or cold. This issue can be less of a problem when participants are instructed beforehand about the expected room temperature.[15]

The educator should eliminate distractions and try to control or decrease the noise level; ask that pagers and cellular phones be turned to the inaudible range. The sounds of nonparticipants talking or laughing and sound of repairmen, custodial workers, dietary personnel, or competing educational sessions are distressing to those trying to concentrate on the speaker. Provide a designated person at the learning site to troubleshoot these problems should they occur.[16,34]

Provide audiovisual equipment that is in working order and ready for use. It is helpful to provide the speaker with a presenter's packet of information to describe the proper use and types of microphones, the control switches, pointers that are available, and any other mechanical operations that may occur at the podium or teaching area. Many speakers assess the teaching room and actual equipment to be used before their presentation; this prepares and reassures the speaker.

One of the most important roles of the educator is to provide an atmosphere of mutual respect, one that is friendly, informal, and supportive. Eye contact, addressing students by name, listening without interrupting, and acknowledging the validity of problems or opinions expressed are characteristics of an effective teacher. Embarrassing the student or the use of intimidation or sarcasm is counterproductive to sharing information and resolving learning deficiencies.[15,34]

Enhancing Understanding and Learning Retention

The educator facilitates the learning process by making the information understandable and memorable (Fig. 11–2). He/she should define or redefine terms with respect to historical or current thinking and use examples or anecdotes to underscore major points. For material that is especially important, the educator should demonstrate enthusiasm. Major points should be emphasized with variations in voice quality, speed, gestures, or overall body language. Repetition should be used, repeating the same point in different ways.

The educator should engage the student in interaction with the material through dialogue, return demonstration, role-play, or in providing real-life examples. Audiovisual aids, such as slides, models, videos, posters, and chalkboards, are excellent support for the learning environment as well.

At the end of the learning session, summarize and review the major points. Let the students know you enjoyed being with them.

Evaluation Plan

Program evaluation is necessary to measure change and growth in the learner.[18,26,36] Feedback to participants and managers on the progress made increases efficiency and provides direction for further improvement. The evaluation process of assessing and rating objectives assists both the learner and educator to improve. Students need to know the progress being

Copyright © 2005, Association for Professionals in Infection Control and Epidemiology, Inc.

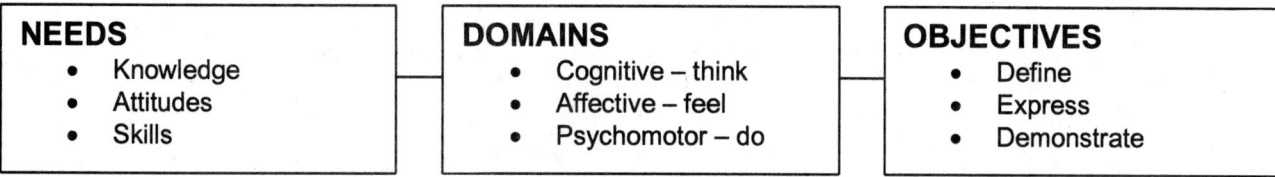

NEEDS	DOMAINS	OBJECTIVES
• Knowledge • Attitudes • Skills	• Cognitive – think • Affective – feel • Psychomotor – do	• Define • Express • Demonstrate

Figure 11–2 Develop learning objectives from learning needs and domains

made, and educators need to know whether objectives have been met.

During the evaluation process, information is provided to the course manager that enables decisions about what to improve, expand, or delete in future presentations. Evaluations indicate what type of programs work best and what has appeal to the learner, as well as measure response to innovative or controversial ideas. Evaluations also serve to provide program justification and accountability, often required by funding agencies, sponsors, or accrediting bodies.

A decision on how evaluation results will be used should be made before the evaluation is done. Specific program elements that should be evaluated include appropriateness of program design, adequacy of teaching and instructional resources, and the knowledge, skills, and attitudes learned by the participants. A representative sample of data from the learner population is necessary to provide evidence of successful learning.

Major types of evaluation include:

- *Formative evaluation* is conducted during the planning of the educational session to provide immediate feedback and to allow appropriate changes to be made. This information guides the development phase of program design.

- *Summative evaluation* occurs after the program is completed to judge effectiveness. It identifies changes to be made before the program is offered again.

- *The Kirkpatrick model* measures the success of training programs at four different levels[4,44,47]:
  - Level 1—Reaction: Did they like it? The primary purpose is to measure participant satisfaction. The course facilitator usually conducts this evaluation immediately following the educational intervention with the use of what is commonly referred to as a "smile" sheet. The participants indicate the degree of satisfaction by selecting the smile that most corresponds to the level of satisfaction experienced.
  - Level 2—Learning. What did they learn? A test is given immediately after the training event to assess the participants' ability for immediate recall of the information presented and to determine

whether a skill or knowledge of the topic is improved, or if attitudes have changed as a result of the training. A test is administered at the completion of training; this test is commonly referred to as a "posttest." Sometimes the same test is given as a "pretest" to measure participants' entry knowledge. The value of this type of evaluation is not so much as a measurement of true learning retention, but as another way to verify or reinforce knowledge of major points addressed in the presentation.
  - Level 3—Transfer: Did the learners' behavior change? Surveys and direct observation of behavior are common methods used to retrieve data on the extent of behavioral change as the result of training. Usually participants receive a survey prior to the training to assess current work practices. The job impact survey is usually conducted after the learners are back on the job three months; the long-term behavioral change is assessed six to twelve months after the training event.
  - Level 4—Results: Business impact. What are the results of training? This level measures overall results of training and usually includes financial or "return on investment" (ROI). It is recognized that ROI is a "lagging indicator" and not the ultimate measurement of educational programs because it provides only a "snapshot" of where you have been educationally and is not a predictor of the future. To measure the effect on the "bottom line" or performing a cost benefit analysis is difficult because it may not capture all strategic objectives. The educator may not have this information. The ROI evaluation is more of a measurement of long-term benefits and not a predictor of true outcome.[47,25]

Evaluation Methodology

Various methods can be used to collect appropriate data or information on learning. Measurements can be made at specific times, for instance. These include pretests (given before the educational program to measure entry knowledge) and posttests (given at the end of the program to measure results and effectiveness of learning experiences; the posttest is similar in content

Copyright © 2005, Association for Professionals in Infection Control and Epidemiology, Inc.

to the pretest). The pretest and posttest tools provide for effective instruction by serving as a course outline or guide for teaching the class. Class participation is stimulated with the knowledge of progress being made. The educator can assess the appropriateness of the material presented, level of complexity, and whether learning has occurred.

Additional methods of evaluation include direct observation of behavioral changes, for example, demonstration of proper use of protective barriers. Questionnaires can also be used, as can one-on-one interviews with learners from the target population.

If a change in on-the-job behavior is anticipated as an outcome of the training exercise, the ICP should review with appropriate supervisors, if the learning objectives were met. It may be necessary to review program content and learner reaction to this content with their supervisor. It is the supervisors' responsibility to advise the learner, if their on-the job behaviors do not meet expectation. The ICP may be involved in any additional coaching needed by this learner on the invitation of the specific supervisor.

Whatever evaluation methodology is used, the data must be gathered, arranged, tabulated, and analyzed to assess needed changes and to make recommendations for curriculum revision before the next presentation. Evaluation measurements must be consistent with the objectives established for the educational program. Caution must be exercised when doing evaluations to prevent the development of the Hawthorne Effect.

Innovative Ways to Teach Infection Control Practices

The selection of teaching style and instructional method depends on the resources of the institution and the resourcefulness of the educator. The educator understands and uses the basic principles of adult learning and has the ability to tailor the instructional method and teaching style to the specific type of learner population represented in the education setting (e.g., nonclinical employees, nursing assistants, resident physicians).

Lectures and Similar Activities

In academic circles, teaching by the lecture method is a popular means of instruction. Lecturing has been defined as "telling learners something they could not otherwise read in a book or review article." It is also a means of exploring hypotheses or controversial issues.[15] Lectures allow the exploration of a lot of material in a limited amount of time and can be used with small or large groups. Other styles of lecturing included guided note-taking, that is, outlining major points to be discussed; "chalk-talks," or illustrating key

thoughts on a chalkboard; and using slide-lecture presentations or a combination of lecture, demonstration, and discussion.

The straight lecture is not a method of choice because students need to be involved in the process to enhance retention of the new knowledge. Its success depends on the relevance of the information to the learner. Public speaking skills are necessary to be effective, and there is less probability of learner retention than with discussion

If a lecture has been selected as the presentation method, select an interesting name or title for the lecture. Recognize time as a major factor in the overall planning of the educational sessions. Schedule slides, demonstrations, and group discussions appropriately, keeping within the time allowed for the presentation. Provide participants with a list of references supporting the presentation.

First-time presenters should practice the lecture in front of someone or record and time the presentation for personal critique. The lecturer who avoids wordiness or the use of words that are meaningless or esoteric will hold the interest of their audience better. Humor is sometimes used to "break the ice" to help the audience and, more often, the speaker to relax. If the joke has no relevance or the speaker is not skilled at comedy, it is best left to those who are. As with other types of learning, experience and practical training are associated with increased competence.[15]

The Socratic Method[41] of presentation is more acceptable to adult learners than the standard lecture format. In this method, teaching is carried out by asking questions of the group rather than by telling. A structured dialog is created that encourages participation. With the Socratic Method the educator can help the learners explore the depth of the topic to be presented and evaluate their responses concurrently. The educator's role in this method focuses on keeping the discussion focused on the topic for discussion, stimulating the discussion, and summarizing what has been dealt with and what has not, and to draw as many learners into the discussion as possible. As previously mentioned, this method will take experience and practice for the educator to successfully present.

More complex or voluminous materials can be presented in a symposium format, where three to six lectures are presented in turn by resource persons on various phases of a single subject or problem. This activity includes open discussion with the audience. Forum or panel formats can also be used. In a forum, one or more speakers engage in free and open discussion about the subject. A Panel is usually comprised of four to seven resource people with special knowledge

Copyright © 2005, Association for Professionals in Infection Control and Epidemiology, Inc.

on the subject. Both of these styles of presentations can be combined to create an interesting program.

Computer-Based Training

Computer-based training is an interactive instructional system in which the computer functions as the "master teacher." The computer program presents the curriculum content in a logical sequence and guides the student to achieve specific learning objectives. This high quality instruction combines the multidisciplinary expertise of the subject matter experts, instructional design, and educational process.

Computer learning is self-paced and designed to meet individual needs and interests. The method is learner friendly and nonjudgmental and provides positive reinforcement. Participant self-esteem stays intact because mistakes are private and there is no risk for wrong answers. Learner participation, immediate feedback, and colorful graphics hold the student's attention and reduce the possibility of boredom. Lack of computer skills may be a distracter for some learners.[26]

This method is versatile in that it can be used independently by individual learners or by groups in a classroom setting with an educator available to answer questions. Screens may be modified to include institution-specific information. This methodology provides a learning alternative for persons unable to attend scheduled classes.[26] This method requires sufficient computer hardware for the anticipated number of learners and learning sessions. Its value is limited in instruction and evaluation of psychomotor skills.

Games

Well-structured games can facilitate learning. Many adult learners perceive games as being childish and are reluctant to participate. Games can be used as a "gathering tool" to introduce a concept or as a testing tool to access learning. Examples of simple games are table top quizzes during safety presentations and word search/word scramble puzzles.

Mass Training Delivery Systems

The "train-the-trainer" method is used for wide-scale institutional education. Leader guides or "how-to" educational modules are used in the training/coaching of persons responsible for staff in-service and continuing education. The train-the-trainer method fosters creativity among staff and makes learning and teaching more enjoyable. In situations where large numbers of staff must be educated over a twenty-four-hour period and in a relatively short span of time, the educational activities of the institution can be maximized by the use of additional educators. Managers responsible for these educational and staff development programs often do not see themselves in the role of educator, however.

With this method, area or unit managers may function as course presenters, reviewing the objectives and studying the training materials. Leader guides are simply written and presented in a concise, systematic format, providing curriculum goals and objectives, course outline, instructional methods, references, and evaluation. A team-teaching approach with staff members may be used, or the manager may elect to teach the course independently. If the team approach is selected, curriculum objectives are assigned to individual staff members, and all staff members may be asked to prepare for the educational session by viewing certain videos or engaging in some other learning activity. As with other methods, a contingency plan is developed for employees who are absent from the training session. Training records and employee educational profiles are by the unit manager.

Role Play/Reenactment

This dramatic teaching strategy uses a situational learning experience and the technique of simulation to allow the learner to experience firsthand a professional dilemma as a spectator or as a participant.[18] It can be used as a springboard for discussion in conjunction with a forum, panel, or symposium or as a building block for conferences and seminars with a focus on problem-solving methods. It can also be used in the development of an educational video production. In diverse cultural settings, this method may increase the discomfort of learners and may actually impede the learning process.

Case Studies

Case studies can be used as a training method to help bridge the learning gap between theory and actual practice. The hypothetical but real-life scenario varies in complexity and style and depends upon learning objectives. The method builds upon a variety of learner skills: analytical, critical, and interactive. Learners explore multiple solutions and enhance creativity and problem solving approaches.

The most common format is the written presentation, but the use of live demonstrations, videos, and simulations are popular. To be effective they require participation of all learners.

Anecdotes: Personal, Clinical Experiences

With this teaching strategy, the learner relates to the experience of a peer, one who has "been there," and recognizes the implication of the information provided.[38] Data on healthcare workers' experiences are

Copyright © 2005, Association for Professionals in Infection Control and Epidemiology, Inc.

collected, analyzed, and used in educational sessions to facilitate group discussion.

As an example, the ICP might interview workers about occupational injury or exposure to bloodborne or airborne pathogens. Healthcare providers recount unique work experiences that present a danger or threaten the personal health in the occupational setting. The goal is to determine how the incident could have been prevented.

This method might be used, for instance, during orientation of new resident physicians by using the personal case histories of colleagues.

Mentoring Programs

Mentoring is one of the oldest forms of guided human development and learning. In Homer's *Odyssey*, Odysseus, King of Ithaca, asked his trusted friend Mentor to care for his family while he was away fighting in the Trojan War. Odysseus was gone for ten years; during that time Mentor protected, guided, taught, and advised Odysseus's young son, Telemachus. Though Mentor was a lowly swine herder by trade, his name became synonymous with "teacher," "advisor," "sage," and "trusted friend." Mentors are recognized as those special people who protect us and help us to reach our potential as human beings.[39]

In modern times, government leaders frequently endorse mentoring initiatives that link responsible adults with children and young people in our communities. In the business world, mentoring is often the means used to preserve "institutional memory" to ensure the implementation of corporate mission, vision, and values. Mentoring is seen as a cost-effective way to upgrade and cross-train the workforce. In some organizations, there are formalized programs in which respected senior managers advise and groom promising candidates who are pursuing upper level positions. Candidates are assisted in dealing with internal forces that influence decision making. Some employers encourage volunteer mentors from within the organization to assist with employee development and learning. Regardless of the program, mentoring is seen as a process in which the mentor and candidate work together to discover and develop the protégé's abilities.[11, 39]

Mentors may be nominated, but, in general, the mentoring relationship is voluntary in nature and remains active as long as it is beneficial. With correct preparation and managerial support, virtually anyone can become a mentor. Mentor/learner matching should be done by linking persons with assessed developmental needs with leaders in the organization having the needed expertise. Mentors and their charges may complete a self-assessment of leadership skills to identify areas of expertise and growth opportunities.

Mentors should be good listeners, focus on learner needs, be willing to share knowledge and expertise, and be capable of brutal honesty, if it is indicated. Mentoring is practiced in partnership with an attitude of generosity, openness, and trust with both parties contributing freely.[11] The mentor may be at the same or a higher level than the learner, but is recognized as seasoned or experienced in the area or subject matter. The participants maintain confidentiality. The information revealed in the mentoring relationship is considered privileged and does not influence performance appraisals. Mentoring is closely related to coaching. They teach, explore alternatives, inspire, act as a sounding board, build confidence and capability, facilitate learning, ask questions, listen with compassion, develop skills, create ownership, provide a challenge, act as a model, and explore potential. A coach often acts as a partner, providing the learner with tools, support, and structure to achieve more than what they might be able to do otherwise.

Training Tools and Aids

Simulation

A mock isolation room was created as a learning station at a large metropolitan hospital. The goal was to increase the awareness of the nursing staff regarding common infection control infractions occurring during the use of medical devices and isolation procautions.[28]

Infection control infractions were staged in an airborne isolation room using a resuscitation mannequin "patient" complete with IV fluids, Foley catheters, tube feeding, suction machine, and ventilator. The simulation method provides for self-learning, participation, and problem-solving effort in a way that is fun and effective.

Flyers advertised educational sessions, participants are provided with the patient case history, and a survey form was used to identify breaches in infection control practices. Problem-solving time was limited to twenty minutes. An "answer station" provided posters with information on the correct practice and rationale. ICPs were available to discuss major issues.

Examples of infection control infractions included:

- urinary catheter system on the floor

- no dressing at the site of an IV line

- the patient lying flat for tube feeding at 100 mL/hr

- saline in a bowl to irrigate suction tubing

APIC Text of Infection Control and Epidemiology

Copyright © 2005, Association for Professionals in Infection Control and Epidemiology, Inc.

- a paper mask

- no soap or alcohol gel available for hand washing.

Educational Cart

Construction of a demonstration cart provides a portable means of displaying educational materials on a specific situation for diverse employee populations working various shifts.[7] For example, the unit could be designed to display and store materials, such as handouts, from the American Lung Association and the Centers for Disease Control and Prevention (CDC) and various types of masks that are available for use. Other types of information available on the cart included tuberculosis epidemiology and transmission, skin testing protocol, diagnosis and treatment regimens, a patient teaching checklist, and an algorithm of control measures.

A prearranged schedule of the touring portable display "TB On the Move" to nursing units and other at-risk departments was announced. The cart ensured that handouts, algorithms, and other written materials were clear, easy to read, and in adequate numbers. An attendance roster and a knowledge assessment tool for evaluation before and after use of the cart was provided.

Multimedia

The multimedia, multisensory educational approach uses a combination of educational stimuli and may incorporate entertaining, fun activities. The development of this type of program usually requires creative thinkers and a multidisciplinary approach. The role and potential for the use of media and technology continues to expand (e.g., print, transparencies, radio and television, slides and types, video, videodisks, computer-based systems, and simulators). A systems approach is indicated to effectively coordinate media equipment, instructional method, and personnel.[46]

The focus of this method is on learner participation and the use of various audiovisual aids to stimulate learning; the more learners sense that they are involved in the educational training session, the more likely learning will occur and be remembered. The CDC education department may be able to assist ICPs from facilities without education or audiovisual departments or those with limited financial resources. The Public Health Training network has become a major provider of distance learning programs and training products for the CDC. Educational offerings range from self-instructional modules and computer-based training to satellite videoconferences, audio conferences, and videotapes. ICPs and other learners may remain at home or in the workplace and receive the latest quality training with nationally recognized continuing education credits (Continuing Education Units [CEUs], Continuing Medical Education [CMEs], and Continuing Nursing Education [CNE]). Call 1–800–41-TRAIN (1–800–418–7246) to receive program information. The Public Health Training Network is on the World Wide Web at: http://www.phppo.cdc.gov/phtn/default.asp. One can browse the catalogue of distance learning courses and resources and view the calendar of upcoming distance learning events.[44]

Audiovisual Aids

Chalkboards/whiteboards are available in most facilities either in portable or installed models. They are inexpensive and easy to use in small to medium-sized groups. The educator writes during class, which consumes time; major concepts can be written in advance. Colored chalk is helpful to augment key thoughts. White boards are alternatives however special markers and erasers are indicated for this type of board. Some colors may have a pungent odor. The boards are easily cleaned.

Overhead projectors are a popular training aid. These devices are a recognized training staple. Projectors enlarge material written on transparent film-like sheets so that a large group can easily read information in a well-lit classroom. The class facilitator can write on the transparencies using special markers for this purpose. Notations can be erased or wiped clean and the transparency is ready for the next class. Transparencies are inexpensive and easily transported. Transparencies tend to stick together; sheet protectors are used to avoid this problem. Number the transparencies to keep them organized. Position the equipment to ensure maximum visibility. It is wise to check the equipment before the class begins to ensure a sharp, clear focus. The equipment is easy to use and requires little maintenance. Keep a spare bulb handy, and learn how to change it. Turn the projector off when not in use. Participants find it bothersome to look at a blank screen or listen to the fan motor run.[34]

The slide projector is noted for being able to produce vivid images and graphics. This projector is easy to operate using remote control, allowing the speaker to move freely about the room. Slide projectors are usually available in most facilities or can be rented if necessary. The slides are prepared in advance and loaded into a carousel or a compact box. Experienced speakers will load the carousel tray themselves to ensure that the slides are in the proper order and right-side up; it is advised to number the slides. A "slide show" is presented in a darkened room and is best for medium to large audiences. A laser pointer is helpful in identifying major points or important data. It is important for the speaker to periodically review the slides so that the information presented is current and appropriate.[34] Visual support should be evaluated to ensure

Copyright © 2005, Association for Professionals in Infection Control and Epidemiology, Inc.

visual impact is heightened and does not distract the learner. Keep visuals strong and simple. It is best to say more than you show.

Computer projection technology provides for powerful multimedia presentations. The projectors may be installed or used as lightweight, portable equipment. The system has enhanced video, high-resolution graphic imagery, and stereophonic sound. It is suitable for large groups, such as employee orientation. Depending upon the computer expertise of the presenter, technical support from the institutional Information Systems Department may be necessary to link the computer systems together. A special cable may be necessary for the computers to communicate with one another. Additionally, the computer programs will need to be compatible for the two systems to work together.

Power Point slides have become one of the most popular and powerful ways to present data in a clear concise method. When stored on a disk they can be easily taken from on learning situation to another. Other advantages for this method include cost of reproduction, ease of editing and customization. Formatting of the slides require both care and consideration. Practice the KISS (Keep it Sweet and Simple) method when designing this style of presentation. In general, the rule of 666 should be applied to this format:

- no more than 6 words per bullet point

- no more than 6 bullet points per slide

- no more than 6 text slides without a visual slide.[14]

Unlike slide presentations, this medium can be presented in a lower light setting and allow for note taking by the learners. Speakers notes can be produced to increase the comfort of the educator and participant notes can be produced that will allow the learners to have exact copies of the projected material. If using preprinted participant notes, print them no more than three per page. This can be used to enhance the learner participation because they will not be dependent upon their ability to write as fast as the educator speaks. Always face the audience, and do not read the slide to the audience. The use of a wireless mouse will allow the educator to walk about the room in a limited fashion and still change the slide. End with a simple thank-you slide so that the learners know that the presentation is finished.

Other considerations with this medium:[14,3]

- Colors:
  - Warm colors (reds, orange, yellows) come forward and command attention. They are difficult to look at in large quantities.

  - Cool colors (blues, green and some purples) recede from your eyes and are more difficult to see at a distance.

  - Cool background colors provide good contrast with text. If you use a warm background color, you may distract the learners from the text message and they will pay attention to the background.

- Contrast: To keep from losing text in the background you have to use color contrast. It is best to pick one or two colors and vary their tints or shades to create the needed contrast.

- Font:
  - Size: 28 point fonts will show well in a large room. Special accommodations can be made for persons of low vision. In this setting headings should be 32 point, subheadings 30 point, text 28 point.[20]

  - Color of fonts can be changed from black to white to improve their contrast with the slide background.[20,3]

- Style: Pick fonts from the same family of fonts. Verdana, Tahoma, and Georgia fonts were designed specifically for online viewing. Arial and Times New Roman are clean fonts that make good titles and headlines.

Videotapes are helpful with self-learning projects and can be obtained from most facility education and staff development departments, libraries, or resource rooms. Videotapes are inexpensive, easily transported, and user-friendly. Mobile units are helpful for on-site "just-in-time" learning situations. Unlike slides, the video may be viewed in a room with normal lighting. Professionally produced videotapes may not be cost-effective depending on facility usage and how fast the information becomes outdated. It is wise to have several subject matter experts review tapes before purchase to ensure the information presented reflects the infection control practices of the facility. It is a burden for the educator to have to "unteach" concepts and confusing to the participant to "unlearn." Short video "snippets" are helpful to the speaker to demonstrate a point or to open the door for group discussion.[34]

Tape recorders, used as a tool for creating classroom ambiance with appropriate music, are an excellent way to relax participants. Music during course registration, at breaks, and at the end of the program can influence mood and induce positive feelings among participants. Tape recorders are also helpful in preparing for presentations. A speaker can study the method of delivery, flow of information, and the time necessary for different segments.[34]

Copyright © 2005, Association for Professionals in Infection Control and Epidemiology, Inc.

Flip charts are frequently used in small group training sessions. They are easily used and inexpensive. If necessary, some pages may be prepared ahead of time. Use contrasting colored markers to project energy and imagination. A speaker can identify participant learning needs on the flip chart and record results of brainstorming exercises. Participants can use flip charts in work groups to show problem-solving activity, action plans, or consensus. Flip charts are an excellent tool for enhancing group interaction and communication. Each work group can demonstrate their work to the group at large and elicit feedback from a group of their peers, for example, management of occupational exposures to bloodborne exposures.[34]

Self-Instructional Modules

Self-instructional modules are written to provide another alternative for the visual learner. They provide a self-paced approach to allow the learner to explore new/old information autonomously or in small groups. Modules are user-friendly and simply written. Subject matter experts usually review the content to provide content validity. ICPs should assist in the development of modules specific to infection control. An example of this technique was developed by McCalla and colleagues[27] to accommodate complicated work schedules and identified knowledge gaps in infection control policies and practices. A pre- and post-test format was used to assess the nursing staff's knowledge on infection control.

Managers are responsible for employee safety education. Self-instructional modules provide the manager or the area educator the approved curriculum for unit training.

Distance Learning[44]

Interactive audio, graphic, and video conferencing systems allow for the exchange of medical information from one location to another through electronic communications. This innovative technology links healthcare providers in remote or underserved areas to specialty patient care services for fast medical consultation. It is also valuable in providing for ongoing employee education, training, and collaboration with other health professionals.[45]

Users must allow ample preparation time in the program-planning phase, especially if this is a new experience. The overall effectiveness of the educational intervention depends upon training and knowledge of equipment use. Onsite communication experts or technologists should be available to provide speaker tips for success, "hands-on" instruction, and written materials for facilitating an effective presentation. Meet with a teleconference representative to assess the services offered and discuss the best way to prepare. If possible, observe distance learning in session and garner advice from experienced presenters.

Some points to remember when arranging a distance learning session:

- Determine the number of sites that will be "online" for your presentation.

- Know the number and location of necessary equipment such as cameras, monitors, microphones, or telephones. Practice using the equipment.

- Introduce at least one spokesperson at each teleconference site. Try to call participants by name.

- Create a group comfort level and mutual regard for participants. Overcome the intimidation of electronic equipment by assisting each other.

- Engage participants in a balanced discussion. Involve on-site and off-site participants equally. Avoid side discussions.

- Ask a representative from each site to report transmission difficulties with sound or vision. If there will be a delay, it is best to announce it. If an off-site group must disengage for any reason, provide an explanation and continue with the presentation or discussion.

- Allow for breaks and questions. The speaker voice quality and the ability to pace and pause during the presentation are important skills to master for an effective delivery.

- Use every opportunity during the presentation to experience or practice the skill of involving the group and eliciting participation. Conversation is the most effective style; humor is appreciated and helps participants to relax, respond to questions, and enjoy the event. Facilitation, like any other public speaking skill, takes thought, preparation, and practice to be effective.

- Plan for a debriefing sessions after the conference to assess program strengths and areas for improvement.

- Provide evaluations for off-site participants. Ask their assistance in providing feedback information to improve the quality of the program.

PREPARING THE ENVIRONMENT FOR LEARNING

It is the responsibility of the educator to ensure facilities are set up appropriately. Environmental factors, such as room temperature, lighting, and training equipment, are checked for proper working order and safety. The physical environment of the training classroom can facilitate the learning process or obstruct it.

Copyright © 2005, Association for Professionals in Infection Control and Epidemiology, Inc.

There is not an ideal setup, but there are many options available.[34]

General Characteristics

The room should be large enough to handle registered participants and "walk-ins." If possible, allow two spaces per person to allow space for materials and personal belongings. A separate table and chairs are provided for the speaker(s). The room should be orderly and look and smell clean. The interior decorating of the classroom should be inviting and stimulating in terms of color and comfort. A resource table, appropriate posters, and separate registration and food areas enhance the setting. Appropriate background music can be pleasant and energizing, especially during registration and breaks.[34]

Common Classroom Settings

The traditional classroom setup with straight rows of desks does not promote interaction. Better ways to arrange the classroom exist.[40]

The horseshoe shape is an all-purpose setup. It allows face-to-face participant contact and provides a writing surface. The educator and training equipment are positioned for easy visibility. Participants can be positioned inside the U for group activity.

Team style is achieved by arranging small tables and chairs around the room. It facilitates group activity and interaction. Some participants will have to turn their chairs around when the class reconvenes, but this is acceptable.

Conference table style is best if the arrangement is circular or square; if it is rectangular, it creates a "person's table" effect and a sense of formality. The facilitator is placed at the head of the table in the power position.

The *circle arrangement* with chairs and no tables allows for direct face-to-face contact.

This is excellent for open group discussion without the barriers of furnishings. If table surface is needed, place tables on the outside of the circle, but within reach of the participants.

Chevron or *fishbone style*, a repeated V arrangement, creates less distance between participants and provides greater visibility of the educator. If the traditional classroom style is the only choice available, then group the chairs in pairs to promote partnering. Provide enough space between rows to allow for the formation of quartets.

Stadium or auditorium style is a limiting environment for active training. Participants can be paired for brief activities requiring a learning partner, though it may seem awkward to participants.[39]

THE INFECTION CONTROL PROFESSIONAL AS A LEARNER

Development of Self

The continual expansion of the mind and knowledge base is vital to one's growth and renewal. The proactive ICP reads extensively, seeks association with keen, value-centered thinkers, and incorporates self-education into a plan for professional development.[13]

Self-assessment is a valuable tool for discovering one's inner compass. Review courses, such as the Certification Study Guide, can be used to identify areas of needed improvement. People must start from where they are by examining personal values and learning needs and having the courage to change. Learning is not something that happens only in the head; it involves the whole being as we interact with our fast-shifting environment. Learning demands that we cope with the intensity of high-speed change and take responsibility for our own performance.[42]

Strive for a deeper level of thinking; make the pursuit of excellence a habit. In conflict resolution or when engaged in problem solving activities, try to first understand and then to be understood. The work of seeking, finding, and analyzing data is driven by the desire to learn and the need for the wisdom to protect those in our charge. For the ICP, learning is not a must but a given.[13]

In today's fast-paced healthcare environment, self-directed learning is a major force for the adult learner. Though organizations will continue to mandate workplace learning, there is a growing awareness of the need for workers who are knowledge-seekers and motivated to learn on their own.[17]

- Motivation to change or learn rarely comes from inspirational teachers, but from a personal need to do something useful to make a difference in life and to establish one's identity.[22]

- Working in a heterogeneous group with those who do not think alike increases personal development. Embracing diversity and seeking to understand conflicting opinions and different ways to solve problems leads to innovation and creative solutions.[10]

- The educator is a perpetual learner and is a role model for others to emulate; educators set the example for effective learning as well as effective teaching.

- The educator assists the learner to claim deficiencies and suggests ways to correct them.[18]

Copyright © 2005, Association for Professionals in Infection Control and Epidemiology, Inc.

- Guidance in self-directed learning is provided through the assessment of goals, needs, and interests and in brainstorming ways to expand professional knowledge base.

- Cognitive strategies used to facilitate the learning process include linking new knowledge to prior knowledge, mind mapping or comparing the relationship of major ideas, questioning facts and validating answers, developing an action plan for self-improvement.[48]

Professional Learning Needs

Continuing education is a professional need of the ICP, who seek it out for a variety of reasons.

Expertise is a job requirement. A Certification Board of Infection Control (CBIC) analysis of job tasks performed by ICPs in the United States and in Canada identified six major areas of knowledge or basic learning needs that are essential to the practice of infection control:

- Identification of infectious disease processes

- Surveillance and epidemiological investigations

- Preventing/controlling the transmission of infectious agents

- Program management and communication

- Education and research

- Infection control aspects of an Employee Health/ Occupational Health Program[30]

The Delphi project[31] was carried out to identify those activities the experienced ICP identified as necessary components of a successful infection control program. Over a series of ten surveys, a job analysis was accomplished. Functions identified as necessary are as follows: IC Communication (13%), Education (16%), Identifying infections (12%), Surveillance/Epidemiological investigations (27%), Prevent transmission (14%), Control outbreaks (8%), and Manage IC Program (10%). Tasks identified as necessary components of the education activities are as follows: developing educational materials (35%), presenting educational materials (35%), assessing educational needs (25%) and evaluation (5%).

In addition, the regulatory and consulting groups that oversee healthcare require that infection control programs be managed by capable, trained individuals. Joint Commission on Accreditation of Healthcare Organizations (JCAHO), for instance, requires that the management of the infection control program be assigned to a qualified person.[23] The intent of this recommendation is to ensure that persons who manage infection control programs are properly trained in surveillance, prevention, and control functions and have knowledge or job experience in the areas of epidemiological principles and infectious disease as well as sterilization, sanitation, and disinfection practices. Certification in infection control is one example of a "qualified individual" that satisfies this JCAHO standard.

A major purpose of CBIC is to maintain a certification process for the protection of the public. CBIC itself encourages professional growth and study among infection control professionals and recognizes those who meet the requirements for certification. The certification examination measures the current standard of knowledge needed to practice infection control and epidemiology. Testing is available in two formats: computer based tests for all first-time certifiers and an optional take-home format (SARE) for recertifiers. Questions in both formats are equivalent to one another.[30]

APIC also sets a standard for continued learning for ICPs. Education that includes developing programs ICPs can use to teach healthcare workers infection control and to promote wellness among patients and the general public is a major goal within APIC's strategic plan. APIC offers a range of training programs beginning with ICE 1, ICE 2, and ICE 3. Many local APIC chapters offer continuing education for their members. ICPs also have a personal investment in competence.[30] In 2003 76% of the ICPs completing the SARE listed "recertification" as their reason for taking this test. Alvin Toffler, *Future Shock* warns, "the illiterate in the year 2000 will not be persons who cannot read or write, but those who cannot learn, unlearn, and relearn."[43] ICPs are aware that they can never stop learning. They are aware that mental toughness, job competencies, and skills are required for effective workplace performance.

Establishing performance improvement goals that are SMART will help the professional meet the continuing education challenge:

- Specific and clear

- Measurable indicators for success

- Appropriate to the job and in sync with organizational mission

- Realistic but challenging. Focus on where you can add value.

- Time activated with short- and long-term objectives.[16]

Copyright © 2005, Association for Professionals in Infection Control and Epidemiology, Inc.

EDUCATIONAL CHALLENGES

Satisfying Facility-Mandated Education

With healthcare becoming one of the most heavily regulated of American industries, employees can anticipate an increase in institutionally mandated education. With a lack of coordination among regulatory bodies, conflict between the various regulations will need to be resolved and communicated clearly to Administration and the healthcare workers. Healthcare facility administrators must ensure organizational compliance to minimize the threat of litigation and/or heavy fines for code violations. For the employer and employee alike, the business side of operations must be balanced with a clear understanding of organizational ethical principles and values. Corporate Compliance emphasizes that actions reflect the fabric of the organizational value system.[12] As new problems evolve, new solutions will occur.

Tracking Performance Outcomes

The positive influence of educational intervention on worker performance will be demonstrated. Educators will routinely use benchmarks to guide learning achievement and responses to change. Educators will be proactive in the anticipation of changes in learner populations and in organizational needs. Tracking performance outcomes and measuring effectiveness of training has become the norm.[38] Leaders recognize that to succeed in the new millennium, the goal for healthcare institutions will be to develop employees to their highest level of performance, to bring out the best in each person. Workers will be encouraged to acquire new knowledge and, in turn, share their expertise or "know how" with others, that is, "each one, teach one." Developing the skills for creativity and innovation in the application of knowledge will be the challenge for the educator who must balance employee and organizational needs.

Maximizing Facilitation Skills

ICPs will become adept in the art of classroom facilitation and the promotion of unbounded thinking among learner populations. The Socratic teaching method[48] reemerges as ICPs strive to help others think critically. The educator asks the appropriate question to provoke and stimulate the learner in identifying and solving problems. This is a time-consuming task that requires both patience and skill, but one which will reap rewards with its impact on critical problem-solving skills.

Maximizing the Use of Training Technology

Technology is the major impetus in the educational change process; it is revolutionizing the way people are taught. Computers enable employees to manage time more effectively and are excellent study aids. Since 1990, computer literacy is a major training focus of workplace education. Web search engines have expanded the traditional methods used for research and increased the availability of innovative thinking. Self-directed learning is more easily accomplished with the computer than at any previous time. Self-directed teams will become the norm in healthcare. The goal will be to assess and make recommendations for needed changes.[22,26]

Recognizing Learner Population Diversity

Because of reengineering and reorganization, healthcare organizations are experiencing an increase in the growth on part-time or temporary staff, contract labor, students, and volunteers. Coupled with increasing average age, learner audiences will include a more diverse group with a wider array of worker expertise.

As part of performance improvement, the healthcare worker will assume more responsibility for workplace learning. Currently, performance appraisals in some facilities indicate the expectations for mastery of certain infection control skills. With increased emphasis on facility report cards and public reporting of hospital-acquired infections, the expectation is that more facilities will include compliance with infection control policies and procedures in employee performance appraisals.

Implementing Competency-Based Training

Workplace training initiatives will be directly linked to the implementation of professional and regulatory standards as well as facility policies and procedures. ICPs will become more focused on skill development and the worker competencies necessary to meet the infection control objectives, for example, sterilization and disinfection and specimen handling. Competencies describe worker skills, knowledge, and the mindset necessary to achieve effective job performance. These elements detail the specific outcomes or job expectations as indicated by role work setting and professional standards and facility accepted benchmarks or "best practices" in the field. The focus is on the demonstration of competence by benchmarking rather than a comparison to fellow workers or peers. The benchmarking process ensures ongoing evaluation and monitoring.

Developing Flexibility in Training Methods

With the recognition that adults learn in a variety of ways, ICPs will expand their teaching skills beyond the traditional lecture/slide show method. The impact of bioterrorism, new and unusual disease presentations, such as West Nile disease, Monkey pox, SARS, and

Copyright © 2005, Association for Professionals in Infection Control and Epidemiology, Inc.

Avian flu, have increased the need for timely thorough education activities. To address these increasing demands ICPs will need to develop new strategies based on evidence-based practices to readily adapt to the learning needs of their audiences and their facilities.

IV.   SUMMARY AND CONCLUSIONS

Adults bring life experiences into the learning situation. Life changes can motivate adults to engage in new learning experiences. Learning new skills and knowledge takes time for integration to occur. Action plans, accountability and follow-up all increase the likelihood that learning will take place. Theories of education are only a guide to the instructor. Effective instructors will be flexible, eclectic and creative in the instructional presentations they make. Presentations must be perceived as interesting, useful and relevant for the adult learner to willingly participate in the activity. Measurements of learning should be made over time to identify future training needs.

V.   FUTURE TRENDS/RESEARCH

Increasing demands for mass staff education to address a complex and rapidly changing healthcare environment will additional skills and resources for ICPs. Reliance on outside sources of creditable education will become more necessary as more unusual disease processes become evident. Collaboration with outside sources of education will also need to be enhanced. Non-traditional formats for education will have to be utilized to accommodate the changing needs for timely information on infection control practices and procedures.

VI.   INTERNATIONAL PERSPECTIVES

Concepts of trans-cultural care need to be incorporated into successful educational activities. Cultural backgrounds will affect the ability of the learner to participate in learning activities and accommodate new skills and ideas. Trans-cultural education will encompass different perceptions based on geography, gender, religion, social status, age, sexual orientation, and ethnic diversity. Care must be taken to minimize miscommunication when the instructor and the learners do not speak the same language. The development of a mentor relationship as a cultural quality control will help guide the instructor to develop appropriate educational activities.

REFERENCES

1. Andragogy (M. Knowles): Available online at http://tip.psychology.org/knowles.html
2. Becker R: Taking the misery out of experimental training, *Training* February 1998.
3. Beretta G: *Understanding color,* Palo Alto, 2000, Hewlett-Packard Company.
4. Bernthal PR: Evaluation that goes the distance, *Train Dev J* 41–45, 1995.
5. Bhola HS: *World trends and issues in adult education.* London, 1989, Zed Books.
6. Bloom's Taxonomy: Learning domains or Bloom's taxonomy. Available online at http://www.nwlink.com/donclard/hrd/bloom.html
7. Borella A, Hixon F, Yahl M: TB education on the move [poster], 21st Annual Education Conference, APIC: The next generation, Cincinnati, 1994.
8. Buzan, Tony: *Make the most of your mind,* 1984, Fireside Books.
9. Caffarella RS: Preparing for the transfer of learning. In *Planning programs for adult learners: a practical guide,* San Francisco, 1994, Josey-Bass.
10. Canaday H: Rising price, *Selling Power* 17:22, 1997.
11. Cohen N: *Mentoring adult learners,* Malabar, FL, 1995, Krieger Publishing.
12. Compliance officers: Pandoras they're not, *Hosp Health Netw* 1998.
13. Covey, SR: *The seven habits of highly effective people,* New York, 1989, Simon & Schuster.
14. Designing Guidelines for Creating a Quality Power Point Presentation. Available online at http://education.umn.edu/tel/itfellows/power_point_designs/index_design.htm
15. Dorek PM, Huang S, Chan-Yan C: A lecturing skills course for residents, *Train Learn Med* 6:2, 1994.
16. Fine A, Sachs M: Setting goals, *Soccer Psychol* 14–15, 1998.
17. Fitchett J: Managing your organization's key asset-knowledge [poster], *Healthc Forum J* 1998.
18. Hinson P: Education. In Olmsted RN, editor: *2002 Infection control and applied epidemiology, principals and practice,* Washington, DC, 2002, Mosby, Association for Professionals in Infection Control and Epidemiology.
19. Hinson P: Education for the adult learner. In Gurevich I, Tafura P, Cunha B, editors: *The theory and practice of infection control,* New York, 1984, Praeger.
20. Hollingsworth CD: Making effective presentation/using color effectively. Available online at http://www.iupui.edu/webtrain/tutorials/effective_visual_aids_files/htm
21. Hyerle D: *Designs for thinking connectively,* ed 3, Lyme, NH, 1990, Innovative Science.
22. Industry report, 1997. *Training* October 1997.
23. Joint Commission on Accreditation of Healthcare Organizations: *Accreditation Manual for Hospitals,* Chicago, 2003, Joint Commission on Accreditation of Healthcare Organizations, IC1.2.
24. Kitchel E: Guidelines for the development of PowerPoint presentations for audiences that may include persons with low vision. American Printing House for the Blind. Available online at http://www.aph.org/tc/ppguide.html
25. Kirkpatrick DL: *Evaluating training programs: the four levels,* ed 1, San Francisco, 1994, Berrett-Koehler.
26. Lancaster D, Willis MA: Computer-assisted instruction (CAI): a time-saving, individualized teaching methodology, *Am J Infect Control* 22:3, 1994.
27. McCalla, Koll, et al. Improving Infection Control Education for Nurses Using Self-Learning Modules: An Infection Control Project. [Poster]. 31st Annual Educational Conference and International Meeting: APIC, 2004, Phoenix.
28. Moralego D, Gaese C: The mock isolation room: a fun way to review infection control, *J Contin Educ Nurs* 24:4, 1993.
29. Needs Assessment. Available online at http://www3.edc.org/NTP/needsassessment.htm
30. Nutty CJ: 2003 APIC Certification study guide, Washington, DC, APIC, 2003.
31. O'Boyle C, Jackson M, Henly S: Staffing requirements for infection control programs in US health care facilities: Delphi project, vol 30, no 3, Washington, DC, 2002, AJIC, Mosby, pp 321–333.

Copyright © 2005, Association for Professionals in Infection Control and Epidemiology, Inc.

32. Parry S: 10 ways to win more management support for training, *Training Director's Forum Newsletter* December 1995.
33. Pavlov's dog. Available online at http://www.nobel.se/medicine/educational/pavlov/readmore.html
34. Powers B: Training aids to enhance learning. In *Instructor excellence,* San Francisco, 1992, Josey-Bass.
35. Ricks DM: Challenging assumptions that block work, *Training* August 1997.
36. Ryatt A, Lohan K: *Creating training miracles,* San Francisco, 1997, Pfeiffer & Company.
37. Self-directed learning. Available online at http://home.twcny.r-r.com/hiemstra/sdlearn.html
38. Shandler D: *Reengineering the training function: how to align training with the new corporate agenda,* Delray, FL, 1996, St. Lucie Press.
39. Shea G: *Mentoring—a practical guide,* Menlo Park, CA, 1992, Crisp Publications.
40. Silberman M: Layouts for setting up a training classroom. In *101 ways to make training active,* San Diego, 1995, Pfeiffer & Company.
41. Socratic teaching. Available online at http://lonestar.texas.net/mseifert/crit3.html
42. Toffler A: *Learning for tomorrow,* New York, 1974, Vintage.
43. Toffler A: *Future shock,* New York, 1970, Bantam.
44. *Training Director's Forum Newsletter:* Evaluation, July 1997.
45. US Department of Health and Human Services: *Distance learning courses and resources,* Public Training Network, 1998.
46. Visconti T, Irby B, Escano A: Infection control can be fun: a creative approach to infection control education in the pharmacy [poster].Presented at 21st Annual Educational Conference: APIC—the next generation, Cincinnati, 1994.
47. Willyerd KA: Balancing your evaluation act, *Training* 53–58, 1997.
48. Zemke R: In search of self-directed learners, *Training* 60–68, 1998.
49. Zemke R and Zemke S. 30 Things we know for sure about adult learning, *Innovation Abstracts* 6:8, 1984.

SUPPLEMENTAL RESOURCES

Downloadable wordsheets and crossword puzzles: http://www.qualin-t.com/index.html.

Issues related to cultural diversity: http://www.culturediversity.org

Cross-cultural resources and clinical practice guidelines: http://medicine.ucsf.edu/resources/guidelines/culture.html

Copyright © 2005, Association for Professionals in Infection Control and Epidemiology, Inc.

12

REVISED 2004

Patient Safety

Denise M. Murphy, RN, BSN, MPH, CIC*
Chief Safety and Quality Officer
Barnes-Jewish Hospital at Washington University
Medical Center
St. Louis, Missouri

ABSTRACT

"If you know how to prevent infections, you know how to protect patients from most adverse events."[1] The patient safety movement in this country is thought to have begun in 1999, with the publication of the Institute of Medicine's report *To Err is Human.*[1] In fact, formal efforts to keep patients safe began in the United States with the development of hospital infection control programs in the 1960s, and globally, even as far back as the mid-1800s, when Hungarian physician Ignaz Semmelweis and British nurse Florence Nightengale publicized the value of hand hygiene as an infection prevention technique. However, the so-called epidemic of medical errors plaguing our nation's healthcare system and eroding the public's trust in providers is a reality.

There are almost 90,000 deaths annually linked to healthcare-acquired infections, a problem that dedicated infection control professionals (ICPs) attack daily. Although the statistics on medical errors have been widely scrutinized, one cannot cast a blind eye to the additional 50,000–100,000 deaths caused annually by medication errors, falls, wrong site surgeries, missed diagnoses, or misidentified patients. There has been a public outcry and a national call to action to stop this epidemic and focus on preventing all healthcare-related adverse events. Every healthcare professional, in every institution and at every level, has been challenged to develop and implement programs to actively seek out risk and document harm (surveillance/reporting), to proactively design error-proof processes and systems (prevention), and to create a culture where everyone, with every action, is responsible and accountable for patient safety (control). This chapter provides an overview for professionals in surveillance and disease prevention and control of the broader patient safety challenges and their role in national patient safety efforts.

KEY CONCEPTS

- Patient safety terminology and definitions

- Theories on accident causation

- Creating a culture of safety

- Teamwork and communication

- Human factors in patient safety (and HR engineering)

- Surveillance for patient safety events/patient safety event reporting

*The author would like to acknowledge the work of the BJC Patient Safety Council, specifically, those members who participated in the development of the Patient Safety Curriculum: Trish Hill, RN, Barbara Caleca, RN, and Laurie Wolf, Human Factors Engineer.

Copyright © 2005, Association for Professionals in Infection Control and Epidemiology, Inc.

- The learning organization

- Targeted intervention to reduce medical errors and evidence-based prevention measure and control

- Role of ICP in patient safety

I.   BACKGROUND

The Institute of Medicine (IOM) defines *medical error* as the failure of a planned action to be completed as intended or the use of a wrong plan to achieve an aim.[1] Two large studies, one conducted using 1984 data from over 30,000 hospitalized patients in New York State and another using 1992 data on patients in Colorado and Utah, found that 2.9% to 3.7% of inpatient admissions experienced an adverse event.[2] (See Figure 12–1.) These alarming statistics led to the publication of the IOM report, *To Err is Human,* on the epidemic of medical errors in the United States in November 1999.[1]

That report stated that 44,000 to 98,000 people die in hospitals each year as a result of human errors. It prompted examination of the "human" aspect of human error, specifically to look at faulty systems, processes, and conditions that lead people to make mistakes or fail to prevent them from doing so. This signified a move away from a more traditional medical and nursing school model which looked to blame mistakes on individuals, or their lack of adequate training. The most common adverse errors affecting patients include: medication and transfusion errors, infections, complications of surgery (including wrong-site surgery), suicide, restraint-related injuries, falls, burns, pressure ulcers, misidentification, and wrong diagnosis or treatment.

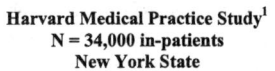

Harvard Medical Practice Study[1]
N = 34,000 in-patients
New York State

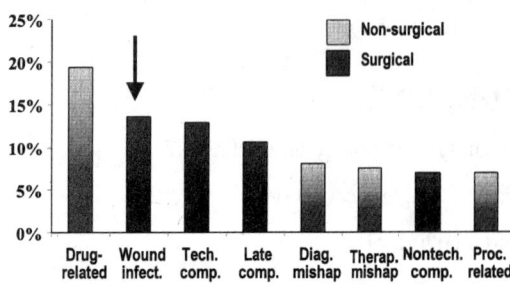

Source: Brennan, 1991

Figure 12–1   Most frequent adverse events in hospitalized patients.

Reported medical error-related deaths exceed the combined numbers of deaths and injuries from motor and air crashes, suicides, falls, poisoning, and drownings, despite the fact that such events are still seriously under-reported. Most errors occur in intensive care units, operating rooms, and emergency departments. The Agency for Healthcare Research and Quality (AHRQ) summarizes the underlying causes of medical error[4] to be related to:

- Communication problems

- Inadequate information flow

- Human problems

- Patient-related issues

- Organizational transfer of knowledge

- Staffing patterns/work flow

- Technical failures

- Inadequate policies and procedures

In addition to the high cost in morbidity and mortality linked to medical errors, AHRQ estimates that medical errors cost a large hospital about $5 million per year and total $17 — $29 billion per year in the United Sstates.[5] Costs include the expense of additional care required to treat medical errors, lost income and household productivity, and the cost of long-term or permanent disability. The additional costs of societal mistrust in the healthcare system and diminished satisfaction of patients and health professionals is hard to quantify but could be very damaging.

In terms of lives lost, the IOM report estimates that medication errors alone, either in or out of the hospital, account for over 7,000 deaths per year. Studies show that about two of every 100 admissions experience a preventable adverse drug event, resulting in average excess hospital costs of $4,700 per admission, or $2.8 million annually for a 700-bed teaching hospital. The report states that, if these findings are generalizable, the increased hospital costs alone of preventable in-patient adverse drug events are about $2 billion per year.[1]

CDC estimates that 2 million patients/year are infected in U.S. hospitals and that approximately 90,000 die (1 death every 6 minutes). Healthcare-acquired infections are estimated to cost at least $6.7 billion annually in 2002 dollars.[8] The Harvard Medical Practice study listed surgical site infections as the second most common adverse event experienced by in-patients in New York hospitals.[6] The literature reports that up to 350,000 hospitalized patients acquire bloodstream infections each year, and these infections cost a minimum of about $38,703 per episode.[9] Bloodstream infections are associated with a

APIC Text of Infection Control and Epidemiology

Copyright © 2005, Association for Professionals in Infection Control and Epidemiology, Inc.

mean attributable mortality of 15–20%.[10] The impact of these two types of healthcare-acquired infections alone underscores the importance of infection prevention in reducing adverse outcomes from hospitalization. Between 1995 and July 2004, 2,768 sentinel events in hospitals were reported to JCAHO; 75% of them resulted in a patient's death.[11] Fourteen percent of these events were wrong site surgeries. The Association of Operating Room Nurses (AORN) defines wrong site surgery broadly as any surgical procedure done on the wrong body part or the wrong patient. It is considered a sentinel event under the JCAHO definitionthat a sentinel event is any unanticipated event resulting in death or permanent disability, or risk thereof. JCAHO encourages voluntary reporting of sentinel events and requires that a root cause analysis (RCA) be conducted and results reported. During the 2004 National Patient Safety Conference, a JCAHO representative reported that in fully 100% of RCAs submitted to them for wrong site surgery, someone in the room at the time of the error admitted knowing that something wrong was about to happen but was too intimidated to speak up or stop the error. The data support this claim, given that the top root cause of *all* medical errors is a breakdown in communication among healthcare workers.

In addition to wrong site surgeries, wrong site errors are a risk with any invasive procedure, such as performing a thoracotomy, inserting chest tubes, or placing central line catheters. The excess costs of hospitalization and prolonged lengths of stay associated specifically with wrong site errors has not been reported in the literature, but may be significant.

The overall cost of medical errors cited in the IOM report ($17 to $29 billion) doesn't include lost opportunity costs — money spent for diagnostic tests, to treat medication errors, or to return patients to the operating room for drainage of surgical site infections with is then unavailable for other, potentially more valuable activities. The costs to insurers, providers, and patients are inflated by services that would have been unnecessary if proper care had been provided. In many parts of the United States, clinicians are abandoning their medical practices due to the rising cost of malpractice premiums. Yet no amount of money in damages or settlements can make up for the physical and psychological damage experienced by patients and families as a result of serious medical error.

II. BASIC PRINCIPLES

The IOM report cites the categories or types of medical errors reported by Leape et al.,[3] as diagnostic, therapeutic, preventive, or related to failures of communication, equipment or other system. Diagnostic errors are defined as those related to:

- error or delay in diagnosis
- failure to employ indicated tests
- use of outmoded tests or therapy
- failure to act on results of monitoring or testing.

Treatment-related errors are:

- errors in performance of an operation, procedure, or test
- errors in administering treatment
- errors in the dose or method of using a drug
- avoidable delay in treatment or in responding to an abnormal test result
- inappropriate (not indicated) care.

Preventive errors are:

- failure to provide prophylactic treatment
- inadequate monitoring or follow-up of treatment

Some terms that appear frequently in the patient safety literature are defined in Table 12–1.

III. PATIENT SAFETY

Theories on Accident Causation

Much has been written about accident causation and many lessons learned from other high-risk industries where consequences of human or technological failures are grave. Although there may not be total congruence of comparisons made between healthcare and the airline or manufacturing industries, everyone can agree that healthcare is a complex environment in which systems fail and people suffer.

The two most common models of accident causation in the patient safety literature come from James Reason and from David D. Woods. The human tendency to remember events with "hindsight bias" has been explored by Richard Cook.

The "Swiss Cheese" Model

Reason's "Swiss Cheese" model[12] demonstrates how complex systems fail because of the combination and timing of multiple small failures. Reason contends that any one failure or situation alone would be insufficient to cause an accident, but that the combination and timing of small failures look much like the alignment of holes in a piece of Swiss cheese (see Figure 12–2).

An example of the Swiss cheese concept follows. An intensive care unit (ICU) nurse is floated to an

Copyright © 2005, Association for Professionals in Infection Control and Epidemiology, Inc.

Table 12-1. Patient safety terminology

Term	Meaning (Source)
Patient Safety	Freedom from accidental injury (IOM)
Adverse Event	An injury caused by medical management rather than the underlying disease (Brennan)
Error	Failure of a planned action to be completed as intended (e.g., error of execution) or use of a wrong plan to achieve an aim (e.g., error of planning). (IOM)
Near Miss or Close Call	Situation in which a medical error has been found and stopped before affecting a patient
Active Failures	Unsafe acts or omissions committed by those whose activities can have immediate adverse consequences (e.g., pilots, air traffic controllers, physicians, nurses) (Vincent)
Latent Errors	Errors in design, organization, training, or maintenance that lead to operator errors and the effects of which typically lie dormant in the system for a lengthy period of time (IOM)
Intentional Unsafe Acts	Events that pertain to patients and result from: (1) a criminal act, (2) a purposefully unsafe act, (3) an act related to alcohol/substance abuse, and/or (4) events involving alleged or suspected patient abuse of any kind (Veteran's Administration)
Human Factors Engineering (HFE)	Discipline concerned with design of tools, machines, equipment, and systems that are safe, comfortable, and effective for human use, taking into account human capabilities, limitations, and characteristics. HFE is used synonymously with ergonomics, usability engineering, and user-centered design. (Gosbee)
Sentinel Event	An unexpected occurrence involving death or serious physical or psychological injury, or risk thereof (JCAHO)
Root Cause Analysis (RCA)	A process for identifying the basic or causal factors that underlie variation in performance. This process should be used to identify risk that led to a sentinel event.
Failure Mode and Effects Analysis (FMEA)	A systematic, proactive method for evaluating a process to identify where and how it might fail and to assess the relative impact of different failures, in order to identify the parts of the process that are most in need of change (Institute for Healthcare Improvement)

oncology unit due to a staffing shortage. She administers a wrong dose of chemotherapy. This nurse fails to have an experienced oncology nurse doublecheck the physician's order against the prepared medication before giving it to the patient. The experienced oncology nurse who anticipates being asked to assist with the doublecheck, is unexpectedly involved in a

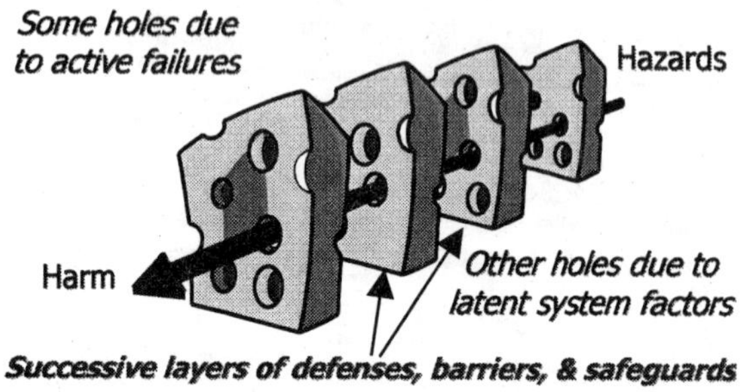

Figure 12-2 "Swiss Cheese" model of accident causation.[12]

crisis and forgets to "check in" with the float nurse prior to the incident. The holes in the Swiss cheese lined up, and the patient was harmed.

In this case, the active failure was the nurse's noncompliance with the medication administration policy and delivery of the wrong chemotherapeutic agent. Other failures — other holes in the Swiss cheese — are considered latent or hidden. The floating nurse is probably uncomfortable with her lack of experience dealing with oncology patients, as well as her stress level related to being pulled from her assigned unit. Both of these factors likely distract her and contribute to the mistake. What neither nurse sees are the budget cuts that led to the staffing shortages and allowed organizational safety systems (safe staffing levels) to fail both the staff and the patient.

The "Blunt End/Sharp End" Model

David Woods writes about a second model of accident causation called the "Blunt End/Sharp End" model.[13]

Copyright © 2005, Association for Professionals in Infection Control and Epidemiology, Inc.

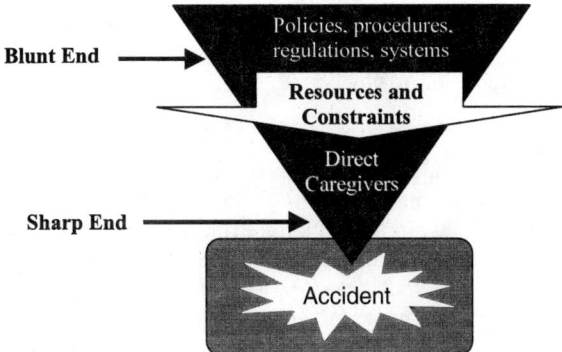

Figure 12–3 "Blunt End/Sharp End" model of accident causation.[13]

This model assumes that healthcare workers at the "sharp end," where patient care is delivered, are affected by decisions, policies, and regulations made at the "blunt end" of the system, which represents, in broad terms, hospital administration of any kind. This administrative end generates resources, defines constraints, and createsconflicts that shape the world of technical work and produce latent failures (see Figure 12–3). At the sharp end, constraints can place pressure on providers who, in turn, develop coping mechanisms (healthy) or shortcuts (often risky) that impact the patient and family.

"Hindsight Bias"

Richard Cook, an anesthesiologist who has dedicated his career to understanding the cause and reaction to accidents in healthcare, reminds us that investigations into accidents usually stop with the identification of human error and of practitioners as the cause of the event. There is often no evaluation of systems or processes that may have contributed, just the blaming of people.

This type of people-centered investigation often leads to something Cook calls "hindsight bias."[13] Knowledge about the outcome of an event makes the path to failure seem to have been foreseeable or predictable, although it was actually not foreseen. Hindsight bias can occur when we make a judgment or choice and are later asked to recall that judgment or recount behaviors and actions. If, after an accident, it becomes evident what the right action or judgment should have been, the memory of our own actions may become biased toward the new or right information. Thinking back on an accident, we often remember things a little differently than the way they actually happened, and we tend to fill in any gaps with information we feel is closer to what should have happened.

Creating a Just Culture of Safety

Theories and models about patient safety raise our awareness about the complexity of the system in which patients receive care and providers work. The patient safety literature is filled with recommendations for organizational leaders to become "systems thinkers" and to eliminate the "blame-and-shame" mentality of the past. A culture of safety must prevent punitive reactions to mistakes, and staff members must feel confident that if they speak out about risk, their leaders will respond. Providers involved in medical errors must know that leaders will look beyond the obvious and drill down until the root causes of accidents and errors are found and that they will routinely evaluate systems and processesduring any accident investigation. Until such a major culture change is embraced and front line staff members are more involved in the decision-making that affects the delivery of care, we will never get to the true etiology of medical errors, and our efforts at prevention and elimination may be futile.

Before we can envision a culture of safety, we must understand the culture of complex organizations. Organizational culture can be described as the set of values, guiding beliefs, or ways of thinking that are shared among members of an organization. It is the feel of an organization which is quickly picked up by new members. Culture is "the way we do things around here." Culture is powerful and is perhaps most noticeable when new strategies or programs are implemented that go against the embedded organizational culture. People often resist changing the way they do things, or changing the culture in which they live or work.

How do we define a culture of safety? It is well expressed by Tom Hellmich, a physician member of the Patient Safety Council at Children's Hospital and Clinics in Minneapolis. Dr. Hellmich states,

> The medical culture that silently taught the ABCs as *Accuse, Blame* and *Criticize* is fading. Rising in its place is a safety culture emphasizing blameless reporting, successful systems, knowledge, respect, confidentiality and trust.[14]

Schools of medicine, nursing, and allied health, previously taught providers to ask, when things went wrong, "Who did it?" The focus was on individuals' failures. This is referred to as the traditional medical model. In a safety culture, we must ask, "What happened?" Leaders are obliged to discover where systems broke down, leaving both patients and staff at risk for accidents and errors. The traditional culture reacts to harm after it occurs. In a safety culture, we try to anticipate accidents and errors, to be proactive and identify risks before they result in harm.

Copyright © 2005, Association for Professionals in Infection Control and Epidemiology, Inc.

A punitive culture reacts to bad behaviors; a just culture looks at the system: the environment, the knowledge, the tools, and other stressors that may affect behavior. In a just culture, top-down communication is replaced with bi-directional communication, with information flowing down to the front line from leadership and back up to leadership from those providing patient care on the front line. Silence about harmful events is discouraged. Instead, open, honest disclosure about serious patient safety events builds a learning organization and a safer place to work and provide care.

David Marx, an attorney whose career in human resources and organizational development has focused on responding to employees involved in adverse events, differentiates between a non-punitive and a just response to error. He also describes a just culture of safety in terms of a set of beliefs and a set of duties.[15] Our beliefs must:

- Recognize that professionals make mistakes.

- Acknowledge that even professionals develop unhealthy norms (shortcuts).

- Support zero tolerance for reckless behaviors.

Marx adds that we also have a set of duties to:

- Openly admit we have made a mistake.

- Call out when we see risk.

- Participate in the learning culture, by sharing mistakes and near-misses with others so they can prevent similar situations.

- Absolutely avoid reckless behaviors.

When the patient safety movement in our country began, many referred to the establishment of a non-punitive culture as a solution for medical errors. This raised concerns that people who acted recklessly would not be held accountable for their behaviors. Lucien Leape, a surgeon at Harvard, often identified as the leader of the patient safety movement, says that a just culture "doesn't mean there is no role for punishment. Punishment is indicated for willful misconduct, reckless behavior and unjustified, deliberate violation of rules . . . but not for human error."[16]

Types of Organizational Culture

To participate in creation of a just culture of safety, it may help to understand the different types of organizational culture. Literature on organizational culture describes three distinct types of culture: pathologic, bureaucratic, and generative. Table 12–2 describes the differences in these three cultures.

A safety culture has also been described as generative, uneasy about risk, constantly seeking out best practices, always looking for where the next mistake is going to happen, and then working to prevent it. A safety culture fosters a "learning organization," where

Table 12-2. How organizational vultures handle patient safety information[18]

Pathologic Culture	Bureaucratic Culture	Generative Culture)
Powerful people are honored	Silos vs. collaborative	Teamwork expected
Code of silence; don't want to know about risk or harm	Failures known by few	Near-misses/errors openly shared
Communication very limited	Top-down communication	Bi-directional communication
Failure is concealed	Risk and harm not emphasized	Actively seeking out risk and share information about errors
Blame and shame mentality	Reactive, crisis-oriented	Proactive, systems focus
Punitive response to mistakes	Focus on individuals	Committed to fixing broken systems and processes
What is not known does not have to be acted upon	Failure leads to local repairs	Failures lead to far- reaching reforms
Messengers are "shot"	Messengers listened to, if they report	Messengers are trained and rewarded
Change extremely difficult	Forced change creates anxiety	Change is embraced
New ideas actively discouraged	New ideas often present problems	New ideas welcome
Leaders command and control	Bureaucratic; allusion that leaders listen and collaborate	Leaders listen and act, coach and mentor

Source: Adapted from Jean Reeder, 2001

APIC Text of Infection Control and Epidemiology

Copyright © 2005, Association for Professionals in Infection Control and Epidemiology, Inc.

staff members share information about mistakes and errors in order to prevent them from recurring. This type of organization emphasizes reciprocal account-ability, meaning that everyone holds each other accountable for patient safety. The leadership can expect staff members to call out or stop the line when they see risk, and staff can expect leadership to listen and act, even if that involves dealing with problem professionals who display intentionally reckless behaviors. Patients and family members must be included as respected partners and must understand their own responsibility for keeping themselves safe. Examples include keeping written records of medications and allergies or reminding busy healthcare workers to perform hand hygiene.

The National Patient Safety Foundation outlines five attributes of a safety culture that all healthcare organizations should strive to operationalize through implementation of strong safety management systems:[17]

1. All workers (including front line staff, physicians, and administrators) accept responsibility for the safety of themselves, their co-workers, patients, and visitors

2. Safety has priority over financial and operational goals.

3. The organization encourages and rewards the identification, communication, and resolution of safety issues.

4. There are provisions for organizational learning from accidents.

5. The organization allocates appropriate resources, structure, and accountability to maintain effective safety systems.

Once errors occur, it is important to analyze the contributing factors and categorize the errors according to underlying causes. This helps determine how to respond. Skills-based errors should lead to an evaluation of training. Knowledge-based errors might trigger more education. Rules-based errors may indicate that policies and procedures are too complex, especially if there has been a trend toward employees repeatedly making the same types of errors. Managers should ask themselves whether errors are the result of an active failure or a latent failure – with underlying causes more hidden – which may indicate the need for a broader discussion of the systems that failed.

Communication and Teamwork

A failure to communicate effectively is the cause of the vast majority of avoidable accidents. This is true also outside of healthcare. The aviation industry reports that communication failures were at the root of

70–80% of all the jet transport accidents over a 20-year timeframe. The industry has made great strides toward improving its safety record by focusing on optimizing crew resource management techniques and removing communication barriers among pilots and members of the flight team. The industry also instituted a non-punitive method for reporting errors and near misses, allowing for team learning and interventions aimed at improvement.

In an effort to force healthcare organizations to more seriously address communication gaps as a key patient safety issue, JCAHO has incorporated requirements for improved communication in several of the National Patient Safety Goals (refer to Table 12–5 later). These include read-backs on verbal orders and critical lab values; identification of patients using two sources; site marking using the word "YES" on operative/procedure sites; checklists to verify correct patient, site, and procedure; and calling a "time-out" before procedures and operations to ensure that healthcare team members are all in agreement. Healthcare systems are complex and require communication among many individuals in different roles and typically under a great deal of stress. Team members must keep in mind that communication does not simply include what we say but how we say it, what we don't say, and what our body language conveys. Communication about things that do not go as planned can promote learning and can hopefully encourage proactive discussions about risk reduction and mistake-proofing our systems.

There are many barriers to effective communication and team work. Some barriers are the result of pathologic or bureaucratic organizational cultures, and breaking them down takes time and an active commitment from leadership, middle-management, and the front-line workers. Differences in culture, age, gender, race, and religious background may also act as barriers to effective team work and communication. The use of jargon when speaking to non-clinicians may also prevent important information from being shared and understood. Other barriers include: hierarchy, past experiences, conflicting patient care goals, and rapid changes in the healthcare environment.[20]

Michael Leonard and his colleagues offer a list of basic key elements to effective communication:

• Get the person's attention.

• Make eye contact; face the person .

• Introduce yourself.

• Use person's name — familiarity is key.

• Ask for easily accessible information, things you know the people you are talking with can answer.

• Be explicit when asking for input.

Copyright © 2005, Association for Professionals in Infection Control and Epidemiology, Inc.

- Provide information.

- Talk about next steps.

- Encourage ongoing monitoring and cross-checking.

Despite the importance of clear, concise communication, in some healthcare cultures it may be frightening to be assertive. Assertiveness can also be difficult for individuals who have been raised in cultures where speaking up and/or questioning is discouraged, especially when authority is involved. Assertiveness does not mean being aggressive. It is the responsibility of every healthcare worker to respectfully challenge authority while advocating for patient safety. Patients' lives may depend on our ability to be respectfully assertive and persistent until it is clear that we are understood and that the right thing is being done for the patient. Some factors that can make it hard to be assertive include a strong hierarchy, lack of a common mental model, lack of a supportive "safety climate," and a fear of looking unsure or foolish.

Some organizations have "stop the line" policies that empower everyone to respectfully call out and stop any risky process or procedure until team members are in agreement and all preventable risks are removed.[20]

Situational Briefing Model

One means of removing barriers to effective communication is the use of a standardized situational briefing model. This allows members of the healthcare team to communicate information in a clear, concise, and consistent manner. S-B-A-R communication is one such method. S-B-A-R is an acronym for Situation, Background, Assessment, and Recommendation.[20] This method helps nurses, technicians, and therapists to use a brief, effective approach to managing critical healthcare information.

Before using S-B-A-R communication and calling a physician, it is important to:

- Assess the patient.

- Review the chart for the appropriate physician to call.

- Know the admitting diagnosis.

- Read most recent progress notes and assessments from clinicians on prior shift.

- Have available when speaking with the physician: the medical record, patient allergies, medications, IV fluids, and laboratory and other diagnostic test results.

Situation

- State your name, position, and unit .

- "I am calling about [patient name and room number]."

- "The problem I am calling about is . . ."

Background

- State the admission diagnosis and date of admission.

- State the pertinent medical history.

- A brief synopsis of the treatment to date.

Assessment

Begin with outlining any changes from prior assessments. Include changes in:

- Mental status

- Pain

- Respiratory rate or quality; retractions/use of accessory muscles

- Pulse and blood pressure rate and quality; rhythm changes

- Skin color; wound drainage

- Neurological changes

- Gastrointestinal, genitourinary, or bowel changes (nausea, vomiting, diarrhea, increased or decreased output)

- Musculoskeletal weakness, joint deformity

Recommendation

State clearly what you think the patient needs urgently. Examples may include:

- "Transfer the patient to ICU or PICU."

- "Come to see the patient immediately."

- Talk to the patient and/or family about the code status.

- Ask for a consultant to see the patient now.

- Suggest tests or laboratory studies needed (e.g., chest x-ray, arterial blood gases, EKG).

Note: If a change in treatment is ordered, ask how often vital signs should be checked and when the physician would like to be contacted again. Document any changes in patient status, what intervention was completed, and whether or not the intervention was effective. Include any contact you have made with the physician.

Copyright © 2005, Association for Professionals in Infection Control and Epidemiology, Inc.

Tips for Effective Communication

In conclusion, a breakdown in communication among healthcare team members is the primary root cause in most errors and is associated with low measurers of patient and physician satisfaction. It is important to remember the following facts about communication:

- Just because you said it and understand it, doesn't mean you were heard and/or understood.

- Communication is not accomplished unless both parties are on the same page.

- Patient safety depends on use of a standard method of communication that gives the right amount and type of useful information to the healthcare team.

- Be assertive — your patients are counting on you.

- Ask clarifying questions if you don't understand.

- Share information, especially about problems and mistakes. It is the only way we will ever be able to improve systems and prevent medical errors.

Human Factors and Patient Safety

Patient safety programs are beginning to take advantage of tools that have been used in industry and manufacturing for years to study the cause and effects of human error. Three such tools are human factors engineering, human factors analysis, and ergonomics.

- Human factors engineering (HFE) involves research in human psychological, social, physical, and biological characteristics and is concerned with design of tools, machines, and systems that take into account human capabilities, limitations, and characteristics. The goal is to create designs that are safe, comfortable, and effective for humans to use.

- Human factors analysis is the systematic study of elements involving a human-machine interface with the intent of improving working conditions or operations.

- Ergonomics is the science of studying people at work, then designing tasks, jobs, information, tools, equipment, facilities, and the working environment so that people can be safe, effective, productive and comfortable. In the highly complex healthcare environment, understanding how humans interface with technology and equipment is crucial to understanding and preventing errors.

The concepts associated with human factors engineering can help healthcare workers, especially those involved with patient safety, to analyze events and develop workable and effective countermeasures, eliminating the use of dangerous shortcuts that lead to medical errors. [21]

Ideally, those analyzing critical or sentinel events are also working on proactively identifying risk and putting measures in place to prevent recurring mistakes. When planning to bring new technology or equipment to the patient care setting, or when evaluating work flow, there are several questions that one should ask about the expectations of the operator (human), the tools and equipment, and the environment in which the operator is expected to function. When conducting a human factors analysis relating to patient safety, Carayon, Alvarado, and Hundt recommend including the following questions: [22]

- What are the characteristics of the individual performing the work? Does the individual have the musculoskeletal, sensory, and cognitive abilities to do the required tasks? If not, can any of these gaps in ability be accommodated in the design of the task?

- What tasks are being performed, and what characteristics of those tasks may contribute to unsafe patient care? What in the nature of the tasks allows the individual to perform them safely or assume risks in the process?

- What tools and technologies are being used to perform the tasks, and do they increase or decrease the likelihood of untoward events?

- What aspects of the physical environment can be sources of error or promote safety? What in the physical environment ensures safe behavior or allows room for unsafe behavior?

- What is in the organization prevents or allows exposures to hazard, and what promotes or hinders patient safety? What allows for assuming safe or unsafe behavior by the individual?

Components of human factors assessment should also include:

- Evaluating the work: What is the work/rest ratio?

- Evaluating the workers: What are their physical and mental capabilities?

- Evaluating the environment: Do noise levels, lighting, and work-flow inhibit or or facilitate successful completion of the teask? (See Figure 12–4.)

We all experience the interplay of human factors in our everyday life. For example, we may encounter double doors on which the handles on each are made to pull the door open, despite the fact that one door opens in and should be pulled, and the other opens out and should be pushed. A good design makes actions of the user intuitive; there should be no need to apply signs or stickers to indicate proper usage or give instructions. An example of another bad design, which is obvious to most infection control professionals, are the paper towel dispensers found in many hospital

---

Patient Safety

Copyright © 2005, Association for Professionals in Infection Control and Epidemiology, Inc.

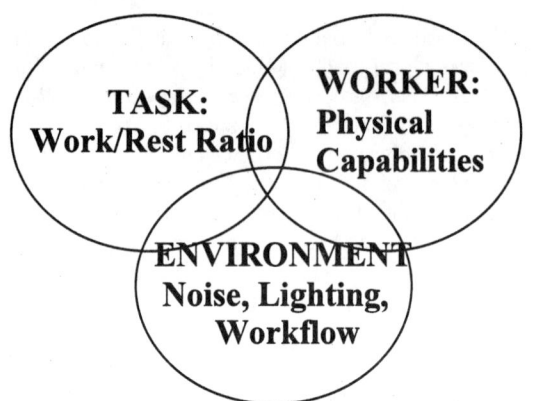

Figure 12-4 Components of a human factors assessment.[23]

bathrooms in which the mechanism that holds the clean towels is connected to the dirty paper towel disposal unit. This design makes it easy to contaminate freshly cleaned hands with dirty towels that overflowout of the dispenser.

The study of human factors helps us more easily identify and assess technology, equipment, systems, and processes that are (unintentionally) designed to allow mistakes. Conversely, understanding human factors helps us think of methods for mistake-proofing the environment, making it harder to do the wrong thing. All healthcare workers should be aware of the impact of human factors on reducing medical errors.

Patient safety experts tell us that to create a culture of safety, we must become "system thinkers." It helps to be able to define a system. A system is a combination of elements organized in a structure to achieve goals and objectives. System elements can be seen as the interaction of:

- elements (personnel, equipment, procedures)

- environment (physical, social, organizational)

- inputs and outputs

- structure

- purpose and goals.

When evaluating a system you must understand the reliability of the system and the human using it. System reliability depends on the reliability of each individual component. Components can be in series, parallel, or in combination. Parallel systems are redundant and can increase reliability. Parallel redundancy is often provided for human functions because the human component in a system is the least reliable. Mistakes by humans have been reported as the cause of serious accidents the majority of the time.(80% of industrial accidents; 50% of pilot accidents; 50–70% of nuclear power accidents).

Failure Modes and Effects Analysis

The best way to assess the likelihood of human error is through a "failure modes and effects analysis" (FMEA). This helps predict the effect of human error on system performance and to identify possible improvements needed to design a safer system.[22] Although human error seems to be responsible for a large percentage of accidents, there is often more to story. Once we find someone to blame for an error, we may fail to see the environmental (lack of equipment or bad design), or administrative (bad policies or procedures) components that contributed.

In healthcare, the patient is at the center of the system. Patient factors can include unique patient reactions (an intervention that works on one patient may not work on another) and unstable conditions within the same patient. For healthcare workers, the mental workload involved in patient care is tremendous. A recent study looking at the working memory of a nurse indicates that he/she is thinking of an average of 16 things simultaneously during a work shift. It is not hard to imagine errors of omission when the typical working memory holds a seven-digit telephone number without strain. In addition to mental capabilities, healthcare providers should be evaluated for:

- Physical size (anthropometry)

- Endurance / fatigue (physiology)

- Force (biomechanics)

- Hand and arm coordination (kinesiology)

- Sensory (hearing, vision, touch)

Environmental issues that impact safe care delivery include:

- Noise, light (glare), vibration, temperature, force

- Work space or supplies layout

- Equipment and environment match tasks

To illustrate the importance of the interface of human factors and the environment, consider the issue of clinical alarms as a safety measure. There are alarms on ventilators, cardiac monitors, IV pumps, and other equipment and computerized technology. Clinical alarms are designed to alert providers about danger, and slightly different sounds and pitches indicate need for an urgent, intermediate, or slower response. In a typical intensive care unit, it is easy to become desensitized to so many similar sounds, rhythms, and pitches. Unfortunately, alarms may simply become background

APIC Text of Infection Control and Epidemiology

Copyright © 2005, Association for Professionals in Infection Control and Epidemiology, Inc.

noise, with the result that a patient in real need may be overlooked for just a minute too long.

Administrative and organizational issues are another component of the care delivery system. Internal and external constraints and regulations have an impact on development of policies, procedures, and processes. Shift work is often associated with sleep deprivation. Staffing levels are influenced by shortages of professional staff, budgetary constraints, and patient acuity.

Communication may be the most important component of the patient care system. Communication about technology, equipment, processes, and procedures must be clearly delivered, and there must be confirmation that it is understood by healthcare providers. In an already complex environment, communications processes should be as simple as possible, with little or no calculations required or opportunities for misinterpretation. In addition to verbal communication, visual cues (posters, signs, pictorials) can also clarify steps in a process to ensure safety.

Patient safety experts and human factors engineers should work in partnership with manufacturers and distributors of medications. Since medication mishaps account for the majority of medical errors in most organizations, it is important to understand the dangers associated with look-alike and sound-alike medications. "TALL man lettering" and color-coding, both on medication vials and in storage areas, is one human factors solution to a serious patient safety problem. TALL man lettering uses capital letters to distinguish the critical aspects of a particular drug name, leaving more generic aspects in lower case.

Outcomes in complex work depend on the integration of individual, team, technical, and organizational factors. Using the traditional epidemiologic model (host, agent, environment), the infection control professional can be an integral part of assessing systems and identifying situations where human factors problems are responsible for increased risk and helping to design the solution.

Risk and Incident Reporting

If the current rate of harm in healthcare is to be reduced, we need to identify how and why adverse events occur, and, in particular, how system defects may contribute to their occurrence. The only way to do this is for individuals to report.[24] The aviation industry provides an excellent model for how "no blame reporting" can improve safety. In the 30 years since its inception, the Federal Aviation Administration (FAA) safety reporting system has logged over 500,000 confidential near-miss reports, with over 30,000 incidents reported each year.[25]

The Agency for Healthcare Research and Quality (AHRQ) defines near miss as "events in which the unwanted consequences were prevented because there was a recovery by planned or unplanned identification and correction of the failure." The effectiveness of a patient safety program can, to some degree, be measured by increased near-miss reporting — employees openly admitting to mistakes and identifying broken systems before they result in patient harm.

Similar to surveillance for healthcare-associated infections, especially post-discharge surveillance programs, adverse event or incident reporting can only be as effective as providers' willingness to report. The organization must set the expectation upon hire that safety event reporting is a priority. Individual employees have a responsibility to know and follow policies and procedures applicable to assigned duties, to use sound judgment and be aware of potential hazards before taking action, and to promptly report events or situations of actual or *potential* harm.

Management has a set of responsibilities that include educating staff on event reporting, making continuous safety improvements, and identifying system flaws and potential corrective actions. Managers must focus on the "how" not the "who" of an event, while underscoring individual accountability and responsibility. This is the foundation of a just culture of safety. Individual performance, as well as process and systems evaluation, is critical to ensure safe practice. Hiring managers must make clear the expectations about patient safety responsibilities, asking employees to "call out" about risk and make a commitment to act upon the concerns voiced by their staff members.

Clinical (medical staff) and administrative leaders also have a set of duties to ensure a safety culture and climate. Senior leaders must promote development and support implementation of recommended safety improvements. Allocating resources to safety initiatives and devoting as much individual time or oversight as possible can ensure the success of patient safety efforts. Proactive mindfulness about safety means leaders must not only encourage reporting of critical incidents but must actively enlist front-line staff in identifying real or potential hazards, before they result in harm. Providing necessary support (time, money, personnel) for continuing education regarding safety issues and practices and actively taking part in safety education programs spreads the message that the organization is committed to patient safety. The governing body, or hospital board, must be included in leadership activities that promote patient safety, especially those that involve ongoing monitoring of critical or sentinel events and the effectiveness of action plans or prevention efforts. Most governing boards have patient care

---

Copyright © 2005, Association for Professionals in Infection Control and Epidemiology, Inc.

quality committees responsible for overseeing clinical quality and safety of patient care delivery.

After a medical error occurs, the organization has a responsibility to both the patient and the healthcare workers involved in the event. The patient wants an honest explanation, the facts about the occurrence. Additionally, they want an apology for the situation, to know the plan for fixing their problem, and some assurance that efforts are being made to prevent recurrence. The healthcare workers involved in a medical error want a system assessment, the support of colleagues, a sense of shared responsibility for the error (with leadership), the preventive action plan, a commitment to fix system problems, and, often, psychological counseling.[26]

Reporting programs are generally designed to target problem areas through trend analysis, to create an information base to assist in creation of corrective and prevention measures, to spread knowledge about risk, and to promote open communication. Until we know the scope of any problem and stratify risk and harm into categories, it is difficult to plan for improvement. Improved risk/event reporting should lead to higher-quality patient care delivery. As with surveillance for healthcare-associated infections, raising awareness and putting in place a just culture will initially *increase* the error or incident rates, and it is important to educate leadership and staff to expect this from improved surveillance and reporting. Eventually, the success of the patient safety program can be measured to some degree by increased reporting *and* decreased incidents that result in patient harm. Better reporting is only the first step. It is a challenge to engage clinicians and others who have demanding jobs and competing priorities in performance improvement and intervention efforts, but this is the key to improved clinical outcomes.

Criteria for successful reporting systems were outlined by John Eisenberg, the first director of the AHRQ, when he opened the Fourth Decennial Conference on Nosocomial Infections by stating that the CDC's National Nosocomial Infection Surveillance (NNIS) program was an excellent model for patient safety programs. Eisenberg outlined reasons for the success of the NNIS reporting system: (1) it is voluntary and confidential; (2) it utilizes standardized definitions, numerators, denominators, and protocols; (3) it targets high-risk populations (ICU, surgical); (4) it demands that an adequate number of staff members are dedicated to data collection; (5) it provides a large sample size; (6) it disseminates data back to care providers; and (6) it monitors rates and links to prevention efforts.

Patient safety event or incident reporting systems also need to stratify data whenever possible. Systems should include a method for categorizing harm to patients, sometimes referred to as a "harm score." Harm scores can include broad categories such as: no error, error but no harm, error with harm, and error with death as outcome. The Medication Errors Reporting Program (MERP), operated by the United States Pharmacopeia (USP) in cooperation with the Institute for Safe Medication Practices (ISMP), is a confidential national voluntary reporting program that uses a harm score to categorize medication errors. MERP provides expert analysis of the system causes of medication errors and disseminates recommendations for prevention. Regulatory agencies and manufacturers are notified of needed changes in products when safety is of concern. Without reporting, such events would unrecognized and thus important epidemiological and preventive information would be unavailable. Errors, near misses, or hazardous conditions may be reported to the program. These include but are not limited to administration of the wrong drug or the wrong strength or dose of medication; confusion over look-alike/sound-alike drugs; incorrect route of administration; calculation or preparation errors; misuse of medical equipment; and errors in prescribing, transcribing, dispensing, and monitoring of medications. Case studies are published by ISMP and/or USP to alert healthcare professionals and others about recommendations to prevent errors.

In addition to medication errors, educating employees about what to report should begin with the JCAHO list of sentinel events. Sentinel events require root cause analyses, and voluntary reporting to JCAHO at the time of event is strongly encouraged (although voluntary). Sentinel events include[27]:

- Any patient death, paralysis, coma, or other major permanent loss of function associated with a medication error

- Any suicide of a patient in a setting where the patient is housed around-the-clock, including suicides following elopement i.e., unauthorized departure, from such a setting

- Any elopement of a patient from an around-the-clock care setting resulting in a temporally related death (suicide or homicide) or major permanent loss of function

- Any procedure on the wrong patient, wrong side of the body, or wrong organ

- Any intrapartum (related to the birth process) maternal death. Any perinatal death unrelated to a congenital condition in an infant having a birthweight greater than 2500 grams

- Assault, homicide, or other crime resulting in patient death or major permanent loss of function

Copyright © 2005, Association for Professionals in Infection Control and Epidemiology, Inc.

- A patient fall that results in death or major permanent loss of function as a direct result of the injuries sustained in the fall

- Hemolytic transfusion reaction involving major blood group incompatibilities.

Note: An adverse outcome that is directly related to the natural course of the patient's illness or underlying condition, e.g., terminal illness present at the time of presentation, is not reportable except for suicide in, or following elopement from, a 24-hour care setting.

Examples of events that are *not* reportable to JCAHO includethe following:[27]

- Any "near miss"

- Full return of limb or bodily function to the same level as prior to the adverse event by discharge or within 2weeks of the initial loss of said function

- Any sentinel event that has not affected a recipient of care (patient, client, resident)

- Medication errors that do not result in death or major permanent loss of function

- Suicide other than in an around-the-clock care setting or following elopement from such a setting

- A death or loss of function following a discharge "against medical advice (AMA)"

- Unsuccessful suicide attempts

- Unintentionally retained foreign body without major permanent loss of function.

- Minor degrees of hemolysis with no clinical sequelae

Note: In the context of its performance improvement activities, an organization may choose to conduct intensive assessment, e.g., root cause analysis, for some non-reportable events. (Refer to the "Improving Organization Performance" chapter of your JCAHO standards manual.)

Aside from sentinel events, critical patient safety events should also be reported, whether they actually resulted in harm or the potential for harm existed (near miss).[27] These may include, but not be limited to:

- Inpatient or outpatient injuries

- Unsafe medication practices (violation of the five "rights": right patient, medication, time, route, and dose)

- Violation of patient rights (i.e., confidentiality)

- Patient falls (with or without injury)

- Unexplained or unexpected medical/surgical outcome or mishap

- Equipment problems (related or not to a particular patient).

While creating a just culture of safety and convincing staff to increase reporting, we may run across some myths or unspoken rules that need to change if decreasing medical error is the goal. These unspoken rules have developed over time because of the stigma attached to errors. Due to short staffing and other restraints, shortcuts become common practice. Fear of embarrassment, or even punishment, may drive staff members to protect themselves and their colleagues by independently changing practice when they feel it is in their patients' best interest. As a result, important information about the cause of errors is lost and system problems cannot be addressed. Some of these unspoken rules and examples are listed below.[28]

- If I can make it right, it is not an error (e.g., when a dose is omitted, a nurse changes the subsequent drug administration scheduled to "get back on track")

- If it's not my fault, it is not an error (e.g., late administration or an omission when the prescribed drug was not available on the unit)

- If another patient's needs are more urgent than accurate medication/treatment, it is not an error (e.g., medication delivery is omitted or delayed by dealing with urgent situations arising with another patient)

- A clerical error is not a real medical error (e.g., a nurse on a previous shift fails to document drug administration or documented in the wrong section of the record)

- If my actions prevent something worse, it is not an error (e.g., a nurse knows that he/she would be busy later due to planned admissions, discharges, etc., and administers medication early rather than risk omitting doses)

- If everyone knows (or does it), it is not an error (e.g., nurses give medications early or withhold medications at night so that patients suffering from sleep deprivation can rest uninterrupted for longer periods of time)

For the current rate of harm in healthcare to be reduced, we need to identify how and why adverse events occur, how system defects contribute to the events, and then make the commitment to better reporting.The most common barriers to reporting include lack of knowledge about what to report or how to report, lack of trust, extra work, skepticism about the likelihood that things will change, desire to forget the event, and fear of reprisal or punishment.[20]

Risk identification and patient safety reporting programs can collect data using paper incident forms, on-line report entry, card-based information, and tele-

Copyright © 2005, Association for Professionals in Infection Control and Epidemiology, Inc.

phone hotlines. Reporting systems must be readily available and accessible by all members of the healthcare team, and they must be user-friendly and secure. The best reporting programs keep information confidential, which is often the greatest driver to improved safety event reporting.

Risk analysis of reported aggregate data must look at trends in type of errors, people, systems, and processes involved; place and time of occurrence; and risk factors identified. This information should be shared with key stakeholders and used to drive improvements that reduce risk of harm to patients (and employees).

Interventions to Reduce Adverse Events in Healthcare

"Patients should not be harmed by the care that is intended to help them, nor should harm come to those who work in health care."[1] It is impossible to reduce medical errors and adverse outcomes by focusing in isolation on any one aspect of the healthcare system. As Wood's blunt-and-sharp-end model of accident causation implies, patient safety must be analyzed from the national level, where health policy and legislation is created, down to the front line of patient care delivery. The second IOM report, "Crossing the Quality Chasm: A New Health System for the 21st Century,"[29] examines the reasons why, as a nation, we are far from offering world class healthcare. The report indicates that "all health care organizations should adopt as their explicit purpose to continually reduce the burden of illness, injury and disability, and to improve the health and functioning of the people of the United States."[29] To close the quality chasm between what we know our consumers deserve and what the system is able to consistently deliver, the chasm report suggests that the healthcare system focus on six aims:

1. Patient safety, the fundamental cornerstone of the healthcare system: care provided in a safe manner, in a safe environment, recognizing that humans will make mistakes and that errors do occur. The goal must be to prevent harm before it reaches the patient and affects the healthcare worker adversely (the "second victim" of medical errors). Everyone is involved in seeking out risk and identifying opportunities to make care safer, learning from medical errors and near misses.

2. Patient-centeredness: We must focus on the patient's experience of illness and receiving healthcare and on systems that work or fail to work to meet individual patient's needs. Patient's values, preferences, and expressed needs should be at the center of decisions made. Coordination and integration of care, information, communication, education, physical comfort, emotional support, and involvement of family and friends must be factored into care plans and actions. Finally, every patient must have access to high-quality care.

3. Effectiveness: The IOM defines effectiveness as "care that is based on the use of systematically acquired evidence to determine whether an intervention produces better outcomes than alternatives – including the alternative of doing nothing." This premise is the foundation upon which evidence-based medicine rests. Effective care depends on the triad of (1) the best research evidence from well designed experiments, trials, and studies; (2) clinical expertise; and (3) the patient's values, preferences, concerns, and expectations.

4. Efficiency: The efficiency of the system can be improved through two primary methods: reducing quality waste, and reducing administrative or production costs. Quality waste refers to the overuse of services (where a healthcare service is provided when the potential risks outweigh the benefits) and the elimination of medical errors. Administrative and production waste can be reduced by eliminating duplicative work processes (especially paperwork), redundant testing, and multiple re-entries of various types of practitioner orders.

5. Equity: Simply stated, the benefits of the healthcare system should be available to all. All disparities in providing healthcare must be removed, at the population and individual levels, that are based on race, ethnicity, gender, or ability to pay.

6. Timeliness: At all levels of the organization, focus must be on ensuring that patient care processes flow smoothly. This means that long waits to access care, to receive diagnostic testing and treatments, and to obtain test results upon which to base decisions, must be decreased or eliminated.

Table 12–3 outlines current approaches to patient care that should be discarded in favor of new and more beneficial strategies that can improve patient safety and the quality of care.

In healthcare organizations, surveillance, reporting, and analysis are the foundation of risk prevention programs, but targeted interventions must be deployed if patient safety programs are to be successful in reducing harm from medical errors and other adverse events. Several organizations have analyzed the effectiveness of guidelines, standards of care, and prevention measures in order to recommend evidence-based measures for improving patient safety. These include Agency for Healthcare Research and Quality (AHRQ), National Quality Forum, Centers for Disease Prevention and Control and Prevention (CDC), National Patient Safety Foundation, JCAHO, and Center for Medicare and Medicaid Services (CMS). Although not an

Copyright © 2005, Association for Professionals in Infection Control and Epidemiology, Inc.

Table 12-3. Current versus safer, higher-quality approaches to patient care delivery

Current Approach to Patient Care	→	Safer, Higher-Quality Patient Care
Care is primarily based on visits.		Care is based on continuous healing relationships.
Professional autonomy drives variability.		Care is customized according to patient's needs and values.
Professionals control care.		The patient is the source of control.
Information is a record		Knowledge is shared and information flows freely.
Decision-making is based on training and experience.		Decision-making is evidence-based.
"Do no harm" is an individual responsibility.		Safety is a system property.
Secrecy is necessary.		Transparency is necessary.
The system reacts to needs.		Needs are anticipated.
Cost reduction is sought.		Waste is continuously decreased.
Preference is given to professional roles over the system.		Cooperation among clinicians is a priority.

Source: Adapted from Crossing the Quality Chasm IOM Report.[29]

exhaustive list, some of these measures are outlined here. (The CDC guidelines for the prevention of nosocomial or healthcare-associated infections are not discussed here, although these are some of the best evidence-based and scientifically tested guidelines focused on prevention of adverse events.)

In 2002, the first attempt was made by regulatory and accreditation agencies to develop and publish national standards for healthcare institutions to adopt in order to improve the most common types of medical errors. Organizations accredited by JCAHO were expected to be fully compliant with the first set of National Patient Safety Goals by January 2003. Each year, a multi-disciplinary expert advisory board reviews current trends in medical errors and attempts to expand prevention efforts through updated versions of these patient safety goals (see Table 12–4 for a summary of the 2005 National Patient Safety Goals).

Of interest is the fact that, in 2004, infection control processes were included. Goal #7 was created to address healthcare worker education and compliance with hand hygiene and the inclusion of healthcare-associated deaths and disability as sentinel events, requiring root cause analysis and follow up.

The National Quality Forum (NQF) published a document, entitled *Safe Practices for Better Heath Care*, to begin addressing the lack of standardization and prioritization of evidence-based measures to improve patient safety. The NQF report outlines 30 priority healthcare safe practices that should be implemented in all clinical settings to reduce the risk for harm.[30] These "voluntary consensus standards" were selected from over 200 practices reviewed based on the practice's specificity, effectiveness, potential benefit, generalizability, and readiness for implementation. The practices are organized in five broad categories:

- Creating a culture of safety

- Matching healthcare needs with service delivery capability

- Facilitating information transfer and clear communication

- Increasing safe medication use

Implementation of the recommended practices at healthcare facilities will depend on the organization's own priorities and circumstances, such as, availability of resources, practices already implemented, environmental constraints, and patient mix/population needs. The report also recommends specific actions related to dissemination and implementation of the safe practices, measuring their implementation, and updating and improving the set of practices. The 30 safe practices are detailed in Table 12–5.

The patient safety literature citing evidence-based prevention measures credits the field of hospital epidemiology and infection control with successful interventions to reduce risk and adverse outcomes. AHRQ recommends that all healthcare organizations focus on the following infection prevention initiatives:

- Improving hand hygiene

- Utilizing barrier precautions to prevent transmission of infection

- Prudent antibiotic use to reduce *Clostridium difficile* & vancomycin-resistant enterococcus (VRE)

- Preventing urinary tract infections

- Preventing central venous catheter (CVC)-related bloodstream infections (BSIs)

- Preventing ventilator-associated pneumonia (VAP)

- Preventing surgical site infections (SSIs)

Copyright © 2005, Association for Professionals in Infection Control and Epidemiology, Inc.

Table 12-4. 2005 National Patient Safety Goals[19]

On July 9, 2004, the Joint Commission's Board of Commissioners approved the 2005 National Patient Safety Goals. This year, the Joint Commission developed program-specific goals for all accreditation programs. Below are the 2005 NPSGs, which include continuing 2004 goals. New goals for 2005 are included with program applicability indicated in brackets.

Goal 1: Improve the accuracy of patient identification. [All programs]
- Use at least two patient identifiers (neither to be the patient's room number) whenever administering medications or blood products; taking blood samples and other specimens for clinical testing, or providing any other treatments or procedures. [Ambulatory, Assisted Living, Behavioral Healthcare, Critical Access Hospital, Disease-Specific Care, Home Care, Hospital, Laboratory, Long Term Care, Office-Based Surgery]
- Prior to the start of any invasive procedure, conduct a final verification process to confirm the correct patient, procedure, site, and availability of appropriate documents. This verification process uses active—not passive—communication techniques. [Assisted Living, Disease-Specific Care, Home Care, Laboratory, Long Term Care]

Goal 2: Improve the effectiveness of communication among caregivers. [All programs]
- For verbal or telephone orders or for telephonic reporting of critical test results, verify the complete order or test result by having the person receiving the order or test result "read-back" the complete order or test result. [All programs]
- Standardize a list of abbreviations, acronyms and symbols that are not to be used throughout the organization. [All programs]
- Measure, assess and, if appropriate, take action to improve the timeliness of reporting, and the timeliness of receipt by the responsible licensed caregiver, of critical test results and values. [Ambulatory, Behavioral Healthcare, Critical Access Hospital, Disease-Specific Care, Home Care, Hospital, Laboratory, Office-Based Surgery]
- All values defined as critical by the laboratory are reported directly to a responsible licensed caregiver within time frames established by the laboratory (defined in cooperation with nursing and medical staff). When the patient's responsible licensed caregiver is not available within the time frames, there is a mechanism to report the critical information to an alternative response caregiver. [Laboratory]

Goal 3: Improve the safety of using medications. [Ambulatory, Behavioral Healthcare, Critical Access Hospital, Disease-Specific Care, Home Care, Hospital, Long Term Care, Office-Based Surgery]
- Remove concentrated electrolytes (including, but not limited to, potassium chloride, potassium phosphate, sodium chloride >0.9%) from patient care units. [Ambulatory, Critical Access Hospital, Disease-Specific Care, Home Care, Hospital, Long Term Care, Office-Based Surgery]
- Standardize and limit the number of drug concentrations available in the organization. [Ambulatory, Behavioral Healthcare, Critical Access Hospital, Disease-Specific Care, Home Care, Hospital, Long Term Care, Office-Based Surgery]
- Identify and, at a minimum, annually review a list of look-alike/sound-alike drugs used in the organization, and take action to prevent errors involving the interchange of these drugs. [Ambulatory, Behavioral Healthcare, Critical Access Hospital, Home Care, Hospital, Long Term Care, Office-Based Surgery]

Goal 4: Eliminate wrong-site, wrong-patient, wrong-procedure surgery. [Disease-Specific Care]
- Create and use a preoperative verification process, such as a checklist, to confirm that appropriate documents (e.g., medical records, imaging studies) are available. [Disease-Specific Care]
- Implement a process to mark the surgical site and involve the patient in the marking process. [Disease-Specific Care]

Goal 5: Improve the safety of using infusion pumps. [Ambulatory, Assisted Living, Behavioral Healthcare, Critical Access Hospital, Disease-Specific Care, Home Care, Hospital, Long Term Care, Office-Based Surgery]
- Ensure free-flow protection on all general-use and PCA (patient controlled analgesia) intravenous infusion pumps used in the organization. [Ambulatory, Assisted Living, Behavioral Healthcare, Critical Access Hospital, Disease-Specific Care, Home Care, Hospital, Long Term Care, Office-Based Surgery]

Goal 6: Improve the effectiveness of clinical alarm systems. [Disease-Specific Care]
- Implement regular preventive maintenance and testing of alarm systems. [Disease-Specific Care]
- Assure that alarms are activated with appropriate settings and are sufficiently audible with respect to distances and competing noise within the unit. [Disease-Specific Care]

Goal 7: Reduce the risk of healthcare-associated infections. [All programs]
- Comply with current Centers for Disease Control and Prevention (CDC) hand hygiene guidelines. [All programs]
- Manage as sentinel events all identified cases of unanticipated death or major permanent loss of function associated with a healthcare-associated infection. [All programs]

Goal 8: Accurately and completely reconcile medications across the continuum of care. [Ambulatory, Assisted Living, Behavioral Healthcare, Critical Access Hospital, Disease-Specific Care, Home Care, Hospital, Long Term Care, Office-Based Surgery]
- During 2005, for full implementation by January 2006, develop a process for obtaining and documenting a complete list of the patient's current medications upon the patient's admission to the organization and with the involvement of the patient. This process includes a comparison of the medications the organization provides to those on the list. [Ambulatory, Assisted Living, Behavioral Healthcare, Critical Access Hospital, Disease-Specific Care, Home Care, Hospital, Long Term Care, Office-Based Surgery]
- A complete list of the patient's medications is communicated to the next provider of service when it refers or transfers a patient to another setting, service, practitioner or level of care within or outside the organization. [Ambulatory, Assisted Living, Behavioral Healthcare, Critical Access Hospital, Disease-Specific Care, Home Care, Hospital, Long Term Care, Office-Based Surgery]

Goal 9: Reduce the risk of patient harm resulting from falls. [Assisted Living, Critical Access Hospital, Home Care, Hospital, Long Term Care]
- Assess and periodically reassess each patient's risk for falling, including the potential risk associated with the patient's medication regimen, and take action to address any identified risks. [Assisted Living, Critical Access Hospital, Home Care, Hospital, Long Term Care]
- Implement a fall reduction program, including a transfer protocol, and evaluate the effectiveness of the program. [Long Term Care]

Goal 10: Reduce the risk of influenza and pneumococcal disease in institutionalized older adults. [Assisted Living, Disease-Specific Care, Long Term Care]
- Develop and implement a protocol for administration and documentation of the flu vaccine. [Assisted Living, Disease-Specific Care, Long Term Care]
- Develop and implement a protocol for administration and documentation of the pneumococcus vaccine. [Assisted Living, Disease-Specific Care, LTC]
- Develop and implement a protocol to identify new cases of influenza and to manage an outbreak. [Assisted Living, Disease-Specific Care, Long Term Care]

(Continued)

APIC Text of Infection Control and Epidemiology

Copyright © 2005, Association for Professionals in Infection Control and Epidemiology, Inc.

Table 12-4. Continued

Goal 11: Reduce the risk of surgical fires. [Ambulatory, Office-Based Surgery]
- Educate staff, including operating licensed independent practitioners and anesthesia providers, on how to control heat sources and manage fuels, and establish guidelines to minimize oxygen concentration under drapes. [Ambulatory, Office-Based Surgery]

Goal 12: Implementation of applicable National Patient Safety Goals and associated requirements by components and practitioner sites. [Network]
- Inform and encourage components and practitioner sites to implement the applicable National Patient Safety Goals and associated requirements. [Network]

As of January 1, 2005, all Joint Commission accredited healthcare organizations will be surveyed for implementation of applicable 2005 goals and requirements—or acceptable alternatives (see below)—as appropriate to the services the organization provides. An organization's compliance with applicable requirements (or an acceptable alternative) will be scored as an element of performance if the requirement is in the standards. Otherwise, they will be scored at the level of the National Patient Safety Goal as an Accreditation Participation Requirement, which are separately described in the JCAHO accreditation manual.

Source: Failure Mode and Effects Analysis in Health Care: Proactive Risk Reduction, JCAHO[35]

Kennedy et al. discuss infection control interventions that provide the strongest evidence for prevent healthcare-associated infections that should be implemented, especially among critical care populations. These include: (1) use of maximum sterile barriers in CVC insertion; (2) appropriate use of antimicrobial prophylaxis to prevent SSI; (3) the continuous aspiration of subglottic secretions to prevent VAP; and (4) antibiotic-impregnated CVCs to prevent catheter-related infection. [30]

Sentinel Event Investigation: Root Cause Analysis and Failure Mode and Effects Analysis

After each critical or sentinel event occurs, whether resulting in harm or not, an intensive investigation should occur. Root cause analysis (RCA) is a process for identifying the basic or causal factors that underlie variation in performance. RCA is done if, after a fact-gathering debriefing with the team involved in the critical event, a determination is made that the event meets the definition of a sentinel event. Timely communication and making sure a patient is protected from additional/ongoing harm must be the priority.

In 2004, JCAHO added to the National Patient Safety Goals a requirement that healthcare organizations manage as sentinel events all identified cases of unanticipated death or major permanent loss of function associated with a healthcare-associated infection (HAI).[19] This means that if a patient with a healthcare-acquired infection (1) dies or is permanently disabled, (2) and the death or disability is unanticipated, or (3) if the patient was placed at risk for death or permanent disability, it should be considered a sentinel event. A credible RCA must then be conducted within 45 days of the event.

This goal compels us to create a system for identifying possible HAI-related deaths. Methods may include working with health information management (medical records) personnel to identify all deaths, comparing hospital deaths with HAI database to identify potential HAI-related deaths, and working with the hospital epidemiologist or infection control committee chair to review records to determine if death or disability is "unanticipated." Knowing expected mortality rates associated with each type of HAI is critical for managing this new book of work. For example, VAP is associated with a high anticipated mortality rate (up to 60%), and so it may be hard to consider a VAP death as unanticipated. On the other hand, patients having elective surgery with few risk factors for surgical site infection are not expected to die of SSI-related complications. Since all unanticipated deaths should be considered sentinel events and be investigated, JCAHO is asking organizations to no longer exclude those deaths related to infection.

In most organizations, experts in risk management or performance improvement departments are responsible for facilitating the RCA process and can assist infection control professionals with an intense investigation. The ICP can be seen as a content expert and, after some experience, would be an excellent team leader. The steps in conducting RCA are similar to those used to do outbreak investigation or even FOCUS PDSA. A crosswalk displaying similarities in these tools and methods for identifying causality and planning improvements is included in Table 12–6. [32] JCAHO created a framework to use to make sure all elements of RCA are addressed. Table 12–7 provides an example of how this framework might be used to investigate an infection-related sentinel event.[33] Teams should tackle each area of content on the framework to help identify root cause and put effective control measures in place to reduce risk or recurrence.

Part of the sentinel event investigation process includes conducting a Failure Modes and Effects Analysis (FMEA). FMEA is a systematic, proactive method for evaluating a process to identify where and how it might fail and to assess the relative impact of different

Copyright © 2005, Association for Professionals in Infection Control and Epidemiology, Inc.

Table 12-5. The National Quality Forum-Endorsed Set of Safe Practices*31

1. Create a healthcare culture of safety.

2. For designated high-risk, elective surgical procedures or other specified care, patients should be clearly informed of the likely reduced risk of an adverse outcome at treatment facilities that have demonstrated superior outcomes and should be referred to such facilities in accordance with the patient's stated preferences.

3. Specify an explicit protocol to be used to ensure an adequate level of nursing based on the institution's usual patient mix and the experience and training of its nursing staff.

4. All patients in general intensive care units (both adult and pediatric) should be managed by physicians having specific training and certification in critical care medicine ("critical care certified").

5. Pharmacists should actively participate in the medication-use process, including, at a minimum, being available for consultation with prescribers on medication ordering, interpretation and review of medication orders, preparation of medications, dispensing of medications, and administration and monitoring of medications.

6. Verbal orders should be recorded whenever and immediately read back to the prescriber (i.e., a healthcare provider receiving a verbal order should read back the information that the prescriber conveys in order to verify the accuracy of what was heard).

7. Use only standard abbreviations and dose designations.

8. Patient care summaries or other similar records should be should not be prepared from memory.

9. Ensure that care information, especially changes in orders and new diagnostic information, is transmitted in a timely and clearly understandable form to all of the patient's current healthcare providers who need the information to provide care.

10. Ask each patient or legal surrogate to recount what he or she has been told during the informed consent discussion.

11. Ensure that written documentation of the patient's preference for life-sustaining treatments is prominently displayed in his or her chart.

12. Implement a computerized prescriber order entry system.

13. Implement a standardized protocol to prevent the mislabeling of radiographs.

14. Implement standardized protocols to prevent the occurrence of wrong-site procedures or wrong-patient procedures.

15. Evaluate each patient undergoing elective surgery for the risk of an acute ischemic cardiac event during surgery, and provide prophylactic treatment of high-risk patients with beta blockers.

16. Evaluate each patient upon admission, and regularly thereafter, for the risk of developing pressure ulcers. This evaluation should be repeated at regular intervals during care. Clinically appropriate preventive methods should be implemented consequent to the evaluation.

17. Evaluate each patient upon admission, and regularly thereafter, for the risk of developing deep vein thrombosis (DVT)/venous thromboembolism (VTE). Utilize clinically appropriate methods to prevent DVT/VTE.

18. Utilize dedicated anti-thrombotic (anti-coagulation) services that facilitate coordinated care management.

19. Upon admission, and regularly thereafter, evaluate each patient for risk of aspiration.

20. Adhere to effective methods of preventing central venous catheter-associated bloodstream infections.

21. Evaluate each pre-operative patient in light of his or her own planned surgical procedure, for the risk of surgical site infection, and implement appropriate antibiotic prophylaxis and other preventive measures based on that evaluation.

22. Utilize validated protocols to evaluate patients who are at risk for contrast media-induced renal failure, and utilize a clinically appropriate method for reducing risk of renal injury based on the patient's kidney function evaluation.

23. Evaluate each patient upon admission, and regularly thereafter, for the risk of malnutrition. Employ clinically appropriate strategies to prevent malnutrition.

24. Whenever a pneumatic tourniquet is used, evaluate the patient for the risk of an ischemic and/or thrombotic complication, and utilize appropriate prophylactic measures.

25. Decontaminate hands with either a hygienic hand rub or by washing with a disinfectant soap prior to and after direct contact with the patient or objects immediately around the patient.

26. Vaccinate healthcare workers against influenza to protect both them and patients from influenza.

27. Keep work spaces where medications are prepared clean, orderly, well lit, and free of clutter, distraction, and noise.

28. Standardize the methods for labeling, packaging, and storing medications.

29. Identify all "high-alert" drugs (e.g., intravenous adrenergic agonists and antagonists, chemotherapeutic agents, anti-coagulants and anti-thrombotics, concentrated parenteral electrolytes, general anesthetics, neuromuscular blockers, insulin and oral hypoglycemics, narcotics, and opiates).

30. Dispense medications in unit dose or, when appropriate, unit-of-use form, whenever possible.

*See full NQF report for applicable care settings for each practice, detailed specifications, and additional background and reference material.

APIC Text of Infection Control and Epidemiology

Copyright © 2005, Association for Professionals in Infection Control and Epidemiology, Inc.

Table 12-6. Crosswalk Demonstrating Similarities Among FOCUS PDCA, Root Cause

FOCUS-PDCA		Step in Preparing for a Root Cause Analysis	Outbreak Investigation
F ind An Opportunity			
O rganize a Team	Step 1	Organize a Team	1. Confirm existence f outbreak
	Step 2	Define the Problem	2. Confirm diagnosis of cases
C larify the Current Process	Step 3	Study the Problem	3. Prepare or investigation
	Step 4	Determine What Happened	4. Create case definition
U nderstand Variation	Step 5	Identify Contributing Process Factors	5. Search for additional cases
	Step 6	Identify Other Contributing Factors	6. Characterize epidemic by person,
	Step 7	Measure – Collect and Assess Data on Proximate and Underlying Causes	place, time (line list)
	Step 8	Design and Implement Interim Changes	7. Generate tentative hypothesis
	Step 9	Identify Which Systems Are Involved – Root Causes	8. Test hypothesis
	Step 10	Prune the List of Root Causes	9. Institute additional studies
	Step 11	Confirm Root Causes	10. Iimplement interventions
S elect the improvement solution	Step 12	Explore and Identify Risk Reduction Strategies	11. Communicate findings
P lan the Improvement	Step 13	Formulate Improvement Actions	12. Move to process improvement!
	Step 14	Evaluate Proposed Improvement Actions	
	Step 15	Design Improvements	
	Step 16	Ensure Acceptability of the Action Plan	
D o the Improvement and Collect Data	Step 17	Implement the Improvement Plan	
C heck and Study the Results	Step 18	Develop Measures of Effectiveness and Ensure Their Success	
	Step 19	Evaluate Implementation of Improvement Efforts	
A ct and Hold the Gain	Step 20	Take Additional Action	
	Step 21	Communicate the Results	

failures, in order to identify the parts of the process that are most in need of change. [34]

FMEA includes review of the following:

- Steps in the process

- Failure modes (What could go wrong?)

- Failure causes (Why would the failure happen?)

- Failure effects (What would be the consequences of each failure?)

Teams use FMEA to evaluate processes for possible failures and to prevent them by correcting the processes proactively rather than reacting to adverse events after failures have occurred. This emphasis on prevention may reduce risk of harm to both patients and staff. FMEA is particularly useful in evaluating a new process prior to implementation and in assessing the impact of a proposed change to an existing process.[34] The greatest strength of failure mode and effects analysis lies in its ability to focus users on the process of redesigning potentially problematic process to prevent the occurrence of failures.

The focus on before-the-fact process design/redesign through FMEA is a relatively new one for healthcare. Articles on the application of FMEA to healthcare processes started appearing in the healthcare literature in the 1990s. Some of the earliest articles focused on the application of FMEA to the medication administration process in hospitals and to drug product development in the pharmaceutical industry. The increasing national focus on the safety of individuals served by healthcare organizations is adding new impetus to the application of FMEA in all types of healthcare settings. The continuing efforts of the ISMP, NCPS, and other organizations join with those of JCAHO in raising awareness of FMEA throughout healthcare. One of JCAHO's new patient safety and medical/healthcare error reduction standards requires leaders to define and implement a proactive system for identifying risk and reducing the risk of healthcare process or system failures the cause harm, and it outlines the use of FMEA. Proactive risk reduction processes that encompass the basic steps included in an FMEA approach may be used to comply with Joint Commission requirements. The requirement went into effect for hospitals on July 1, 2001.

If a particular failure cannot be prevented, FMEA then focuses on protections that can be put in place to prevent the failure from reaching the patient, or, in the worst case, mitigate its effects if it reaches the patient. The major components are outlined below:[35]

- Failure (F) means lack of success, nonperformance, nonoccurrence, or breaking down or ceasing to function. It takes place when a system or part of a

Copyright © 2005, Association for Professionals in Infection Control and Epidemiology, Inc.

Table 12-7. APIC Framework for Conducting Root Cause Analysis on Infection-related Sentinel Events[33]

	Level of Analysis	Questions	Findings
What happened?	Sentinel Event	What are the details of the event? (Brief description)	What type of infection did the patient have that caused the death or permanent loss of function?
		When did the event occur? (Date, day, time)	
		What area/service was impacted?	Surgery? ICU? Pulmonary Services? Transplant unit?
Why did it happen?	The process or activity in which event occurred	What are the steps in the process, as designed? (flow diagram helpful)	Sterilization process? Skin preparation process? Prophylactic antibiotic administration? Environmental cleaning? *The process should be flowcharted "as is," so critical steps can be identified.*
What were the most proximate factors?		What steps were involved in (contributed to) the event?	Were instruments cleaned adequately before putting in the sterilizer? Was the cycle allowed to complete? Was the skin prep rushed because everyone was in a hurry to start the case? Was the antibiotics given at the right time pre-op (or at all)? *Analyze the flowchart and determine the gaps.*
(Typically "special cause" variation)	Human factors	What human factors were relevant to the outcome?	Did staff feel pressured to get the job done quickly? Were critical steps missed because they thought they weren't important? Have shortcuts been built into the system? *Participants have to be painfully honest without fear of retribution!*
	Equipment factors	How did the equipment performance affect the outcome?	Was the appropriate preventive maintenance done? Was the staff oriented appropriately to equipment? *Types of equipment may be autoclaves, sterilizers, ventilators, all types of tubing's connected to the patient, etc.*
	Controllable environmental factors	What factors directly affected the outcome?	Was the staff in a hurry? Is clean equipment stored near contaminated equipment? Does the staff have what they need when they need it? Were there distractions that interrupted the process? *Are work area/work conditions conducive to the process?*
	Uncontrollable external factors	Are they truly beyond the organization's control?	Are there productivity standards for MDs that force them to hurry through processes? *Having physicians involved in investigation is critical to success.*
	Other	Are there any other factors that have directly influenced this outcome?	*This is the time for the group to brainstorm other systems or processes that they feel contributed to the outcome*
		What other areas or services are impacted	
Why did that happen? What systems and processes underlie those proximate factors?	Human Resources issues	To what degree is staff properly qualified and currently competent for their responsibilities?	Is the right skill level person performing the function? Is orientation adequate? Have the staff demonstrated competency on the equipment they are using? Has competency with the *process* been demonstrated? Are the learning needs of the individual taken into consideration when training/orienting new employees? *This is the time to ask all relevant questions about adequate education and training for the process.*

Continued

APIC Text of Infection Control and Epidemiology

Copyright © 2005, Association for Professionals in Infection Control and Epidemiology, Inc.

Table 12-7. Continued

Level of Analysis	Questions	Findings
(Common cause variation here may lead to special cause variation in dependent processes)	How did actual staffing compare with ideal levels?	Was the department running short that day? Did the therapists have time to do their rounds? Were tubing changes let go due to inadequate staff? Are there enough people to do the job? *Ideal staffing levels are difficult to determine. Comparison with industry standards, if available, can be helpful.*
	What are the plans for dealing with contingencies that would tend to reduce effective staffing levels?	What does the department do if they are "short-staffed" for the day? Who prioritizes? *What realistic options for replacement personnel are available to the manager?*
	To what degree is staff performance in the operant process(es) addressed?	How do we know the staff is competent to do the procedure? Is there adequate supervision? Are the staff allowed to find creative shortcuts? *Does staff understand their role in reducing infectious complications as part of the process they work in?*
	How can orientation and in-service training be improved?	*Brainstorm and listen carefully to the front-line caregiver that knows best what will and will not work. Once an event of this nature occurs, staff really think about their role and what could be done better. They don't want a repeat incident!*
Information management issues	To what degree is all necessary information available when needed? Accurate? Complete? Unambiguous?	Are there procedures available to the staff? What information about the patient was passed on in report? Any critical information omitted? Did the therapist know they had to see the patient? Is the procedure for sterile dressing changes complete? Did the pre-op nurse know the pre-op antibiotic had not been given? *This information can be found in documents, on-line, direct communications, shift reports, etc*
	To what degree is communication among participants adequate?	Was the technician comfortable telling the physician that the skin prep was not complete or that the equipment had been rushed through the sterilization process? *This is a critical question when doing a root cause analysis – communication breakdown has been the root cause of most events*
Environmental management issues	To what degree was the physical environment appropriate for the processes being carried out?	Is the staff member able to work uninterrupted? Is the sink placed in such a way that it makes hand washing cumbersome? Are fans blowing through dirty work areas? Is the ventilator equipment stored appropriately? Are the surgical supplies in a clean, dry area, away from contamination? *This sometimes requires a site visit by the team to the area in question.*
	What systems are in place to identify environmental risks?	Does the hospital have a process for content experts to make assessments of environmental risks? Is the ICP a welcome visitor in Surgery? Are the issues identified acted upon and is there accountability?
	What emergency and failure-mode responses have been planned and tested?	*The group can brainstorm all potential failure modes associated with the process and determine what interventions would be most helpful to prevent that potential failure mode? This is a very labor-intensive process.*

Continued

Copyright © 2005, Association for Professionals in Infection Control and Epidemiology, Inc.

Table 12-7. Continued

Level of Analysis	Questions	Findings
Leadership issues: – Corporate culture	To what degree is the culture conducive to risk identification and reduction?	Is the staff comfortable in reporting risks? Is their manager responsive? Does the staff know what to do if no action is taken? *Asking this question may reveal some serious systems issues or management issues that leadership should be aware of and must act on.*
– Open communication ab about risk	What are the barriers to communication of potential risk factors?	Is the manager available to the staff? Are all opinions respected, regardless of skill level? *Processes may need to be developed to allow free and open communication*
– Clear communication of priorities	To what degree is the prevention of adverse outcomes communicated as a high priority? How?	Has the staff been educated on patient safety and prevention of adverse outcomes? Do they understand the rationale for each step in a process to reduce risk of infectious outcomes? Does the Environmental Services employee understand how critical their role is in infection prevention and control? How is the department-specific orientation to infection prevention and control communicated to the staff?

system performs in a way that is not intended or desirable.

- Mode (M) means the way of operating or using a system or process, or a way or manner in which a thing is done. A mode is the way or manner in which something, such as a failure, can happen. Combining the words failure and mode, a *failure mode* is the manner which something can fail. A failure mode generally describes the way the failure occurs and its impact on a process. Any step in a process can fail, and each failure may have many failure modes.

- Effects (E) is defined as the results or consequences of an action. Effects are the results of failure modes. They might be direct or indirect, long- or short-term, likely or unlikely. In any case, they are the result of the impact of a particular failure mode on the stability of the entire process or a portion thereof. A failure effect is the consequence(s) a failure mode has on the operation, function, or status of a process step. In healthcare, effects generally are classified according to the outcome of the process — the impact on the care recipient.

- Analysis (A) is defined as the detailed examination of the elements or structure or something, perhaps a process, substance, or situation. An FMEA team performs an analysis to determine possible failure modes and effects, how serious the possible effects could be, and ways to eliminate or reduce failure risk and prevent harm.

FMEA can be used to improve many types of processes or subprocesses. High-risk patient care processes provide the natural staring place. High-risk processes are those in which a failure of some type is most likely to jeopardize the safety of the individuals served by the healthcare organization. Processes that will benefit from FMEA may be new to the organization or they may be existing and potentially (or actually) problematic. A subprocess may be singled out for an FMEA, or the analysis might cover the entire process. FMEA can be use proactively either before a new process is put in place or before a process that has been redesigned "goes live" following a root cause analysis due to a sentinel event.[35]

In summary, FMEA can improve the safety of individuals receiving care by preventing failures and preventing injury and harm from near misses when, despite an organization's best efforts, failures do occur. FMEA can narrow or eliminate gaps in quality and performance and yield improved outcomes. It is an easy-to-learn performance improvement method that enhances organization-wide collaboration and understanding. In short, its use is good business practice. FMEA's sole limitation is that it involves a commitment of human resources and time.

The Role of the Infection Control Professional in Patient Safety

Most people associate going to a hospital with being in a clean, often sterile, environment, and did not expect infection to be a possible outcome of hospitalization.

Copyright © 2005, Association for Professionals in Infection Control and Epidemiology, Inc.

But the reality is that healthcare-associated infections are the 4th leading cause of death in the United States, after heart disease, cancer, and stroke. Most people can imagine the devastation of an infection, even those who have not read the Harvard Medical Practice Study, which pointed to surgical site infections as the number-two adverse event experienced by hospitalized patients. The statistics in the literature are largely made of up infections that occur in hospitals, accounting for only part of the problem. Infection control professionals track infectious adverse events within and outside of the traditional healthcare environment — in long-term care, home health, and outpatient surgery and dialysis units. Few clinicians have the widespread, comprehensive view of adverse events that ICPs bring to the patient safety arena. In addition to experience, the history of ICPs dates back to professionals such as Florence Nightingale (1854) tracking mortality rates among soldiers in the Crimean war and Dr. Ignaz Semmelweis (1865) suggesting that hand disinfection would end puerperal sepsis.

Surveillance, prevention, and control measures are the foundation of any program whose aim is to identify and categorize risk, using problem-solving techniques and critical thinking skills to eliminate injury and harm. These fundamental skills and core competencies are what ICPs bring to patient safety programs. Marketing these skills and competencies is how ICPs can demonstrate their value to healthcare leaders interested in improving the safety and quality of clinical care. Volunteering to participate in, and if possible lead, an organization's patient safety efforts may include: active membership on the patient safety committee, offering training and courses in the principles of epidemiology, assisting with the set up or evaluation of surveillance programs for medication errors or falls, or guiding a team through the process of developing interventions to reduce the incidence of pressure ulcers in high-risk population. But program participation should be driven by individual interests and abilities. If an ICP's strength is statistics and/or data analysis, the performance measurement aspect of the patient safety program may find this experience invaluable. If the ICP's talents lie more in education and training, she or he can offer to be part of organization-wide efforts, especially for education targeting medical staff or teams of professionals with whom they already have critical relationships. Since infection prevention and control is such an important aspect of any patient safety program, staying focused on doing that well may be the best use of organizational infection control resources. For individuals, keeping options open to move into a generalist role, tracking any adverse outcome of care, provides a safety net for the ICP in times of budgetary constraints and staffing reduction.

If an ICP can prevent infections, he or she can prevent almost any other adverse outcome and should have confidence that a patient safety program depends on their skills and experience.

APIC's own professional practice standards[36] outline the skills and competencies that ICPs need in order to be effective managers and leaders in the hospital epidemiology and infection control program. These practice standards should be part of the position description and performance appraisal of every ICP, since they demonstrate the valuable assets brought to the organization's patient safety program. These include:

- Infection prevention and control practice
- Epidemiology
- Surveillance
- Education
- Consultation
- Performance improvement
- Program management and evaluation
- Fiscal responsibility
- Research

The most valuable asset ICPs bring to patient safety is a practice based on the science of epidemiology: the study of populations, characterized by time, place, and risk factors; use of proper definitions and measurements; and use of appropriate study designs depending on the questions to be answered:

- Do we know the outcome and have to find the risk factors? *Case-control*
- Do we know the risk factors and want to find out what the outcome will be? *Cohort*
- Can we alter either the risk factors or the outcome? *Randomized-controlled trials/intervention study*

Epidemiologic skills used to reduce endemic infection rates through surveillance and prevention activities can be applied to the study of any adverse outcome of healthcare. Once indicators are selected to measure adverse outcomes, the same competencies are needed:

- Data management: collection, organization, analysis, reporting
- Feedback of data and information to key stakeholders
- Education of healthcare workers about risks and reduction strategies
- Development and implementation of interventions to reduce risk and improve processes

Copyright © 2005, Association for Professionals in Infection Control and Epidemiology, Inc.

- Evaluation of interventions based on data (improved rates or processes)

- Continued surveillance and prevention activities

Performance improvement skills are another valued asset the ICP brings to the patient safety table. These include:

- Change management

- Customer focus

- Systems thinking

- Team leading and facilitation

- Measurement and evaluation skills

- Knowledge and experience with tools and methods to support performance and process improvement

Peter Pronovost, medical director of the Johns Hopkins Hospital (JHH) Patient Safety program, has shared the 12 steps they use to build and evaluate the success of the patient safety program. These competencies all within the realm of infection control practice:

1. Evaluate the culture of safety.

2. Employ leadership in safety efforts.

3. Educate staff about culture of safety.

4. Address staff's concerns; involve them.

5. Select, define, measure safety indicators.

6. Measure compliance with safety practices.

7. Focus on improving systems that support compliance with safety practices.

8. Plan and prioritize improvement efforts.

9. Implement improvements.

10. Share successful outcomes and stories — disseminate results.

11. Celebrate staff that identify mistakes openly.

12. Know that errors result from faulty systems, not bad people.

IV. SUMMARY AND CONCLUSIONS

The ICP's responsibilities toward the patient safety program include reviewing IOM, NPSF, and AHRQ reports, always looking for evidence-based practices. Once identified, the ICP can help facilitate the integration of evidence-based research into practice. We must constantly monitor responses from APIC, Society for Healthcare Epidemiology of America (SHEA), CDC, and other professional associations to the latest trends or hot topics in patient safety. The ICP must stay

focused, despite many competing priorities, on developing and facilitating the implementation of interventions to reduce healthcare-associated infections. Demonstrate improvement through process measures (e.g., on-time pre-op antibiotics), as well as outcome measures (e.g., infection rates). Promoting infection control program success will not only market the ICP's skills and competencies, but will share ideas and information with others who are tackling non-infectious adverse outcomes. Additionally, the ICP promote her o rhis role as an internal consultant – as are a program manager and organizational leader – by learning performance improvement and risk management language, tools, and methods. Root cause analysis and performance improvement action plans are an expectation of the job, and so the ICP should volunteer to participate on teams addressing patient safety and lead them as often as possible. Despite a strong background in epidemiology, fear of being overstretched to the point of incompetence is often what keeps many qualified ICPs from voluntarily taking on more responsibility. After the immediate reaction ("how can I possibly expand my responsibility?"), a wise question to ask might be, "How can I share my expertise most effectively while protecting my limited time and resources?" The ICP should ask organizational decision-makers for help in re-aligning time and resources to allow for broader involvement in patient safety. ICPs are the organization's internal patient safety experts and must remain closely aligned with initiatives to reduce any and all adverse outcomes of healthcare.

The publication and enforcement of the National Patient Safety Goals has helped to elevate the importance of hospital epidemiology and infection control programs and the ICP. The critical role of hand hygiene in the prevention of HAIs has now become an enforceable safety standard. ICPs have shared data and information about the positive effects of hand hygiene for years. Now we are challenged to creatively use limited resources to observe, measure, and improve compliance. This is in addition to required involvement in sentinel event investigation! As professionals, we can consider this an overwhelming expansion of our work, or as an opportunity to expand skills and increase our value.

ICPs bring a wealth of knowledge and expertise to patient safety. With a large and strong national organization and many invaluable partnerships, ICPs provide strength in numbers and confidence from teamwork. The epidemic of medical errors must be stopped. In collaboration with partners such as SHEA, CDC, AORN, ASHRM, and others, APIC can offer a more effective voice for organizational, community, political, and business leaders to hear. Together, we have a better chance of success at creating cultures where

Copyright © 2005, Association for Professionals in Infection Control and Epidemiology, Inc.

everyone's safety is a priority, a commitment and a passion.

V. FUTURE TRENDS

The issues of patient safety will not go away, and will instead receive increasing attention both from those who pay for healthcare as well as those who consume it. Public reporting of outcomes and the linking of reimbursement to outcomes will continue to challenge systems.

VI. INTERNATIONAL PERSPECTIVES

Although regulatory requirements differ, patient safety is a global issue with a global impact. This has been evidenced through outbreak investigations involving pharmaceuticals and single-use and reprocessed medical supplies. In addition, the safety issues involving multidrug-resistant organisms and emerging infections that affect multiple countries continue to be a large part of safety initiatives. Patient safety initiatives will continue to be part of both strong and weak relationships among healthcare providers worldwide.

REFERENCES

1. Kohn LT, Corrigan JM, Donaldson MS, eds. To err is human: building a safer health system. Washington, D.C., 2000, National Academy Press. Available at: http://books.nap.edu/books/0309068371/html/index.html or *http://www.ahrq.gov/news/focus/ptsafety.pdf*
2. Leape LL, Brennan TA, Laird N, Lawthers AG, Barnes BA, Herbert L, Newhouse JP, Weiler PC and H Hiatt. The Nature of Adverse Events in Hospitalized Patients: Results of the Harvard Medical Practice Study. *N Engl J Med* 324(6): 377084, 1991.
3. Leape LL, Lawthers AG, Brennan TA, et al.: Preventing Medical Injury. *Qual Rev Bull* 19(5):144–49; 1993.
4. Agency for Healthcare Quality and Research. Patient Safety Initiative: *Building Foundations, Reducing Risk*. Interim Report to the Senate Committee on Appropriations. AHRQ Publication No. 04-RG005, Rockville, MD, December 2003, Agency for Healthcare Research and Quality. http://www.ahrq.gov/qual/pscongrpt/ (accessed 12/6/04).
5. Agency for Healthcare Quality and Research. Focus on Research: Patient Safety. AHRQ Publication number 02-M021. Rockville, MD, March 2002, Agency for Healthcare Research and Quality. Available at:http://www.ahrq.gov/news/focus/ptsafety.pdf Accessed 12/6/04.
6. Brennan TA, Leape LL, Laird NM, et al.: *Harvard Medical Practice Study I. Qual Saf Health Care.* 13(2):145–51; discussion 151–2, 2004.
7. Brennan, TA: The Institute of Medicine Report on Medical Errors — Could It Do Harm? *N Engl J Med* 342:1123–1125, 2000.
8. Graves N: Economics and preventing hospital-acquired infection. *Emerg Infect Dis* 2004. Available from:http://www.cdc.gov/ncidod/EID/vol10no4/02–0754.htm Accessed 10/3/02.
9. Stone PW, Larson E, Kawar LN: A systematic audit of economic evidence linking nosocomial infections and infection control interventions: 1990–2000. *Am J Infect Control.* 30(3):145–52, 2002.
10. Wenzel RP, and Edmond MB: The Impact of Hospital-Acquired Bloodstream Infections. *Emerging Infectious Diseases* 7(2), 2001. Available at: http://www.cdc.gov/ncidod/eid/vol7no2/wenzel.htm
11. Joint Commission on Accreditation of Healthcare Organizations. Sentinel Event Statistics. July 31, 2004. Available at: http://www.jcaho.org/accredited + organizations/hospitals/sentinel + events/sentinel + event + statistics.htm Accessed 10/1/04.
12. Reason J:. Human error: models and management. *BMJ* 320: 768–770. 2002.
13. Cook RI, and Woods DD: Operating at the sharp end: the complexity of human error. In: Bogner MS, ed.: *Human error in medicine.* Hinsdale, NJ, 1994, Lawrence Erlbaum Associates, pp. 255–310. Available at: http://www.ctlab.org/, accessed 6/6/2004 and http://www.ctlab.org/properties/pdf%20files/operating%20at%20the%20sharp.pdf Accessed 10/01/04.
14. Morath, J: Presentation at BJC HeatlhCare, Patient Safety Forum, St. Louis, MO, 2003.
15. Marx D. *Patient safety and the "just culture": a primer for health care executives.* New York, Columbia University, 2001. Available at: http://www.mers-tm.net/support/Marx_Primer.pdf, accessed 3/20/2003
16. Leape LL: Presentation at Missouri Hospital Association, Patient Safety Seminar. St. Louis, MO, 2002.
17. National Patient Safety Foundation. *Safety Culture.* Available at: http://search.freefind.com/find.html?id = 28648537&t = s& nsb = &pageid = r&mode = ALL&s = definitions& query = Safety + Culture Accessed 9/24/04.
18. Reeder, JM: *Patient Safety: Cultural Changes, Ethical Imperatives.* Healthcare Quarterly.Volume 2, No. 1. *Healthcare Papers.* New York, 2001, Longwood Publishing.
19. Joint Commission on Accreditation of Healthcare Organizations. National Patient Safety Goals. Available at: http://www.jcaho.org/accredited + organizations/patient + safety/05 + npsg/npsg_facts.htm Accessed 10/3/04.
20. Leonard M: Presentation. BJC HealthCare, Patient Safety Forum, St. Louis, MO. September 2002.
21. Gosbee J: Human Factors Engineering and Patient Safety. *Qual Saf Health Care* 11: 352–354, 2002. Available at https://qhc.bmjjournals.com/cgi/content/full/11/4/353 Accessed 9/6/04.
22. Carayon P, Alvarado C, Hundt A: *Reducing Workload and Increasing Patient Safety through Work and Workspace Design.* Paper Commissioned by the Institute for Medicine Commission on the Work Environment for Nurses and Patient Safety. In *Keeping Patients Safe: Transforming the Work Environment for Nurses.* Ann Page, ed., Madison, WI, 2004, Center for Quality and Productivity Improvement and the Department of Industrial Engineering, University of Wisconsin – Madison.
23. Wolf L: BJC HealthCare, Patient Safety Curriculum. Human Factors Module. 2004.
24. Leape LL: Error in Medicine, *JAMA* 272:1151–7, 1994.
25. Baker, SP, O'Neill, B., Ginsburg M., Guohua L. The Injury Fact Book, 2 ed., New York, 1992, Oxford University Press.
26. Leape LL, Berwick DM: Safe health care: are we up to it? *BMJ* 320:725–726, 2000.
27. The Joint Commission on Accreditation of Healthcare Organizations. Sentinel Events in Hospital Settings. Available at http://www.jcaho.org/accredited + organizations/hospitals/sentinel + events/voluntarily + reportable + sentinel + even ts.htm Accessed 10/5/04.
28. Caleca B: BJC HealthCare Patient Safety Curriculum. Importance of Reporting Module. 2004.
29. The Institute of Medicine. *Crossing the Quality Chasm: A New Health Systetm for the 21st Century.* Washington, DC, 2001, National Academy of Sciences. Available at www.iom.edu/report.asp?id = 5432 Accessed: 10/20/04.
30. Kennedy V, O'Heron S, Jaloway J, Steinfeld C: Nosocomial infections in intensive care patients. *Crit Care Nurs Clin N Am.* 14(4):417–426, 2002.
31. The National Quality Forum. *Safe Practices for Better Healthcare: A Consensus Report.* 2003. Available @ www.qualityforum.org/txsafeexecsumm Accessed 9/24/04.
32. Murphy DM: Crosswalk Demonstrating Similarities Between FOCUS PDSA, Root Cause Analysis and Outbreak Investigation. Available @ www.apic.org
33. Frain J, Murphy DM, Dash GP, Kasai M:. Association for Professionals in Infection Control and Epidemiology. Integrating Sentinel Event Analysis Into Your Infection Control Practice. Available @ www.apic.org Accessed 9/24/04.
34. The Institute for Health Care Improvement. Failure Mode and Effects Analysis: Overview. Available at: www.qualityhealthcare.com Accessed: 10/15/04.

Copyright © 2005, Association for Professionals in Infection Control and Epidemiology, Inc.

35. Joint Commission on Accreditation on HealthCare Organizations. Failure Mode and Effects Analysis in Health Care: Proactive Risk Reduction. 2002. Available at: www.jcaho.org Accessed 10/17/04.
36. Horan-Murphy T, Barnard B, Chenowith C, et al.: APIC/CHIC-Canada infection control and epidemiology: Professional and practice standards. *Am J Infect Control* 27:47–51, 1999.

SUPPLEMENTAL RESOURCES

Agency for Healthcare Research and Quality (AHRQ): www.ahrq.gov

American Hospital Association (AHA): www.hospitalconnect.com

American Society for Healthcare Risk Management (ASHRM): www.a-ha.org/ashrm

Association of Health Care Pharmacists (AHCP): www.ashp.org

Association of Operating Room Nurses (AORN): www.aorn.org

Association for Professionals in Infection Control and Epidemiology (APIC): www.apic.org

Centers for Disease Control and Prevention (CDC): www.cdc.gov

Institute for Healthcare Improvement (IHI): www.qualityhealthcare.org

Institute for Safe Medication Practices (ISMP): www.ismp.org

Joint Commission for Accreditation of Healthcare Organizations (JCAHO): www.jcaho.org

Society for Healthcare Epidemiology of America (SHEA): www.shea-online.org

Premier Safety Institute (PSI): www.premierinc.com

National Patient Safety Foundation (NPSF): www.npsf.org

National Quality Forum (NQF): www.qualityforum.org

Haley R. Measuring the costs of nosocomial infections: methods for estimating economic burden on the hospital. Am J Med 1991;ZS91:32S–8S.

Haley RW. Incidence and nature of endemic and epidemic nosocomial infections. In: Bennett JV, Brachman P, editors. Hospital infections. Boston: Little, Brown; 1985. p. 359–7.

Copyright © 2005, Association for Professionals in Infection Control and Epidemiology, Inc.

Risk Factors for Infection Transmission

Loretta L. Fauerbach, MS, CIC
Shands Hospital at the University of Florida
Gainesville, Florida

ABSTRACT

A lack of standardized infection criteria and surveillance methods makes comparison of infection rates among healthcare facilities difficult. Nosocomial infection surveillance data that adjust for specific infection risks should be used for interhospital comparison of infection rates.[1-5]

KEY CONCEPTS

- Infection control professionals (ICPs) should consult a variety of sources for updated information on infection risks, including the National Nosocomial Infections Surveillance System (NNIS), the Joint Commission on Accreditation of Healthcare Organizations (JCAHO)'s ORYX monitoring system, relevant studies published in the professional medical literature, and recommendations from the Hospital Infection Control Practices Advisory Committee (HICPAC).

- The risk of nosocomial or iatrogenic infection during patient care is related to the mode of transmission of the infectious agent, the type of patient care activity or procedure being performed, and the patient's underlying host defenses.

- Some of the patient factors that increase the risk of infection include immunosuppressive disease and disorders, malignant disorders, poor nutritional status, age, diabetes, extensive burn wounds, or trauma. Additionally, particular medical interventions have been shown to have an influence on the patient's risk of infection: the presence of invasive devices, placement in an intensive care unit, exposure to antibiotics, immunosuppressive therapy, length of hospitalization, and an increased number of healthcare worker examinations/procedures.

- Healthcare personnel (i.e., employees, medical staff, students, and volunteers) are at risk for exposure to microorganisms in the healthcare facility or in the home setting during home care activities.

- Visitors and family are at risk for exposure to microorganisms when they visit healthcare facilities. When they provide direct patient care, visitors and families have the same risk as healthcare providers for transmission of infectious disease via direct contact with blood, body fluids, excretions, and secretions.

- Prevention of infection in patients, staff, and visitors requires attention to both human and environmental factors. In partic-

Copyright © 2005, Association for Professionals in Infection Control and Epidemiology, Inc.

ular, infection risk can be reduced by adherence to appropriate infection control measures (e.g., hand-washing, barrier precautions).

I.   BACKGROUND

The National Nosocomial Infections Surveillance System (NNIS) is a nationwide voluntary surveillance network for nosocomial infections. It was established by the Centers for Disease Control and Prevention (CDC) in 1970 to help create a national database of nosocomial infections and improve surveillance methods in hospitals. In 1985, the goals of NNIS were broadened, and the type of information collected was increased to more completely characterize infections and permit identification of potential risk factors. An imminent change in NNIS involves expanding the concept to include a variety of patient safety issues—not only those related to infection. The vision for the new system, National Healthcare Safety Network (NHSN), involves the development of an Internet-based knowledge system for accumulating, exchanging, and integrating relevant information and resources among private and public stakeholders that would support local efforts to protect patients and promote healthcare safety. This system is expected to be operational during 2005. Until then, NNIS remains operational and represents the gold standard for infection benchmarking for healthcare facilities.

Currently, NNIS is the only source of national surveillance data on nosocomial infections in the United States.[6] Hospitals participating in NNIS must meet certain eligibility criteria related to average census, infection control staffing, and availability of the required computer hardware and software. NNIS periodically publishes nosocomial infection rate data to allow for interhospital comparison. These data address nosocomial infection rates in adult (surgical, medical, and cardiothoracic) and pediatric intensive care units (overall and device-associated[3,7]); nosocomial infections in the high-risk nursery (overall, birthweight-stratified, and device-associated[7]); and surgical wound infection rates by wound class, operative procedure, and patient-risk index.[1,8] NNIS has also published a study on the accuracy of reporting nosocomial infections in the intensive care units.[9]

II.   BASIC PRINCIPLES

The Joint Commission on Accreditation of Healthcare Organizations (JCAHO), through its Agenda for Change, initiated a system to facilitate continuous monitoring of healthcare organizational performance. Specifically, it adopted an indicator monitoring system known as ORYX, which includes infection control indicators. This reporting system, however, may include

and compare data from administrative reports as well as data collected by traditional surveillance methodologies. An expansion of ORYX now involves the evaluation of current disease states and evaluates compliance with documented best practices. These measurements are termed *core measures*. Currently, the core measure that has specific relevance to infection prevention and control is the one that deals with community-acquired pneumonia (CAP). Specific performance indicators for this core measure include adherence to rapid antimicrobial administration and vaccination measures. Additional information about core measures can be obtained by visiting the JCAHO website (http://www.jcaho.org).

Studies published in professional journals are an important source of relevant information. Keeping current with the medical literature in infection control will provide references to obtain specific rates of nosocomial infection. As noted above, the lack of standard methodologies and definitions must be considered. Computer-assisted literature searches (e.g., MEDLINE, Paradigm) allow for efficient access to pertinent studies published in the professional literature.[3] Recommendations from the Hospital Infection Control Practices Advisory Committee are also a source of information about risk factors.[10-13]

III.   RISK FACTORS FOR INFECTION TRANSMISSION

Exposure Risks

The risk of nosocomial or iatrogenic infection during patient care is related to the mode of transmission of the infectious agent, the type of patient care activity or procedure being performed, and the individual's underlying host defenses. The duration of exposure, the inoculum, and the pathogenicity of the infectious agent also significantly influence the infectious risk.[4] An increased risk of infection has been associated with stays in the intensive care unit, prolonged hospitalization, and antimicrobial use.[14,15] Patients are at risk for exposure to and colonization with microorganisms through various routes of transmission, which may lead to nosocomial or iatrogenic infection. Patients may also represent an infectious risk for other patients, healthcare workers, and visitors because of their infectious process.

Airborne Transmission

Airborne transmission of microorganisms can occur in the following situations:

1. A patient with a respiratory disease is not isolated on airborne precautions, or personnel or visitors have a respiratory illness such as tuberculosis, chickenpox, or measles.[16,17]

Copyright © 2005, Association for Professionals in Infection Control and Epidemiology, Inc.

2. A negative-air-pressure room is not used for airborne precautions or to house the patient during emergency department or clinic visits.[18]

3. The ventilation system is contaminated with microorganisms. Levels of potentially pathogenic microorganisms may vary and present varying risks according to the immune competency of the host; for example, *Aspergillus* species do not produce disease in the immunocompetent patient but are potentially life threatening for the bone marrow transplant patient.[19]

4. The air conditioning or water systems become contaminated with waterborne bacteria that become aerosolized and inhaled by the patient (e.g., *Legionella* species in the water supply, which is aerosolized through shower heads).[20-25]

Direct Contact

Direct contact with microorganisms from healthcare workers has occurred during patient care activities. Direct contact with infectious material of another patient most commonly occurs in pediatric and geriatric settings. Visitors and volunteers may also be a source, depending on the activities in which they engage with the patient. Direct contact leading to contact with blood, body fluids, excretions, and secretions may occur in the following instances[26-29]:

1. During patient care by the healthcare worker or a visitor or family member, or

2. During interactive activities in playrooms or lounges between patients, for example, children with lesions touching each other or drooling on each other, transferring organisms (e.g., adenovirus causing epidemic keratoconjunctivitis or transmission of respiratory syncytial virus from patient to staff via respiratory secretions).[13,30-32]

Indirect Contact

Indirect contact with contaminated equipment, food, water, or supplies may occur in the following situations:

1. Inadequate handwashing is performed by a care provider.[33]

2. Equipment is not cleaned, disinfected, or sterilized adequately between patients, leading to colonization and infection (e.g., contaminated endoscopes, contaminated urine receptacles for emptying urinary catheter drainage bags, or unsterilized surgical equipment from a faulty autoclave).[34]

3. Food and water supplies are not prepared and maintained according to sanitation standards (e.g., raw eggs are used to mix formula, ice machines are not cleaned, or meat that harbors *Salmonella* is undercooked).[35]

4. Sharps and biohazardous waste are not disposed of properly, allowing percutaneous injuries or mucous membrane exposures to occur.[36,37]

5. Pharmaceutical supplies are not prepared, stored, and administered according to industry standards (e.g., contaminated parenteral or irrigation fluids cause nosocomial infections).[38,39]

Occupational Exposure

Healthcare personnel (i.e., employees, medical staff, students, and volunteers) are at risk for exposure to microorganisms in the healthcare facility or in the home setting during home care activities.[13,40-45] Airborne transmission is a concern, because personnel need not be in immediate contact to become infected and may still be exposed, even if they are not providing direct patient care. Airborne transmission of microorganisms is a potential for personnel in the following situations:

1. A patient with an airborne transmitted disease is not promptly recognized and isolated in a negative-air-pressure isolation room (e.g., tuberculosis transmission).[46]

2. An employee does not use an appropriate mask (i.e., a 95 N respirator) when caring for a patient in an isolation room.[47]

3. Another healthcare worker has an unrecognized airborne infection (e.g., incubating chickenpox) and reports to work.[13,16]

4. A visitor is infected with an airborne-transmitted disease, such as measles.[17]

5. Ventilation is inadequate and carries air from an isolation room to other areas of a facility, resulting in airborne transmission of diseases (see Chapter 93, Mycobacteria).

6. The ventilation system is contaminated with an infectious agent, such as *Legionella* species.[20-25,48]

The potential for contact with blood, body fluids, secretions, and excretions most often occurs for the healthcare worker during direct patient contact (by the medical and surgical staff or during nursing care, respiratory care, radiology, and physical therapy) or in the laboratory. Other employees, such as those in social services and pastoral care, recreational therapy, or volunteers, are at minimal risk for exposure based on their routine job tasks and activities. Direct contact can occur in the following situations:

Copyright © 2005, Association for Professionals in Infection Control and Epidemiology, Inc.

1. Contact with blood and body fluids occurs without appropriate barrier precautions (e.g., for hepatitis C or herpes simplex virus [from oral secretions]).[13,49]

2. Personal protective equipment malfunctions or breaks.

3. The healthcare worker fails to identify risk and the need for personal protective equipment (e.g., a patient has herpes zoster on the back and the need for gloves is not communicated to the respiratory therapist before initiating chest physical therapy, resulting in an exposure; or the therapist fails to use gloves to prevent transmission of vancomycin-resistant *Enterococcus*).[50,51]

4. Inadequate handwashing allows transmission of enteric illnesses, such as hepatitis A or methicillin-resistant *Staphylococcus aureus* (MRSA) via the hands of healthcare workers.[41]

Indirect contact with contaminated food, water, or supplies may occur for the healthcare provider and potentially result in disease transmission in the following situations:

1. Sharps and biohazardous waste are not disposed of properly, allowing percutaneous injuries or mucous membrane exposures to occur.[13,42] The risk of transmission of bloodborne pathogens associated with needlestick exposures also increases if appropriate postexposure prophylaxis is not appropriately initiated.[52]

2. Food and water supplies used by the employees are not prepared and maintained according to sanitation standards.

3. Inadequate handwashing or proper personal protective equipment is not used during handling of contaminated equipment by healthcare workers.[53]

Visitors and Family Members

Visitors and family are at risk for exposure to microorganisms when they visit healthcare facilities or provide care in the home. Airborne transmission of disease is a concern, since the risk is difficult to minimize because the agents are hard to detect. The visitor may not have had direct contact with the infected person or source; therefore, no one recognizes that an airborne exposure may have occurred and the appropriate prophylaxis is not given. Airborne transmission of microorganisms is a potential for visitors in the following situations:

1. A patient with a respiratory-transmitted disease is not promptly recognized and isolated in a negative-air-pressure room (e.g., a child with measles is not triaged quickly in an emergency care setting and remains in the area, exposing others in the waiting room).[17]

2. A visitor does not use a mask when entering an isolation room.[47]

3. Another visitor has an unrecognized airborne-transmitted disease, such as a child in the prodromal stage of chickenpox in an outpatient pediatric clinic.

4. Ventilation is inadequate and carries air from an isolation room to other areas of facility, as has been reported in multidrug-resistant tuberculosis outbreaks.[18]

5. The ventilation system harbors an infectious agent.

When they provide direct patient care, visitors and families have the same risk as healthcare workers for transmission of infectious disease via direct contact with blood, body fluids, excretions, and secretions. The potential for exposure during these activities would be similar to that for healthcare providers. Visitors and families have a risk similar to that of healthcare providers for transmission of an infectious agent through indirect contact if: they handle contaminated patient care equipment, or if they ingest contaminated food or water while in the healthcare setting.[35]

Practices to Decrease the Risk of Transmission

An infection control committee should establish and monitor compliance with and effectiveness of the facility's infection control policies and procedures. Patient care practices, including specific patient care procedures, should be monitored. The infection risk of certain patient care procedures can be reduced by adherence to appropriate infection control measures (e.g., hand washing, barrier precautions).[10-13,27,32,48,52-56] High-risk procedures include:

1. Intravascular access, especially central lines

2. Mechanical ventilation

3. Surgical and invasive procedures

4. Intracranial monitoring

5. Parenteral nutrition (e.g., hyperalimentation)

6. Urinary tract instrumentation, especially indwelling catheterization

7. Extracorporeal membrane oxygenation.[57]

For more information, the reader is invited to refer to chapters addressing specific high-risk procedures, including: Chapter 24, Intravascular Device Infections; Chapter 23, Surgical Site Infections; Chapter 25, Urinary Tract Infections; Chapter 48, Endoscopy.

Copyright © 2005, Association for Professionals in Infection Control and Epidemiology, Inc.

Surveillance Activities

The 1985 Study on the Efficacy of Nosocomial Infection Control (SENIC) found that active nosocomial infection surveillance and the reporting of infection rate data back to associated healthcare workers resulted in a reduction in the occurrence of nosocomial infections. For example, surgical site infections (SSIs) are reduced when a surgeon-specific, nosocomial, SSI rate is provided to the surgeon; similarly, the urinary tract infection (UTI) rate is decreased when the unit-specific nosocomial UTI rate is reported back to the nursing unit.[58-60]

Patient Placement

The physical space requirements for patient care areas and hospital rooms set by state and federal codes mandate adequate spacing between patients to prevent crowding and reduce the risk of microorganism transmission. Policies should exist to ensure assessment of unique patient needs regarding patient placement based on their risk for exposure. Patients who are at increased risk for infection because of immunosuppression[19,61,62] may require separation by private room or cohorting from infected patients, e.g., patients with draining lesions. Patients infected or colonized with epidemiologically significant organisms, such as vancomycin-resistant enterococci (VRE) or MRSA, may be separated from other patients as part of an overall control plan.[48,63-65] Patients with airborne diseases such as tuberculosis should be cared for in a negative-air-pressure isolation room.[18] A private room is desirable; however, patients with the same airborne disease may share a room if there is no clinical contraindication.

Cohorting of patients infected or colonized with a common organism by room and/or personnel assignments can reduce the risk of transmission of infectious agents to other noninfected patients.[31,55] Criteria for cohorting patients is based on:

1. Common risk factors, such as infants born during same time frame or patients admitted with similar infection (e.g., *Salmonella*)

2. Common exposure to a communicable disease, such as a ward for those exposed to varicella, if individual private rooms are not available and patients are not immunosuppressed

3. Prevention of contact between patients known to be infected or colonized with patients who are newly admitted or not harboring the organism; cohorting in this manner is often used as an outbreak-control measure.

Patient Hygiene

One goal of personal hygiene for the patient is related to infection control: reduction of the microbial load of the skin and maintenance of the well-being of mucous membranes such as the mouth and vagina. The following are examples of activities that may reduce the bioload:[66]

1. Washing from clean to less-clean areas using clean washcloths

2. Preoperative showering using antimicrobial soap[67]

3. Washing with antimicrobial soaps, such as chlorhexidine gluconate, to reduce carriage of resistant organisms such as MRSA

4. Encouraging or assisting patient in maintaining good oral hygiene[68]

5. Encouraging good genital-area cleansing

Patient Education

Patients should be taught the concept of standard barrier precautions to educate them concerning exposure to blood and body fluids, including excretions and secretions. They should also be instructed about the proper disposal of contaminated items, such as tissues and sanitary napkins. Basic hygiene should be taught to patients who need it, including the use of toilet facilities. This is particularly important for children, for patients with an altered mental status, and often for recent immigrants from developing countries. Patients can participate in their own care and lower their infection risk through an increased understanding and improved practice of aseptic principles. When indicated, patients should be taught the following:

1. Handwashing and hygiene

2. Barrier techniques to prevent exposure to blood and body fluids, and proper handling of sharps

3. Mode of transmission of microorganisms from one area of the body to another

4. Location of portals of bacterial entry that are associated with therapeutic and diagnostic measures to reduce the risk of inadvertent contamination of intravenous sites, dialysis sites, or surgical sites

5. Symptoms associated with infection and the need to report them to their healthcare providers

6. Effective breathing and coughing techniques to be used postoperatively to reduce pulmonary complications

7. Cough containment to reduce transmission of airborne pathogens

Copyright © 2005, Association for Professionals in Infection Control and Epidemiology, Inc.

8. Principles and methods for disposal of sharps and medical waste

9. Specific patient care procedures that the patient will be performing

10. Discharge planning

Patients are also being discharged from the acute care setting more rapidly than in the past. Coordination of the discharge process, including education of the patient and family, the home care agency, and the long-term-care facility, is essential to reduce infection risk and ensure the continuation of consistent care. Invasive devices and surgical sites may require postdischarge care. When indicated, information should be provided on:

1. The care of respiratory devices, including (a) cleaning and disinfection of reusable respiratory-care equipment (including humidifiers), and (b) care of tracheostomies and suctioning techniques

2. The care of intravascular catheters, including (a) site care and maintenance, (b) line changes, and (c) medication storage and administration

3. The care of urinary catheter systems, including (a) indwelling and suprapubic catheterization techniques and maintenance, (b) self-catheterization, (c) cleaning and disinfection of urinary catheterization equipment, and (d) other urinary management techniques

4. The preparation, care, and storage of enteral tube feedings

5. Wound care and sterile dressing techniques

6. Standard barrier precautions for the patient and care providers

7. The management and handling of biohazardous waste, including sharps

8. Special precautions for specific communicable diseases, such as tuberculosis, and the role of the public health department in patient follow-up and administration of direct observation therapy[18]

9. Adherence to and importance of completion of treatment modalities, including antimicrobial therapies

10. Signs and symptoms that should be reported to the healthcare provider.

Personnel Practices

Employee health policies designed to reduce the risk of infection transmission to patients, fellow employees, and visitors should establish the following guidelines:[13]

1. Immunization of personnel must be required and available.[13,69]

2. Work should be restricted for employees with a communicable disease or infectious process, such as diarrhea, group A streptococcal infections, conjunctivitis, draining dermatitis or exudative lesions, active tuberculosis, and possible infectious rashes.

3. Patients can be assigned to specific employees based on employees' immunity (e.g., only employees with immunity to varicella should be assigned to work with patients who have chickenpox).

4. Protocols should be created for evaluation and follow-up of employee exposure to infectious diseases.[13,70,71] These include: (a) employee hygiene practices, such as proper handwashing, proper attire, and general cleanliness; (b) employee education to increase understanding and knowledge of their role in infection control and specific patient care practices that may decrease risks for patients;[27] (c) monitoring of compliance with established infection control protocols and provision of feedback to promote an effective infection control program; and (d) appropriate patient/nursing staff ratios.[72,73]

Environmental, Engineering, and Dietary Practices

Housekeeping procedures designed to reduce bioload and remove contaminated blood or body fluids can reduce the risk of transmission of an infectious agent from an environmental reservoir. Selection and use of products appropriate for the task is important[34] (see Chapter 21, Cleaning, Disinfection, and Sterilization). Examples of these practices include safe handling and removal of biohazardous trash and sharps, cleaning procedures for patient rooms, operating room end-of-case cleaning, routine cleaning of ice machines, and removal of food from patient care areas after meals.

Engineering procedures to establish and maintain water, ventilation, and sewage systems that meet regulatory standards can reduce the risk of infections. Preventive maintenance is an important part of ensuring the quality of these systems. Thorough infection control risk assessments for construction and renovation projects will provide measures to prevent and/or reduce infection risk (see Chapter 108).

Dietary procedures to establish sanitary practices for the preparation, distribution, and storage of food reduce the risk of foodborne infectious-agent disease. Basic components should address local public health regulations, including maintenance, temperature documentation, and cleaning of freezers and refrigerators; cleaning and sanitization of eating and cooking utensils; and food preparation standards.

Copyright © 2005, Association for Professionals in Infection Control and Epidemiology, Inc.

Patient care equipment standards should include standards for cleaning, disinfection, and sterilization of reusable items to reduce risk of transmission of microorganisms from patient care items to the patient. Standards must also include procedures for distribution and storage of patient care equipment, as well as recall procedures for products identified as unsafe or inadequately processed or sterilized.

Visitor Guidelines

Each facility should establish and teach the following guidelines to minimize the risk of disease transmission:

1. Areas of the facility where visiting is allowed

2. Precautions that visitors must take if visiting a patient in a high-risk area or isolation (e.g., handwashing, wearing personal protective equipment), or if they are being trained to assist in providing care

3. Exclusion of visitors with communicable disease, and, possibly, additional visitor restriction during times of high levels of community illness, such as influenza epidemics

4. Sibling visitation guidelines, including screening for active or potentially incubating communicable diseases.

Relationship between Patient Care Requirements and Infection Risk

Host factors that influence infection risk are related to specific and nonspecific immune system components and to the number and type of microorganisms introduced into a body system. An increased need for healthcare provider intervention is also associated with an increased risk for infection. Some of the patient factors that increase the risk of infection include immunosuppressive disease and disorders, malignant disorders, poor nutritional status, age, diabetes, extensive burn wounds, or trauma.[74] Additionally, particular medical interventions have been shown to have an influence on the patient's risk of infection: the presence of invasive devices (e.g., indwelling urinary catheters and intravenous equipment), placement in an intensive care unit, exposure to antibiotics, immunosuppressive therapy, length of hospitalization, and an increased number of healthcare worker examinations/procedures (e.g., increased number of vaginal exams during labor).[75-77]

Care requirements, as measured by severity-of-illness classifications, may be useful in nosocomial risk stratification and are influenced by the following patient conditions:[74]

1. Ability to ambulate

2. Mental alertness

3. Ability to perform routine basic activities of daily living

4. Need for assistance to maintain normal body system functions.

Readers are advised to consult general medical and nursing textbooks for specific information on activities designed to support normal body function.

IV. SUMMARY AND CONCLUSIONS

Prevention of infection in patients, staff, and visitors requires attention to both human and environmental factors. Clear and comprehensive protocols, with regular monitoring for compliance, can promote a safe patient care environment and optimal outcomes. Nursing staff ratios per patient have also been shown to influence the risks of infection during patient care. Clearly more data and research are needed to provide staffing ratios and other measures that establish the optimal care setting for reducing infection risk.

V. FUTURE TRENDS/RESEARCH

The forthcoming National Healthcare Safety Network will provide new opportunities to promote patient and healthcare worker safety by providing protocols for monitoring adverse events associated with devices, procedures, and medications; feedback of comparative data for performance improvement; and access to prevention tools, lessons learned, and best practices.

VI. INTERNATIONAL PERSPECTIVES

Although many risk factors may be specific to a country as well as the environment of care, compliance with best practices can promote improved outcomes regardless of the environmental or organizational constraints. Expansion of benchmarking to international audiences and aggressive sharing of best practices and lessons learned will provide wider access to sharing of experiences.

REFERENCES

1. Gaynes RP, Martone WJ, Culver DH, et al: U.S. Department of Health and Human Resources. Centers for Disease Control and Prevention: Nosocomial infection rates for interhospital comparison: limitations and possible solutions, *Infect Control Hosp Epidemiol* 12(10): 609–21, Oct 1991.
2. Emori TG, Culver DH, Horan TC, et al: U.S. Department of Health and Human Resources. Centers for Disease Control and Prevention: National Nosocomial Infections Surveillance System (NNIS): description of surveillance methods, *Am J Infect Control* 19(1): 19–35, Feb 1991.
3. Keita-Perse OJ, Edwards JR, Culver DH, Gaynes RP: Comparing nosocomial infection rates among surgical intensive-care units: the importance of separating cardiothoracic and general surgery intensive-care units, *Infect Control Hosp Epidemiol* 19(4): 260–1, 1998.

Copyright © 2005, Association for Professionals in Infection Control and Epidemiology, Inc.

4. Archibald LK, Gaynes RP: Hospital-acquired infections in the United States. The importance of interhospital comparisons, *Infect Dis Clin North Am* 11(2): 245–55, 1997.

5. Keita-Perse O, Gaynes RP: Severity of illness scoring systems to adjust nosocomial infection rates: a review and commentary, *Am J Infect Control* 24(6): 429–34, 1996.

6. Horan TC, Emori TG: Definitions of key terms used in the NNIS System, *Am J Infect Control* 25(2): 112–6, 1997.

7. Gaynes RP, Edwards JR, Jarvis WR, Culver DH, Tolson JS, Martone WJ: Nosocomial infections among neonates in high-risk nurseries in the United States. National Nosocomial Infections Surveillance System, *Pediatrics* 98(3 Pt 1): 357–61, 1996.

8. Delgado-Rodrigues M, Sillero-Arenas M, Medina-Cuadros M, Martinez-Gallego G: Nosocomial infections in surgical patients: comparison of two measures of intrinsic patient risk, *Infect Control Hosp Epidemiol* 18(1): 19–23, 1997.

9. Emori TG, Edwards JR, Culver DH, et.al: Accuracy of reporting nosocomial infections in intensive-care-unit patients to the National Nosocomial Infections Surveillance System: a pilot study, *Infect Control Hosp Epidemiol* 19(5): 308–16, 1998.

10. Centers for Disease Control and Prevention, HICPAC: Guidelines for prevention of nosocomial pneumonia, *MMWR* 46(RR-1): 1–79, 1997.

11. Centers for Disease Control and Prevention, HICPAC: Draft Guidelines for the Prevention of Surgical Site Infection, 1998, *Fed Register* (63/116): 33168–92, 1998.

12. Pearson, M: Hospital Infection Control Practices Advisory Committee: Guideline for prevention of intravascular device-related infections, *Am J Infect Control* 24: 262–93, 1996.

13. Centers for Disease Control and Prevention; HICPAC: Guidelines for infection control in health care personnel, 1998, *Am J Infect Control* 26: 289–354, 1998.

14. Gaynes R: The impact of antimicrobial use on the emergence of antimicrobial-resistant bacteria in hospitals, *Infect Dis Clin North Am* 11(4): 757–65, 1997.

15. Archibald L, Phillips L, Monnet D, McGowan JE Jr, Tenover F, Gaynes R: Antimicrobial resistance in isolates from inpatients and outpatients in the United States: increasing importance of the intensive care unit, *Clin Infect Dis* 24(2): 211–15, 1997.

16. Lund J: Varicella zoster virus in the health care setting: risk and management, *AAOHN* 41(8): 3699–773, Aug 1993.

17. Raad II, Sherertz RJ, Rains CS, et al: The importance of nosocomial transmission of measles in the propagation of a community outbreak, *Infect Control Hosp Epidemiol* 10(4): 161–66, Apr 1989.

18. Centers for Disease Control and Prevention: Guidelines for preventing the transmission of Mycobacterium tuberculosis in healthcare facilities, 1994, *MMWR Recomm Rep* 43(RR-13): 1–132, Oct 28, 1994.

19. Sherertz RJ, Belani A, Kramer BS, et al: Impact of air filtration on nosocomial *Aspergillus* infections: unique risk of bone marrow recipients, *Am J Med* 83(4): 709–18, Oct 1987.

20. Benz-Lemoine E, Delwail V, Castel O, et al: Nosocomial legionnaires' disease in a bone marrow transplant unit, *Bone Marrow Transplant* 7(1): 61–63, Jan 1991.

21. Carratala J, Gudiol F, Pallares R, et al: Risk factors for nosocomial *Legionella pneumophila* pneumonia, *Am J Respir Crit Care Med* 149(3 Pt 1): 625–29, March 1994.

22. Goetz A, Yu VL: Screening for nosocomial legionellosis by culture of the water supply and targeting of high-risk patients for specialized laboratory testing, *Am J Infect Control* 19(2): 63–66, Apr 1991.

23. Hart CA, Makin T: Legionella in hospitals: a review, *J Hosp Infect* 18 Suppl A: 481–89, Jun 1991.

24. Mastro TD, Fields BS, Breiman RF, et al: Nosocomial legionnaires' disease and use of medication nebulizers, *J Infect Dis* 163(3): 667–71, Mar 1991.

25. Vincent-Houdek M, Muytjens HL, Bongaerts GP, et al: Legionella monitoring: a continuing story of nosocomial infection prevention, *J Hosp Infect* 25(2): 117–24, Oct 1993.

26. Bennett RG: Diarrhea among residents of long-term care facilities, *Infect Control Hosp Epidemiol* 14(7): 397–404, Jul 1993.

27. Daly PB, Smith PW, Rusnak PG, et al: Impact on knowledge and practice of a multiregional long-term care facility infection control program, *Am J Infect Control* 20(5): 225–33, Oct 1992.

28. Harkness GA, Bentley DW, Mottley M, et al: *Streptococcus pyogenes* outbreak in a long-term care facility, *Am J Infect Control* 20(3): 142–48, Jun 1992.

29. Niederman MS: Nosocomial pneumonia in the elderly patient: chronic facility and hospital considerations, *Clin Chest Med* 14(3): 479–90, Sep 1993.

30. Buffington J, Chapman LE, Stobierski MG, et al: Epidemic keratoconjunctivitis in a chronic care facility: risk factors and measures for control, *J Am Geriatr Soc* 41(11): 1177–81, Nov 1993.

31. Isaacs D, Dickson H, O'Callaghan C, et al: Handwashing and cohorting in prevention of hospital acquired infections with respiratory syncytial virus, *Arch Dis Child* 66(2): 227–31, Feb 1991.

32. Garcia R, Raad I, Abi-Said D, et al: Nosocomial respiratory syncytial virus infections: prevention and control in bone marrow transplant patients, *Infect Control Hosp Epidemiol* 18(6): 412–16, 1997.

33. Ehrenkranz NJ, Alfonso BC: Failure of bland soap handwash to prevent hand transfer of patient bacteria to urethral catheters, *Infect Control Hosp Epidemiol* 12(11): 654–62, Nov 1991.

34. Rutala WA: APIC guideline for selection and use of disinfectants, *Am J Infect Control* 18(2): 99–117, Apr 1990.

35. Levine WC, Smart JF, Archer DL, et al: Foodborne disease outbreaks in nursing homes, 1975 through 1987, *JAMA* 266(15): 2105–09, Oct 16, 1991.

36. Gentry EM, Nowak G, Salmon CT, et al: Addressing the public's concerns about human immunodeficiency virus transmission in health-care settings, *Arch Intern Med* 153(20): 2334–40, Oct 25, 1993.

37. Kelen GD: Human immunodeficiency virus and the emergency department risks and risk protection for health care providers, *Ann Emerg Med* 19(3): 242–48, Mar 1990.

38. Fernandez-Crehuet-Navajas M, Jurado-Chacon D, Guillen-Solvas JF, et al: Bacterial contamination of enteral feeds as a possible risk of nosocomial infection, *J Hosp Infect* 21(2): 11–20, Jun 1992.

39. Freeman J, Goldman DA, Smith NE, et al: Association of intravenous lipid emulsion and coagulase-negative staphylococcal bacteremia in neonatal intensive care units, *N Engl J Med* 323(5): 301–08, Aug 2, 1990.

40. Buesching WJ, Neff JC, Sharma HM: Infectious hazards in the clinical laboratory: a program to protect laboratory personnel, *Clin Lab Med* 9(2): 351–61, Jun 1989.

41. Doebbeling BN, Li N, Wenzel RP: An outbreak of hepatitis A among health care workers: risk factors for transmission, *Am J Public Health* 83(12): 1679–84, Dec 1993.

42. Friedland G: Risk of transmission of HIV to home care and health care workers, Part 2, *J Am Acad Dermatol* 22(6): 1171–74, Jun 1990.

43. Centers for Disease Control and Prevention: Case-control study of HIV seroconversion in health-care workers after percutaneous exposure to HIV-infected blood—France, United Kingdom, and United States, January 1988–August 1994, *MMWR* 44: 929–33, 1994.

44. Centers for Disease Control and Prevention: Transmission of HIV possibly associated with exposure of mucous membrane to contaminated blood, *MMWR* 46: 620–23, 1997.

45. Bell DM: Occupational risk of human immunodeficiency virus infection in healthcare workers: an overview, *Am J Med* 102 (suppl 5B): 9–15, 1997.

46. Dutt AK, Stead WW: Tuberculosis, *Clin Geriatr Med* 8(4): 761–75, Nov 1992.

47. Pettinger A, Nettleman MD: Epidemiology of isolation precautions, *Infect Control Hosp Epidemiol* 12(5): 303–307, May 1991.

48. Centers for Disease Control and Prevention; HICPAC: Recommendations for preventing the spread of vancomycin resistance. Recommendations of the Hospital Infection Control Practices Advisory Committee (HICPAC), *MMWR Recomm Rep* 44(RR12): 1–13, 1995.

49. Centers for Disease Control and Prevention: Recommendations for prevention and control of hepatitis C virus (HCV) infection and HCV-related chronic disease, *MMWR Recomm Rep* 47 (RR19): 1–39, Oct 1998.

50. Gerner HM, Staab AS, Ivey FD, et al: Controlling the spread of varicella zoster in the hospitalized patient, *J Am Acad Nurse Pract* 4(4): 156–59, Oct–Dec 1992.

51. Slaughter S, Hayden MK, Nathan C, et al: A comparison of the effect of universal use of gloves and gowns with that of glove use alone on acquisition of vancomycin-resistant enterococci in a medical intensive care unit, *Ann Intern Med* 125(6): 448–56, 1996.

Copyright © 2005, Association for Professionals in Infection Control and Epidemiology, Inc.

52. Centers for Disease Control and Prevention: Public Health Service guidelines for the management of health-care worker exposure to HIV and recommendations for post exposure prophylaxis, *MMWR* 47(RR-7): 1–33, 1998.
53. Hughes JM: Universal precautions: CDC perspective, *Occup Med* 4 (suppl): 13–20, 1989.
54. Lofgren RP, MacPherson DS, Granieri R, et al: Mechanical restraints on the medical wards: are protective devices safe? *Am J Public Health* 79(6): 735–38, June 1989.
55. Galner J: Hospital Infection Practices Advisory Committee: Guidelines for isolation precautions in hospitals, *Infect Control Hosp Epidemiol* 17: 53–80, 1996.
56. Larson E: APIC guideline for handwashing and hand antisepsis in health care settings, *Am J Infect Control* 23: 251–69, 1995.
57. Coffin SE, Bell LM, Manning M, Polin R: Nosocomial infections in neonates receiving extracorporeal membrane oxygenation, *Infect Control Hosp Epidemiol* 18(2): 93–96, 1997.
58. Haley RW: Surveillance by objective: a new priority-directed approach to the control of nosocomial infections, *Am J Infect Control* 13(2): 78–89, Apr 1985.
59. Haley RW, Culver DH, White JW, et al: The nationwide nosocomial infection rate: a need for vital statistics, *Am J Epidemiol* 121(2): 159–205, Feb 1985.
60. Jackson MM, Fierer J, Barrett Connor E, et al: Intensive surveillance for infections in a three-year study of nursing home patients, *Am J Epidemiol* 135(6): 685–96, Mar 15, 1992.
61. Carlisle PS, Gucalp R, Wiernik PH: Nosocomial infections in neutropenic cancer patients, *Infect Control Hosp Epidemiol* 14(6): 320–24, 1993.
62. Smith PW. Nosocomial infections in the elderly, *Infect Dis Clin North Am* 3(4): 763–77, Dec 1989.
63. Karanfil LV, Murphy M, Jospehson A, et al: A cluster of vancomycin-resistant *Enterococcus faecium* in an intensive care unit, *Infect Control Hosp Epidemiol* 13(4): 195–200, Apr 1992.
64. Mylotte JM, Karuza J, Bentley DW: Methicillin-resistant *Staphylococcus aureus*: a questionnaire survey of 75 long-term care facilities in western New York, *Infect Control Hosp Epidemiol* 13(12): 711–18, Dec 1992.
65. Sexton DJ, Harrell LJ, Thorpe JJ, et al: A case-control study of nosocomial ampicillin-resistant enterococcal infection and colonization at a university hospital, *Infect Control Hosp Epidemiol* 14(11): 629–35, Nov 1993.
66. Frost L, Pedersen M, Seiersen E: Changes in hygienic procedures reduce infection following caesarean section, *J Hosp Infect* 13(2): 143–148, Feb 1989.
67. Mangram A, Horan T, Pearson M, Silver LC, Jarvis WR, Hospital Infection Control Practices Advisory Committee: Guideline for prevention of surgical site infection, 1999, *Am J Infect Control* 27(2): 97–132, 1999.
68. Scannapieco FA, Mylotte JM: Relationships between periodontal disease and bacterial pneumonia, *J Periodontol* 67(10 Suppl): 1114–22, 1996.
69. Centers for Disease Control and Prevention; HICPAC: Immunization of health-care workers: recommendations of the Advisory Committee on Immunization Practices (ACIP) and the Hospital Infection Control Practices Advisory Committee (HICPAC), *MMWR Recomm Rep* 46(RR-18): 1–42, 1997.
70. Moore RM Jr, Kaczmarek RG: Occupational hazards to health care workers: diverse, ill-defined, and not fully appreciated, *Am J Infect Control* 18(5): 316–27, Oct 1990.
71. Haiduven D, Hench C, Simpkins S, Steven D: Standardized management of patients and employees exposed to pertussis, *Infect Control Hosp Epidemiol* 19: 861–64, 1998.
72. Fridkin SK, Pear SM, Williamson TH, Galgiani JN, Jarvis WR: The role of understaffing in central venous catheter-associated bloodstream infections, *Infect Control Hosp Epidemiol* 17(3): 150–58, 1996.
73. Archibald LK, Manning ML, Bell LM, Banerjee S, Jarvis WR: Patient density, nurse-to-patient ratio and nosocomial infection risk in a pediatric cardiac intensive care unit, *Pediatr Infect Dis J* 16(11): 1045–48, 1997.
74. Bueno-Cavanillas A, Rodriguez-Contreras R, Lopez-Lugue A, et al: Usefulness of severity indices in intensive care medicine as a predictor of nosocomial infection risk, *Intensive Care Med* 17(6): 336–39, 1991.
75. Broderick A, Mori M, Nettleman MD, et al: Nosocomial infections: validation of surveillance and computer modeling to identify patients at risk, *Am J Epidemiol* 131(4): 734–42, Apr 1990.
76. Craven DE, Steger KA, Hirschhorn LR: Nosocomial colonization and infection in persons infected with human immunodeficiency virus, *Infect Control Hosp Epidemiol* 17(5): 304–18, 1996.
77. Stroud L, Edwards J, Danzing L, Culver D, Gaynes, R: Risk factors for mortality associated with enterococcal blood stream infections, *Infect Control Hosp Epidemiol* 17(9): 576–80, 1996.

SUPPLEMENTAL RESOURCES

Antonelli M, Moro ML, D'Errico RR, Conti G, Bufi M, Gasparetto A: Early and late onset bacteremia have different risk factors in trauma patients, *Intensive Care Med* 22(8): 735–41, 1996.

Arbo MJ, Fine MJ, Hanusa BH, et al: Fever of nosocomial origin: etiology, risk factors, and outcomes, *Am J Med* 95(5): 505–12, Nov 1993.

Archibald LK, Corl A, Shah B, et al: *Serratia marcescens* outbreak associated with extrinsic contamination of 1% chloroxylenol soap, *Infect Control Hosp Epidemiol* 18(10): 704–9, 1997.

Asensio A, Guerrero A, Quereda C, et al: Colonization and infection with methicillin-resistant *Staphylococcus aureus*: associated factors and eradication, *Infect Control Hosp Epidemiol* 17(1): 20–28, 1996.

Avila-Figueroa C, Goldmann DA, Richardson DK, et al: Intravenous lipid emulsions are the major determinant of coagulase-negative staphylococcal bacteremia in very low birth weight newborns, *Pediatr Infect Dis J* 17(1): 10–17, 1998.

Beaujean DJ, Blok HE, Vandenbroucke-Grauls CM, et al: Surveillance of nosocomial infections in geriatric patients, *J Hosp Infect* 36(4): 275–84, 1997.

Bhattacharyya N, Kosloske AM, Macarthur C: Nosocomial infection in pediatric surgical patients: a study of 608 infants and children, *J Pediatr Surg* 28(3): 338–43; discussion 343–44, Mar 1993.

Borger MA, Rao V, Weisel RD, et al: Deep sternal wound infection: risk factors and outcomes, *Ann Thorac Surg* 65(4): 1050–56, 1998.

Boscarino JA, Chang J: Commentary: inaccurate data on quality care may do more harm than good—an alternative approach is required, *Am J Med Qual* 12(4): 196–200, 1997.

Caballero-Granado FJ, Cisneros JM, Luque R, et al: Comparative study of bacteremias caused by Enterococcus spp. with and without high-level resistance to gentamicin, *J Clin Microbiol* 36(2): 520–25, 1997.

Campion FX, Rosenblatt MS: Quality assurance and medical outcomes in the era of cost containment, *Surg Clin North Am* 76(1): 139–59, 1996.

Cook PP, Hecht DW, Syndman DR: Nosocomial *Branhamella catarrhalis* in a paediatric intensive care unit: risk factors for disease, *J Hosp Infect* 13(3): 299–307, Apr 1989.

Craven DE, Barber TW, Steger KA, et al: Nosocomial pneumonia in the 1990s: update of epidemiology and risk factors, *Semin Resp Infect* 5(3): 157–72, Sep 1990.

Craven DE, Steger KA, Barber TW: Preventing nosocomial pneumonia: state of the art and perspectives for the 1990s, *Am J Med* 91(3B): 44S–53S, Sep 16, 1991.

D'Aquila NM; Habegger D, Wilwerth EJ: Converting a QA program to CQI, *Nurs Manage* Oct 25 (010): 68–71, 1994.

Dean DA, Burchard KW: Fungal infection in surgical patients, *Am J Surg* 171(3): 374–82, 1996.

Dean DA, Burchard KW: Surgical perspective on invasive Candida infections, *World J Surg* 22(2): 127–34, 1998.

Delgado-Rodriguez M, Medina-Cuadros M, Martinez-Gallego G, Sillero-Arenas M: Total cholesterol, HDL-cholestrol, and risk of nosocomial infection: a prospective study in surgical patients, *Infect Control Hosp Epidemiol* 18(1): 9–18, 1997.

Copyright © 2005, Association for Professionals in Infection Control and Epidemiology, Inc.

Durand-Zaleski I, Delaunay L, Langeron O, et al: Infection risk and cost-effectiveness of commercial bags or glass bottles for total parenteral nutrition, *Infect Control Hosp Epidemiol* 18(3): 183–88, 1997.

Elting LS, Khardori N, Bodey GP, et al: Nosocomial infection caused by *Xanthomonas maltophilia*: a case-control study of predisposing factors, *Infect Control Hosp Epidemiol* 11(3): 134–38, Mar 1990.

Ferguson JK, Gill A: Risk-stratified nosocomial infection surveillance in a neonatal intensive care unit: report on 24 months of surveillance, *J Paediatr Child Health* 32(6): 525–31, 1996.

Flanagan A: Ensuring health care quality: JCAHO's perspective. Joint Commission on Accreditation of Healthcare Organizations, *Clin Ther* 19(6): 1540–4, 1997.

Fridkin SK, Jarvis WR: Epidemiology of nosocomial fungal infections, *Clin Microbiol Rev* 9(4): 499–511, 1996.

Fridkin SK, Welbel SF, Weinstein RA: Magnitude and prevention of nosocomial infections in the intensive care unit, *Infect Dis Clin North Am* 11(2): 479–96, 1997.

Garrouste-Orgeas M, Marie O, Rouveau M, et al: Secondary carriage with multi-resistant *Acinetobacter baumannii* and *Klebsiella pneumoniae* in an adult ICU population: relationship with nosocomial infections and mortality, *J Hosp Infect* 34(4): 279–89, 1996.

Girou E, Stephan F, Novara A, Safar M, Fagon JY: Risk factors and outcome of nosocomial infections: results of a matched case-control study of ICU patients, *Am J Respir Crit Care Med* 157(4 Pt 1): 1151–58, 1998.

Goldstein EJ: Anaerobic bacteremia, *Clin Infect Dis* 23 Suppl 1: S97–101, 1996.

Gross PA: Striving for benchmark infection rates: progress in control for patient mix, *Am J Med* 91(3B): 16S–20S, 1991.

Haley RW, Culver DH, White JW, et al: The efficacy of infection surveillance and control programs in preventing nosocomial infections in U.S. hospitals, *Am J Epidemiol* 121(2): 182–205, 1985.

Holmberg RE Jr, Pavia AT, Montgomery D, et al: Nosocomial *Legionella* pneumonia in the neonate, *Pediatrics* 92(3): 450–53, Sep 1993.

Horwitz JR, Chwals WJ, Doski JJ, Suescun EA, Cheu HW, Lally KP: Pediatric wound infections: a prospective multicenter study, *Ann Surg* 227(4): 553–58, 1998.

Kobs A: Infection control, *Nurs Manage* 28(8): 17–19, 1997.

Korinek AM: Risk factors for neurosurgical site infections after craniotomy: a prospective multicenter study of 2944 patients. The French Study Group of Neurosurgical Infections, the SEHP, and the C-CLIN Paris-Nord, *Neurosurgery* 41(5): 1073–79; discussion 1079–81, 1997.

Lai KK, Melvin ZS, Menard MJ, Kotilainen HR, Baker S: Clostridium difficile-associated diarrhea: epidemiology, risk factors, and infection control, *Infect Control Hosp Epidemiol* 18(9): 628–32, 1997.

Linden PK, Pasculle AW, Manez R, et al: Differences in outcomes for patients with bacteremia due to vancomycin-resistant *Enterococcus faecium* or vancomycin-susceptible E. faecium, *Clin Infect Dis* 22(4): 663–70, 1996.

Lucet JC, Chevret S, Decre D, et al: Outbreak of multiply resistant enterobacteriaceae in an intensive care unit: epidemiology and risk factors for acquisition, *Clin Infect Dis* 22(3): 430–36, 1996.

McGowan JE Jr: Success, failures and costs of implementing standards in the USA—lessons for infection control, *J Hosp Infect* 30 Suppl: 76–87, Jun 1995.

Medina-Cuadros M, Sillero-Arenas M, Martinez-Gallego G, Delgado-Rodriguez M: Surgical wound infections diagnosed after discharge from hospital: epidemiologic differences with in-hospital infections, *Am J Infect Control* 24(6): 421–28, 1996.

Moreland J: Quality assurance to quality improvement: the impact of the agenda for changes. *AACN Clin Issues Crit Care Nurs* 2(1): 82–89, 1991.

Mulin B, Rouget C, Clement C, et al: Association of private isolation rooms with ventilator-associated *Acinetobacter baumanii* pneumonia in a surgical intensive-care unit, *Infect Control Hosp Epidemiol* 18(7): 499–503, 1997.

Papanicolaou GA, Meyers BR, Meyers J, et al: Nosocomial infections with vancomycin-resistant *Enterococcus faecium* in liver transplant recipients: risk factors for acquisition and mortality, *Clin Infect Dis* 23(4): 760–66, 1996.

Patel R, Badley AD, Larson-Keller J, et al: Relevance and risk factors of enterococcal bacteremia following liver transplantation, *Transplantation* 61(8); 1192–97, 1996.

Penzak SR, Abate BJ: Stenotrophomonas (Xanthomonas) maltophilia: a multidrug-resistant nosocomial pathogen, *Pharmacotherapy* 17(2): 293–301, 1997.

Petri MG, Konig J, Moecke HP, et al: Epidemiology of invasive mycosis in ICU patients: a prospective multicenter study in 435 non-neutropenic patients. Paul-Ehrlich Society for Chemotherapy, Divisions of Mycology and Pneumonia Research, *Intensive Care Med* 23(3): 317–25, 1997.

Rebollo MH, Bernal JM, Llorca J, et al: Nosocomial infections in patients having cardiovascular operations: a multivariate analysis of risk factors, *J Thorac Cardiovasc Surg* 112(4): 908–13, 1996.

Rello J, Rue M, Jubert P, et al: Survival in patients with nosocomial pneumonia: impact of the severity of illness and the etiologic agent, *Crit Care Med* 15(11): 1862–67, 1997.

Singh-Naz N, Sprague BM, Patel KM, Pollack MM: Risk factors for nosocomial infection in critically ill children: a prospective cohort study, *Crit Care Med* 24(5): 875–78, 1996.

Spankin S, Trupl J, Havska I, et al: Bacteremia and fungemia occurring during antimicrobial prophylaxis with Ofloxacin in cancer patients: risk factors, etiology and outcome, *J Chemother* 8(5): 387–93, 1996.

Steinberg JP, Clark CC, Hackman BO: Nosocomial and community-acquired *Staphylococcus aureus* bacteremias from 1980 to 1993; impact of intravascular devices and methicillin resistance, *Clin Infect Dis* 23(2): 255–59, 1996.

Stroud L, Srivastava P, Culver D, et al: Nosocomial infections in HIV-infected patients: preliminary results from a multicenter surveillance system (1989–1995), *Infect Control Hosp Epidemiol* 18(7): 479–85, 1997.

Talon D, Mulin B, Rouget C, Bailly P, Thouverez M, Viel JF: Risks and routes for ventilator-associated pneumonia with *Pseudomonas aeruginosa*, *Am J Respir Crit Care Med* 157(3 Pt 1): 978–84, 1998.

Tran LT, Auger P, Marchand R, et al: Epidemiological study of Candida spp. colonization in cardiovascular surgical patients, *Mycoses* 40(5–6): 169–73, 1997.

Velasco E, Thuler LC, Martins CA, Dias LM, Goncalves VM: Nosocomial infections in an oncology intensive care unit, *Am J Infect Control* 25(6): 458–62, 1997.

Vidal F, Mensa J, Almela M, Martinez JA, et al: Epidemiology and outcome of *Pseudomonas aeruginosa* bacteremia, with special emphasis on the influence of antibiotic treatment. Analysis of 189 episodes, *Arch Intern Med* 156(18): 2121–26, 1996.

Voss A, Le-Noble JL, Verduyn-Lunel FM, Foudraine NA, Meis JF: Candidemia in intensive care unit patients: risk factors for mortality, *Infection* 25(1):8–11, 1997.

Weber, JM; Sheridan, RL; Pasternack, MS; Tompkins, RG: Nosocomial infections in pediatric patients with burns, *Am J Infect Control* 25(3): 195–201, 1997.

Weinstein JW, Ros M, Towns M, et al. Resistant enterococci: a prospective study of prevalence, incidence and factors associated with colonization in a university hospital. *Infect Control Hosp Epidemiol* 17(1): 36–41, 1996.

Copyright © 2005, Association for Professionals in Infection Control and Epidemiology, Inc.

14

Principles of Microbial Pathogenicity and Host Response

Charles P. Craig, MD, FACP, FIDSA, FCCP
Medical Director Infection Control Services,
St. Joseph Mercy Health System, Ann Arbor,
Michigan
Clinical Professor of Medicine, Wayne State
University
Ann Arbor, Michigan

ABSTRACT

Infection results when an imbalance occurs between the mechanisms that microorganisms employ to induce infection and the complex physiological response systems that are employed by a host to prevent such infections. These can be altered to restore vigorous natural immunity and terminate or prevent infection. Understanding these mechanisms is essential to the design and implementation of effective infection control programs in healthcare settings.

KEY CONCEPTS

- Virulence, commonly recognized as the measure of a microbe's ability to invade and create disease in a host, is determined by characteristics that relate to the favored site of invasion, disease induction, and avoidance of host resistance.

- The initial element in virulence is the ability of an organism to survive in the external environment during transit between hosts.

- The second element in virulence is a mechanism for transmission to a new host.

- When a microorganism reaches a favorable site for inducing disease, it must adhere to the structure that it will infect.

- Once a pathogen has attached successfully to a site for infection, it must have mechanisms for proliferation.

- Following local proliferation by a pathogen, elements of virulence favor invasion and dissemination.

- One limb of the immune response is called the *cell mediated immune* (CMI) *system*, which is induced, mediated, or regulated by T lymphocytes and mononuclear phagocytes. If the CMI system is altered, defense against virus, mycobacterial, and fungal infections, among others, can be seriously compromised; antibody production may even be indirectly adversely affected.

- A cellular immune response is initiated when a foreign substance, such as a bacterium, virus, or other foreign antigen, is taken up by large phagocytic cells of various types (macrophages in tissues, Langerhans cells in skin, and follicular dendritic cells in lymph node germinal centers).

Copyright © 2005, Association for Professionals in Infection Control and Epidemiology, Inc.

- T lymphocytes comprise a number of families that are highly specific in function.

- Cytokines (including lymphokines from lymphocytes) are substances liberated by various cell lines that have specific structures and biological activities.

- In contrast with CMI, humoral immunity is expressed by proteins called *antibodies*. These are principally within the bloodstream, but secretory antibody is also present in oral secretions, tears, intestinal contents, breast milk, prostate, and the female reproductive tract.

I. BODY[1-6]

Virulence, commonly recognized as the measure of a microbe's ability to invade and create disease in a host, is determined by characteristics that relate to the favored site of invasion, disease induction, and avoidance of host resistance.

The initial element in virulence is the ability of an organism to survive in the external environment during transit between hosts. Successful pathogens possess ecological niches in the environment, such as blood in the case of bloodborne pathogens (e.g., hepatitis B and C, human immunodeficiency virus (HIV), cytomegalovirus). *Mycobacterium tuberculosis* possesses a lipid coating in its cell wall and collects dried proteins from sputum to protect it against death by drying in air. *Pseudomonas* has the capacity to extract minute quantities of nutrients from water, including dead microorganisms, and survive in aqueous environments for months. Many organisms are carried successfully from host to host within vectors, such as West Nile virus, yellow fever virus, and plasmodia (malaria) in mosquitoes, and *Borellia burgdorferi* and *Rickettsia rickettsiae* (Rocky Mountain spotted fever) in ticks.

The second element in virulence, as it is understood, is a mechanism for transmission to a new host. Effective insect vectors transmit pathogens by injecting material from salivary glands or defecation into sites of penetration of host skin. A few viruses, such as respiratory syncytial virus, can survive and be transmitted to hands and hence to mucous membranes from environmental surfaces, such as bed rails. Some bacteria possess mechanisms of motility, such as *Escherichia coli,* which enables it to ascend a flowing stream of urine from urinary bladder to the kidney and cause pyelonephritis. When a microorganism reaches a favorable site for inducing disease, it must adhere to the structure that it will infect. Electrostatic negative charges on most bacteria favor adherence to human cells, and specific adhesions on bacterial surfaces favor attachment to sites of infection. Such attachment may be complex, such as the interaction between CD4 receptors on HIV and CD4-bearing lymphocytes, then subsequent attach-

ment of glycoprotein (GP) 120 to a specific site on the lymphocyte, followed by attachment of GP41 on HIV to its respective receptor on the lymphocyte. Each step is followed by conformational changes in the virus coat or capsid to facilitate the next step. Binding to foreign bodies, such as intravenous catheters by bacteria, often involves a bacteria-secreted glycocalyx (slime).

Once a pathogen has attached successfully to a site for infection, it must have mechanisms for proliferation. HIV, after going through the steps cited previously, elaborates a conformation-inducing peptide that actuates GP41 like a spring, bringing the virus and lymphocyte membranes into close approximation and permitting the entry of virus RNA into the lymphocyte for subsequent transcription into DNA and integration of the produced DNA into the lymphocyte chromosomes, where it can begin to produce new viral components. Bacteria often secrete enzymes that enhance spread through tissues. The classic example of enzyme secretion and rapid spread through tissues is *Streptococcus pyogenes*. This mechanism is responsible for the fact that the most promptly occurring operative site infections, beginning in less than twenty-four hours from incision, are from *S. pyogenes*. Bacteria may secrete exotoxins that kill or immobilize cellular host defenses, such as those of *Clostridium perfringens*, the causative agent of gas gangrene. *Streptococcus pneumoniae* and *Hemophilus influenzae* possess capsules that inhibit ingestion by neutrophils or protect them after ingestion into phagocytes. The glycocalyx that facilitates attachment of certain bacteria to implanted plastic devices is also hydrophobic and interferes with penetration of water soluble antibiotic to embedded bacteria. Secreted enzymes from some bacteria dissolve tissue proteins to provide nutrients for pathogenic bacteria. Many, if not most, bacteria concentrate iron from the environment, which is an essential factor for enhancing virulence factors for growth and toxin production. Following local proliferation by a pathogen, elements of virulence favor invasion and dissemination. These can be the same factors that enhance local proliferation, such as capsules, toxins, digestive enzymes, and hydrophobicity. Others include (1) a rigid cell wall, which is a physical barrier to host defenses; (2) cell surface components, other than capsules, that inhibit phagocytosis; (3) the ability to alter its cell surface and thus avoid host-created specific antibodies, such that occurs in influenza A virus; and (4) deterrents to intracellular killing after phagocytosis. Some that have been identified are those that prevent superoxide production by pathogens that can kill bacteria and mechanisms that avoid fusion of lysosomes within phagocytes that contain bactericidal elements and ingested organisms (e.g., *M. tuberculosis*).

Copyright © 2005, Association for Professionals in Infection Control and Epidemiology, Inc.

Bacterial Toxins

Bacterial toxins are extensively studied virulence factors. Exotoxins, those secreted by bacteria, particularly gram-positive bacteria, are often heat inactivated, neutralized by specific antibody, and may possess enzymatic activity. Such toxins have sometimes been altered to create effective vaccines, such as diphtheria toxin. Endotoxins are complexes of bacterial proteins, lipids, and polysaccharides that remain firmly within bacteria. They are surface components of gram-negative bacteria, resist inactivation by heat, are only partially neutralized by antibody, and possess the capability of interacting with host systems to set off cascades of responses that can induce fever, swelling, vascular leaking, pain and shock, such as the complement cascade, kinins, and cytokine release.

Types of Bacterial Toxins

Examples of significant bacterial toxins include (1) diphtheria toxin of *Corynebacterium diphtheriae* (toxic to myocardial cells); (2) tetanospasmin of *Clostridium tetani,* which interferes with nerve conduction at the neuromuscular junction; (3) botulinum toxin from *Clostridium botulinum,* which also interferes with neuromuscular transmission; (4) cholera toxin from *Vibrio cholerae,* which increases secretion of fluids into the gastrointestinal (GI) tract, causing profuse diarrhea and fluid and electrolyte loss; (5) enterotoxins of *Staphylococcus aureus,* which stimulate GI peristalsis, activate complement and induce shock, as in toxic shock syndrome; (6) *Clostridium difficile* toxin, which creates ulcers in the mucosa of the colon; and (7) gram-negative bacterial endotoxin, which, through its key lipid A moiety, can produce fever, activate blood clotting and fibrinolysis, and inhibit vasoconstriction, causing shock. A variant *E. coli* strain, J5, produces an atypical lipid A that induces antibody when used as a vaccine that is protective against many activities of endotoxin.

The Cellular Immune System[7-11]

One limb of the immune response is called the *cell mediated immune* (CMI) *system,* which is induced, mediated, or regulated by T lymphocytes and mononuclear phagocytes. CMI interacts with antibody mediated humoral immune system via effects of CD4 T lymphocytes, B lymphocytes, and granulocytes. All-important T lymphocytes are derived from precursors that originate in bone marrow during fetal life, migrate to the thymus where they mature, then populate lymph nodes, spleen, and bone marrow as the thymus undergoes involution early in life. CMI is highly specific, as is humoral immunity, and is thought to owe its specificity to surface components of T lymphocytes called *major histocompatibility complexes* (MHCs) (see later).

A cellular immune response is initiated when a foreign substance, such as a bacterium, virus, or other foreign antigen, is taken up by large phagocytic cells of various types (macrophages in tissues, Langerhans cells in skin, and follicular dendritic cells in lymph node germinal centers). Sometimes B lymphocytes can directly ingest foreign antigens without prior processing. The initial binding of foreign substances to these receptor cells occurs to immunoglobulin G (IgG) receptors fixed on the surface of these cells. After the adherent foreign materials are ingested by the receptor cells, they are processed intracellularly to small molecules and then bound to MHCs, genetically coded surface proteins with terminal antigen-binding sites. Larger microorganisms are processed intracellularly with compartments called *phagosomes,* and their small molecule products are bound to class II MHCs then presented to CD4 lymphocytes. Small microorganisms, principally viruses, are processed free in cytoplasm of the phagocytic cells, bound to class I MHCs, and presented to CD8 cytotoxic lymphocytes. Transfer of class II MHC bound materials to CD4 lymphocytes is associated with release of various lymphokines, including interleukin-1 (IL-1), interleukin-6 (IL-6), and, as recently reported, perhaps interleukin-12 (IL-12) and interleukin-16 (IL-16) (see later). If the CMI system is altered, defense against virus, mycobacterial, and fungal infections, among others, can be seriously compromised; antibody production may even be indirectly adversely affected.

T lymphocytes comprise a number of families that are highly specific in function. All T lymphocytes are thought to bear the CD3 surface marker. The CD4 marker is on a subset of CD3 cells and identifies a population of helper lymphocytes. Their functions include promotion of phagocytosis of invading pathogens, enhancement of activity of other T and B lymphocytes through released lymphokines (cytokines), and preservation of immunological memory, such as that used in vaccine boosters to induce protective immunity. CD8 cells are another subset of CD3 cells and may be cytotoxic or suppressive in function. Cytotoxic lymphocytes kill cells in which viruses are replicating, and they sometimes kill tumor cells. Suppressor CD8 cells control the intensity of T and B lymphocyte activity by suppressing their reproduction and metabolism, thus avoiding an excessively robust response that might be harmful to the host. *Natural killer* (NK) cells are neither CD4 nor CD8 cells, and they have the ability to lyse and kill tumor cells and virus-infected cells. They bear on their surfaces CD16 and CD56 markers. Certain CD4 lymphocytes are noncommitted ("naive" or "virgin") cells that are not yet specifically antigen committed and thus can respond to novel pathogens and amplify the host's immune response to them.

Copyright © 2005, Association for Professionals in Infection Control and Epidemiology, Inc.

Cytokines (including lymphokines from lymphocytes) are substances liberated by various cell lines that have specific structures and biological activities. Among them are IL-1, IL-2, IL-4, IL-6, IL-12, IL-16, the interferons, lymphotoxin, granulocyte macrophage colony-stimulating factor (GMCSF), and monocyte colony-stimulating factor. These families of cytokines may possess various physiological properties:

- priming and stimulating antibody production

- stimulating reproduction of cell lines (mast cells, eosinophils, macrophages)

- promoting differentiation of B-lymphocytes or T-lymphocytes, cytotoxic T lymphocytes, macrophages, and neutrophils

- fever induction

- interference with intracellular virus reproduction

- involution and death of tumor cells

- protein catabolism

- inflammation promotion

- reproduction of granulocytes

- reproduction of monocytes

For detailed descriptions of these functions of interleukins, the reader is referred to several extensive review articles on the subject (see references).

Components and Function of the Humoral Immune System[12]

In contrast with CMI, humoral immunity is expressed by proteins called *antibodies*. These are principally within the bloodstream, but secretory antibody is also present in oral secretions, tears, intestinal contents, breast milk, prostate and, to a small degree, urine. Antibody is also secreted from mucosal surfaces of the female reproductive tract. Antibody is produced by B lymphocytes, which originate in the fetal liver and bone marrow, then populate the spleen and lymph nodes. In other animal species B lymphocytes originate from the bursa of Fabricius, a structure analogous to the human appendix. B lymphocytes, stimulated by native or macrophage-processed soluble antigen, divide and mature into antibody-producing cells called *plasma cells* or *plasmacytes*. B lymphocytes have IgM immunoglobulin receptors on their surfaces, which function in early immune recognition and response, and IgD immunoglobulin, which functions in later immune responses. Both classes of surface antibodies are specific to individual foreign antigens.

All antibody molecules possess structural sites referred to as *Fab* (fragment, antigen-binding), which react with specific antigens, and another structural site called Fc

(fragment, crystallizable), which distinguishes among the antibody classes (Fig. 14–1) .

Immunoglobulin G (IgG) is the major circulating and extravascular (interstitial) antibody, a protein molecule of approximately 160,000 molecular weight, which possesses two Fab reactive sites linked to one Fc component. IgG is the late-occurring immunoglobulin in an immune response and is the longest lived. Because it enters interstitial tissue relatively easily, it is the major antibody to protect "tissue." There are four subclasses of IgG (IgG1 to IgG 4). Immunoglobulin M (IgM) consists of five limbs, each containing two Fab sites, linked to an Fc molecule. Thus, an intact IgM molecule has ten reactive Fab sites. IgM is the first reacting immunoglobulin in an immune response to an infection and is generally produced for no more than six months after the onset of the infection. Exceptions include antibody to polysaccharides, which are IgM and long-lived, and antibody to blood group substances in the ABO blood group system. Because of its very large molecular weight, IgM is largely contained within the vascular tree.

Immunoglobulin A (IgA) is the principal secretory antibody in humans, is principally produced in plasma cells residing in mucous membranes, and is commonly secreted as a dimmer of two IgA molecules, each with two Fab fragments and one Fc, and linked together to T-piece (secretory protein). Smaller quantities of IgA, as monomers and without T-piece, circulate in the bloodstream. When IgA reacts with antigen, it may cause the release of histamine from mast cells and basophilic neutrophils leading to an allergic clinical response.

Immunoglobulin D (IgD) is an immunoglobulin of characteristic structure with two Fab sites and one Fc piece, which is present principally on the surface of lymphocytes, where it serves to bind specific antigens. Trace amounts circulate free in plasma.

Immunoglobulin E (IgE) is the principal allergy-inducing immunoglobulin, known as *regain*. It consists of two Fab fragments linked to an Fc piece, and, when it reacts with antigen, stimulates release of histamine and other inflammatory substances from basophils and mast cells. IgE-producing plasma cells are found in large numbers on the mucous membranes of individuals with significant seasonal allergies. Its activity in the GI tract may aid in protection against intestinal parasites.

The functions of immunoglobulins relate to events subsequent to their binding to their respective specific antigens. When two molecules of IgG bind to an antigen, such as a bacterium, they activate the complement system and thus facilitate phagocytosis, intracellular killing of pathogens, and lysis of cells and bacteria. A single molecule of IgM, presumably because of its

Copyright © 2005, Association for Professionals in Infection Control and Epidemiology, Inc.

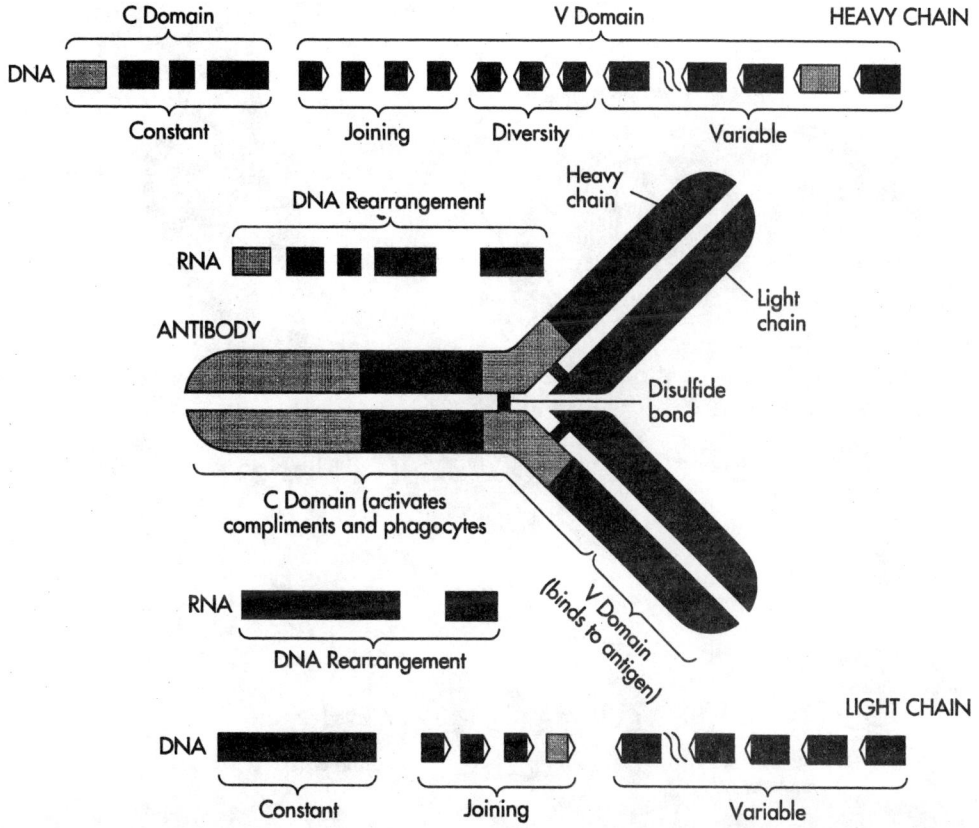

Figure 14–1 Antibody molecule is made up of a pair of heavy chains and a pair of light chains. The chains are encoded by genes that consist of different DNA segments. These segments rearrange to make genes for chains that are different in each B cell. The joining is variable, so only a few gene segments generate the estimated 100 million antibodies the body is capable of producing. (From Nossal JV. Life, death and the immune system. Sci Am 1993;269:55.)

numerous reactive Fab sites, can activate complement when it reacts with its antigen. IgA binds to organisms attempting to invade mucous membranes, interfering with motility of the organisms, adhesion to the membrane, and phagocytosis. IgA is highly effective in preventing virus infections of the respiratory and intestinal mucosa, such as rhinovirus, influenza virus, coronavirus, and enteroviruses, such as poliovirus and Coxsackie virus. Functions of IgD and IgE are described earlier. Figure 14–2 presents a summary of defense against infection provided by the immune system.

Nonspecific Host Defenses[13-15]

The human host possesses a range of naturally occurring obstacles to invasion by a broad range of potentially pathogenic organisms. Caucasians and Africans possess vigorous natural resistance to deep mycoses, including *Histoplasma capsulatum* and *Coccidioides immitis* and to rubeola virus, whereas Asians lack resistance to the former two, and Alaskan and Hawaiian natives to the latter. Successive epidemics of fatal rubeola swept both Alaska and Hawaii after introduction by European colonists. Skin and mucous membranes are important mechanical barriers to infection. The normal flora deplete the environment of nutrients essential for pathogens, compete for tissue-binding sites, and secrete naturally occurring antibiotics that kill potential pathogens. Skin secretes short chain fatty acids lethal for many pathogens.

Host physiology may help prevent infection. Fever, naturally regulated in the hypothalamus, may be beneficial to the host. Fever is induced through the hypothalamus by endogenous pyrogenic substances, including IL-1, IL-2, IL-6, IL-8, TNF, IFN, and colony-stimulating factors also effect the hypothalamus. Likewise, endogenous antipyretics prevent dangerously high fevers. These include arginine vasopressin, melanocyte-stimulating hormone, and TNF. Whether fever is beneficial or harmful to the host continues to be debated, despite years of research attesting to probable benefit.[15,17] Phylogenetic studies indicate that fever is an evolutionally determined protective mechanism. Animals lacking

Copyright © 2005, Association for Professionals in Infection Control and Epidemiology, Inc.

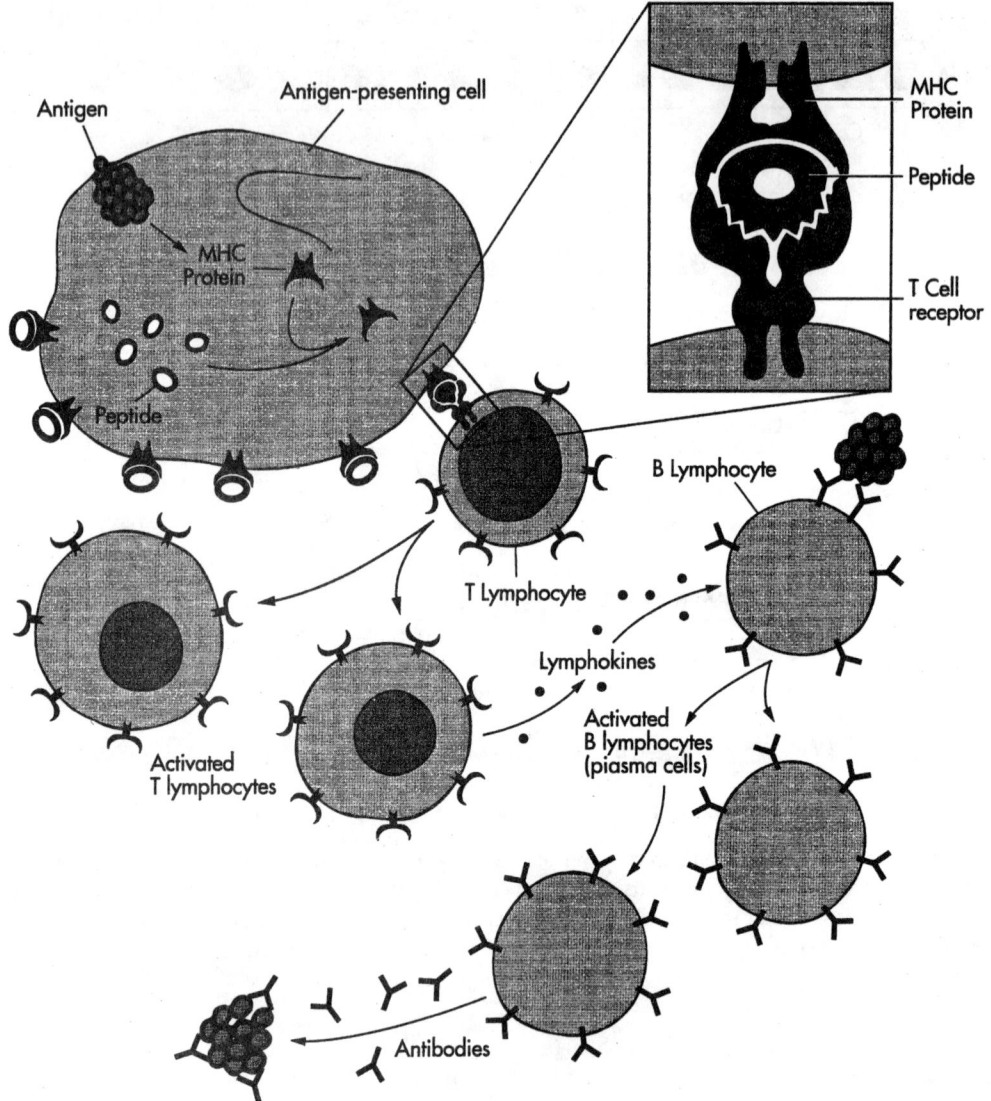

Figure 14–2 How the immune system defends the body. The body is protected by a diverse army of cells and molecules that work in concert. The ultimate target of all immune responses is an antigen, which is usually a foreign molecule from a bacterium or other invader. Specialized antigen-presenting cells, such as macrophages, roam the body, ingesting the antigens they find and fragmenting them into antigenic peptides. Pieces of these peptides are joined to major histocompatibility complex (MHC) molecules and are displayed on the surface of the cell. Other white blood cells, called T lymphocytes, have receptor molecules that enable each of them to recognize a different peptide-MHC combination. T cells activated by that recognition divide and secrete lymphokines, or chemical signals, that mobilize other components of the immune system. One set of cells that responds to those signals comprises the T lymphocytes, which also have receptor molecules of a single specificity on their surface. Unlike the receptors of T cells, however, those of B cells can recognize parts of antigens free in solution, without MHC molecules. When activated, the B cells divide and differentiate into plasma cells that secrete antibody proteins, which are soluble forms of their receptors. By binding to antigens they find, the antibodies can neutralize them or precipitate their destruction by complement enzymes or by scavenging cells. Some T and B cells become memory cells that persist in the circulation and boost the immune system's readiness to eliminate the same antigen if it presents itself in the future. Because the genes for antibodies in B cells mutate frequently, the antibody response improves after repeated immunizations. (From Janeway CA. How the immune system recognizes invaders. Sci Am 1993;269:75.)

Copyright © 2005, Association for Professionals in Infection Control and Epidemiology, Inc.

the ability to generate fevers naturally seek warmer environs in the face of infections, and, when they are prevented from doing so, they have higher mortality than permitted cohorts. In vitro studies indicate that many host defenses are more efficient against pathogens at higher physiological temperatures. Some organisms, such as *Cryptococcus*, will not grow above 38°C. Conversely, certain responses to fever may be deleterious. Febrile convulsions, frequently triggered by reactivation of latent herpes virus 6 in the central nervous system (CNS) by fever, are one example of possible adverse effect of fever.[16] Persons with underlying heart disease and reduced stroke volume may develop worsening CHF in the face of tachycardia induced by fever. It is probably safe to generalize that a low grade fever, between 38°C and 38.5°C, enhances natural defenses. Higher body temperature in persons with cardiovascular disease or history of febrile convulsion should be considered for treatment.

Secretions, especially from mucous membranes, help protect against infection, both from antibacterial contents and flow. Lysozyme is a low-activity enzyme secreted by mucous membranes and kills a narrow range of gram-positive bacteria. Gastric acid is a major barrier to infection of the intestinal tract with swallowed pathogens. Antacids or acid secretion blockade markedly increases the susceptibility of experimental animals to intestinal pathogens. Some secreted enzymes from salivary glands, pancreas, and intestinal mucosal cells partially digest invading pathogens. Bile salts are inhibitory to a range of pathogenic bacteria. The addition of ciliary sweeping, which is both unidirectional and coordinated, to secretions helps wash the nose, mouth, respiratory tract, and pharynx of bacteria, which are then swallowed and inactivated by gastric acid. Motility in the alimentary and urinary tracts expels many invading pathogens and toxic substances.

The vascular tree contains circulating defenses that are naturally occurring. Natural antibody, formed in response to normal flora, cross reacts with pathogens and helps expel them. Fibronectin is a circulating protein that binds to pathogen receptors and prevents their adherence to cells. Hormones, such as estrogens, control secretions and characteristics of mucous membrane cells and thus the nature of bacteria inhabiting their surfaces. Circulating phagocytic neutrophils and monocytes, without aid of humoral elements, can ingest and kill many pathogens.

Components and Activities of the Complement System[18,19]

The complement system consists of eleven sequentially reacting serum proteins that, in their activated forms, possess biological activities essential to host defenses against many invading microorganisms and tumor cells.

Activation of the complement system may occur in either the classical or alternate pathway. When antigens, including pathogenic organisms, interact with IgG or IgM antibody, they activate complement in the classical pathway. Certain microorganisms spontaneously activate the alternate pathway. The net effect of activation through either pathway is enhancement of phagocytosis, increase in vascular permeability, blood vessel dilatation, chemoattraction of neutrophils into an area of inflammation, smooth muscle contraction, and lysis of certain pathogens, especially the *Neisseriacea* family, by the terminal components.

The components of the human complement system include C1q, r, and s; C4; C2; C3; C5; C6; C7; C8; and C9. This is also the sequence of activation in the classical pathway. The alternate pathway begins with direct activation of C3, without the necessity of activation of the C1 complex, C4, or Cs (Fig. 14–3). In the process of alternate pathway activation a fragment of

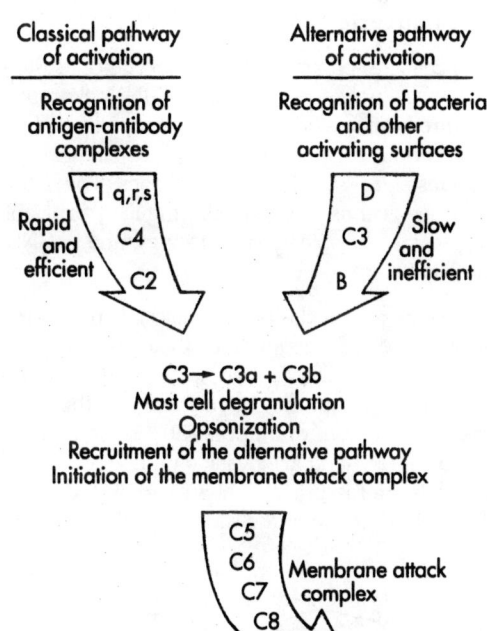

Figure 14-3 The complement system. The complement system consists of three families of proteins. Two of these, the classical pathway of activation and the alternative pathway of activation, cause the cleavage of C3 into two fragments, C3b and C3a. These fragments have important biologic activities. In addition, C3b, together with elements of the classical pathway (Bb, properdin), forms enzymes (C5 convertases) that cleave C5, the initial member of the terminal family of proteins. Cleavage of C5 leads to the formation of the membrane attack complex that can result in osmotic lysis of cells. (From Paul WE. Fundamental Immunology. New York: Raven; 1993.)

Copyright © 2005, Association for Professionals in Infection Control and Epidemiology, Inc.

C3, termed *C3b,* is created, which generates a positive feedback loop to amplify complement activation.

To enhance destruction of foreign cells, these cells protect host cells; host cells possess complement regulatory proteins that block complement activation on their surfaces, which could be destructive. Alternatively, foreign cells possess on their surfaces components not present on host cells, which facilitate complement activation. These components are essential for complement to distinguish between host and foreign cells.

Some rare individuals are genetically deficient in certain complement components. These may result in congenital illnesses, such as angioneurotic edema associated with deficiency of C1, recurrent bacterial infections in those deficient in C2 or C3, and recurrent bacteremia with pathogenic Neisseriae in individuals deficient in C7, C8, or C9. These naturally occurring deficiencies have helped define the roles of complement in natural resistance and host homeostasis.

The Phagocytic Cell System[20,21]

Several cell lines comprise the phagocytic cell system. Granulocytes (polymorphonuclear [PMN] leukocytes) are of three classes: neutrophils, eosinophils, and basophils. Mononuclear phagocytes occur as circulating monocytes and tissue fixed macrophages. The latter occur in the liver as Kuppfer cells, the lung as alveolar macrophages, the spleen as histiocytes, and in CNS as dendroglia.

Granulocytes have inclusions (granules) within their cytoplasm that are recognized by their stain properties and give the three classes their names. These granules contain elements that may be released into the environment of an infection, or intracellularly into a phagosome, to degrade and kill invading pathogens. Neutrophils are the principal antibacterial PMNs and the first cells to arrive at the site of an inflammatory

focus. Basophils, which have no defined role in resistance to infection, are related to mast cells, contain large quantities of histamine, and participate in allergic responses. Eosinophils are important in hypersensitivity reactions and defense against pathogens and are early arrivals at the site of a primary exposure to an antigenic substance. See Figures 14–3 and 14–4 for stages of neutrophil development. Note that left–right orientation (immature cells to the left) has given rise to the common but often misused term "left shift" in clinical jargon. In reality it implies an abundance of immature neutrophils in the peripheral blood.

Mononuclear phagocytes (circulating and fixed) are effector cells in inflammation, arriving after neutrophils. They are major defenses against intracellular pathogens, such as *Brucella, Toxoplasma* and *Trypanosoma cruzi.* They also function as antigen processing and presenting cells for induction of the immune response (see previous text) and ingest and dispose of effete, damaged or nonfunctional cells. They help in the process of tissue repair and lessen cellular response that occurs in inflammation.

Neutrophils: Opsonization and Phagocytosis

Neutrophils function through migration opsonization, phagocytosis, and intracellular killing. Migration is directed into a site of infection by chemical gradients of microbial elaborated substances or activated complement components. Opsonization occurs when antibody and complement coat a pathogen. Their presence on the surface of the pathogen promotes phagocytosis, the attachment and engulfment of a microbe, and enclosure of it with a vacuole (phagosome). Phagocytosis initiates a burst of neutrophil metabolism, resulting in generation of hydrogen peroxide and superoxides, which, when released into phagosomes, are microbicidal. The process of release of microbicidal

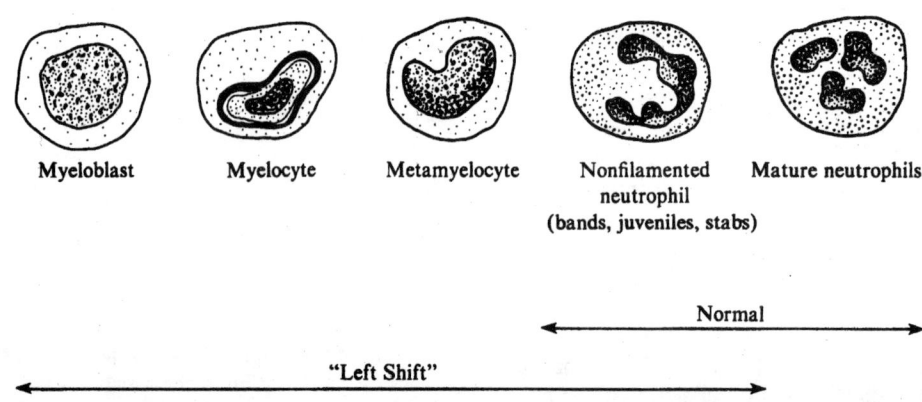

| Myeloblast | Myelocyte | Metamyelocyte | Nonfilamented neutrophil (bands, juveniles, stabs) | Mature neutrophils |

Normal

"Left Shift"

Figure 14–4   Stages of neutrophil development. A laboratory finding of increased numbers of immature neutrophils in the peripheral blood is referred to as a "left shift."

Copyright © 2005, Association for Professionals in Infection Control and Epidemiology, Inc.

and digestive materials from lysosomes of neutrophils into phagosomes is enhanced by opsonization. Granule contents released into the extracellular environment function as attractants for more neutrophils. The normal number of white blood cells (WBCs) in peripheral blood is between 4000 and 10,000 cells/cu mm. WBC numbers in excess of 10,000 are termed *leukocytosis*. Total WBC count less than 4000 is called *neutropenia*. If the absolute number of neutrophils is falling below 1000/cu mm or resides below 500, there is significant danger of fatal infection. Absolute neutrophil count is derived by multiplying the cumulative percent of mature and immature PMN times the total WBC count.

II. SUMMARY AND CONCLUSIONS

Infection results when an imbalance occurs between the mechanisms that microorganisms employ to induce infection and the complex physiological response systems that are employed by a host to prevent such infections. ICPs must understand those mechanisms in order to design and implement effective infection control and prevention programs.

REFERENCES

1. Hewlitt EL: Toxins. In Mandell GL, Bennett JE, Dolan R, editors: *Principles and practice of infectious diseases*, ed 5, New York, 2000, Churchill Livingstone, pp 21–30.
2. Wiedermann BL, Kaplan SL: Microbial virulence factors. In Feigin RD, Cherry TD, editors: *Textbook of pediatric infectious diseases*, ed 4, Philadelphia, 1998, WB Saunders, pp 192–214.
3. Gibbons RJ: Bacterial attachment to host tissues. In Gorbach SL, Bartlett JG, Blacklow HR, editors: *Infectious diseases*, Philadelphia, 1992, WB Saunders, pp 7–17.
4. Thorne GM: Toxins. In Gorbach SL, Bartlett JG, Blacklow HR, editors: *Infectious diseases*, ed 2, Philadelphia, 1998, WB Saunders, pp 9–17.
5. Joiner KA: Other virulence factors. In Gorbach SL, Bartlett JG, Blacklow HR, editors: *Infectious diseases*, ed 2, Philadelphia, 1998, WB Saunders, pp 18–27.
6. Tompkins LS: Molecular epidemiology in infectious diseases. In Gorbach SL, Bartlett JG, Blacklow HR, editors: *Infectious diseases*, ed 2, Philadelphia, 1998, WB Saunders, pp 28–34.
7. Johnson RM, Brown EJ: Cell-mediated immunity in host defense against infectious diseases. In Mandell GL, Bennett JE, Dolan R, editors: *Principles and practice of infectious diseases*, ed 5, New York, 2000, Churchill Livingstone, pp 112–145.
8. Tosi MF, Cates KL: Immunologic and phagocytic responses to infection. In Feigin RD, Cherry TD, editors: *Textbook of pediatric infectious diseases*, ed 3, Philadelphia, 1998, WB Saunders, pp 14–54.
9. Romani L, Pucetti P, Bistoni F: Interleukin-12 in infectious diseases, *Clin Microbiol Rev* 10(4):611–636, 1997.
10. Yoshikai Y, Nishimura H: The role of interleukin-15 in mounting an immune response against microbial infections, *Microbes Infect* 2(4):381–389, 2000.
11. Markham RB: Cell-mediated immunity. In Gorbach SL, Bartlett JG, Blacklow HR, editors: *Infectious diseases*, ed 2, Philadelphia, 1998, WB Saunders, pp 66–81.
12. Heinzel FP: Antibodies. In Mandell GL, Bennett JE, Dolan R, editors: *Principles and practice of infectious diseases*, ed 5, New York, 2000, Churchill Livingstone, pp 45–66.
13. Tramont EC, Hoover DL: Innate (general or nonspecific) host defense mechanisms. In Mandell GL, Bennett JE, Dolan R, editors: *Principles and practice of infectious diseases*, ed 5, New York, 2000, Churchill Livingstone, pp 31–38.
14. Smith AL: Indigenous flora. In Feigin RD, Cherry TD, editors: *Textbook of pediatric infectious diseases*, ed 4, Philadelphia, 1998, WB Saunders, pp 95–98.
15. Lorin MI: Fever: pathogenesis and treatment. In Feigin RD, Cherry TD, editors: *Textbook of pediatric infectious diseases*, ed 3, Philadelphia, 1992, WB Saunders, pp 130–134.
16. Kazuhiro K, Hiroshi N, Atsuko H, et al: Association of human herpesvirus 6 infection of the central nervous system with recurrence of febrile convulsions, *J Infect Dis* 167:1197–1200, 1993.
17. Kluger MJ: Fever revisited, *Pediatrics* 90:846–850, 1992.
18. Densen P: Complement. In Mandell GL, Bennett JE, Dolan R, editors: *Principles and practice of infectious diseases*, ed 5, New York, 2000, Churchill Livingstone, pp 67–88.
19. Winkelstein JA: The complement system. In Gorbach SL, Bartlett JG, Blacklow HR, editors: *Infectious diseases*, ed 2, Philadelphia, 1998, WB Saunders, pp 35–40.
20. Nauseef WM, Clark RA: Granulocytic phagocytes. In Mandell GL, Bennett JE, Dolan R, editors: *Principles and practice of infectious diseases*, ed 5, NewYork, 2000, Churchill Livingstone, pp 89–111.
21. Klempner MS, Malech HL: Phagocytes: normal and abnormal neutrophil host defenses. In Gorbach SL, Bartlett JG, Blacklow HR, editors: *Infectious diseases*, ed 2, Philadelphia, 1998, WB Saunders, pp 41–65.

Copyright © 2005, Association for Professionals in Infection Control and Epidemiology, Inc.

15

REVISED 2004

The Immunocompromised Host

George F. Risi, Jr., MD, FACP, FIDSA
Infectious Disease Specialist, Director, Infection
Control Department
St. Patrick Hospital
Missoula, Montana

ABSTRACT

Infectious diseases are a major cause of morbidity and mortality in immunocompromised patients. Infections are often predictable and may also be preventable. This chapter provides a practical overview of the broad topic of the immune compromised host and prevention of infection, focusing on specific types of immune compromise and the types of infection associated with them. Methods of strengthening host resistance are discussed, as well as techniques to avoid exposures to potential pathogens. Topics have been chosen to include areas of care that differ from the immune competent patient, including immunizations, augmentation of host resistance, and antimicrobial prophylaxis. National practice guidelines are cited, when available, and, where no consensus exists, practical recommendations based on available literature are provided. A systematic approach to care of the immunocompromised host, tailored to the needs of each individual patient, will reduce the risk of infection.

KEY CONCEPTS

- Several categories of immune function exist.

- Thorough history taking and detailed physical examination may reveal areas of potential problem.

- Host resistance to infection can often be augmented.

- Avoidance of hospitalization is desirable, whenever feasible.

- Rigorous implementation of handwashing and standard isolation guidelines are the most important of all interventions.

I.   BACKGROUND

The immunocompromised host is a person with impairments in the body's normal mechanisms of defense against infection. A review of normal host defenses is beyond the scope of this chapter, but references to recent discussions of the topic can be found in the supplemental resources section of this chapter. Several categories of host defects that are commonly associated with impaired resistance exist. Within these categories, broad variations in immunologic function are recognized. Often the degree of abnormality may wax or wane with time and therapy. Comprehensive management of the immunocompromised host entails all of the following elements: (1) recognition of the categories of host defects that are associated with impaired resistance, (2) understanding of the

Copyright © 2005, Association for Professionals in Infection Control and Epidemiology, Inc.

opportunistic organisms and their source that are most often associated with the compromised host, (3) what kind of infection to anticipate in each kind of immune compromise, (4) the most common portals of entry for opportunistic organisms, (5) the fact that clinical manifestations of illness may be different in the immunocompromised host, and (6) an understanding of the broad array of modalities for prevention of infection.

II. BASIC PRINCIPLES

Recognition and Characterization of the Immunocompromised Host

The immunocompromised host is an individual who has one or more defects in the body's normal defense mechanisms that predisposes him or her to infections, often life threatening, that would otherwise not occur. These individuals continue to be at risk for common infections as well, and these may pursue a more aggressive course than they might otherwise. The number and type of immunocompromised hosts is constantly increasing for several reasons, including the aging of the U.S. population, medical advances that have kept alive persons who previously would have died from their underlying disease, pandemic infection by human immunodeficiency virus (HIV) and hepatitis B (HBV) and C (HCV) viruses, increasing homelessness and resultant lack of basic hygiene and good nutrition, increased rates of malignancy of a variety of types, and immigration of persons from developing parts of the world where exotic and potentially immunocompromising infectious agents are endemic.

The categories of host defects that are commonly associated with impaired resistance are listed in Table 15–1.

Within these categories, broad variations in immunological function are recognized. Most patients have abnormalities that may wax or wane with time and therapy. For this reason, the individual patient's risk of infection is best evaluated by defining his or her net state of immunosuppression.

The net state of immunosuppression is determined by the interaction of several variables, including: (1) host-defense defects caused by the disease process itself; (2) the dose, duration, and temporal sequence of immunosuppressive therapy; (3) presence or absence of neutropenia and/or lymphopenia; (4) the state of humoral and cellular host defenses; (5) the integrity of the skin (to include presence or absence of an indwelling intravenous catheter) and mucosal surfaces of the body; (6) metabolic factors, such as malnutrition, uremia, hyperglycemia, and hepatic dysfunction; (7) abnormalities of the reticuloendothelial system, most notably the absence of splenic function; and (8) the presence or absence of immunomodulating infections, such as HIV,

Table 15-1. Categories of Host Defect that are Associated with Impaired Resistance

Defects in the cutaneous barrier to invasion of endogenous or acquired organisms

1. Surgical incisons
2. Thermal or chemical burns
3. Traumatic damage to skin
4. Severe dermatological conditions
   - Poorly controlled advanced eczema or psoriasis
   - Scleroderma
   - *Mycosis fungoides*
   - Chronic fungal infections of skin or nail beds
5. Indwelling intravenous (IV) lines, either temporary or long term
6. Injections, either legal/medicinal or illicit
7. Ulcers: decubitus, diabetic, others
8. Vascular insufficiency, either arterial or venous

Mucous membrane barrier defects

1. Mucositis induced by irradiation or chemotherapy
2. Trauma to the head and neck
3. Smoking (tobacco, recreational drugs)
4. Inhalation injuries (heat, smoke, caustic chemicals, recreational drugs)
5. Poor oral hygiene
6. Erosions from nasogastric or endotracheal tubes or indwelling Foley catheter
7. Antacids, proton pump inhibitors, etc.
   - Decrease the number of ingested organisms needed to cause gastroenteritis
   - Allow a reservoir of bacteria to develop in the stomach, which can be regurgitated and aspirated

Conditions that cause obstruction of a natural body passage

1. Tumors of the lung, gastrointestinal tract, pancreatic head, elsewhere
2. Aspiration of a foreign body
3. Renal stones, enlargement of the prostate
4. Gallstones
5. Cystic fibrosis

Abnormal number or function of granulocytes

1. Leukemia
2. Chemotherapy for malignant disease
3. Aplastic anemia
4. Granulocytopenia as an adverse drug reaction (interferon, others)
5. Dysfunctional granulocytes, despite normal numbers
   - Diabetes mellitus, especially if poorly controlled
   - Corticosteroid administration
   - Rheumatoid arthritis
   - Renal failure
   - Congenital disorders of phagocyte function: Chediak-Higashi syndrome,
   - Chronic granulomatous disease, hypereosinophilic syndrome (Job syndrome), others

(Continued)

Copyright © 2005, Association for Professionals in Infection Control and Epidemiology, Inc.

Table 15-1. Continued

Abnormalities of cell-mediated immunity
1. Bone marrow transplantation
2. HIV infection
3. Chemotherapy • For malignancy • For rheumatological disorders
4. Aging
5. Hodgkin's disease
6. Corticosteroid administration
7. Third trimester of pregnancy
8. Severe malnutrition

Abnormal humoral immunity
1. Bone marrow transplantation
2. HIV infection
3. Chronic lymphocytic leukemia
4. Multiple myeloma and Waldenstrom's macroglobulinemia
5. Aging
6. Childhood immunoglobulin deficiencies
7. Acquired hypogammaglobulinemia (common variable immunodeficiency)

Patients with defects in multiple arms of immunity
1. Aging
2. Severe trauma
3. Alcoholism or chemical dependency
4. Homelessness
5. Splenectomy
6. Organ failure (cirrhosis, chronic renal failure with or without hemodialysis)
7. Spinal cord injury
8. High dose corticosteroid administration
9. Chemotherapy

hepatitis viruses, cytomegalovirus (CMV), Epstein-Barr virus (EBV), and human herpesvirus 6 (HHV-6).[1, 2, 3] Additional stressors include smoking,[4] injecting drug use,[5] obesity,[6] and alcoholism.[7, 8] The net state of immunosuppression determines not only the risk of infection and the need for prevention, but it also influences the likelihood of effectiveness of attempts at intervention.

Opportunistic organisms that most often cause disease in the immunocompromised host

In the immune-intact individual only a relative handful of pathogens are able to cause disease. These have been called "true pathogens" and include, for example, such organisms as influenza, *Salmonella typhi*, *Yersinia pestis*, *Bacillus anthracis*, as well as several others. As the host becomes progressively more immunocompromised, progressively less virulent organisms are able to become pathogenic. Thus patients with major immune defects are subject to a larger number and greater variety of infectious diseases.

It is important to recall that although the classic pathogens also cause disease in the immunocompromised host, often their presentation is different than would be seen in the healthy individual.

Table 15–2 lists the organisms that are commonly considered opportunistic.

Opportunistic organisms encountered internationally

Increasing numbers of individuals reside in the United States who were born in another country, importantly, from parts of the developing world. A significant variety of organisms that are uncommon in the United States are endemic and may reactivate in the setting of immunosuppression.[9]

Internationally acquired infections that may lie dormant for prolonged periods

- *Strongyloides stercoralis*
- *Schistosoma* spp.
- *Pseudomonas pseudomallei*
- Hydatid disease (*Echinococcus* spp.)
- *Trichinella spiralis*
- Tapeworms, especially *Taenia solium*
- Nematodes (*Onchocerca volvulus*)

The source of the infection may be endogenous, exogenous, or both.

Isolation of a specific microorganism may at times allow its source of origin to be determined (Table 15–3). This is helpful in determining the optimal way to proceed with individual patients. Note that organisms that arise from an endogenous source in one patient may be then transmissible to healthcare workers or other patients.

Most important portals of entry for opportunistic organisms

The skin is an important portal, especially for individuals with long-term IV access devices of all types as well as patients with major defects in skin integrity, such as burns. The microbiology of burn infections has been recently reviewed.[10] *Staphylococcus aureus* and *Pseudomonas aeruginosa* continue as the two dominant organisms, representing 23% and 19% of all isolates from burn wounds, respectively. The majority of the remainder of isolates fall into seven genera (Table 15–4).

Copyright © 2005, Association for Professionals in Infection Control and Epidemiology, Inc.

Table 15-2. Most Common Infections Expected in Certain Types of Immune Defect

Breaks in cutaneous integrity: invasion by skin flora

A. *Staphylococcus aureus*, coagulase negative Staphylococci

B. *Streptococcus pyogenes*

C. *Corynebacterium* spp.

D. Malassezia furfur, if lipid containing intravenous solutions are being given

Defects in mucous membranes, with invasion by resident flora

A. Anaerobic bacteria (*Clostridium perfringens, Clostridium septicum, Bacteroides fragilis*)

B. Aerobic gram-negative bacilli

C. *Candida* spp. and *Torulopsis. glabrata*

D. *Enterococcus* spp. and *Streptococcus bovis*

Obstruction of a natural body passage: overgrowth or invasion or both by resident flora

A. Lung: oral flora; if patient hospitalized, nosocomial gram negatives

B. Biliary and pancreatic system: aerobic gram negative bacilli, *Enterococcus* sp. anaerobes

C. Colon: aerobic gram-negative bacilli, anaerobes, *S. bovis*

Granulocytopenia (defined as absolute neutrophil count <500/mL)

A. Duration less than 2 weeks; most common
- Aerobic gram-negative bacilli
- *S. aureus* and coagulase negative Staphylococci

Duration of greater than two weeks: above PLUS
- *Candida* spp. and *T. glabrata*
- *Aspergillus* spp.

Dysfunction of cell-mediated immunity

A. Bacteria: primarily the intracellular pathogens
- *Listeria monocytogenes*
- *Salmonella* spp.
- *Mycobacterium* spp.
- *Nocardia asteroides*
- *Legionella pneumophila*, other *Legionella* spp.
- *Rhodococcus equi*
- *Pseudomonas pseudomallei*

B. Fungi
- *Cryptococcus neoformans*
- *Candida* spp. and *T. glabrata*
- *Coccidioides immitis*
- *Histoplasma capsulatum*
- *Penicillium marneffei*
- *Pneumocystis jiroveci*

C. Herpes group viruses

D. Protozoa
- *Toxoplasma gondii*
- *Cryptosporidium parvum*

E. Helminths
- *Strongyloides stercoralis*

Humoral dysfunction—encapsulated bacteria

A. *Streptococcus pneumoniae*

B. Encapsulated strains of *Haemophilus influenzae*

C. *Neisseria meningitidis*

Table 15-3. Source of Opportunistic Infection

Opportunists that are more commonly (but not exclusively) endogenous

A. *Mycobacterium tuberculosis* (lung, lymphatics, others)

B. Coagulase negative staphylococci (skin)

C. *Corynebacterium* spp. (skin)

D. *Enterococcus* spp. and *S. bovis* (gastrointestinal tract)

E. *Clostridium septicum* (gastrointestinal tract)

F. *Candida* spp. and *Torulopsis glabrata* (oropharynx and gastrointestinal tract)

G. *Coccidioides immitis* (lung, liver, spleen, others)

H. *Histoplasma capsulatum* (lung, liver, spleen)

I. *Malassezia furfur* (skin)

J. *Pneumocystis jiroveci* (lungs, rarely elsewhere)

K. *Toxoplasma gondii* (central nervous system)

L. Herpesvirus group (primarily skin and mucous membranes)

Opportunists that are more commonly but not exclusively exogenous

A. *Clostridium difficile* (hands of personnel, fomites)

B. *Legionella pneumophila* (contaminant of tap water, spread by aerosols)

C. *Rhodococcus equi* (soil)

D. *Aspergillus* spp. (ventilation systems, especially during construction or demolition)

E. Zygomycetes (ubiquitous in environment)

F. Rapidly growing mycobacteria (*M. fortuitum, M chelonei,* others, from environmental sources)

G. *Cryptosporidium parvum* (water supplies)

H. Viruses other than the herpes group (hands, droplet nuclei)

Opportunists that can be either endogenous or exogenous

A. Aerobic gram negative bacilli
1. Endogenous from oropharynx and gastrointestinal tract
2. Exogenous from aerosols, contaminated food, fomites

B. *Staphylococcus aureus*
1. Endogenous as resident skin flora, nasal carriage
2. Exogenous from hands of personnel

From the oropharynx affected by chemotherapy, thermal burn, radiation, or the presence of a nasogastric tube, local invasion into the bloodstream can occur by the members of the normal oropharyngeal flora (see previous table). The presence of a nasogastric tube has been shown to change the oropharyngeal ecosystem with increased presence of *P. aeruginosa*.[11] Additionally, hospitalization is associated with acquisition of nosocomial organisms within the oropharynx that replace the normal flora.[12] The lung is the common portal of entry for *Mycobacterium tuberculosis, Aspergillus* spp., and regionally important fungi, such as *Coccidioides immitis, Histoplasma capsulatum, Penicillium marneffei,* and *Paracoccidioides brasiliensis*. Within the gastrointestinal tract the stomach serves as a reservoir for bacteria that can be aspirated, especially if gastric acid is neutralized.[2] In the neutropenic host the

APIC Text of Infection Control and Epidemiology

Copyright © 2005, Association for Professionals in Infection Control and Epidemiology, Inc.

Table 15-4. Bacteria and Fungi that Constituted 1,830 Isolates Recovered from 1,234 Burn Wound Infections: NNIS System CDC, 1980–1998

Pathogen #	Isolates (%)
Staphylococcus aureus	420 (23)
Pseudomonas aeruginosa	353 (19.3)
Enterococci	202 (11.0)
Enterobacter spp.	176 (9.6)
Escherichia coli	131 (7.2)
Coagulase negative staphylococci	78 (4.3)
Candida albicans	64 (3.5)
Serratia marcescens	64 (3.5)
Klebsiella pneumoniae	48 (2.6)
Others	294 (16)

gastrointestinal tract is the most important source for bacteremia as the result of transmigration across the mucosal barrier.

Clinical manifestations of disease may be different in the immunocompromised host versus the intact host

The immunocompromised host may present with a very different picture compared to the intact host. The pace of disease may be much more rapid than in the competent host. This is especially true for instance in the asplenic patient presenting with bacterial infection or the neutropenic patient. Seemingly trivial problems may rapidly become life threatening. Granulocytopenic patients have little purulence at the site of infection and less obvious chest radiographical findings. Elderly patients may have confusion or incontinence as their only manifestation of infection. Patients receiving corticosteroids may have diminished or absent fever response. Patients who are sedated or have central nervous system dysfunction perceive pain less well and are less able to articulate a problem to the examiner. Finally, the white-blood-cell count may be in the normal range but demonstrate an increased number of immature (band) forms.

III. PREVENTING INFECTION IN THE IMMUNOCOMPROMISED HOST

Identify and address specific problems before the patient is subjected to immunocompromising procedures

A thorough history and a detailed physical examination are essential in the care of the immunocompromised patient. Potential problems can be identified in a careful interview, which may be supplemented with a printed questionnaire for consistency (Fig. 15–1).

The patient may provide information about previous infections that imply specific types of immune dysfunction. Examples of such potential sentinel organisms are listed in Table 15–5.

A complete listing of all medications should include all over-the-counter medications. Additionally, patients may seek dual services with traditional as well as alternative healthcare providers and may be taking substances in the forms of teas, food additives, or pills that, although "natural," may still affect the immune system.[13] These substances should also be noted on the intake form.

Birthplace and geographical areas of residence or extensive travel are important clues to potential latent infections. Hobbies and recreational activities, such as spelunking, hiking and camping, hunting or fishing, may expose the patient to zoonotic infections. The patient's sexual history should be obtained, including the incidence of sexually transmitted diseases and their treatments, as well as the history of drug use, including quantity of alcohol consumption, oral, inhaled or injectable illicit substances, and misuse of prescription drugs. Finally, a meticulous systems review and physical examination should be performed.

Routine lab work should include a complete blood count with differential, a chemistry panel that includes a measurement of liver enzymes, renal function, and electrolytes. A reasonable estimate of nutritional status can be obtained by the use of serum albumin, transferring, and total lymphocyte count.

Patients requiring long-term venous access should have such devices placed well in advance of any immunosuppressive therapy. Detailed protocols for skin prep, catheter placement, and catheter care have been published.[14, 15] A review of the literature regarding use of antimicrobial-impregnated catheters to reduce the rate of catheter-related bloodstream infection failed to demonstrate any significant benefit.[16] Any needed dental work should be completed before therapy is administered. Patients who smoke should be strongly encouraged to quit or at least reduce their consumption[4] since smoking can increase the severity of a variety of respiratory viral illnesses and can exacerbate mucositis induced by chemotherapy or radiation. Any chronic skin, scalp, or nail bed condition should be addressed and brought under control as much as possible before rendering the immune system more compromised.

Potential recipients of solid organ transplant should be screened in advance of the transplant for latent infection. The aims of such screening are fourfold[17]:(1) to determine the immune status of the recipient against

Copyright © 2005, Association for Professionals in Infection Control and Epidemiology, Inc.

Infectious Disease Specialists, P.C.

Patient Medical History

Name_____ Date of Birth_____

Reason for your visit today _____
_____

How long has this been going on?

Other physicians (include alternative health care providers seen recently
Doctor_____ Reason_____
Doctor_____ Reason_____
Doctor_____ Reason_____

List all medications (prescription, non-prescription, herbal/organic products, etc.)
_____ _____ _____ _____
_____ _____ _____ _____
_____ _____ _____ _____

Medication Allergies _____

If possible describe the type of reaction_____
_____

Circle any illnesses you have had and specify the year
Cancer_____ Heart Disease _____ Diabetes _____
Hypertension_____ Abnormal bleeding _____ Blood clots_____
 Asthma_____ Pneumonia_____ Rheumatic Fever _____
Kidney trouble _____ Jaundice/hepatitis _____ Blood infection _____
Cellulitis/skin condition_____ Sexually transmitted disease_____
Depression/mental illness _____ Tuberculosis _____
Other medical illnesses not listed above_____
_____

List all previous surgeries (include date, hospital, surgeon name) _____
_____

Have you ever had a blood transfusion? Y/N if yes, how many and when? _____

Copyright © 2005, Association for Professionals in Infection Control and Epidemiology, Inc.

Vaccination history. List yes or no and year
    Tetanus Y/N year_____   Influenza Y/N year(s)_____
    Pneumonia Y/N year_____   MMR Y/N year _____
    Varicella (chickenpox) Y/N year_____
    Hepatitis A Y/N year   Hepatitis B Y/N year _____

Family History

	Living/Deceased	Age/Age at death	Present health/cause of death

Father _____
Mother_____
Spouse_____
Brothers
    No. living _____ Health _____
    No dead _____ Cause of death_____
Sisters
    No. living _____ Health _____
    No dead _____ Cause of death_____
Children
    No. living _____ Health _____
    No dead _____ Cause of death_____

List any other known family illnesses and in whom _____
_____

Social History
Place of Birth_____   Religious Affiliation_____
Occupation   _____   Place of residence _____
Travel history
    Outside US _____
    Within US _____

Do you smoke (cigarettes, pipe, cigar) or chew tobacco? Y/N Daily amount _____
Did you use tobacco in the past? Y/N Daily amount_____When stopped _____
Do you consume alcohol? Y/N Type _____ Amount in a typical week _____
Sexual orientation (circle one)   N/A Opposite Sex Same Sex Both Neither
Do you own house pets?   Y/N Type_____
Do you hunt or eat game meat?   Y/N
Are you exposed to "farm" animals? Circle all that apply:
    Horses Cattle Sheep Pigs Poultry Llamas Other_____

Do you or have you in the past consumed fish, meat or dairy products that are raw, very
rare or unpasteurized? Y/N If yes, please elaborate _____
_____

Figure 15-1. (Continued)

Copyright © 2005, Association for Professionals in Infection Control and Epidemiology, Inc.

Is your diet what you would consider typical or average? Y/N If no, please elaborate

_____

Review of Systems: Check all that apply

Headaches_____ Seizures/blackouts_____ Sinusitis _____ Nosebleeds_____
Ringing/Buzzing in ears _____Pain on swallowing_____ Dental problems _____
Cold sores _____ Chest pains _____ Shortness of breath _____ Chronic cough ____
Change in appetite _____ Change in bowel habits _____Change in weight_____
If weight has changed, is it up or down and how much? _____
Difficulty urinating _____Genital ulcers or vaginal discharge _____
Chronic skin condition _____ Athletes foot _____
Arthritis_____ Ankle swelling_____
Weakness ,numbness or tingling of a body part (specify) _____

Other issues not covered in the questionnaire:

_____
_____
_____
_____
_____
_____

Figure 15-1. (Continued)

common pathogens that can be transmitted by transplants. This is because established immunity against pathogens, such as cytomegalovirus, *Toxoplasma gondii,* and possibly HBV, protects the recipient from severe sequelae of infection with these agents; (2) to permit the allocation of organs from donors infected with a certain pathogen to recipients who are already carriers of this agent, such as HCV infection; (3) to recognize and possibly treat infections that can be expected to exacerbate or reactivate after immunosuppression, such as tuberculosis, the endemic mycoses histoplasmosis and coccidioidomycosis, or parasites, such as *Strongyloides stercoralis*; and (4) to avoid transplantation in patients with a poor prognosis after transplantation, such as HIV infection or colonization with certain pan-resistant bacteria.

Augmentation of Host Resistance

Gastric acidity

Gastric acid is an important defense mechanism against bacterial pathogens, and, in general, should not

be neutralized in an immunocompromised patient. With a normal gastric acid barrier, the majority of ingested pathogens never reach the intestinal tract to cause disease. Neutralization of this barrier may increase the susceptibility to and severity of a variety of bacterial and parasitic diseases.[18-25] In the hospitalized patient, the stomach can serve as a reservoir for overgrowth of nosocomial gram-negative bacteria when acidity is neutralized.[26] These bacteria serve as a reservoir for aspiration after regurgitation.[2]

An association has been found between elevated gastric pH and increased incidence of pneumonia.[26, 27] Cook et al.[28] performed a meta-analysis of 63 randomized clinical trials and concluded that the use of H2 antagonists tends to increase the risk of pneumonia compared with no prophylaxis. The use of sucralfate may lower the risk of pneumonia compared with the risk associated with the use of antacids and H2 antagonists. Because sucralfate is as effective as antacid preparations in prevention of stress ulceration,[29] this agent should be preferentially used for the immunocompromised patient.

APIC Text of Infection Control and Epidemiology

Copyright © 2005, Association for Professionals in Infection Control and Epidemiology, Inc.

Table 15-5. Common Opportunistic Organisms

Opportunistic bacteria

A. Bacteria that commonly cause disease in immunocompetent hosts as well as in immunocompromised individuals (partial list)
1. *Staphylococcus aureus*
2. *Streptococcus pneumoniae*
3. *Haemophilus influenzae*
4. *Escherichia coli*
5. *Mycobacterium tuberculosis*

B. Coagulase negative staphylococci

C. *Corynebacterium* spp. (aka "diphtheroids")

D. Enterococci (*E. faecalis* and *E. faecium*) and *Streptococcus bovis*

E. *Listeria monocytogenes*

F. Aerobic gram-negative bacilli (only most common listed)
1. *Pseudomonas aeruginosa*
2. *Klebsiella pneumoniae, K. oxytoca*
3. *Enterobacter aerogenes, E. cloacae*
4. *Legionella pneumophila*

G. *Nocardia asteroides*

H. Anaerobic bacteria
1. *Bacteroides* spp., especially *B. fragilis*
2. *Clostridium* spp. (*C. perfringens, C. septicum, C. difficile*)

Opportunistic fungi

A. Candida spp. (*C. albicans, C. krusei, C. parapsilosis*, others)

B. *Torulopsis* (aka *Candida*) *glabrata*

C. *Aspergillus* spp.

D. *Cryptococcus neoformans*

E. Zygomyctes (*Mucor, Rhizopus, Absidia, Rhizomucor*)

F. *Malassezia furfur*

G. *Trichosporon begelii*

H. *Pneumocystis jiroveci* (formerly *P. carinii*)

I. Regionally in U.S., *Coccidioides immitis, Histoplasma capsulatum*

Opportunistic viruses

A. Herpesvirus group (CMV, Varicella, herpes simplex, EBV, human herpes virus 6 (HHV 6) and HHV 7 (Kaposi sarcoma virus)

B. Measles virus

C. Adenovirus

D. Enteroviruses

E. Respiratory syncytial virus (RSV)

Opportunistic protozoa

A. *Toxoplasma gondii*

B. *Cryptosporidium parvum*

Opportunistic Helminths

Strongyloides stercoralis

Immunizations

Patients should be up to date on all routine immunizations.[3, 30] The Advisory Committee on Immunization Practices (ACIP) divides patients with immunocompromising disorders into three practical categories: (1) patients with HIV infection, (2) patients with severe immunosuppression not caused by HIV, and (3) patients with other conditions that cause limited immune deficits, such as asplenia, renal failure, diabetes, and alcoholism. In general, inactivated vaccines can be administered to patients in all three categories. Live virus vaccines are generally contraindicated in all patients in group 2, in some patients in group 1, and in no patients in group 3. The ACIP has recently published a recommended immunization schedule by age group and medical condition.[31]

Vaccines will likely play an increasingly important role in disease prevention in the future. A variety of investigational uses for vaccines are under study, including vaccination for *S. aureus* in chronic hemodialysis patients,[32] vaccination against *P. aeruginosa* infections for patients with cystic fibrosis,[33] immunization against the endotoxin of gram-negative bacteria,[34] and vaccination of trauma victims against *Klebsiella* and *Pseudomonas*.[35] Better protection for the immunocompromised patient will likely require the development of more effective adjuvants as well.[36]

Immunization in recipients of transplanted organs (autologous or allogeneic bone marrow transplants, solid organ transplants)

In general, vaccines are more likely to be effective in persons whose immune system is functioning normally compared to the compromised host. The more compromised the host, the less effective the vaccine is likely to be. For transplant patients of all types, therefore, it is desirable to update all immunizations in advance of a transplant. [37]

Recipients of transplanted marrow or stem cells suffer severe immunosuppression for several months after transplantation. This immunosuppression occurs regardless of the type of graft (autologous, syngeneic, or allogeneic), the underlying disease, the conditioning and preparative regimens, and whether graft versus host disease (GVHD) develops. Even in the absence of GVHD, reconstitution of a fully functioning immune system occurs slowly during the course of several months to years. Thus interest is considerable in modalities to prevent infection during the period after transplantation. The literature supports the use of vaccinations, and standard preparations can be used effectively. The optimal timing of administration has not been precisely defined, but poor responses to vaccination can be expected for at least the first 6 months after transplantation. Detailed recommendations have recently been published for immunization of hematopoietic stem cell transplant recipients.[38] Recommendations include the use of tetanus/diphtheria, *Haemophilus influenzae* type B, Hepatitis B, 23 valent *Streptococcus pneumoniae* vaccine, inactivated polio vaccine, annual influenza, and at 24 months

---

Copyright © 2005, Association for Professionals in Infection Control and Epidemiology, Inc.

post-transplant use of measles, mumps, and rubella (MMR) vaccine (assuming no ongoing immunosuppression)

Because of the ongoing use of immunosuppressive medications, solid organ transplant recipients are at risk of life-threatening infections indefinitely. Specific vaccinations have been recommended for these patients, to include pneumococcal, influenza, and hepatitis A and B. Also indicated, in select cases, are tetanus, diphtheria, and *Haemophilus influenzae* type B. Specific vaccination recommendations for solid organ transplant recipients have recently been published.[39]

Passive immunization with either intramuscular or intravenous immune globulin

The administration of preformed donor antibody by either the intramuscular or intravenous route has a role in the prevention of infection in the compromised host; it is indicated as postexposure prophylaxis in susceptible patients exposed to hepatitis A, HBV, or measles virus. A variety of immunohematological disorders have been successfully treated with intravenous immune globulin (IVIG) to include immune thrombocytopenia, autoimmune hemolytic anemia, and others.[40] Many other potential uses are currently under investigation[40-43] to include treatment of recurrent sinopulmonary infection,[41] low birth weight infants,[42] multiple myeloma,[41] trauma, burns, high risk surgical patient,[41, 43] and even insulin-dependent diabetes mellitus.[44, 45, 46] IVIG is not generally recommended for routine oncology patients but may be indicated in selected patients with chronic lymphocytic leukemia, humoral immunodeficiency syndromes, and B cell defects.[47, 48]

Granulocyte transfusions

The transfusion of donor leukocytes to augment resistance in chemotherapy-induced neutropenia was once commonly used. However, minimal benefit was gained, primarily because of the small numbers of granulocytes that could be harvested from donors. In addition, adverse reactions were common, including fever, alloimmunization, and transmission of CMV.[49] For these reasons, granulocyte transfusion has become relatively uncommon.

Recent developments, including improved donor screening and use of colony stimulating factors to improve the harvest from donors, may lead to increased use of granulocyte transfusion in a subset of the neutropenic population. The patients most likely to benefit from this would be those with profound and sustained neutropenia or neutropenic patients with infection not responding to antimicrobial therapy.[50]

Colony-stimulating factors

Two hematopoietic growth factors are currently available. Granulocyte colony-stimulating factor (GCSF) and granulocyte/macrophage colony-stimulating factor (GMCSF) have been shown to reduce the duration of neutropenia in patients receiving chemotherapy.[51] Some studies have shown that treated patients had fewer febrile episodes, fewer hospitalizations, and shorter hospital stays but did not have fewer severe infections or improved survival.[51] In 1996 a panel convened by the American Society of Clinical Oncology concluded that treatment with GCSF or GMCSF is unnecessary in patients with neutropenia of short duration (less than 1 week) but that it may benefit patients with prolonged neutropenia.[52] Others have argued that shorter hospital stays and fewer days of antimicrobial therapy represent important quality of life improvements justifying the use of these agents, even if the duration of neutropenia is expected to be brief.[53] Although the ASCO guidelines do not recommend the routine use of colony stimulating factors in treatment of febrile neutropenia, a recently published survey revealed that the majority or surveyed physicians do use these agents in this situation.[54] Thus, the precise role of colony stimulating factors in the setting of chemotherapy-induced neutropenia is in evolution.

The use of GCSF and GMCSF in the non-neutropenic host to augment neutrophil function in established infection is a topic of great interest.[55] Although growth factors are not approved for this indication, augmentation of host defenses and improved survival have been demonstrated in animal models, with ongoing trials in humans.[56, 57] Other types of cytokines, such as interleukins and interferons, may also find uses in the immunocompromised host in the future.[58]

Reduction of Exposure to Pathogens

Isolation and hand hygiene

In the majority of circumstances standard isolation guidelines[59] are sufficient for protection of most immunocompromised hosts, if they are followed strictly and are accompanied by good hand hygiene. Hand hygiene has been the focus of extensive research recently, summarized in the CDC's Guideline for Hand Hygiene in Health Care Settings.[60] Compliance among healthcare workers with guidelines for isolation and hand hygiene continues to pose a challenge[60, 61, 62]; adherence to published guidelines is especially important when dealing with the immunocompromised host.

Reverse isolation has been extensively studied in the granulocytopenic patient. Most studies that showed improved outcomes for patients in reverse isolation did not adequately control for other variables. When

Copyright © 2005, Association for Professionals in Infection Control and Epidemiology, Inc.

careful handwashing is enforced and food and supplies are handled appropriately, reverse isolation offers no additional benefit in reducing infection in the typical granulocytopenic patient,[63, 64] and there no longer appears to be a role for this modality.

Protective isolation or the total protective environment is a regimen that was designed to both reduce the patient's endogenous microbial burden and prevent the acquisition of new organisms. The patient is kept in a single room with positive air pressure, and all air that enters the room is passed through a high efficiency particulate (HEPA) filter. Only sterile products, food, and water are allowed to enter the room. Personnel entering the rooms must dress in sterile gowns and gloves. A number of studies have documented that the total protective environment can reduce the number of infections in profoundly granulocytopenic individuals, but it is both expensive and inconvenient for both the patient and the healthcare workers . Because of improvements in the past several years in the treatment of established infections, protective isolation is not necessary for the routine care of cancer patients with granulocytopenia.[65]

Prophylactic antimicrobials

Patients at risk for development of pneumonia caused by *Pneumocystis jiroveci* should receive prophylaxis with trimethoprim-sulfamethoxazole (TMP/SMX) for the duration of that risk. Alternatives for allergic patients include dapsone by mouth and pentamidine given by inhalation.

Multiple studies have demonstrated the efficacy of prophylactic antibiotic administration to patients with neutropenia.[66] The overall benefit of this modality, however, has been called into question for three reasons. First, antibiotic prophylaxis has not been shown to consistently reduce mortality rates. Second, the potential exists for deleterious effects from toxicity and fungal overgrowth. Finally, use of antimicrobials has been shown to cause the emergence of antibiotic resistant bacteria.[66, 67, 68] Thus, whereas the evidence for use of prophylaxis would be enough to warrant an A-I recommendation (good evidence to support a recommendation for use based on evidence from one or more properly randomized, controlled trials), the guidelines for the past several years[66, 69] have not recommended the routine use of antimicrobials for prophylaxis against bacterial infection.

Subsets of patients, however, may be candidates for this modality. Specifically, antimicrobial prophylaxis may be reasonable for patients with profound neutropenia (<100 neutrophils/mm^3), especially if coupled with any of the following: lesions that break the mucous membranes or skin, the use of indwelling intravenous catheters, use of invasive instrumentation (i.e.,

endoscopy), presence of severe periodontal disease, history of invasive dental procedures, or post-obstructive pneumonia. The status of the underlying malignancy should be taken into consideration, and if the patient is the recipient of an organ transplant, the status of organ engraftment. Finally, personal factors such as willingness to comply with prescribed prophylaxis, personal hygiene habits, and environmental (hospital or home) circumstances should be considered.[66] If prophylaxis is considered, TMP/SMX and fluoroquinolones (ciprofloxacin, levofloxacin, others) have been studied the most extensively. Antibiotics, if given, should be given for as short of a period as possible.[66]

The antifungal drugs, fluconazole and itraconazole, have been investigated for prevention of invasive fungal infections in neutropenia. Routine use of these agents for all cases of neutropenia is not recommended.[66] Similarly to the argument made above for antibiotic prophylaxis, some special circumstances may exist where the benefits of antifungal prophylaxis outweigh the risk of emergence of resistant organisms.

Prevention of healthcare-associated pneumonia

Recognition in advance of the patients who are at greatest risk for development of pneumonia is critical to prevention. Intubation and mechanical intubation alter first-line defenses. Therefore, such patients are at the highest risk of development of nosocomial pneumonia. Other risk factors are extremes of age, severe underlying disease, immunosuppression, depressed sensorium, cardiopulmonary disease, and thoracoabdominal surgery.

Most cases of healthcare-associated pneumonia occur by aspiration of bacteria colonizing the oropharynx or upper gastrointestinal tract of the patient. Factors that tend to increase the colonization of the oropharynx include coma, hypotension, acidosis, azotemia, alcoholism, diabetes mellitus, leukocytosis, leukopenia, pulmonary disease, nasogastric or endotracheal tubes, and receipt of antimicrobials.[12]

The Hospital Infection Control Practices Advisory Committee (HCIPAC) has published detailed recommendations for prevention of nosocomial pneumonia.[12, 70] Recommended measures include decreasing aspiration by the patient, preventing cross-contamination or colonization via hands of personnel, appropriate disinfection or sterilization of respiratory therapy devices, use of available vaccines to protect against particular infections, and education of hospital staff and patients. New measures under investigation involve reducing oropharyngeal and gastric colonization by pathogenic organisms[2] and vaccinations against nosocomial pathogens.[34, 35]

Copyright © 2005, Association for Professionals in Infection Control and Epidemiology, Inc.

Water

Water is a reservoir and a source for healthcare associated infections.[71] Several commonly encountered pathogens are able to replicate in tap water, to include aerobic gram-negative bacteria, such as *Pseudomonas* spp., *Legionella* spp., and nontuberculous mycobacteria. The reservoirs of concern include drinking water, sinks, faucet aerators, showers, tubs, toilets, dialysis water, ice and ice machines, flower vases (see later), eyewash stations, and dental unit water stations. Those of at least moderate or high concern for infection in the immunocompromised host include potable water, ice and ice machines, tubs for immersion, and in hospitals with high rates of *Legionella* spp., faucet and shower aerators.[71] Highly immunocompromised patients should drink sterile water, use ice made from sterile water, and avoid immersion in tubs.

Food

Fresh fruit and vegetables carry several species of gram-negative rods as part of their natural flora.[65, 72] Shooter et al.[73] performed cultures on a variety of foods from eight hospitals in the London area. Foods sampled included salads, cold meat, cold sweets, other cold foods, hot food, and pureed food. A significant proportion of salads were found to carry *P. aeruginosa*, *Escherichia coli*, and *Klebsiella* spp. Furthermore, the majority of positive cultures yielded greater than 1,000 colonies per gram of food.

Organisms colonizing fruits and vegetables have been shown to colonize the gastrointestinal tract of neutropenic patients after ingestion[72] and may lead to invasive disease. The neutropenic diet,[74] also called the cooked food diet or the low-bacterial diet, has been advocated by some to reduce the exposure of patients to these potential pathogens. Although this modality has not been studied alone, when combined with skin cleansing, topical and oral nonabsorbable antibiotics, and a laminar airflow room, serious bacterial infections have been avoided.[75] The neutropenic diet is a reasonable modality to employ for the neutropenic patient, especially if the duration of neutropenia is expected to be prolonged. Its use in hematopoietic stem cell transplant recipients has also recently been recommended.[38]

Although a hospital kitchen occasionally may be the source of food contamination,[76] agents of gastroenteritis and hepatitis A are much more likely to be encountered in food purchased in a restaurant. Thus, for hospitalized immunocompromised patients, food should not be brought in from outside the hospital.

Gamma irradiation can be successfully applied to a variety of foods, including fresh fruits and vegetables, with virtual complete elimination of viable bacteria and no health hazard to the patient.[77] Although currently infrequently used, irradiation has the potential to allow a much more liberal diet for the immunocompromised patient.

Plants and fresh flowers

It is well established that plants and fresh flowers carry microbial flora that are pathogenic for the immunocompromised host. Kates et al.[78] examined the microbial flora of vase water from cut flowers obtained from hospital environments, restaurants, and flowers grown in private gardens. A total of 41 different bacterial species were identified, including many common nosocomial bacterial species. Overall, 90% of the isolated organisms were known as causative agents of infection. High levels of resistance to multiple antimicrobials were found in the organisms irrespective of their source, indicating that multiple-resistant microbial flora found in vase water is indigenous to flowers, rather than originating from the healthcare environment.

The colony count of water from vases rose steadily over time. The authors postulated that the hands of healthcare personnel becoming transiently colonized while changing vase water could serve as a potential source for infection. Their recommendations therefore are reasonable; ban flowers from high-risk areas, such as cancer wards and burn units, designate the handling of flowers to support staff with no patient contact or when this is not feasible, wear gloves when handling flowers, wash hands after contact with plant material, change the vase water at least every 48 hours, dispose vase water into designated sinks that are not in the immediate environment of the patient, and thoroughly disinfect vases after use.

Potted plants also carry gram-negative rods as normal flora.[79] However, they would seem to pose less risk of transmission because no large water reservoir exists and less manipulation is involved. The immunocompromised patient, nevertheless, should avoid direct contact with living potted plants of any type.

Visitors

The healthcare team should ensure that visitors are properly screened for infections and instructed about the importance of proper infection control precautions, especially proper handwashing in advance of interacting with the patient. All visitors should be instructed to follow the same standard precautions as healthcare workers.[59] Visitors who are currently suffering either from a diagnosed illness that is communicable by airborne, droplet nuclei, or contact routes, or who have symptoms of upper respiratory infection or diarrhea should be discouraged from visiting the patient. If visitation does take place, appropriate precautions should be employed.[59]

Copyright © 2005, Association for Professionals in Infection Control and Epidemiology, Inc.

Pediatric visitors may carry and transmit disease unknowingly,[80] and thus it is advisable that visitors under the age of 12 years be permitted only with physician approval, even if they appear healthy. Children should be screened for known illness or exposure in the previous 4 weeks to: varicella, rubella, rubeola, mumps, hepatitis A, group A streptococcal pharyngitis, pertussis, viral respiratory infection, undifferentiated diarrhea, vomiting, fever, rash, or live virus immunization (MMR or polio).[81] Patients should wash hands carefully after interaction with any pediatric visitors.

Pets

Pet therapy has been advocated as psychologically beneficial to hospitalized patients.[82, 83] However, pets in the hospital setting pose potential serious infection control hazards because of the number of microorganisms that may be transmitted to humans (Table 15–6).[84]

If pets are allowed to visit a patient, the pet should be housebroken (i.e., no puppies or kittens), tame, docile, clean, up to date on all vaccinations, and pronounced disease free by a veterinarian.[82]

Certain circumstances argue against allowing pet visitation. Patients who have had a splenectomy are at high risk for invasive infection by *Capnocytophaga canimorsus*, a gram-negative bacterium that is part of the normal oral flora of dogs. Because pets can act as fomites for the transmission of bacteria between patients, patients who are placed in contact isolation should not be allowed to interact with animals. Some animals pose an unacceptable risk of diseases, such as rabies (skunks, raccoons, and bats) or *Salmonella* carriage (turtles), and should not routinely be part of a pet therapy program. As a result of asymptomatic urinary excretion of *Leptospira* spp. (dogs and others) and lymphocytic choriomeningitis virus (mice and hamsters), careful hand cleansing is necessary after exposure to the urine of these animals.[85]

Table 15-6. Diseases Transmitted from Pets (Goldstein)

Infectious Disease	Cats	Dogs	Birds	Rodents	Rabbits
Anthrax (*Bacillus anthracis*)	X	X			
Bartonella spp.	X				
Brucella spp.		X			
Campylobacter spp.	X	X			
Cryptosporidium	X	X			
Dirofiliriasis		X			
Echinococcosis		X			
Erysipeloid (*Erysipelothrix rhusiopathiae*			X		
Histoplasma capsulatum	X	X			
Leptospira spp.		X		X	
Listeria monocytogenes		X	X		X
Murine typhus (*Rickettsia typhi*)			X		
Ornithosis (*Chlamydia psittaci*)			X		
Lymphocytic choriomeningitis virus				X	
Mycobacterium marinum					X
Pasteurella multocida	X	X			
Plague (*Yersinia pestis*)		X		X	X
Q fever (*Coxiella burnetti*)		X			
Rabies	X	X			
Rat bite fever (*Streptobacillus moniliformis*)				X	
Rickettsia rickettsii		X			
Salmonella spp.	X	X	X	X	X
Toxocariasis	X	X			
Tularemia (*Francisella tularensis*)	X	X	X		X
Viral encephalitis			X		
Yersiniosis (Yersinia spp.)		X		X	

Copyright © 2005, Association for Professionals in Infection Control and Epidemiology, Inc.

Table 15-7. Dormant Organisms and Their Geographical Distribution

Organism	Distribution
Mycobacterial	
M. tuberculosis	Worldwide, especially in urban centers and developing countries
M. avium complex	Ubiquitous
Fungal	
Histoplasma capsulatum	Central river valleys of U.S.
Coccidioides immitis	Desert southwest
Blastomyces dermatiditis	Mississippi and Ohio river basins
Pneumocystis jiroveci	Worldwide distribution
Penicillium marneffei	Southeast Asia
Bacterial	
Pseudomonas pseudomallei	Southeast Asia, south pacific
Protozoal	
Strongyloides stercoralis	Tropics and southern U.S.
Toxoplasma gondii	Worldwide
Viral	
Herpes group viruses	Worldwide
JC papovavirus	Worldwide

Prophylaxis against the emergence of endogenous infections

A variety of organisms have the capacity to establish latency within the body once an infection has been established. This establishment may occur with symptomatic clinical illness (i.e., primary varicella, herpes simplex, others) or without clinical illness (i.e., *M. tuberculosis, P. jiroveci*). Some clinically apparent infections become latent and reactivate during immune compromise. Table 15–7 lists the most important microorganisms that establish latency, as well as their geographic distribution. Some agents can be detected serologically (*C. immitis, T. gondii*) or by skin testing (*M. tuberculosis*). Under certain circumstances it is appropriate to offer prophylaxis against these infections to reduce the incidence of their reactivation to cause clinical disease.

IV.   SUMMARY AND CONCLUSIONS

Care of the immunocompromised host poses tremendous challenges. Those challenges include identification of the compromised patient and determining their net state of immunosuppression, anticipating the microbial pathogens of unique concern for their type of immune deficit, augmenting their innate resistance to opportunistic infection, and early identification of infection such that appropriate therapy can be instituted. The infection control issues include both prevention of acquisition of potential pathogens as well as prevention of reactivated infection from affecting other individuals. New therapies continue to evolve, and novel pathogens continue to be discovered.[86, 87] Well-supported

guidelines now exist for care of patients in a variety of circumstances as described previously. Optimal approaches to other circumstances are yet to be defined completely, leading to the need for extrapolation and use of clinical experience. Effective methods for overcoming such obstacles as emerging drug resistance and failure of HCW to adhere to basic hygiene techniques also remain. Cost-effectiveness and appropriate situations for healthcare delivery will be additional areas of study.

Treatment decisions often need to be made in situations where no formal guidelines yet exist. In such situations, the recommendations discussed herein are reasonable based on the literature that currently exists. In the individual patient they should be applied carefully, taking into consideration the specific situation and the net state of immunosuppression of the patient. Careful follow-up of the immunocompromised patient is important because infection can become fulminant.

V.   FUTURE TRENDS/RESEARCH

Probiotics

The term *probiotics* refers to the medicinal use of viable organisms to restore microbial balance within a host. The Food and Agriculture Organization (FAO) of the United Nations and the World Health Organization (WHO) have stated that there is adequate scientific evidence to indicate that there is potential for probiotics to provide health benefits and that specific strains are safe for human use.[88] Whereas the comprehensive review of the literature by the FAO and WHO demonstrated a relatively small number of areas in which probiotics have proven antidisease effects, preliminary investigations have been promising for their use in enhancing mucosal immunity, treatment of surgical wound infection, reduction in the incidence of certain malignancies, and reducing the duration of diarrhea. The interested reader is referred to the review by Reid[89] as well as the online posting of the Working Group report of the FAO and WHO for a discussion of the potentials of this modality.[88]

Vaccinations

Tremendous advances in vaccine technology have been made in the past decade. And although many of these advances have been directed toward the traditional definition of a vaccine, namely the prevention of an infectious disease, new technologies have extended the scope of vaccinations to include both prevention and treatment of autoimmune diseases and malignancy. Additionally, vaccination as part of a therapeutic strategy for established infection, cancer, autoimmune disease, and allergy is now on the horizon. The implications of this line of research for

APIC Text of Infection Control and Epidemiology

Copyright © 2005, Association for Professionals in Infection Control and Epidemiology, Inc.

the immunocompromised patient are immeasurable. A detailed discussion of these issues provides fascinating reading.[90]

Irradiation of Food Products

Despite ongoing efforts of public health agencies and food growers, processors and manufacturers to reduce the risk of foodborne diseases, every year in the United States foodborne diseases cause approximately 76 million illnesses, 225,000 hospitalizations, and 5,000 deaths.[91] A substantial portion of those illnesses are borne by immunocompromised patients. Food irradiation or "cold pasteurization" of solid foods with low doses of γ rays, X rays, and electrons can effectively control bacterial and parasitic pathogens even at extremely low levels of contamination.[77, 91] Consumption of foods prepared in these ways has been shown to be safe.[77] Despite this, food irradiation for the general public or for the immunocompromised host has yet to be embraced fully. This is an area for which sound scientific basis for proceeding already exists. Thus, the major impediment to its use is education of healthcare providers as well as the general public.

REFERENCES

1. Fishman JA, Rubin RH: Infection in organ-transplant recipients, N Engl J Med 338:1741–1751, 1998.
2. Rubin RH, Greene R: Clinical approach to the compromised host with fever and pulmonary infiltrates. In Rubin RH, Young LS, editors: Clinical approach to infection in the compromised host, ed 4, New York, 2002, Kluwer Academic, pp 111–162.
3. American College of Physicans Task Force on Adult Immunization. Guide for adult immunization, ed 3, Philadelphia, 1994, American College of Physicians.
4. Murin S, Bilello KS, Matthay R: Other smoking-affected pulmonary diseases, Clin Chest Med 21:121–137, 2000.
5. Tuazon CU, Sheagren JN: Increased rate of carriage of Staphylococcus aureus among narcotic addicts, J Infect Dis 129:725–727, 1974.
6. Marti A, Marcos A, Martinez JA: Obesity and immune function relationships, Obes Rev 2:131–140, 2001.
7. MacGregor RR: Alcohol and immune defense, J Am Med Assoc 256:1474–1479, 1986.
8. Szabo G: Alcohol's contribution to compromised immunity, Alcohol Health Res World 21:30–41, 1997.
9. Walker PF, Jaranson J: Refugee and immigrant health care, Med Clin North Am 83(4):1103–1120, 1999.
10. Mayhall CG: The epidemiology of burn wound infections: then and now, Clin Infect Dis 37:543–550, 2003.
11. Leibovitz A, Dan M, Zinger J, et al: Pseudomonas aeruginosa and the oropharyngeal ecosystem of tube fed patients, Emerg Infect Dis 9:956–959, 2003.
12. Tablan OC, Anderson LJ, Arden NH, et al: Guideline for prevention of nosocomial pneumonia, Infect Control Hosp Epidemiol 15:587–627, 1994.
13. Eisenberg DM: Advising patients who seek alternative medical therapies, Ann Intern Med 127:61–69, 1997.
14. Centers for Disease Control and Prevention. Guidelines for the prevention of intravascular catheter-related infections, MMWR 51/ RR-10:1–32, 2002.
15. McGee DC, Gould MK: Preventing complications of central venous catheterization, N Engl J Med 348:1123–1133, 2003.
16. McConnell SA, Gubbins PO, Anaissie EJ: Do antimicrobial–impregnated central venous catheters prevent catheter related bloodstream infections? Clin Infect Dis 37:65–72, 2003.
17. Schaffner A: Pretransplant evaluation for infections in donors and recipients of solid organs, Clin Infect Dis 33(suppl 1):S9-S14, 2001.
18. Hornick RB, Musik SI, Wenzel R, et al: The Broad Street Pump revisited: response to volunteers to ingested cholera vibrios, Bull N Y Acad Med 47:1181, 1971.
19. Giannella RA, Broitman SA, Zamcheck N: Influence of gastric acidity on bacterial and parasitic enteric infections: a perspective, Ann Intern Med 78:271, 1973.
20. Littman A: Potent acid reduction and risk of enteric infection, Lancet 335:222, 1990.
21. Wingate DL: Acid reduction and recurrent enteritis, Lancet 335:222, 1990.
22. Howden CW, Hunt RH: Relationship between gastric secretion and infection, Gut 28:96–107, 1987.
23. Larner AJ, Hamilton MI: Review article: infective complications of therapeutic gastric acid inhibition, Aliment Pharmacol Ther 8(6):579–584, 1994.
24. Neal KR, Brij SO, Slack RCB, et al: Recent treatment with H2 antagonist and antibiotics and gastric surgery as risk factors for salmonella infection, Br Med J 308:176, 1994.
25. Neal KR, Scott HM, Slack RCB, et al: Omeprazole as risk factor for Campylobacter gastroenteritis: a case control study, Br Med J 312:414–415, 1996.
26. Driks MR, Craven DE, Celli BR, et al: Nosocomial pneumonia in intubated patients given sucralfate as antacids or histamine type 2 blockers, N Engl J Med 317:1376–1382, 1987.
27. Niederman MS, Craven DE: Editorial response: devising strategies for preventing nosocomial pneumonia: should we ignore the stomach? Clin Infect Dis 24:320–323, 1997.
28. Cook DJ, Reeve BK, Guyatt GH, et al: Stress ulcer prophylaxis in critically ill patients. Resolving discordant meta-analyses, J Am Med Assoc 275:308–314, 1996.
29. Prod'hom G, Leuenberger P, Koerfer J, et al: Nosocomial pneumonia in mechanically ventilated patients receiving antacid, ranitidine, or sucralfate ad prophylaxis for stress ulcer, Ann Intern Med 120:653–662, 1994.
30. Centers for Disease Control and Prevention. General recommendations on immunization. Recommendations of the Advisory Committee on Immunization Practices and the American Academy of Family Physicians, MMWR 51(RR-2):1–35, 2002.
31. Advisory Committee on Immunization Practices. Recommended adult immunization schedule by age group and medical conditions, United States, 2003–2004. Web site available at www.cdc.gov/nip/recs/adult-schedule.pdf
32. Shinefield H, Black S, Fattom A, et al: Use of a Staphylococcus aureus conjugate vaccine in patients receiving hemodialysis, N Engl J Med 346:491–496, 2002.
33. Cryz SJ, Wedgwood J, Lang AB, et al: Immunization of non-colonized cystic fibrosis patients against Pseudomonas aeruginosa, J Infect Dis 169:1159–1161, 1994.
34. Stutz P, Liehl E: Lipid A analogs aimed at preventing the detrimental effects of endotoxin, Infect Dis Clin North Am 5:847–873, 1991.
35. Campbell WN, Hendrix E, Cryz S, et al: Immunogenicity of a 24 valent Klebsiella capsular polysaccharide vaccine and an eight valent Pseudomonas O-polysaccharide conjugate vaccine administered to victims of acute trauma, Clin Infect Dis 23:179–181, 1996.
36. Hibberd PL, Rubin RH: Immunization strategies for the immunocompromised host: the need for immunoadjuvants, Ann Intern Med 110:955–956, 1989.
37. Avery RK, Ljungman P: Prophylactic measures in the solid organ recipient before transplantation, Clin Infect Dis 33(suppl 1):S15-S21, 2001.
38. Centers for Disease Control and Prevention. Guidelines for preventing opportunistic infections among hematopoietic stem cell transplant recipients. Recommendations of CDC, the Infectious Disease Society of America, and the American Society of Blood and Marrow Transplantation, MMWR 49:1–125, 2000.
39. Duchini A, Goss JA, Karpen S, et al: Vaccinations for adult solid-organ transplant recipients: current recommendations and protocols, Clin Microbiol Rev 16:357–363, 2003.
40. Dwyer JM: Manipulating the immune system with immune globulin, N Engl J Med 326:107–116, 1992.
41. Siber GR, Snydman DR: Use of immune globulins in the prevention and treatment of infections. In Remington JS, Swartz MN, editors: Current clinical topics in infectious diseases, vol 12, Boston, 1992, Blackwell Scientific, pp 208–256.

Copyright © 2005, Association for Professionals in Infection Control and Epidemiology, Inc.

42. Baker CJ, Melish ME, Hall RT, et al: Intravenous immune globulin for the prevention of nosocomial infection in low birth weight neonates, *N Engl J Med* 327:213–219, 1992.

43. Cometta A, Baumgartner JD, Lee WL, et al: Prophylactic intravenous administration of standard immune globulins compared with core lipopolysaccharides in patients at high risk of post surgical infection, *N Engl J Med* 327:234–240, 1992.

44. Pocecco M, DeCampo C, Cantoni L, et al: Effect of high doses of intravenous IgG in newly diagnosed diabetic children, *Helv Paediatr Acta* 42:289–295, 1987.

45. Heinze E, Thon A, Vetter U, et al: Gamma globulin therapy in 6 newly diagnosed diabetic children, *Acta Pediatr Scand* 74:605–606, 1985.

46. Leong GM, Thayer Z, Antony G, et al: High dose intravenous immunoglobulin therapy for insulin dependent diabetes mellitus. In Imbach P, editor: *Immunotherapy with intravenous immunoglobulins,* London, 1991, Academic Press, pp 269–282.

47. Buckley RH, Schiff RI: The use of intravenous immune globulin in immunodeficiency diseases, *N Engl J Med* 325:110–117, 1991.

48. Yap PL: Prevention of infection in patients with B cell defects: focus on intravenous immunoglobulin, *Clin Infect Dis* 33(suppl):S80-S89, 1993.

49. Winston DJ, Winston GH, Howell CL, et al: Cytomegalovirus infection associated with leukocyte transfusions, *Ann Intern Med* 93:671–675, 1980.

50. Lucas KG: Another look at granulocyte transfusions in neutropenic patients with cancer, *Infect Med* 13:79–92, 1996.

51. Hoelzer D: Hematopoietic growth factors—not whether but when and where, *N Engl J Med* 336:1822–1824, 1997.

52. American Society of Clinical Oncology. Update of recommendations for the use of hematopoietic colony stimulating factors: evidence based clinical practice guidelines, *J Clin Oncol* 14:1957–1960, 1996.

53. Mitchell PL, Morland B, Stevens MC, et al: Granulocyte colony stimulating factor in established febrile neutropenia: a randomized study of pediatric patients, *J Clin Oncol* 15:1163–1170, 1997.

54. Bennett CL, Smith TJ, Weeks JC, et al: Use of hematopoietic colony stimulating factors: the American Society of Clinical Oncology survey, *J Clin Oncol* 14:2511–2520, 1996.

55. Dale DC: Potential role of colony stimulating factors in the prevention and treatment of infectious diseases, *Clin Infect Dis* 18(suppl 2):S180-S188, 1994.

56. Nelson S: Role of granulocyte colony stimulating factor in the immune response to acute bacterial infection in the non-neutropenic host: an overview, *Clin Infect Dis* 18(suppl 2):S197-S204, 1994.

57. Alcid DV, Mathew P: Colony stimulating factors in the therapeutic approach to sepsis, *Curr Infect Dis Rep* 1:218–223, 1999.

58. Ballow M: Symposium. Future directions of cytokine and immunoglobulin therapy, *Clin Immunol Immunopathol* 62(1):SS1–2, 1992.

59. Garner JS and the Hospital Infection Control Practice Advisory Committee. Guideline for isolation precautions in hospitals, *Infect Control Hosp Epidemiol* 17:54–80, 1996.

60. Centers for Disease Control and Prevention. Guideline for Hand Hygiene in Health Care Settings. Recommendations of the Healthcare infection control practices advisory committee and the HICPAC/SHEA/APIC/IDSA Hand hygiene task force, *MMWR* 51(RR-16):1–48, 2002.

61. Pittet D, Mourouga P, Perneger TV, et al: Compliance with handwashing in a teaching hospital, *Ann Intern Med* 130:126–130, 1999.

62. Boyce JM: It is time for action: improving hand hygiene in hospitals, *Ann Intern Med* 130:153–154, 1999.

63. Nauseef WM, Maki DG: A study of the value of simple protective isolation in patients with granulocytopenia, *N Engl J Med* 304:448, 1981.

64. Pizzo PA: Considerations for the prevention of infectious complications in patients with cancer, *Rev Infect Dis* 11(suppl):S1551-S1563, 1989.

65. Pizzo PA: Empirical therapy and prevention of infection in the immunocompromised host. In Mandell GL, Bennett JE, Dolin R, editors: *Principles and practice of infectious diseases,* ed 5, Philadelphia, 2000, Churchill Livingstone, pp 3102–3112.

66. Hughes WT, Armstrong D, Bodey GP, et al: 2002 Guidelines for the use of antimicrobial agents in neutropenic patients with cancer, *Clin Infect Dis* 34:730–751, 2002.

67. Weber SG, Gold HS, Hooper DC, et al: Fluoroquinolones and the risk for methicillin resistant *Staphylococcus aureus* in hospitalized patients, *Emerg Infect Dis* 9:1415–1422, 2003.

68. Zervos MJ, Hershberger E, Nicolau DP, et al: Relationship between fluoroquinolone use and changes in susceptibility to fluoroquinolones of selected pathogens in 10 United States teaching hospitals, 1991–2000, *Clin Infect Dis* 37:1643–1648, 2003.

69. Hughes WT, Armstrong D, Bodey GP, et al: 1997 Guidelines for the use of antimicrobial agents in neutropenic patients with unexplained fever, *Clin Infect Dis* 25:551–573, 1997.

70. Centers for Disease Control and Prevention. Guidelines for prevention of nosocomial pneumonia, *MMWR* 46(RR-1):1–78, 1997.

71. Weber DJ, Rutala WA: The environment as a source of nosocomial infections. In Wenzel RP, editor: *Prevention and control of nosocomial infections,* ed 4, Philadelphia, 2003, Lippincott Williams & Wilkins, pp 575–597.

72. Remington JS, Schimpf SC: Please don't eat the salads, *N Engl J Med* 304:433–435, 1981.

73. Shooter RA, Faiers MC, Cooke EM, et al: Isolation of *Escherichia coli, Pseudomonas aeruginosa* and *Klebsiella* from food in hospitals, canteens and schools, *Lancet* 2:390–392, 1971.

74. Wade JC: Epidemiology and prevention of infection in the compromised host. In Rubin RH, Young LS, editors: *Clinical approach to infection in the compromised host,* ed 3, New York, 1994, Plenum Medical, pp 5–32.

75. Buckner CD, Clift RA, Sanders JE, et al: Protective environment for marrow transplant recipients: a prospective study, *Ann Intern Med* 89:893–901, 1978.

76. Casewell M, Philips I: Food as a source of *Klebsiella* species for colonization and infection of intensive care patients, *J Clin Pathol* 31:845–849, 1978.

77. Monk JD, Beuchat LR, Doyle MP: Irradiation inactivation of food borne microorganisms, *J Food Prot* 58:197–208, 1995.

78. Kates SG, McKinley KJ, Larson EL, et al: Indigenous multiresistant bacteria from flowers in hospital and nonhospital environments, *Am J Infect Control* 19:156–161, 1991.

79. Siegman-Igra Y, Shalem A, Berger SA, et al: Should potted plants be removed from hospital wards? *J Hosp Hyg* 7:82–85, 1986.

80. Goldwater PN, Martin AJ, Ryan B, et al: A survey of nosocomial respiratory viral infections in a children's hospital: occult respiratory infection in patients admitted during an epidemic season, *Infect Control Hosp Epidemiol* 12:231–238, 1991.

81. Ford-Jones EL: The special problems of nosocomial infection in the pediatric patient. In Wenzel RP, editor: *Prevention and control of nosocomial infections,* ed 2, Baltimore, 1993, Williams & Wilkins, pp 812–896.

82. Westbrook GJ, Katz S: Pet-facilitated therapy programs: planning considerations and risk-minimizing procedures, *Clin Manag* 5:26–28, 1985.

83. Anon: Hospital dogs raise spirits, not infection rates, *Hosp Infect Control* 12:162–164, 1992.

84. Goldstein EJC: Household pets and human infections, *Infect Dis Clin North Am* 5:117–130, 1991.

85. Rhame FS: The inanimate environment. In Bennett JV, Brachman PS, editors: *Hospital infections,* ed 3, Boston, 1992, Little, Brown, pp 299–333.

86. Relman DA: Detection and identification of previously unrecognized microbial pathogens, *Emerg Infect Dis* 4:382–389, 1998.

87. Drosten C, Gunther S, Preiser W, et al: Identification of a novel coronavirus in patients with severe acute respiratory syndrome, *N Engl J Med* 348:1967–1976, 2003.

88. Food and Agriculture Organization of the United Nations and World Health Organization. 2001 posting date. Regulatory and clinical aspects of dairy probiotics. Food and Agriculture Organization of the United Nations and World Health Organization Expert Consultation Report. Food and Agriculture Organization of the United Nations and World Health Organization Working Group report. Accessed November 18, 2004: http://www.fao.org/es/ESN/food/foodandfood_probiocons_en.stm

89. Reid G, Jass J, Sebulsky MT, et al: Potential uses of probiotics in clinical practice, *Clin Microbiol Rev* 16:658–672, 2003.

90. Ellis RW: Technologies for making new vaccines. In Plotkin SA, Orenstein WA, editors: *Vaccines,* ed 4, Philadelphia, 2004, WB Saunders, pp 1177–1198.

91. Osterholm MT: Food irradiation: something every clinician should know, *Infect Dis News* 4, 2000.

Copyright © 2005, Association for Professionals in Infection Control and Epidemiology, Inc.

SUPPLEMENTAL RESOURCES

Van Der Meer JWM: Defects in host defense mechanisms. In Rubin RH, Young LS, editors: *Clinical approach to infection in the compromised host,* ed 3, New York, 1994, Plenum Medical, pp 33–66.

Tramont EC, Hoover DL: Innate (general or nonspecific) host defense mechanisms. In Mandell GL, Bennett JE, Dolin R, editors: *Principles and practice of infectious diseases,* ed 5, Philadelphia, 2000, Churchill Livingstone, pp 31–38.

Kotb M, Caladra T, editors: *Cytokines and chemokines in infectious diseases handbook,* Totowa, NJ, 2003, Humana Press.

Raoult D, Foucault C, Brouqui P: Infections in the homeless, *Lancet Infect Dis* 1:77–84, 2001.

Keusch GT: Nutrition-infection interactions. In Guerrant RL, Walker DH, Weller PF, editors: *Tropical infectious diseases,* Philadelphia, 1999, Churchill Livingstone, pp 62–75.

Rubin RH, Young LS, editors: *Clinical approach to infection in the compromised host,* ed 4, New York, 1988, Kluwer Academic.

Shamsuddin HH, Diekema DJ: Opportunistic infections in hematopoietic transplant recipients. In Wenzel RP, editor: *Prevention and control of nosocomial infections,* ed 4, Philadelphia, 2003, Lippincott Williams & Wilkins, pp 385–412.

Andrews T, Sullivan KE: Infections in patients with inherited defects in phagocytic function, *Clin Microbiol Rev* 16:597–621, 2003.

McCullough J: Progress toward a pathogen free blood supply, *Clin Infect Dis* 37:88–95, 2003.

Copyright © 2005, Association for Professionals in Infection Control and Epidemiology, Inc.

Clinical Microbiology

Jaime Ritter, MPH, MT(ASCP), CIC
Infection Control Specialist
CR Bard, Inc.
Atlanta, Georgia

ABSTRACT

Clinical microbiology is the branch of science that is concerned with the study of microorganisms that produce disease, the response of the host to infection, and the control of infectious disease. It plays an integral role in the practice of infection control because it defines one of the major components of the disease process: the agent. Fundamental knowledge of microorganisms, their identification, their significance, and basic laboratory techniques provide the infection control practitioner (ICP) with an understanding of pathogenic organisms. This chapter includes an overview of clinical laboratory methods that are used to evaluate the presence and/or significance of microorganisms, the use of specific techniques to evaluate potential reservoirs within the facility, and methods to analyze the relatedness of microorganisms for epidemiological purposes.

Readers who desire more information regarding the technical laboratory aspects of specific organism identification are encouraged to consult the supplemental resources provided at the end of the chapter. Spending a few days in the microbiology laboratory under the direction of a certified laboratory professional is also an excellent method of developing practical knowledge.

KEY CONCEPTS

- The clinical microbiology laboratory plays an integral role in the practice of infection control.

- The clinical microbiology laboratory can provide culture information on a variety of microorganisms.

- Microorganisms of clinical significance include bacteria, fungus, viruses, and parasites.

- The presence of microorganisms in a clinical specimen does not always indicate the presence of infection.

- A variety of methods can be used to identify bacteria, fungus, and viruses.

- Antimicrobial susceptibility testing is commonly used to assist in the selection of appropriate antimicrobial therapy.

- The clinical microbiology laboratory can be useful during outbreak investigations and situations requiring environmental sampling.

Copyright © 2005, Association for Professionals in Infection Control and Epidemiology, Inc.

I. BASIC MICROBIOLOGY: THE ORGANISMS

The field of microbiology includes the study of bacteria, fungi (molds and yeasts), protozoa, viruses, and algae. The ICP is likely to encounter most types of microorganisms with the exception of algae. Most microorganisms are single cells and exhibit characteristics common to all biologic systems: reproduction, metabolism, growth, irritability, adaptability, mutation, and organization. Microorganisms are traditionally placed in their own kingdom (Protista), since they share characteristics that might cause them to be classified in both the plant and animal kingdoms.

MICROORGANISM CLASSIFICATION

Microorganisms and all other living organisms are classified as prokaryotes or eukaryotes. Prokaryotes are probably the smallest living organisms, ranging in size from 0.15 μm (mycoplasmas) to about 2.0 μm (many of the bacteria). Prokaryotic cells are different from eukaryotic cells in that they have no distinct membrane around their nuclear DNA. The characteristics of prokaryotic cells apply to bacteria and cyanobacteria (formerly known as blue-green algae), as well as rickettsiae, chlamydiae, and mycoplasmsas.

Eukaryotic cells are generally larger and more complex than prokaryotic cells. They contain a distinct nucleus and organelles (compartments for localizing metabolic function). Eukaryotes include microorganisms such as fungi, protozoa, and simple algae.

Viruses and subparticles such as prions are considered neither prokaryotes nor eukaryotes because they lack the characteristics of living things, except the ability to replicate (which they accomplish only in living cells).

Classification Schemes

The subgrouping of microorganisms is based ideally on evolutionary lines of descent. Traditionally these have been inferred on the basis of morphologic or biochemical characteristics. Schemes have recently been revised based on the degree of genetic (DNA, RNA) similarity between different species. Using the example of *Escherichia coli,* the groupings (from most to least inclusive) are as follows:

1. Kingdom: Procaryotae (includes all bacteria)

2. Division: Protophyta

3. Class: Schizomycetes

4. Order: Eubacteriales

5. Family: Enterobacteriaceae

6. Genus: *Escherichia*

7. Species: *coli*

Genus and species are of primary importance in designating a microorganism. The correct format for naming an organism is genus (capitalized, italicized, or underlined), species (lowercase, italicized, or underlined): *Escherichia coli* (abbreviation, *E. coli*).

BACTERIA

Cell Structure

Internal Structures

Bacteria are very small, relatively simple, single-celled organisms. They contain a single long circular molecule of double-stranded DNA. This "bacterial chromosome" is not surrounded by a nuclear envelope and is attached to the plasma membrane. In addition to the bacterial chromosome, bacteria often contain small circular, double-stranded DNA molecules called plasmids. While plasmids are not necessary for cell survival they may carry genes for activities such as antibiotic resistance, production of toxins, and synthesis of enzymes. Plasmids can be transferred from one bacterium to another and genes may move from plasmid to chromosome. These genes are called transposable genetic elements or transposons. Bacteria also contain ribosomes which function as the site of protein synthesis. The plasma membrane encloses the cytoplasm of the cell and provides selective permeability for nutrients to enter.

When essential nutrients are depleted, certain gram-positive bacteria (e.g., *Clostridium* and *Bacillus*), form "resting" cells called endospores. These endospores contain condensed nuclear material and protein and can survive extreme heat, lack of water, and exposure to toxic chemicals. When growth conditions permit, the cell will germinate into a dividing bacterium.

External Structures

The cell wall of bacteria is a complex, semi-rigid structure responsible for the shape of the cell. It surrounds the underlying, fragile plasma membrane and protects it and the interior of the cell from the environment. The cell wall is made up of a macromolecular network called peptidoglycan. In most gram-positive bacteria the cell wall consists of many layers of peptidoglycan forming a thick rigid structure. By contrast, gram-negative cell walls contain only one (or very few) layers of peptidoglycan. Gram-negative cells possess an outer membrane that is composed of lipoproteins, lipopolysaccharides, and phospholipids. This outer membrane helps some organisms evade phagocytosis, provides a barrier to certain antibiotics, and confers properties of

Copyright © 2005, Association for Professionals in Infection Control and Epidemiology, Inc.

virulence (endotoxins). Glycocalyx is a general term used for substances that surround cells. Its chemical composition can vary widely. If this substance is organized and firmly attached to the cell wall it is described as a capsule. Capsules may contribute to bacterial virulence and may offer protection from phagocytosis. If the glycocalyx is unorganized and only loosely attached to the cell wall it is described as a slime layer.

Some bacteria have flagella which are long filamentous appendages that can propel the cell. Many gram-negative bacteria possess hair-like appendages that are used for attachment rather than for motility. These are divided into two types, fimbriae and pili. Fimbriae enable a bacterial cell to adhere to surfaces (including other cells) while pili join bacterial cells in preparation for the transfer of DNA from one cell to another.

Size, Shape, and Arrangement of Bacterial Cells

There are many sizes and shapes among bacteria. Most range from 0.2 μm to 2.0 μm in diameter and 2 μm to 8 μm in length. They have a few basic shapes: spherical coccus (pleural: cocci), rod-shaped bacillus (pleural: bacilli), and spiral. Cocci are usually round but can sometimes be irregularly shaped. Cocci that remain in pairs after dividing are called diplococci; those that remain attached in a chain are called streptococci; and those that remain attached in clusters or broad sheets are called staphylococci. Most bacilli appear as single rods and are fairly uniform in shape. However, some bacilli are oval and look so much like cocci they are called coccobacilli. Spiral bacteria have one or more twists. Bacteria that look like curved rods are called vibrios; others that look like a corkscrew and have a fairly rigid structure are called spirilla; and those that are helical and flexible are called spirochetes. (See Fig. 16–1.)

Bacterial Replication

Bacteria normally reproduce by binary fission. The rate of replication can vary from rapid to slow. For example, E. coli may divide every 15 minutes while Myobacterium tuberculosis may replicate every 12 to 24 hours. The first step in division is cell elongation and replication of chromosomal DNA. The cell wall and cell membrane begin to grow inward from all sides. Eventually the in-growing cell walls meet, forming a cross wall (septation) and two individual cells are formed. These "daughter cells" are essentially identical to the parent cell.

However, it is possible for bacteria to change through either genetic recombination or mutation. Genetic recombination refers to the exchange of genes between two DNA molecules to form a new combination of genes on a chromosome. Exchange of genes happens in one of three ways.

(1) Transformation occurs when genes are transferred from one bacterium to another as "naked" DNA in the environment. The transferring DNA either replaces existing chromosomal DNA or adds to plasmid DNA pool.

(2) Conjugation occurs when all or part of a plasmid is transferred from a donor to a recipient cell. The cells must be in direct contact and transfer occurs via the sex pilus. Conjugation can occur between widely separated species, leading to the rapid dissemination of genetic information (e.g., antibiotic resistance genes).

(3) Transduction occurs when bacterial DNA is transferred from a donor cell to a recipient cell inside a virus that infects bacteria, called a bacteriophage, or phage. Mutation usually results from random mistakes in DNA replication. In bacteria, the spontaneous mutation rate is thought to be about one in a billion reproductions. Many mutations are never expressed and do not significantly impact the bacteria. However, if the mutation offers some type of advantage, such as antibiotic resistance, the mutants will survive when an antibiotic is applied.

Submicroscopic Bacteria

Mycoplasma

Mycoplasmas are extremely small bacteria (0.2 μm to 0.8 μm), below the resolving power of a light microscope. They lack cell walls and are surrounded only by an outer plasma membrane. Since they lack a rigid cell wall they vary in shape and are said to be pleomorphic. Mycoplasmas can be grown on artificial media that provide them with sterols (exogenous cholesterol) and other special nutritional or physical requirements. Since colonies are extremely small, cell culture methods are often used. Organisms associated with human infection include *Mycoplasma pneumoniae* (community-acquired pneumonia), *Ureaplasma* (urinary tract infections), and *M. hominis* (wound infections).

Chlamydiae

Chlamydias are obligate intracellular parasitic bacteria. They are gram-negative coccoid organisms that range from 0.2 μm to 1.5 μm. Chlamydiae display a growth cycle that takes place in host cells. The bacteria invade the cells and differentiate into dense bodies called reticulated bodies. The reticulated bodies reproduce and eventually form new chlamydiae in the host cell called elementary bodies. These elementary bodies lyse the host cell and begin a new infection cycle. Organisms associated with human infection include *Chlamydia trachomatis* (male and female genital tract infection),

Copyright © 2005, Association for Professionals in Infection Control and Epidemiology, Inc.

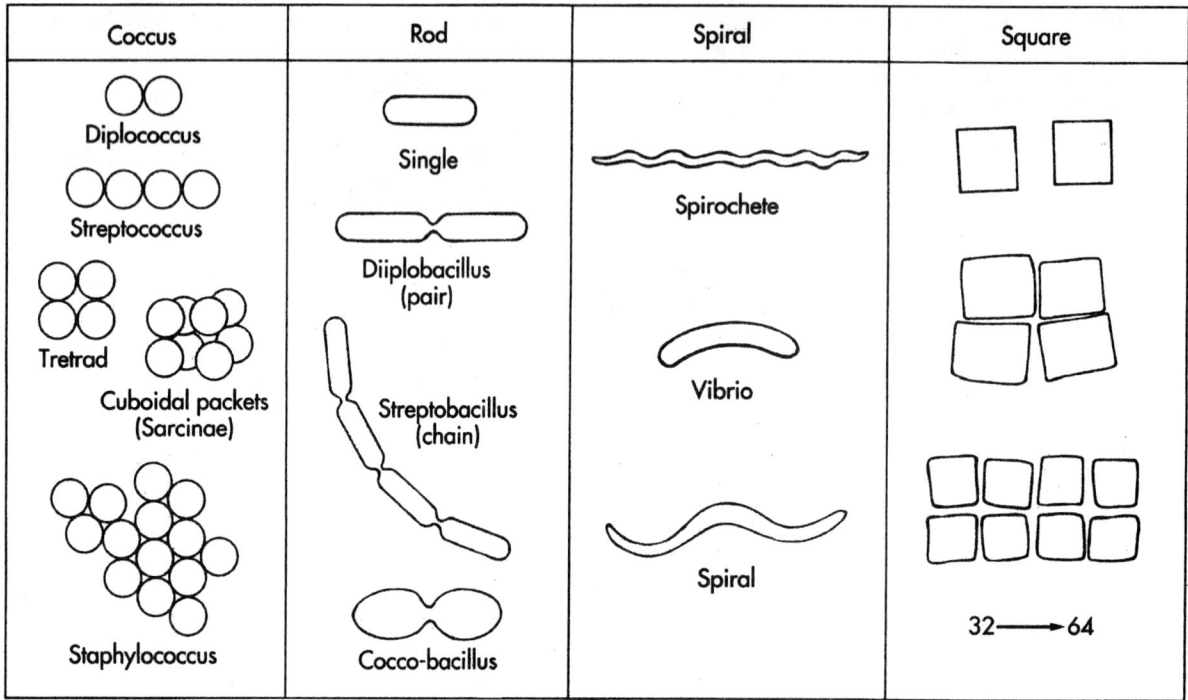

Coccus	Rod	Spiral	Square
Diplococcus	Single	Spirochete	
Streptococcus	Diiplobacillus (pair)	Vibrio	
Tretrad			
Cuboidal packets (Sarcinae)	Streptobacillus (chain)	Spiral	
Staphylococcus	Cocco-bacillus		32 —→ 64

Figure 16–1 Characteristic bacterial cell shapes and arrangements.

C. pneumoniae (atypical pneumonia), and *C. psittaci* (psittacosis).

Rickettsiae

Rickettsiae are obligate intracellular parasitic bacteria. They are gram-negative rod-shaped bacteria or cocco-bacilli (0.8 μm to 2.0 μm long) and divide by binary fission. Rickettsiae infect humans as well as arthropods such as ticks, mites, and lice. Infection is transmitted to humans through the bite of an infected insect. Culture of the organism is rarely attempted in clinical laboratories; therefore, diagnosis is usually achieved using antibody testing or immuno-fluorescent staining of tissue biopsy specimens. Organisms causing human infection include: *Rickettsia rickettsii* (Rocky Mountain Spotted Fever), *R. prowazekii* (epidemic typhus), and *Coxiella burnetti* (Q fever).

FUNGI

Fungi are eukaryotic organisms that derive nutrients from organic materials. They have a cell wall that contains chitin and lack photosynthetic capability. Some fungi are well-adapted human pathogens (e.g., *Candida albicans*). Most, however, are accidental pathogens that humans acquire through contact with decaying organic matter or airborne spores in the environment. Typically fungi are divided into two separate

groups, yeasts and molds, based on the appearance of the organisms.

Yeasts

Yeasts are single celled, microscopic, round-to-oval organisms ranging in size from 2 μm to 60 μm. They have a single nucleus with a nuclear membrane and contain organelles. They typically reproduce by a process of budding. In this process a parent cell forms a "bud" on its outer surface. As the bud elongates the parent cell's nucleus divides and one nucleus migrates into the bud. Eventually the cell wall closes between the parent cell and the bud, and the bud breaks free. Some yeasts reproduce through the process of fission, similar to bacterial reproduction. Commonly pathogenic yeasts include *Candida* species (mucositis, vaginitis, dermatitis, systemic dissemination) and *Cryptococcus neoformans* (meningitis, pneumonia in compromised hosts).

Molds

Molds consist of long, branching filaments of cells called hyphae. A tangled mass of hyphae visible to the naked eye is a mycelium. Some molds reproduce asexually by fragmentation of their hyphae. Additionally, molds may reproduce sexually and asexually by the formation of spores. Asexual spores are formed by the

APIC Text of Infection Control and Epidemiology

Copyright © 2005, Association for Professionals in Infection Control and Epidemiology, Inc.

hyphae of one organism. When these spores germinate they become organisms identical to their parent cell. Sexual spores result from fusion of nuclei from two opposite mating strains of the same species of fungus. Organisms that grow from sexual spores will have characteristics of both parental strains. Common opportunistic pathogenic molds include *Aspergillus* species (necrotizing pneumonia) and agents of mucormycosis (e.g., *Rhizopus* and *Mucor* species)

Dimorphic Fungi

Some fungi exhibit dimorphism. Such fungi can grow as either a mold or as a yeast. The mold-like forms produce vegetative and aerial hyphae; the yeast-like forms reproduce by budding. Typically, dimorphism in fungi is temperature dependent: at 37°C the fungus is yeast-like, and at 25°C it is mold-like. Common pathogenic dimorphic fungi include *Histoplasma capsulatum* (acute pulmonary histoplasmosis, disseminated infection), *Blastomyces dermatitidis* (chronic skin infections, pulmonary lesions), and *Coccidioides immitis* (respiratory tract, meningeal infection). *Pneumocystis carinii*, previously classified as a parasite, was recently reclassified as a fungus based on DNA characteristics. *P. carinii* is a major cause of pneumonia in acquired immunodeficiency syndrome (AIDS) and other immunosuppressive conditions.

VIRUSES

Viruses are obligate intracellular parasites that need living cells to grow and reproduce. Viruses are ultramicroscopic particles containing nucleic acid (either RNA or DNA) surrounded by protein, and in some cases, other components such as a membrane-like envelope. Outside the host cell, the virus particle is known as a virion. The virion is metabolically inert and does not grow or multiply. All viruses multiply in a similar fashion. Multiplication occurs in five steps.

1. Attachment. The virion attaches to a complementary receptor site on the host cell. Certain types of viruses "seek out" specific types of host cells. For example, Epstein Barr virus seeks out receptor sites on B lymphocytes.

2. Penetration. The virion enters the host cell through a process called endocytosis, an active cellular process by which nutrients and other molecules are brought into a cell.

3. Replication. Viral DNA or RNA directs the host cell to begin synthesis of viral components. "Viral" replication uses host cell ribosomes, energy sources and amino acids to produce these viral components.

4. Maturation. The viral components essentially assemble into a viral particle spontaneously; daughter virions are formed.

5. Release. The host cell lyses and the new virions are released. Some viruses will lie dormant in the host cell for months or years. After this latent period new virions form and cause damage to host cells.

Viruses are grouped into families based on nucleic acid type, strategy for replication, and morphology. A viral species is a group of viruses that share the same genetic information and ecological niche. Viral species are designated by descriptive common names based on either the organ system involved (e.g., .*Enterovirus*.), the disease produced (e.g., hepatitis A), or the area in which the disease was first recognized (e.g., Norwalk virus).

PARASITES

Human parasites vary greatly in size and complexity. They may be single-celled microscopic protozoa or complex worms over 10 feet in length. Protozoa are unicellular, free-living eukaryotic organisms. Most protozoan parasites exist in two different forms, the pleomorphic trophozoite stage (feeds, and produces effects in the host) and the cysts stage (most responsible for transmission). Other types of parasites include flukes, tapeworms, roundworms, and ectoparasites such as lice and scabies. Please refer to Chapter 94, Parasites, for more specific information.

II. CLINICAL MICROBIOLOGY

The presence and identification of organisms in a clinical specimen may be indicative of infection. The primary goals of clinical microbiology are to identify the presence of pathogenic organisms in tissues, body fluids, excretions, or secretions and to classify those pathogens to species level based on morphologic and biochemical properties. Additional goals are to predict response to antimicrobial therapy and to assist in epidemiological investigations.

MICROSCOPY

Since microorganisms are invisible to the naked eye, the essential tool in microbiology is the microscope. The microscope permits direct examination of clinical and culture materials and yields information on the presence and relative size, shape, and preliminary identification of microorganisms.

Copyright © 2005, Association for Professionals in Infection Control and Epidemiology, Inc.

Light Microscope

The most commonly used microscope in the clinical laboratory is the light microscope. It is a compound microscope because it contains two types of lenses that function to magnify an object. The lens closest to the eye is called the ocular, while the lens closest to the object is called the objective. Most microscopes of this type have four objective lenses: the scanning lens (4X magnification); the low-power lens (10X); the high-power lens (40X); and the oil emersion lens (100X). With the ocular lens that magnifies 10X, the total magnification will be 40X for the scanning lens and 1000X for the oil immersion lens. Depending on the type of light source used to illuminate the slide (specimen), the compound microscope can be used in several ways.

Bright-field microscopy uses bright light sources (usually incandescent) and is the most common type of microscopy used in the clinical lab. This is the method used to examine specimens that have been stained using the Gram stain method.

Dark-field microscopy is utilized to observe motile organisms that are not able o be stained by common methods (e.g., treponemes, *Borrelia* spp.). This type of microscopy uses a special condenser that scatters light and causes it to reflect off the specimen at an angle. Bright objects appear against a dark background and can offer better resolution than bright-field microscopy.

Phase-contrast microscopy uses a special condenser that throws light "out of phase" and causes it to pass through objects at different speeds. This type of microscopy takes advantage of the different densities of cellular elements and makes them appear to stand out from their backgrounds. Phase-contrast microscopy is typically used for examination of living cells, particularly tissue cultures for viral isolation and identification.

The fluorescent microscope employs an ultraviolet light source. This type of microscopy depends on the ability of naturally fluorescent substances or dyes to absorb energy in non-visible ultraviolet (UV) and short visible wavelengths, become excited, and emit energy in longer visible wavelengths. This method is very popular because of ease of interpretation of stained materials and the speed at which materials can be reviewed. Coupled with specific antibodies (e.g., direct or indirect fluorescent antibody, DFA or IFA, tests), rapid diagnoses of specific organisms can be made.

A fairly recent development in light microscopy is known as confocal microscopy. Specimens are stained with fluorochromes so they will emit or return light. A laser is used to illuminate the specimen. Most confocal microscopes are used in conjunction with a computer to construct three-dimensional images.

Electron Microscope

The energy source in the electron microscope is a beam of electrons produced by an electron-emitting tungsten filament. Since the beam has an extremely short wavelength, it strikes most objects in its path and increases the resolution of the microscope significantly. Viruses and some large molecules can be seen with this type of instrument. Special gold or palladium stains are used to prepare the specimens before viewing. Images are typically viewed on a computer monitor. Transmission electron microscopy (TEM) uses a finely focused beam while scanning electron microscopy (SEM) sends the beam through an electromagnetic lens that allows for three-dimensional views. Due to the significant cost of electron microscopes they are rarely used in clinical laboratories but are useful as research tools.

Specimen preparation

In order to observe clinical or culture materials through a microscope the specimen must be prepared for observation. In some cases the specimen may be placed onto a slide for direct observation. Some fungi and parasites are large and distinct enough to be examined directly (e.g., protozoa, Cryptococcus in India ink). However, most observations are made with stained preparations.

Before the microorganisms are stained they must be fixed (attached) to a microscope slide. A thin film of material is spread over the surface of a slide. This "smear" is then fixed with either heat or chemicals. Fixing the smear not only ensures that the organisms are attached to the slide but also kills the organisms making the slide safe to handle.

Staining Methods

Staining simply means coloring the microorganisms with a dye that emphasizes certain structures. Stains are usually acidic (negatively charged) or basic (positively charged) salts. Basic dyes react with nuclear cell components; acidic dyes react with cytoplasm and granules. Simple staining uses only one dye and may be used to demonstrate the shape, size, arrangement of organisms or the presence of spores. Differential staining uses two or more dyes to demonstrate shape and biochemical color reaction. Differential stains react differently with various microorganisms and thus can be used to distinguish among them. They are used to divide nearly all bacteria into major groups. The most commonly used differential stains are the Gram stain and the acid-fast stain.

Copyright © 2005, Association for Professionals in Infection Control and Epidemiology, Inc.

Gram Stain

The Gram stain was developed in 1884 by the Danish bacteriologist Hans Christian Gram. In this procedure a heat-fixed smear is covered with a basic purple dye, usually crystal violet. After a short time, the purple dye is washed off and the slide is covered with iodine (a mordant that combines with the crystal violet to intensify the stain). When the iodine is washed off, all of the bacterial cells present will be dark violet or purple. The slide is then washed with alcohol or an alcohol-acetone solution. This "decolorizing" solution causes some of the cells to loose their purple color while others maintain their color. At this point some of the cells will have no color and so a counterstain of safranin, a basic red dye, is applied to the smear. The smear is washed again and dried prior to microscopic examination.

Differences in cell-wall structure affect the retention or escape of the combination of crystal violet and iodine complex. Gram-positive bacteria have a thick peptidoglycan cell wall that does not allow the crystal violet/iodine complex to be removed during the alcohol wash. Under the microscope, gram-positive organisms will appear dark violet or purple. Gram-negative bacteria contain a layer of lipopolysaccharide as part of their cell wall. The alcohol wash disrupts this lipopolysaccharide layer and the crystal violet/iodine complex is washed out of the cell wall. As a result, gram-negative cells are colorless until counterstained with safranin. Under the microscope, gram-negative organisms appear pink or red. In addition to bacteria, many fungi and some protozoans and helminthes will stain with the Gram stain process. *Chlamydia*, *Rickettsia*, *Mycobacterium*, and *Nocardia* organisms stain poorly and may require special staining techniques for identification.

The Gram stain is an important tool for the clinical microbiologist. Gram-stain reaction, along with cell shape/arrangement, can be used to determine the type of media that should be used for culture, the appropriate identification procedures that should be done, and the types of antimicrobial testing that should be initiated. The Gram stain is important to clinicians because it may help to determine the quality of a specimen (e.g., presence of epithelial cells or polymorphonuclear leukocytes), the initial direction for therapy (empiric), or the need for isolation precautions (e.g., gram-negative diplococci in cerebrospinal fluid, suggesting meningococci).

Acid-Fast Stain

Cells of certain bacteria and parasites contain long-chain fatty acids (mycolic acids) that make them impervious to crystal violet and other basic dyes. Heat or detergents can be used to force dye into this type of cell. Once this occurs, the cell cannot be decolorized by acid-alcohol, hence the term acid-fast. Acid-fast stains are very useful in identifying *Mycobacterium* spp. (AFB, or acid-fast bacillus), as well as *Nocardia* and *Actinomyces* organisms.

Generally, one of two types of procedures is used for acid-fast stains. The Ziehl-Neelsen procedure uses the red dye carbol fuchsin as the primary stain and methylene blue as the counterstain. Acid-fast organisms will retain the carbol fuchsin and will appear red under the microscope (where the AFB nickname "red-snapper" comes from). The auramine-rhodamine method uses a fluorescent stain as the primary stain. Acid-fast organisms will fluoresce under ultraviolet light.

Miscellaneous Stains

In addition to Gram and acid-fast stains, other staining procedures can be useful in identifying the presence of specific microorganisms. Immunofluorescent staining combines an antibody directed at a specific organism with a dye that converts ultraviolet light into visible light. If the antibody binds with the organism the organism will fluoresce under the microscope. Immunofluorescent stains may be used to detect of *Chlamydia* or *Legionella* sp. from clinical specimens.

The calcofluor white stain (a nonspecific fluorochrome that binds cellulose and chitin in fungi) may be used to detect fungal elements and *Pneumocystis* cysts. The trichrome stain is useful in the identification of many fecal parasites. It is used to enhance the structures of protozoa, cysts, and some ova.

MICROBIAL GROWTH AND IDENTIFICATION

Once a specimen is received in the microbiology laboratory it is assessed for potential microbial pathogens. In most cases, the specimen is placed into or onto special media to cultivate the growth of microbes. Once the microbe grows, further test methods are used to classify/identify the organism.

Bacteria

Like most living organisms, bacteria require the proper type of nutrition, appropriate temperature, and correct atmospheric conditions. In order to cultivate the growth of bacteria, clinical specimens are placed (planted) onto media that provides the nutrients necessary for growth. The choice of media depends on the site being cultured (e.g., throat, blood, urine), the growth requirements of common or suspected pathogens, and the likelihood of normal commensal bacteria

---

Copyright © 2005, Association for Professionals in Infection Control and Epidemiology, Inc.

being present. Most growth media are in agar form (a gelatin-like substance that fills a Petri dish). There are several categories of growth media including (1) nutrient agar, a general-purpose growth medium which supports the growth of a wide variety of bacteria; (2) enrichment medium which contains special nutrients necessary for the growth of hard-to-grow (fastidious) bacteria; (3) selective media which contains chemicals or antibiotics designed to inhibit normal commensals while allowing organisms of interest to grow; and (4) differential media that promotes the differentiation of specific organisms while inhibiting others.

Once the specimen is planted, the media is incubated for at least 24 hours in a warm, moist environment. Most cultures are incubated at human body temperature (35 °C) however some are incubated at room temperature while others are incubated at 42 °C (e.g., *Campylobacter* sp.). Most specimens are incubated for a minimum of 48 hours.

Atmospheric conditions (*i.e.*, the presence or absence of oxygen) are also considered during the incubation process. Organisms that have an absolute requirement for air (oxygen gas) and will not grow in absence of oxygen are called aerobic organisms. Bacteria that grow only in complete or nearly complete absence of ambient atmospheric oxygen and are inhibited or killed by oxygen are known as obligate anaerobes. Facultative anaerobes are organisms that can use oxygen if it is present but can grow without it. Microaerophilic organisms require oxygen in concentrations of 2% to 10%, and in addition, they may also require an increased carbon dioxide concentration.

Once bacterial growth is present, further identification can take place. Initial classification of bacteria is based on Gram's stain characteristics (gram-positive versus gram-negative), morphologic features (cocci versus bacilli), and oxygen utilization. (See Fig. 16–2.) Gram-positive cocci can undergo several types of basic tests to further classify the specific organism. For example, a catalase test can be used to differentiate streptococci (negative) from staphylococci (positive) and a coagulase test can be used to differentiate *S. aureus* (positive) from other staphylococci (negative). For species level identification of gram-positive organisms, a battery of biochemical tests may need to be performed. These tests may be conducted manually (e.g., individual test tubes) or in an automated instrument (e.g., Vitek® or MicroScan®).

Gram-negative bacilli are generally grouped by their ability to ferment lactose as a nutrient. Lactose fermenting Gram-negative bacilli include the Enterobacteriaceae while non-lactose fermenting Gram-negative bacilli include *Pseudomonas* sp. as well as *Proteus* sp. As with gram-positive organisms, species level identification of gram-negative organisms requires a battery

of biochemical tests. These tests may be conducted manually (e.g., individual test tubes) or in an automated instrument (e.g., Vitek®, MicroScan®, or WalkAway®).

Fungi

Depending on the type of organism, some fungus can be identified directly from a clinical specimen. For example, a skin scraping may be directly examined for the presence of fungal hyphae (may require special staining techniques). Additionally, some yeast, especially *Candida* sp., grow on routine blood agar and require no special culture techniques. Yeasts such as *Candida* can be identified to the species level through a series of tests including germ-tube tests (positive – *C. albicans*) and sugar assimilation (done manually or in an automated instrument).

In some cases, cultures need to be done to identify and classify potential fungal pathogens. A selective media such as Sabouraud (suppresses the growth of bacteria) is generally used for culturing fungus. The specimens are usually incubated at room temperature (25° C to 30° C) for several weeks. Identification of fungal isolates is based on the appearance of the colony and on microscopic examination.

In addition to culture, other methods exist to identify the presence of certain fungus. Direct antigen detection methods (e.g., latex agglutination) may be used to identify *C. neoformans*. Serologic test methods can be used to identify coccidiomycosis, histoplasmosis, and *Aspergillus* sp.

Mycobacteria

Mycobacteria require special culture techniques to be isolated. In general, specimens undergo procedures to kill commensal bacteria that may be present (so that the mycobacteria can be isolated). Once the specimen has been processed it is planted on special media and incubated for 4 to 6 weeks. Once the organism grows further testing must be conducted to identify the species.

Since conventional culture techniques may take weeks to recover mycobacteria, other, more rapid techniques have been developed. The Bactec® method utilizes a radiometric culture technique. This technique is used not only to isolate mycobacteria from clinical specimens but also to differentiate *M. tuberculosis* complex from other mycobacteria and for antimicrobial susceptibility testing. Polymerase chain reaction (PCR) methods have also been developed. In this method, genetic chromosomal parts can be detected by DNA probes. DNA probes are usually used after the mycobacteria have been isolated from the culture.

APIC Text of Infection Control and Epidemiology

Copyright © 2005, Association for Professionals in Infection Control and Epidemiology, Inc.

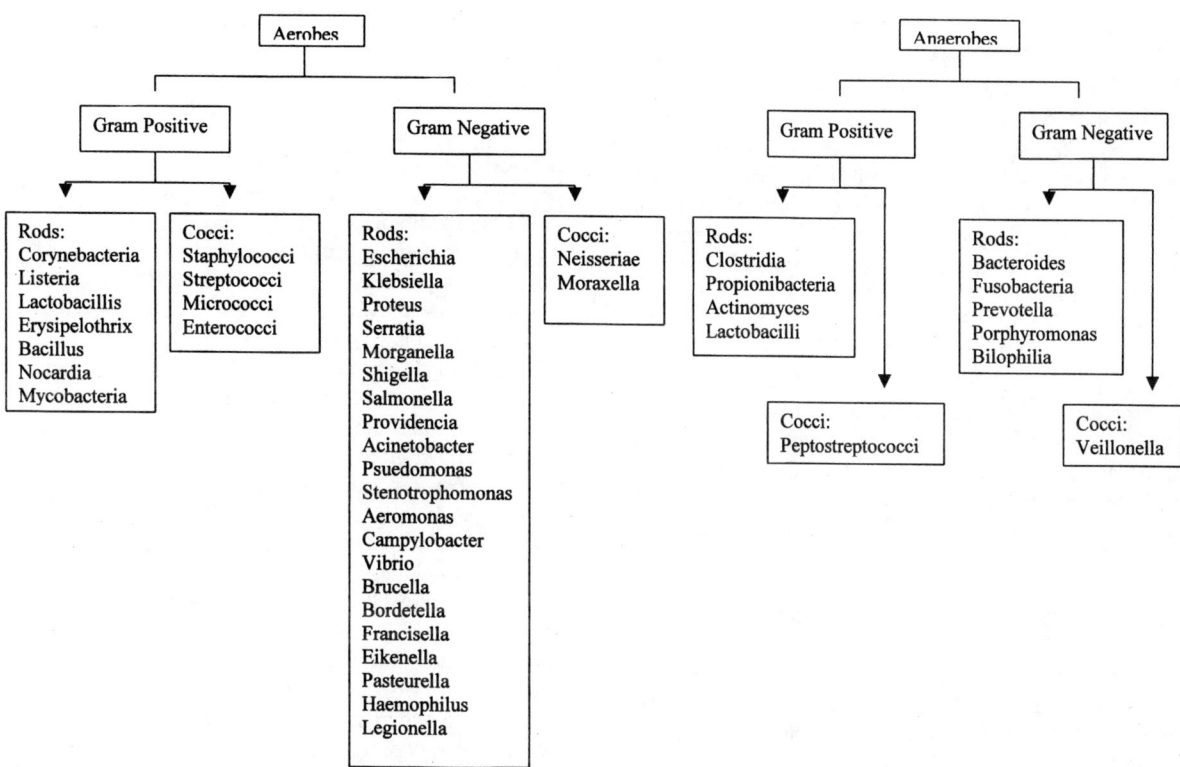

Figure 16–2   Bacteria Identification based on gram stain and cell morphology

Mycoplasma

Due to their fastidious growth requirements, *Mycoplasma* culture is rarely attempted in the clinical laboratory. *M. hominis* may be grown from wounds using special media and from blood using radiometric techniques (e.g., Bactec®). In general, serologic tests are used to diagnose *Mycoplasma* infection.

Chlamydiae

Because of their parasitic nature, Chlamydiae growth requires tissue culture and is not attempted in most laboratories. Direct-detection methods enjoy the greatest popularity for diagnosis. It is now possible to detect the antigen by direct fluorescent antibody slide staining and enzyme-linked immunosorbent assay (ELISA) technique. Invasive infection does produce an immunogenic response. Therefore, *Chlamydia* antibodies can be measured using complement fixation, microimmunofluorescence, and ELISA techniques.

Rickettsiae

Due to their parasitic nature and their host requirements, Rickettsiae are rarely cultured (never in clinical labs). Early diagnosis is usually made on clinical grounds. Currently serologic studies are the most sensitive and specific tests for detection of specific infections (i.e., Lyme disease). ELISA is the best diagnostic test and determines specific levels of antibodies (immunoglobulin M and G, IgM and IgG).

Viruses

Virus culture traditionally requires specialized media containing antibacterial and anti-fungal agents in prepared plastic or glass tubes and flasks. Clinical specimens are cultured on an array of different mammalian cell culture lines depending on the agent suspected clinically. Growth is viewed microscopically and is identified through changes in the host cells rather than as discrete viral "colonies." While tissue cultures are still considered to be the gold standard, many viral infections are diagnosed through other rapid methods. Direct detection methods include (1) electron microscopy, which is used primarily by reference laboratories; (2) ELISA for viruses such as respiratory syncytial virus (RSV), hepatitis B surface antibody, and rotavirus; (3) latex agglutination for viruses such as rotavirus and RSV; (4) DNA probes for viruses such as cytomegalovirus (CMV); and (5) polymerase chain reaction for DNA detection for viruses such as HIV types 1 and 2.

Viral infections cause an immunogenic response and therefore antibody detection methods can be useful in

---

Copyright © 2005, Association for Professionals in Infection Control and Epidemiology, Inc.

the diagnosis of infection. Simple antibody tests can determine the presence or absence of immunoglobulin (Ig). This can be used to determine if a patient has ever been infected with a specific virus (e.g., varicella, adenovirus). Complex antibody systems use a battery of viral antigens and often distinguish IgM (early) from IgG (late) antibodies which may allow conclusions regarding duration and activity of infection. For example, tests for hepatitis B include antibodies to viral surface and core materials.

Parasites

Microscopy is the cornerstone of most parasite diagnosis. Direct or concentrated examination of stool, urine, vaginal secretions, or duodenal aspirates may yield protozoans or eggs of helminths. Specific identification is based on characteristic morphologic appearance. Direct antigen detection methods have been developed for giardiasis and are widely used. Serologic tests methods may be performed when direct examination of tissue is difficult or unrevealing. These tests are usually conducted by reference laboratories and may be useful in diagnosing parasitic infections such as amebiasis, schistosomiasis, cysticercosis, echinococcosis, and malaria.

ANTIMICROBIAL SUSCEPTIBILITY TESTING

Antimicrobial therapy seeks to suppress or kill microorganisms by exploiting biochemical reactions unique to the pathogenic microbe. Ideally, this should be accomplished using the simplest agent with minimal toxicity to the patient. Testing is conducted in order to determine the best antimicrobial therapy for organisms isolated from clinical specimens. The type and extent of antimicrobial testing conducted depends on the organism isolated, the source of the culture (body site), available antimicrobial agents, and typical susceptibility patterns. One of several methods may be used for susceptibility testing.

Disk Diffusion (Kirby-Bauer Method)

A standardized suspension of bacteria is spread in a lawn fashion onto Mueller-Hinton agar. Paper disks impregnated with a standard amount of an antibiotic are placed onto the agar surface and the agar plate is incubated overnight. The zone of inhibition around the disk (area where the organism does not grow) is measured at 10 to 24 hours. Disk diffusion results are reported as susceptible, intermediate or resistant based on the size of the zone of inhibition. Standardized cutoffs for measuring susceptible, intermediate, or resistant by disk diffusion are based on organism and antibiotic.

Broth Dilution

Broth dilution test methods are used to determine the minimal concentration of antibiotic that will inhibit growth (minimal inhibitory concentration, or MIC). This method uses replicate inoculation of a standardized suspension of bacteria in broth into a series of micro-wells containing antibiotics in descending concentration. After a period of incubation, the wells are examined for bacterial growth (seen as turbidity). The first well in the series that shows no bacterial growth contains the minimum inhibitory concentration of the antibiotic that is effective against the organism. Broth dilution test results are reported in micrograms per milliliter (μg/mL). These tests can be conducted and read manually, however, most laboratories use some type of automated or computer assisted instrument. In an automated system the instrument actually reads the test results, in a computer-assisted system a technologist visually assesses bacterial growth and records the results in a computer. Both the automated and computer-assisted systems generate interpretive criteria and cumulative susceptibility profiles. While most instruments require overnight incubation of the test trays, some of the newer systems read growth photometrically and can generate results in as little as 3 to 10 hours (e.g., Vitek®, WalkAway®).

E Test

This is a newer method used for MIC testing. In this method a standardized suspension of bacteria is spread in a lawn fashion onto an agar plate. A non-porous plastic strip impregnated with continuous gradient of concentration of a specific antimicrobial is placed on the agar; the plate is incubated overnight. The strip is marked with a MIC reading scale and is read by noting the area where bacterial growth is inhibited. Results are reported as μg/mL. This test method is limited to certain antibiotics and is typically used for penicillin, ampicillin, and vancomycin.

Special Test Methods

Depending on the organism, some additional tests may be used to evaluate the potential effectiveness of antimicrobial agents. Organisms such as *Haemophilus influenzae* and *Neisseria gonorrhoeae* should be tested for beta lactamase production. Synergy testing, which is used to determine the inhibitory ability of combinations of antibiotics, is often used with *Enterococcus* sp. and *Staphylococcus* sp. Minimal bactericidal concentration (MBC) test methods are used to determine minimal concentration of antibiotic necessary to kill (not merely inhibit growth of) an organism.

Copyright © 2005, Association for Professionals in Infection Control and Epidemiology, Inc.

While MBC testing is infrequently done it may be helpful in certain clinical situations. Susceptibility testing is not commonly conducted for anaerobic organisms. If testing is required MIC agar-based or broth dilution techniques may be used. Likewise, susceptibility testing for viruses and fungi is generally performed in reference laboratories and often is not standardized. Some laboratories can provide MIC testing for *Candida* sp. for amphotericin B and fluconazole.

SPECIMEN COLLECTION AND TRANSPORT

Specimen collection and transport to the laboratory is an essential part of the culture process. Improperly selected, collected, or transported specimens can generate misleading data that may result in inappropriate patient management. In general, all specimens should be collected aseptically and placed in a sterile container. In some cases specimens may be placed directly into culture media (e.g., blood cultures, genital cultures). Special handling techniques may be necessary for some specimens such as those for anaerobic culture. Prompt delivery to the laboratory is essential to prevent the death of pathogenic organisms or the overgrowth of commensal organisms. If transport is delayed, some specimens may be refrigerated (e.g., urine, stool, sputum) while others should be maintained at room temperature (e.g., genital, eye, or spinal fluid).

Specific procedures for specimen collection and transport are institution dependent. Please refer to your institution's laboratory manual for specific procedures and protocols.

III. MICROBIAL PATHOGENESIS

NORMAL FLORA AND COLONIZATION

Microorganisms are ubiquitous in nature and are naturally present in and on our bodies. Normal microbial flora is made up of microorganisms commonly found on healthy human body surfaces. A variety of normal flora organisms can be found on different body sites (see Table 16–1). The term colonization denotes the presence of a microorganism in the absence of symptoms or deep tissue invasion. Normal flora may be described as colonization in most cases (e.g., *E. coli* colonization of stool). Potentially pathogenic organisms may exist as colonizers, which may facilitate transmission (e.g., *N. gonorrhoeae* colonization of pharynx, *Salmonella* sp. colonization of stool).

INFECTION

The term infection refers to a condition in a host resulting from the presence and invasion of microorga-

nisms. Infection implies either recovery of an organism from a normally sterile body site or the production of an inflammatory response by a microorganism. An asymptomatic infection occurs when viable organisms are present in a body site without causing any obvious symptoms (e.g., latent tuberculosis, chronic hepatitis B, latent syphilis). The immune status of the host plays a large role in determining the likely pathogenic potential of a microorganism. Infections with organisms that cause disease primarily in immunodeficient hosts are called opportunistic infections (e.g., *C. neoformans* meningitis in patients with deficient cell-mediated immunity, *Legionella pneumophila* pneumonia in patients with chronic lung disease or transplant recipients). While almost any organism can cause an infection if introduced into a normally sterile body site, certain organisms are commonly associated with specific types of infections. See Table 16–2.

SOURCES OF MICROORGANISMS

Microorganisms can come from a variety of sources. Exogenous organisms are those that come from outside of the host. Exogenous sources include other humans (e.g., *Herpes virus*, *M. tuberculosis*); foodstuffs (e.g., *Salmonella* sp.); contaminated water sources (e.g., *Giardia*, *Enterovirus*); insects (e.g., Lyme disease, malaria); animals (e.g., Brucellosis, *Pasteurella* sp.); and airborne sources (e.g., *Histoplasma*, *Legionella* sp.). Endogenous organisms are derived from the host's own microbial flora (e.g., *S. aureus* carried on skin, *E. coli* carried on the perineum). For some organisms, the distinction is not clear-cut; some pathogens may be acquired first as colonizers, only to cause disease later (e.g., Pneumococcus sp. acquired from another host first causes pharyngeal colonization and then subsequent pneumonia).

IV. ENVIRONMENTAL TESTING

Microbiologic environmental testing is not generally recommended. Environmental culturing can be costly and may require special laboratory procedures. Additionally, in most cases no standards for comparison exist. Because of the lack of standards environmental testing may generate inconclusive data that could result in the implementation of unnecessary procedures. Rationale for special environmental monitoring should be carefully planned and limited to epidemiological investigations. In limited situations "routine" environmental sampling may be indicated.

ROUTINE ENVIRONMENTAL TESTING

Routine microbiologic sampling for quality assurance purposes should be limited to (1) biologic monitoring of

Copyright © 2005, Association for Professionals in Infection Control and Epidemiology, Inc.

Table 16-1. Bacteria commonly found on healthy human body sites

Body Site	Common / Prominent Bacteria	Irregular Bacteria
Conjunctiva	Staphylococci, Corynebacteria, anaerobic Gram (−) cocci	S. viridans, S. pneumoniae, Neisseriae, Haemophilus, Enterobacteriaceae
Genitourinary Tract-External Genitalia	Staphylococci, S. viridans, Enterococci, Corynebacteria, Enterobacteriaceae, Bacteroides, Fusobacteria, anaerobic Gram (+) cocci	Propionibacteria, anaerobic Gram (−) cocci
Genitourinary Tract-Anterior Urethra	Staphylococci, Enterococci, Neisseriae, Corynebacteria, Bacteroides, Fusobacteria, anaerobic Gram (−) cocci	S. viridans, Enterobacteriaceae, Clostridia, Lactobacilli, anaerobic Gram (+) cocci
Genitourinary Tract-Vagina	Staphylococci, S. viridans, Enterococci, Neisseriae, Corynebacteria, Lactobacilli, Bifidobacteria, Bacteroides, anaerobic Gram (+) cocci	Clostridia, Fusobacteria
Mouth	Staphylococci, S. viridans, Enterococci, S. pneumoniae, Neisseriae, Corynebacteria, Haemophilus, Enterobacteriaceae, Actinomyces, Lactobacilli, Bifidobacteria, Fusobacteria, anaerobic Gram (+) cocci, anaerobic Gram (−) cocci	Group A Streptococci, Clostridia, Propionibacteria
Lower Intestine	S. viridans, Enterococci, Corynebacteria, Enterobacteriaceae, Clostridia, Lactobacilli, Bifidobacteria, Fusobacteria, anaerobic Gram (+) cocci	Staphylococci, Propionibacteria, Actinomyces
Upper Respiratory Tract	Staphylococci, S. viridans, S. pneumoniae, Corynebacteria, Haemophilus, Propionibacteria, Actinomyces, Bacteroides, Fusobacteria, anaerobic Gram (+) cocci, anaerobic Gram (−) cocci	Group A Streptococci, Group D Streptococci, Neisseriae, Enterobacteriaceae
Skin	Staphylococci, Corynebacteria, Propionibacteria, anaerobic Gram (+) cocci	S. viridans

Table 16-2. Infections and common organisms

Infection / Site	Common Organisms	Less Common Organisms
Bronchitis	S. pneumoniae, H. influenzae, respiratory viruses	B. pertussis, RSV
Device-Related	Coagulase-negative staphylococci, Corynebacteria sp.	Gram (−) bacilli, Candida sp.
Empyema	S. aureus, Streptococci, anaerobes	S. pyogenes, H. influenzae
Endocarditis	S. viridans, S. aureus, Enterococci	Haemophilus sp., S. epidermidis, Candida sp.
Gastroenteritis	Salmonella sp., Shigella sp., Campylobacter sp., E. coli 0157:H7, viruses	Giardia sp., Yersinia sp., Vibrio sp.
Meningitis	H. influenzae, N. meningitides, S. pneumoniae	L. monocytogenes, C. neoformans, M. tuberculosis, Pseudomonas sp., E. coli
Pelvic Inflammatory Disease	C. trachomatis, N. gonorrhoeae, Bacteroides sp., Enterobacteriaceae	
Peritonitis	Bacteroides sp., anaerobic cocci, Enterococci, Enterobacteriaceae	S. aureus, Candida sp.
Pharyngitis	S. pyogenes, respiratory viruses	C. albicans, N. gonorrhoeae, C. diphtheriae
Pneumonia (Community)	S. pneumoniae, H. influenzae, M. pneumoniae, C. pneumoniae, M. tuberculosis	S. aureus, Gram (−) bacilli, anaerobes, L. pneumophila, P. carinii
Pneumonia (Healthcare-assoc)	Pseudomonas sp., S. aureus, Enterobacteriaceae	Legionella sp., S. pneumoniae
Osteomyelitis	S. aureus	Salmonella sp., Pseudomonas sp., S. agalactiae
Septic Arthritis	S. aureus, N. gonorrhoeae	S. pneumoniae, S. pyogenes
Septicemia	S. aureus, S. pneumoniae, E. coli, Klebsiella sp., Salmonella sp.	Clostridium sp., Candida sp., Listeria sp.
Sinusitis	S. pneumoniae, H. influenzae, S. pyogenes, S. aureus	Gram (−) bacilli
Skin	S. aureus, S. pyogenes, Candida sp., dermatophytes	Gram (−) bacilli, Clostridium sp.
Urinary Tract	E. coli, Enterococci, Candida sp., Klebsiella sp., Proteus sp.	Pseudomonas sp., S. saprophyticus

APIC Text of Infection Control and Epidemiology

Copyright © 2005, Association for Professionals in Infection Control and Epidemiology, Inc.

sterilization processes; (2) monthly cultures of water and dialysate in hemodialysis units; and (3) short-term evaluation of the impact of infection control measures or changes in infection control protocols.[1]

Biologic monitoring of sterilization procedures is designed to provide a maximal challenge to the sterilizer to ensure that other items in the load are sterile without physically opening and culturing a number of items in the load. Standardized preparations of bacterial spores (biologic indicators) are available as a self-contained indicator systems (available from several manufacturers). Different bacterial spores and incubation temperatures are used to test different types of sterilizing procedures. (See chapter 21, Cleaning, Disinfection, and Sterilization. for more details.)

Dialysate and water in hemodialysis units are tested to satisfy local regulations and/or national standards for water quality. These samples are typically tested monthly using standardized protocols and guidelines. (See chapter 49, Dialysis, for more details.)Short-term environmental sampling can be conducted to evaluate the effectiveness of infection control protocols. Examples of this type of testing would be evaluating new cleaning procedures and/or products and for education of employees and staff members.

SPECIAL ENVIRONMENTAL TESTING

Environmental testing may be indicated when epidemiological investigation suggests that a source or reservoir of microorganisms may exist. Testing may involve personnel, medical devices, air, water, food, and/or surfaces. The type of sampling depends on the causative organism, type of infection, and potential sources/reservoirs. Quantitative test methods (determines the amount of an organism present) should be used rather than qualitative methods (determines only if an organism is present).

A variety of methods can be used for solid surface test samples. Swab-rinse sampling uses a template to swab a standardized area. Sponge-rinse and wipe-rinse methods use sterile sponges or wipes rubbed over a large area. Rinse-sampling involves direct immersion of an item if it can be totally exposed to a rinse solution. Impression plating is a method where the culture media is placed directly onto the surface being tested.

Liquid or water testing is generally more difficult to conduct than solid surface testing. There are typically fewer organisms present in liquids and they may be harder to culture. One quantitative test method is the agar spread plate, where a known quantity of the fluid is spread on solid culture media. A second quantitative method is the membrane filter method, where a standard volume of fluid is passed through a membrane filter and placed on a pad containing media. If tests are being conducted to detect *Legionella* sp. special culture media must be used due to the growth requirements of the organism. For more information about environmental testing for *Legionella* sp. (see chapter 76).

Fungal spores are ubiquitous in the environment and generally cause no harm to normal hosts; therefore air sampling should not be initiated lightly. Most facilities have increased concerns about airborne fungus during construction/renovation projects. There are no recommendations regarding routine microbiologic air sampling before, during, or after construction or renovations. However, in cases where there is documented or high potential for healthcare-acquired aspergillosis testing may be indicated. Settling plates (agar plate left open to the environment) should not be used since most fungal spores are too small and buoyant to settle in a consistent fashion. Volumetric air sampling devices, sampling a constant rate of airflow, should be used for testing. Most air sampling devices were originally developed to sample particles rather than fungi and have limitations related to sampling time. While results are difficult to interpret, if total pathogen levels exceed 1.0 colony forming units per cubic millimeter of air on several occasions, evaluation of air systems is needed.

V. THE ROLE OF THE LABORATORY IN OUTBREAK INVESTIGATION

The clinical laboratory plays a pivotal role in both endemic and epidemic epidemiology, but the awareness is heightened during the investigation of an outbreak. The laboratory can assist in the identification of an outbreak by confirming organism identities, recognizing organism clusters, and detecting unusual organisms and/or antimicrobial susceptibility patterns. Additionally, they can retrieve and review archival data to determine background rates of organism isolation and help determine if an outbreak situation actually exists. Finally, the laboratory can save organism isolates from suspected cases and conduct tests to determine if the organisms are the same or related.

DETERMINING ORGANISM RELATEDNESS

Historically, a variety of methods have been utilized to identify pathogenic microorganisms and evaluate their potential epidemiological interrelationships. In general, these methods have primarily relied on phenotypic (i.e., observable) characteristics. However, as test methods have advanced more emphasis has been placed on genotypic methods (i.e., molecular or chromosomal) to determine if organisms are related.

Copyright © 2005, Association for Professionals in Infection Control and Epidemiology, Inc.

Phenotypic Methods

Biotyping characterizes organisms based on the patterns of metabolic activities such as biochemical reactions, colony morphology, or nutritional and environmental requirements. While biotyping can be used with any organism, it has limited ability to distinguish epidemiologically related organisms from unrelated organisms.

Antimicrobial susceptibility testing has also been used to determine if organisms are related. While this type of testing is routinely performed in the clinical laboratory, it is relatively non-specific and has limited usefulness in determining true relatedness.

Serotyping is based on the immunological (i.e., antisera) detection of specific antigenic determinants on the surface of bacterial cells. Serotyping is most commonly used with *Salmonella* sp., *Shigella* sp., and *Pneumococci*. It is not as discriminating as genotypic analysis and requires maintenance of large stocks of typing antisera.

Bacteriophage typing is only useful with bacterial species that are susceptible to infection and lysis by viruses (bacteriophages). The potential interrelationship between different bacterial isolates (i.e., the bacteriophage type) is assessed on the basis of bacteriophage lytic patterns. This methodology is most widely used with *S. aureus* but is no longer recommended as an epidemiological typing method by the CDC.

Electrophoresis may be used to compare the rate of movement of metabolic enzymes or proteins from different isolates. This method assumes that minor differences in enzyme genes or proteins will be reflected in their movement across the test gel. When the test gel is examined related organisms will have the same pattern of movement. While this test method may be used with most common bacterial pathogens it is labor intensive and time consuming.

Genotypic Methods

Plasmid analysis compares bacterial isolates based on the presence of self-replicating extrachromosomal genetic elements (plasmids). Since plasmids often encode antibiotic resistance, clinical bacterial isolates will frequently carry several different plasmid types. The bacterial cells are enzymatically lysed to release the plasmid DNA which can then be analyzed by conventional agarose gel electrophoresis. This type of analysis may be used with common bacterial pathogens which frequently carry plasmids, however, many organisms are "non-typeable" since they do not carry plasmids.

Restriction endonuclease enzymes can subdivide both plasmids and chromosomal DNA into smaller fragments. Using agarose gel electrophoresis, these smaller pieces of genetic material are separated into different sized restriction fragments, which are compared to assess genetic relatedness. Unfortunately, since chromosomal patterns are composed of hundreds to thousands of restriction fragments, interpretation of results may be difficult.

Southern blot analysis of restriction fragment length polymorphisms (RFLPs) is a method in which chromosomal DNA is extracted from clinical isolates and digested with restriction enzymes. Using gel electrophoresis the restriction fragments are separated and transferred to a synthetic membrane. The fragments are then labeled with a homologous piece of DNA that acts as a probe to find complimentary base pairs. Variations in the number and sizes of fragments detected are called RFLPs. This testing method may be used with any organism for which defined probes are available, (e.g., the use of probes derived from genes for ribosomal RNA is termed "ribotyping"). One advantage of this type of testing is that some probes may allow simultaneous assessment of epidemiological interrelationships and definition of other clinically relevant characteristics (e.g., mechanisms of antibiotic resistance; the presence of specific antibiotic resistance genes). Unfortunately, this method is time consuming, labor intensive, and technically difficult.

Pulsed-field gel electrophoresis (PFGE) also begins with the lysis of organisms and digestion of their chromosomal DNA with restriction enzymes. The fragments are separated into a pattern of discrete bands by switching the direction of the electrical current. This pattern serves as a "bar code" of the bacterial chromosome which can be used to assess the relatedness of different clinical isolates. This test method may be used with any organism from which chromosomal DNA can be properly isolated and has been used with a wide variety of bacterial pathogens to assess epidemiological interrelationships. PFGE is probably the most widely used method for "molecular epidemiology" and is generally considered to be the gold standard for most clinically important organisms.

Amplification techniques such as polymerase chain reaction (PCR) are widely used in epidemiological investigation of healthcare acquired pathogens. In PCR, target DNA is extracted from the study organism. Short DNA molecules (primers), which specifically attach to each end of the target sequence, are added to the PCR reaction mixture along with a thermostable DNA polymerase and other reagents essential for DNA synthesis. In the PCR instrument (thermocycler), the target DNA is heated to denature it to single strands. After cooling, the primers attach to each end of the specific target sequence if it is present. DNA polymerase allows duplication (amplification) of the target

Copyright © 2005, Association for Professionals in Infection Control and Epidemiology, Inc.

DNA, resulting in two double-stranded molecules from each original sequence. After many cycles, millions of copies of the target sequence are produced which may be identified by a variety of means (e.g., electrophoresis, reaction with a specific probe, etc.). A number of other amplification methods are variations on the PCR theme and testing methods are continually being developed. As new techniques are developed they must be assessed to determine their usefulness in epidemiological investigations.

VI. FUTURE TRENDS

Clinical microbiology plays an important role in the practice of infection control and epidemiology. Many test methods employed in the clinical microbiology laboratory today are similar to methods used years ago. While these methods are often considered to be the gold standards they are often time consuming and limited (e.g., based on microbial growth, etc.). In an effort to offer clinicians rapid accurate results, research is being directed towards developing new molecular methods and or making existing molecular test methods more widely available.

VII. INTERNATIONAL PERSPECTIVES

The epidemiology and incidence of specific microorganisms can vary widely depending on the environment, commensal flora, and transmission risks. Organisms that may be common in one geographic area may be uncommon in another. However, given the ease of international travel, few microorganisms are "confined" to specific countries or areas. Laboratory techniques are similar in most parts of the world and testing is fairly standard. Additionally, international agencies, such as the Centers for Disease Control and Prevention, can assist with laboratory analysis of unusual or epidemiologically important pathogens. Clinical microbiology laboratories must work closely with clinicians if unusual pathogens are suspected.

REFERENCES

1. Centers for Disease Control and Prevention, Healthcare Infection Control Practices Advisory Committee (HICPAC). *Guidelines for environmental infection control in healthcare facilities*, Atlanta, 2003.

SUPPLEMENTAL RESOURCES

Murray PR, editor: *Manual of clinical microbiology*, ed 7, Washington, DC, 1999, American Society for Microbiology.

Bennett JV, Brachman PS, editors: *Hospital infections*, ed 4, Philadelphia, 1998, Lippincott-Raven.

Wenzel RP, editor: *Prevention and control of nosocomial infections*, ed 4, Philadelphia, 2003, Lippincott, Williams, & Williams.

Tortora GJ, Funke BR, Case CE: *Microbiology, an introduction*, ed 6, Menlo Park, NJ, 1998, Addison Wesley Longman, Inc.

Brooks K, editor: *APIC ready reference to microbes*, APIC, 2002, Washington, DC.

American Society of Microbiology: www.asm.org

APIC TEXT CHAPTERS

Chapter 4: Outbreak Investigation

Chapter 14: Principles of Microbial Pathogenicity and Host Response

Chapter 62: Antimicrobials and Resistance

Copyright © 2005, Association for Professionals in Infection Control and Epidemiology, Inc.

LABORATORY DIAGNOSTICS

Jaime Ritter BS, MT (ASCP), MPH, CIC
Infection Control Specialist
CR Bard, Inc.
Atlanta, Georgia

ABSTRACT

When a patient is being evaluated for infection, it usually requires a thorough history and physical examination, microbiological assessment, as well as other diagnostic tests. In addition to microbiological evaluations, the clinical laboratory can provide other diagnostic measurements that may help to diagnose/identify the infection or to evaluate the stage of an infectious disease or process. This chapter will review some of the more common laboratory tests that may be used in diagnosing and/or staging infections. While this chapter is not all–inclusive, it will offer the infection control professional a better understanding of the type and scope of testing that is available from the clinical laboratory.

KEY CONCEPTS

- Laboratory procedures can be useful tools in the diagnosis of infection.

- Laboratory procedures can be used to assess the stage of infection and/or infectious process.

I.   BACKGROUND

The clinical laboratory can undertake microbiological evaluations and can also provide other diagnostic measurements to assist in the diagnosis and identification of infection or to evaluate the stage of an infectious disease or process.

II.   BASIC PRINCIPLES

In general, there are three types of tests that are helpful in diagnosing or staging infections:

- Microbiologic procedures. Microorganisms may be directly cultured from clinical specimens or directly viewed through microscopy (an overview of clinical microbiology is presented in Chapter 16)

- Procedures used to evaluate the presence of antigens or antibodies to infectious agents

- Procedures that may be helpful in assessing the body's response to infection

Copyright © 2005, Association for Professionals in Infection Control and Epidemiology, Inc.

III. DIAGNOSTIC APPROACHES

Direct Examination

Gram Stain

By far the most common procedure conducted to directly examine a clinical specimen for the presence of microorganisms (i.e., bacteria or fungus) is the Gram stain. This procedure is discussed in detail in Chapter 16, Clinical Microbiology.

Histology/Cytology

Histology or cytology procedures involve gross and microscopic evaluation of a specimen or tissue by a qualified pathologist. Special fixing and/or staining techniques may be used depending on the suspected infectious process. Histological examination is useful for diagnosing infections with agents that are difficult or impossible to culture. The infectious agent may be seen directly in the specimen or indirectly as characteristic cell damage. Histology or cytology examination may be useful in the diagnosis of actinomycosis, *Chlamydia*, cytomegalovirus, genital herpes, giardiasis, histoplasmosis, leprosy (Hansen's disease), lymphogranuloma venereum, and rubeola.

Antigen/Antibody Detection

Antigen Detection

Antigen detection is a direct method for testing for the presence of infectious agents (antigens). These tests differ from direct specimen examination since they generally incorporate the use of immunologic or serologic procedures. These tests may be helpful in early diagnosis when cultures are not yet positive or are not possible. Methods are designed to detect the entire agent (e.g., virus) or part of the agent (e.g., bacterial cell wall structures). Several test methods may be used for antigen detection including agglutination tests, immunofluorescence, and enzyme-linked immunosorbent assay (ELISA). Serum, body fluids, and other clinical specimens may be used for antigen testing.

Antigen tests currently available include but are not limited to: adenovirus, bacterial meningitis (*Haemophilus influenzae, Streptococcus pneumoniae, Neisseria meningitidis*, group B *Streptococcus*), *Brucella spp. Cryptococcus spp.*, hepatitis B e, hepatitis B surface, hepatitis D, human immunodeficiency virus (HIV), influenza virus, *Legionella spp.*, parainfluenza virus, and respiratory syncytial virus.

Antibody Detection

Antibody detection is an indirect method of identifying infection by assessment of the host response (antibody production) to the invading microorganism; sometimes referred to as "serology" or "serologies." Results may be reported qualitatively (positive or negative) or quantitatively (titers) and should be interpreted in consideration of the predictive value of the specific test. A positive antibody titer does not necessarily indicate active infection but may represent a previous infection and should be considered accordingly. Several test methods may be used for antibody detection including agglutination tests, complement fixation, hemagglutination inhibition, indirect immunofluorescence, and radioimmunoassay. Serum is the specimen typically tested, however other specimens may be acceptable depending on the suspected agent.

A multitude of antibody tests exists for detection of infection or exposure to infectious agents. Currently available antibody assays include, but are not limited to: adenovirus, *Chlamydia* group, coxsackie virus, *Cryptococcus spp.*, cytomegalovirus, echinococcus, encephalitis viruses (California, eastern equine, St. Louis, Venezuelan, western equine, West Nile), Epstein-Barr virus, *Entamoeba histolytica* fungus, *Giardia spp., Helicobacter pylori*, hepatitis A, hepatitis B core, hepatitis B e, hepatitis B surface, hepatitis C, hepatitis D, *Herpes simplex*, histoplasma, HIV, *Legionella spp.*, Lyme disease, mumps, pneumocystis carinii, poliomyelitis, psittacosis, rabies, Rocky Mountain spotted fever, rubella, rubeola, *Salmonella spp.*, teichoic acid (a macromolecule present on the cell wall of gram-positive organisms), toxoplasma, treponemal (syphilis), *Varicella zoster*, and *Yersinia enterocolitica*.

Test for Infectious Process

A variety of tests other than microbial assays can be used to assess the body's response to infectious agents. While most of these tests are not used specifically for diagnosis of infection, they may be useful in many cases. Some of the more commonly used tests are described below. See suggested readings at the end of the chapter for information on additional tests or contact your clinical laboratory professional.

Body Fluid Analysis

When infection is suspected in a body fluid (e.g., pleural fluid, peritoneal fluid, synovial fluid) a sample of the fluid is obtained for analysis of its various components and for the detection of the presence of abnormal constituents that may indicate infection. The analysis usually includes total protein, specific gravity, cell count (red blood cells and white blood cells) and Gram stain. Since each body fluid has different "normal levels" chemical analysis results must be compared to the normal values for that fluid. However, in general, the presence of a large number of white blood

Copyright © 2005, Association for Professionals in Infection Control and Epidemiology, Inc.

Table 17-1. Common Findings in CSF Screening for Meningitis

Component	Bacterial	Viral	Fungal
Color/Clarity	Cloudy	Clear/Hazy	Clear/Hazy
Protein	High	Normal-High	Normal-High
Glucose	Low	Normal-Low	Normal-Low
White Blood Cells	High	Normal-High	High
WBC Differential	Polymorphonucleocytes	Lymphocytes	Lymphocytes

cells in any body fluid is an indicator of infection or acute inflammation.

Cerebrospinal Fluid Analysis

When meningitis is suspected it is common to collect a specimen of cerebrospinal fluid (CSF) for analysis. While CSF can be analyzed for a number of components (e.g., calcium, sodium, uric acid), for the purposes of infection diagnosis four basic components are considered. The four components are color and clarity, protein, glucose, and white blood cells including differential. Analysis results will vary depending on the type of infectious agent and may assist in early identification of the type of pathogen present. (See Table 17-1.)

Cold Agglutinins

Cold agglutinins are antibodies that cause clumping or agglutination of type O red blood cells at cold temperatures. The cold agglutinins test is used to detect antibodies that result from *Mycoplasma pneumoniae* infection. In combination with acute respiratory symptoms, a high cold agglutinin titer usually indicates *M. pneumoniae* infection, viral pneumonia, or primary atypical pneumonia.

C-Reactive Protein (CRP)

C-reactive protein is an abnormal serum glycoprotein produced by the liver during acute inflammation. It usually disappears rapidly when inflammation subsides so its detection signifies the presence of a current inflammatory process. This analysis is sometimes used in the diagnosis of meningitis, pneumonia (pneumococcal), sepsis, tuberculosis, and urinary tract infection.

Complete Blood Count

The complete blood count (CBC) is a series of tests of the peripheral blood that evaluate different cellular components. The items commonly evaluated include hemoglobin, hematocrit, red blood cells, red blood cell indices, white blood cells, white blood cell differential, platelets, and microscopic examination of stained blood smears. The CBC is used as a screening tool for

general health assessment as well as to track the progress of many diseases. However, for the purposes of diagnosing or monitoring infection, the white blood cell (WBC) count and differential are most useful.

The WBC count is the total number of WBCs (leukocytes) in 1 mm^3 of peripheral blood. The WBC count has a wide range of normal values depending on the age of the patient. An increased WBC count (leukocytosis, WBC count >10,000), usually indicates infection, inflammation, or leukemic neoplasia. In some infections, especially sepsis, the WBC count can be extremely high and may reach levels associated with leukemia. This is called a "leukemoid" reaction. A decreased WBC count (leukopenia, WBC count <4,000) can occur in cases of overwhelming infection, acquired immune deficiency syndrome (AIDS), viral hepatitis, mononucleosis, and Legionnaires disease.

The WBC differential count measures the percentage of each type of leukocyte present in the blood specimen. Five types of WBCs are found in the blood. In order of frequency, they are neutrophils, lymphocytes, monocytes, eosinophils, and basophils. The primary function of the neutrophil is phagocytosis. Acute bacterial infections stimulate neutrophil production and result in increased WBC counts. When production is stimulated, immature neutrophils, called band or stab cells, may enter the blood system. This occurrence, referred to as "shift to the left" or "left shift," is indicative of an ongoing acute bacterial infection. Eosinophils, typically associated with allergic reactions, can be increased in parasitic infections and occasionally with leprosy and tuberculosis. Increased lymphocytes are associated with cytomegalovirus, infectious mononucleosis, pertussis, syphilis, and toxoplasmosis. Increased monocytes are commonly associated with Epstein-Barr virus.

Fecal Leukocytes

Fecal leukocytes are used to determine the type of diarrhea, invasive or noninvasive, to the mucosa of the colon. The presence of leukocytes in the stool indicates that the cause of diarrhea is an organism or process that is breaking the mucosal barrier of the colon, such as *Salmonella*, *Shigella*, *Amoeba*, *Campylobacter*, *Helicobacter*, or *Yersinia* infections. Leukocytes are usually not present in infectious processes that do not invade the mucosa, such as viral enteritis or toxin mediated diarrhea. *Clostridium difficile* may or may not be associated with leukocytes in the stool.

Lymphocyte Subset

The primary function of lymphocytes is to fight chronic bacterial infections and acute viral infections. Lymphocytes are divided into two types: T cells (mature in the

Copyright © 2005, Association for Professionals in Infection Control and Epidemiology, Inc.

thymus) and B cells (mature in the bone marrow). T cells are involved primarily with cellular-type immune reactions, while B cells participate in humoral immunity (antibody production). T cells are killer cells, CD8 are suppressor cells, and CD4 are helper cells. The differential count does not separate the type of lymphocyte, and further testing is necessary to quantify them in the blood. Of particular interest in monitoring the progression of HIV infection are the CD4 count, CD4 percentage, and the CD4/CD8 ratio. As the CD4 count decreases, the probability of developing AIDS increases.

Sedimentation Rate

When a tube of well-mixed venous blood is positioned vertically, the red blood cells will tend to fall to the bottom. The rate at which they fall is referred to as the erythrocyte sedimentation rate (ESR). While this test lacks sensitivity and specificity for disease processes, it nevertheless is used frequently. An increased ESR is associated with several disease states including acute infection and inflammation.

Weil-Felix Agglutinins

Weil-Felix agglutinin is a test performed to detect and differentiate rickettsial antibodies in the serum. A single high titer or a fourfold rise in titer between acute and convalescent samples is considered diagnostic. This test can be useful in diagnosing Rocky Mountain spotted fever, Q fever, epidemic typhus, murine typhus, scrub typhus, and rickettsialpox.

Urinalysis

Urinalysis is a often-used screening test to assess general health as well as the health of the urinary tract. Total urinalysis involves multiple routine tests and typically includes assessment of color, clarity, presence of proteins, glucose, ketones, blood, nitrite, and leukocyte esterase. Additionally, the urine may be examined microscopically for the presence of red blood cells, white blood cells, casts, crystals, and bacteria or yeast. Of the many components tested, only a few are used to screen for infection. A positive leukocyte esterase test indicates that WBCs are present in the urine (nearly 90% accurate). If the leukocyte esterase is positive, microscopic examination is performed to determine the number of WBCs or WBC casts present. The presence of 10 or more WBCs in the urine may indicate infection; the presence of WBC casts may indicate infection of the kidney. The nitrite test is used to screen for the presence of bacteria in the urine. Many bacteria produce an enzyme that can reduce urinary nitrates to nitrites. If nitrites are present in the urine, it may indicate that bacteria are present (about 50% accurate). During microscopic evaluation, the specimen is also examined for the presence of bacteria and/or yeast. The presence of these microorganisms may indicate infection or colonization of the urinary tract.

IV. SUMMARY AND CONCLUSIONS

The most common procedure for directly examining a clinical specimen for the presence of microorganisms (i.e., bacteria or fungus) is the Gram stain. Histology or cytology procedures which involve gross and microscopic evaluation of a specimen or tissue by a qualified pathologist are useful for diagnosing infections with agents that are difficult or impossible to culture. Antigen detection may be helpful in early diagnosis when cultures are not yet positive or are not possible. Antibody detection does not necessarily indicate active infection but may indicate a previous infection or exposure to infectious agents. A variety of tests other than microbial assays can be used to assess the body's response to infectious agents, including body fluid analysis, cerebrospinal fluid analysis, cold agglutinins test, C-reactive protein analysis, complete blood counts, fecal leukocytes counts, lymphocyte subsets, sedimentation rate tests, Weil-Felix agglutinins, and Urinalysis.

SUPPLEMENTAL RESOURCES

Chernecky, CC, Berger, BJ, editors. *Laboratory Tests and Diagnostic Procedures. 3rd Ed.* Philadelphia, 2001, W.B. Saunders.

Pagana, KD, Pagana, TJ. *Mosby's Manual of Diagnostic and Laboratory Tests. 2nd Ed.* Saint Louis 2002, Mosby.

Copyright © 2005, Association for Professionals in Infection Control and Epidemiology, Inc.

Isolation Systems

Jane D. Siegel, MD
Professor of Pediatrics
University of Texas Southwestern Medical Center
Dallas, Texas

ABSTRACT

Isolation precautions are the foundation for preventing transmission of infectious agents in settings where healthcare is delivered. Incorporation of infection control programs into the institutional safety program is essential. The goal of this chapter is to provide an overview of the principles that support the recommendations for isolation precautions in the most recent guidelines of the Healthcare Infection Control Practices Advisory Committee (HICPAC) and the Centers for Disease Control and Prevention (CDC), scheduled for publication in 2005, and to present some of the key recommendations. The reader is referred to the document, "Guideline for Isolation Precautions: Preventing Transmission of Infectious Agents in Healthcare Settings 2005" (available at www.cdc.gov/ncidod/hip), for specific recommendations and background information. Other guidelines that provide information pertaining to isolation and prevention of transmission of infectious agents are listed in the Supplemental Resources section of this chapter.

KEY CONCEPTS

- Delivery of healthcare in *all* settings—e.g., acute care hospitals, long-term care facilities, ambulatory care centers, and the home—is associated with a risk for transmission of infectious agents, via other patients and healthcare workers or in association with medical devices.

- The patient who has not been identified or is not suspected of being colonized or infected with transmissible infectious agents represents a substantial risk to other patients.

- Risk of transmission of infectious agents is determined by host susceptibility, route of transmission, duration and intensity of exposure, and availability and behavior of healthcare workers with hands-on patient contact.

- Standard precautions are the foundation of all precautions to prevent transmission of infectious agents associated with healthcare, because infectious agents may be present in blood, in all body fluids (except sweat), and on non-intact skin and mucous membranes of all patients; therefore, hand hygiene and personal protective equipment (e.g., gloves, gown, mask, eye/face protection) should always be used if contact with those fluids is likely.

- New Standard Precautions for Patients: Respiratory

Copyright © 2005, Association for Professionals in Infection Control and Epidemiology, Inc.

Hygiene/Cough Etiquette was added in 2004 for the purpose of source containment of respiratory tract pathogens (e.g., severe acute respiratory syndrome (SARS) variant Co-V, avian influenza H5N1, human influenza).

- Transmission-based precautions, which include contact precautions, droplet precautions, airborne precautions, and a protective environment, are required to contain highly transmissible and/or epidemiologically important agents and are based on the mode of transmission of the specific pathogen:

- The following healthcare system components are essential for effective implementation of isolation precautions and prevention of transmission of infectious agents: commitment of organizational leadership to provide necessary fiscal and human resources, incorporation of infection control in the institutional safety climate, appropriate staffing levels for patient care and infection control, clinical microbiology laboratory support, appropriate supplies, and periodic audits of the implementation of Category I recommendations.

- Chemoprophylaxis and pre- and postexposure immunization are effective adjuncts to isolation precautions.

- All institutions must provide education on prevention of transmission of infectious agents for all healthcare workers and track or be prepared to track infection rates for targeted infections, including device-related infections, influenza, and diseases caused by bioweapons, multidrug-resistant organisms (MDROs), especially methicillin-resistant *Staphylococcus aureus* (MRSA) and vancomycin-resistant *Enterococcus* (VRE).

- A multi-component MDRO control program appropriate for the prevalence of MDROs and the risk of transmission and adverse outcome must be implemented and monitored in all healthcare settings.

I.   BACKGROUND

Guidance for isolation precautions in hospitals has been available to infection control professionals since publication of the first document in 1970 (Table 18–1). As more studies of transmission of infectious agents have been published, expanding the evidence base and enhancing our understanding of healthcare epidemiology, the guidelines have evolved to provide recommendations that are applicable across the continuum of care; address appropriate precautions for emerging pathogens, including multidrug-resistant organisms (MDROs); and describe components of

healthcare administration that are required for successful implementation of recommendations.

II.   BASIC PRINCIPLES

At the time of this publication, the Healthcare Infection Control Practices Advisory Committee/Centers for Disease Control and Prevention (HICPAC/CDC) "Guideline for Isolation Precautions: Preventing Transmission of Infectious Agents in Healthcare Settings 2005" is undergoing its final revision after the public comment period and will, when published, update and replace the document published in 1996.[1]

The 2005 document includes a well-referenced 3-part background discussion: (1) review of the scientific data regarding transmission of infectious agents in healthcare settings; (2) description of the fundamental elements to prevent transmission, and (3) a description of the categories of isolation precautions. Appendix A includes an updated alphabetical listing of infectious diseases and the recommended isolation precautions, duration, and pertinent comments. New to this version of the guideline for isolation precautions is Appendix B, which includes a comprehensive review of the relevant published literature to guide development of an MDRO control program appropriate for the conditions within an individual facility. Evidence-based recommendations are provided with specific modifications offered for MDRO control in facilities outside of acute care.

The CDC/HICPAC system for categorizing recommendations is as follows:

- Category IA. Strongly recommended for implementation and strongly supported by well-designed experimental, clinical, or epidemiologic studies.

- Category IB. Strongly recommended for implementation and supported by some experimental, clinical, or epidemiologic studies and a strong theoretical rationale.

- Category IC. Required for implementation, as mandated by federal and/or state regulations or standards.

- Category II. Suggested for implementation and supported by suggestive clinical or epidemiologic studies or a theoretical rationale.

- No recommendation, unresolved issue. Practices for which insufficient evidence or no consensus regarding efficacy exists. This category assists investigators in determining topics that are in need of further study.

It is expected that all Category IA, IB, and IC recommendations will be implemented by healthcare facili-

Copyright © 2005, Association for Professionals in Infection Control and Epidemiology, Inc.

Table 18-1. History of Guidelines for Isolation Precautions in Hospitals[1]

Year/ref	Document issued	Comment
1970[2]	*Isolation techniques for use in hospitals,* ed 1	• Introduced 7 isolation precaution categories with color-coded cards: strict, respiratory, protective, enteric, wound and skin, discharge, and blood • Required no user decision-making • Strong in its simplicity; overisolation prescribed for some infections
1975[3]	*Isolation techniques for use in hospitals,* ed 2	• Same conceptual framework as ed 1
1983[4]	CDC guideline for isolation precautions in hospitals	• Provided two systems for isolation: category-specific and disease-specific • Protective isolation eliminated; blood precautions expanded to include body fluids • Categories included strict, contact, respiratory, AFB [AU: What is meant by AFB? Please spell out.], enteric, drainage/secretion, blood and body fluids • Emphasized decision-making by users
1985–1988[5,6]	Universal precautions	• Developed in response to HIV/AIDS epidemic • Dictated application of blood and body fluid precautions to all patients, regardless of infection status • Did not apply to feces, nasal secretions, sputum, sweat, tears, urine, or vomitus unless contaminated by visible blood • Added personal protective equipment to protect healthcare workers from mucous membrane exposures • Handwashing recommended immediately after glove removal • Added specific recommendations for handling needles and other sharp devices; concept became integral to the OSHA 1991 rule on occupational exposure to bloodborne pathogens in healthcare settings
1987[7]	Body substance isolation	• Emphasized avoiding contact with all moist and potentially infectious body substances except sweat, even if blood was not present • Shared some features with universal precautions • Weak on infections transmitted by large droplets or by contact with dry surfaces • Did not emphasize need for special ventilation to contain airborne infections • Handwashing after glove removal not specified in the absence of visible soiling
1996[1]	Guideline for isolation precautions in hospitals	• Prepared by the Healthcare Infection Control Practices Advisory Committee (HICPAC) • Melded major features of universal precautions and body substance isolation into standard precautions, to be used with all patients at all times • Included 3 transmission-based precaution categories: airborne, droplet, and contact • Listed clinical syndromes that should dictate use of empiric isolation until an etiologic diagnosis is established

ties. Because studies of interventions of MDROs include an average of 7 interventions, combinations of interventions have been assigned a Category IB, but most individual interventions cannot be rated, since the benefit attributable to a single intervention cannot be determined.

It is important to note the use of the term *healthcare-associated infections* (HAIs) in response to the changes that have occurred in the delivery of healthcare in the United States. Infections that develop in association with the delivery of healthcare may not have been acquired in a hospital and therefore cannot be considered nosocomial, or the geographic location where the infection was acquired may not be apparent. However, those infections that develop in association with healthcare may require assessment of healthcare practices to determine whether interventions are indicated to decrease the risk.

III. RECOMMENDATIONS FOR ISOLATION PRECAUTIONS

Reaffirmation and Expansion of Standard Precautions

The 2005 revision reaffirms standard precautions as the foundation of all precautions to prevent transmission of infections associated with healthcare. Because unsuspected infectious agents may be present in blood and all body fluids except sweat and on nonintact skin and mucous membranes of all patients, hand hygiene and personal protective equipment (PPE) (e.g., gloves, gown, mask, eye/face protection) should always be used if contact with those substances is likely. Although this concept was developed initially in response to the need to prevent transmission of bloodborne pathogens (e.g., human immunodeficiency virus [HIV], hepatitis B and C viruses) and termed "universal precautions" or "body substance isolation," it is clear that it is appro-

Copyright © 2005, Association for Professionals in Infection Control and Epidemiology, Inc.

priate for prevention of transmission of other pathogens, most notably respiratory tract pathogens, including severe acute respiratory syndrome-CoV variant (SARS-CoV), influenza, and MDROs. In response to the experience with the SARS outbreaks of 2003, the concept of standard precautions was expanded to patients for the purpose of source containment in the form of *respiratory hygiene/cough etiquette.* The following components are included:

1. Education of healthcare facility staff, patients, and visitors;

2. Posted signs in language appropriate to the population served, with instructions to patients and accompanying family members or friends;

3. Source control measures (e.g., covering the mouth/ nose with a tissue when coughing and disposing of used tissues, using surgical masks on the coughing person when tolerated and appropriate, coughing into the sleeve for individuals who are unlikely to be carrying or cuddling infants and young children);

4. Hand hygiene after contact with respiratory secretions; and

5. Spatial separation, ideally more than 3 feet, of persons with respiratory infections in common waiting areas when possible.

These measures are targeted to patients and accompanying family members or friends but apply to any person with signs of a cold or other respiratory infection (e.g., cough, congestion, rhinorrhea, increased production of respiratory secretions) who enters any healthcare facility[8] (Table 18–2).

Transmission-Based Precautions

Transmission-based precautions includes the following set of precautions, which are recommended to contain highly transmissible and/or epidemiologically important agents and is based on the mode of transmission of the specific pathogen:

1. Contact precautions. Includes use of PPE when contact with the inanimate environment is likely due to demonstrated environmental contamination for vancomycin-resistant *Enterococcus* (VRE), methicillin-resistant *Staphyloccus aureus* (MRSA), *Clostridium difficile,* or respiratory syncytial virus.

2. Droplet precautions. Controversy exists over the potential distance that large respiratory droplets may travel, but recommendations have not changed from the use of surgical masks within 3 feet of the patient.

3. Airborne precautions. These call for an airborne infection isolation room with negative room air pressure relative to corridors, air exhaustion directly to the outside or recirculated through HEPA filtration with 6 to 12 air changes per hour. The SARS outbreaks of 2003 raised a number of questions regarding droplet versus airborne transmission. Although the droplet route was most frequent, there is evidence that airborne transmission occurred when healthcare workerss were exposed to aerosol-producing procedures (e.g., endotracheal intubation). The proposed classification of aerosol transmission as obligated, preferential, or opportunistic is useful to explain the variations observed.[9]

4. Protective Environment. Positive room air pressure is required, relative to corridors, along with HEPA filtration of incoming air at 12 or more air changes per hour. This precaution is recommended only for allogeneic hematopoietic stem cell transplants, since there are no data supporting benefits for other groups. The principle of the protective environment is to provide appropriate engineering controls to prevent exposure to environmental fungal spores.

Recommended procedures for donning and removing PPE are also included. Since studies have demonstrated that isolation of patients is associated with adverse psychological effects as well as decreased attending physician contact and other adverse effects, providers must understand and follow the criteria for initiating and discontinuing isolation precautions.

Influence of Healthcare System Components on the Effectiveness of Recommended Isolation Precautions

Based on published studies, there is a set of recommendations that require administrative commitment of fiscal and human resources for education, supplies, and compulsory auditing to ensure implementation of the recommended practices. Individuals trained in infection control should be available on site or by contract to all healthcare organizations. The number of full-time employees dedicated to infection control will be determined by the ever-expanding scope of infection control responsibilities within an institution (surveillance, education, auditing, prevention of transmission of MDROs, construction, emerging pathogen preparedness, etc.). Levels close to 1 per 100 beds in acute care hospitals have been suggested.[10] Levels of bedside nurse staffing appropriate to the intensity of care required and the number of patients in a unit must be assured as part of an institution's infection control and patient safety program.[11-13] Recommendations are also made for all healthcare institutions to have (on site or by contract) microbiology laboratory services that will support infection control needs, including rapid diagnostic testing, identification of MDROs, performance of surveillance

Copyright © 2005, Association for Professionals in Infection Control and Epidemiology, Inc.

Table 18-2. Recommendations for Application of Standard Precautions for the Care of All Patients in All Healthcare Settings

Activity	Recommendation
Hand hygiene	Perform after touching blood, body fluids, secretions, excretions, contaminated items; immediately after removing gloves; between patient contacts
Personal protective equipment (PPE)	
• Gloves	Use for touching blood, body fluids, secretions, excretions, contaminated items; for touching mucous membranes and non-intact skin
• Mask, eye protection, face shield	Use during procedures and patient care activities likely to generate splashes or sprays of blood, body fluids, secretions
• Gown	Use during procedures and patient care activities when contact of clothing or exposed skin with blood or body fluids, secretions, and excretions is anticipated
Soiled patient care equipment	Handle in a manner that prevents transfer of microorganisms to others and to the environment
Environmental control	Develop procedures for routine care, cleaning, and disinfection of environmental surfaces
Textiles and laundry	Handle in a manner that prevents transfer of microorganisms to others and to the environment
Needles and other sharps	Do not recap, bend, break, or hand-manipulate used needles; use safety features when available; place used sharps in puncture-resistant container
Patient resuscitation	Use mouthpiece, resuscitation bag, other ventilation devices to prevent mouth contact
Patient placement	Prioritize for single-patient room if patient is at increased risk of transmission, is likely to contaminate the environment, does not maintain appropriate hygiene, or is at increased risk of acquiring infection or developing an adverse outcome following infection
Respiratory hygiene/cough etiquette (source containment of infectious respiratory secretions in symptomatic patients, beginning at initial point of encounter, e.g.b emergency department, ambulatory clinics, physician offices)	Instruct symptomatic persons to cover mouth/nose when sneezing/coughing; use tissues and dispose in no-touch receptacle; observe hand hygiene after soiling of hands with respiratory secretions; wear surgical mask if tolerated or maintain spatial separation of at least 3 feet, if possible

Adapted from: Garner 1996[1] and www.cdc.gov/flu/professionals/pdf/resphygiene.pdf.[8]

cultures when indicated, and periodic susceptibility summary reporting.[14,15]

Prevention of Transmission of MRSA, VRE, and Other MDROs

As new multidrug-resistant organisms emerged during the past 10 to 15 years, interim guidelines were issued until the epidemiology was defined. Based on experience with MRSA, VRE, vancomycin-intermediate S. aureus, vancomycin-resistant S. aureus, and extended spectrum beta-lactamase–producing cephalosporins (ESBLs), we have learned that general principles of control apply to all resistant bacteria. Therefore, this revised guideline provides recommendations that call for an assessment of the status of all multidrug-resistant organisms within an institution or a healthcare system

or region and development of an individualized control program using the general principles of prevention of transmission for all resistant pathogens. The following 7 components for an MDRO control program are defined: (1) administrative measures/adherence monitoring, (2) MDRO education, (3) judicious use of antimicrobials, (4) surveillance, (5) infection control (isolation) precautions to prevent transmission, (6) environmental measures, and (7) decolonization. Because MDRO control is a public health crisis demanding implementation of an effective control program in all healthcare settings, there is a baseline set of recommended measures for each of the seven components.

If control is not achieved using these baseline measures, then a set of intensified measures for each com-

Copyright © 2005, Association for Professionals in Infection Control and Epidemiology, Inc.

ponent is recommended. The indications for intensification of the measures are as follows:

1. Evidence that transmission of MDROs is *not* decreasing, despite implementation of routine measures and documentation of adherence (use of control charts or other methods of measurement that account for background variation to track trends in transmission of MDROs targeted in the institution is recommended[16-18])

2. Identification of the first case of an epidemiologically important MDRO within a healthcare facility

3. Evidence that incidence and prevalence of target MDROs have increased beyond the accepted institutional level, despite documented implementation of baseline control measures

These recommendations affirm the usefulness of active surveillance cultures and contact precautions for MRSA and VRE control, which have been recommended in the consensus guideline for prevention of transmission of MRSA and VRE published by the Society for Healthcare Epidemiology of America in 2003.[19] These recommendations acknowledge that the literature does not support application of a single set of recommendations for all healthcare facilities, given the complexity of healthcare systems in the United States and the variation in prevalence of key MDROs, in addition to MRSA and VRE. For example, focusing on MRSA and VRE control may not be appropriate for institutions whose problem MDROs are ESBLs or other multidrug-resistant gram-negative bacilli, whose prevalence is affected by antimicrobial use more than are MRSA and VRE.

Performance Measures

Since 2002, HICPAC/CDC guidelines have identified specific Category IA recommendations as appropriate performance indicators to monitor the effectiveness of the implementation of updated or new guidelines. The importance of monitoring adherence to infection control recommendations is demonstrated most consistently for hand hygiene.[20] It cannot be concluded that recommended measures are ineffective, unless it is known that those practices are followed consistently by healthcare workers who have direct patient contact. Performance indicators are most likely to include:

- Appropriateness and timeliness of initiation of transmission-based precautions based on clinical diagnosis and of discontinuation of precautions

- Appropriateness of use of PPE by healthcare workers caring for patients for whom transmission-based precautions are required

- Adequacy of single-patient rooms and supplies for infection control precautions

- Staffing levels in areas of ongoing transmission of infectious agents

- Preventive measures selected for prevention of MDRO transmission and identification of contributing factors when MDRO transmission is not decreasing

IV. SUMMARY AND CONCLUSIONS

Isolation precautions are the foundation for preventing transmission of infectious agents associated with healthcare. However, as sites for the delivery of healthcare have changed in the United States, and as the importance of human factors in prevention of transmission of infectious agents has been identified, novel strategies are required to assure that the risk of HAI is minimized. The increase in the prevalence of MDROs and in community-associated MRSA infections poses new challenges to the prevention of HAI. Implementation of recommended practices, monitoring adherence to and effectiveness of those practices, changing control plans as needed to fit the unique conditions of each healthcare setting, and monitoring outcomes will optimize patient safety regarding adverse events associated with HAI.

REFERENCES

1. Garner JS: Guideline for isolation precautions in hospitals. The Hospital Infection Control Practices Advisory Committee, *Infect Control Hosp Epidemiol* 17:53–80, 1996.
2. National Communicable Disease Center: *Isolation techniques for use in hospitals,* ed 1 Washington, DC: 1970, US Government Printing Office; PHS publication no 2054.
3. Centers for Disease Control and Prevention: *Isolation techniques for use in hospitals,* ed 2, Washington, DC: 1975, US Government Printing Office; HHS publication no. (CDC) 80–8314.
4. Garner JS, Simmons BP: CDC Guideline for isolation precautions in hospitals, Atlanta, GA, 1983, US Department of Health and Human Services, Public Health Service, Centers for Disease Control; HHS publication no. (CDC) 83–8314, *Infect Control* 4: 245–325, 1983.
5. Centers for Disease Control and Prevention: Recommendations for preventing transmission of infection with human T-lymphotropic virus type III/lymphadenopathy-associated virus in the workplace, *MMWR Morb Mortal Wkly Rep* 34:681–86, 691–95, 1984.
6. Centers for Disease Control and Prevention: Update: universal precautions for prevention of transmission of human immunodeficiency virus, hepatitis B virus, and other bloodborne pathogens in health-care settings, *MMWR Morb Mortal Wkly Rep* 37: 377–82, 387–88, 1988.
7. Lynch P, Jackson MM, Cummings MJ, Stamm WE: Rethinking the role of isolation practices in the prevention of nosocomial infections, *Ann Intern Med* 107:243–46, 1987.
8. Centers for Disease Control and Prevention: Fact sheet: Respiratory hygiene/cough etiquette in healthcare settings, Nov 4, 2004, Available at: www.cdc.gov/flu/professionals/pdf/resphygiene.pdf
9. Roy CJ, Milton DK: Airborne transmission of communicable infection—the elusive pathway, *N Engl J Med* 350:1710–12, 2004.
10. O'Boyle C, Jackson M, Henly SJ: Staffing requirements for infection control programs in US health care facilities: Delphi project, *Am J Infect Control* 30:321–33, 2002.

Copyright © 2005, Association for Professionals in Infection Control and Epidemiology, Inc.

11. Needleman J, Buerhaus P, Mattke S, Stewart M, Zelevinsky K: Nurse-staffing levels and the quality of care in hospitals, *N Engl J Med* 346:1715–22, 2002.
12. Jackson M, Chiarello LA, Gaynes RP, Gerberding JL: Nurse staffing and health care-associated infections: Proceedings from a working group meeting, *Am J Infect Control* 30:199–206, 2002.
13. Lundstrom T, Pugliese G, Bartley J, Cox J, Guither C: Organizational and environmental factors that affect worker health and safety and patient outcomes, *Am J Infect Control* 30:93–106, 2002.
14. Peterson LR, Hamilton JD, Baron EJ, et al: Role of clinical microbiology laboratories in the management and control of infectious diseases and the delivery of health care, *Clin Infect Dis* 32:605–11, 2001.
15. Simor AE: The role of the laboratory in infection prevention and control programs in long-term care facilities for the elderly, *Infect Control Hosp Epidemiol* 22:459–63, 2001.
16. Curran ET, Benneyan JC, Hood J: Controlling methicillin-resistant *Staphylococcus aureus, Infect Control Hosp Epidemiol* 23:13–18, 2002.
17. Benneyan JC: Statistical quality control methods in infection control and hospital epidemiology: Part 1. Introduction and basic theory, *Infect Control Hosp Epidemiol* 19:194–214, 1998.
18. Benneyan JC: Statistical quality control methods in infection control and hospital epidemiology: Part 2. Chart use, statistical properties, and research issues, *Infect Control Hosp Epidemiol* 19:265–77, 1998.
19. Muto CA, Jernigan JA, Ostrowsky BE, et al: SHEA guideline for preventing nosocomial transmission of multidrug-resistant strains of *Staphylococcus aureus* and *Enterococcus, Infect Control Hosp Epidemiol* 24:362–86, 2003.
20. Centers for Disease Control and Prevention: Guideline for hand hygiene in health-care settings: Recommendations of the Healthcare Infection Control Practices Advisory Committee and the HICPAC/SHEA/APIC/IDSA Hand Hygiene Task Force, *MMWR Recomm Report* 51(No. RR-16):1–44, 2002.

SUPPLEMENTAL RESOURCES

American Academy of Pediatrics, American College of Obstetricians and Gynecologists: Guidelines for Perinatal Care, ed 5, Elk Grove Village, IL, 2002, American Academy of Pediatrics; Washington, DC, American College of Obstetricians and Gynecologists.

Boyce JM, Pittet D, HICPAC, et al: Guideline for hand hygiene in health-care settings: recommendation of the Healthcare Infection Control Practices Advisory Committee and the HICPAC/SHEA/APIC/IDSA Hand Hygiene Task Force. Society for Healthcare Epidemiology of America/Association for Professionals in Infection Control/Infectious Diseases Society of America, *MMWR Recomm Rep* 51(RR-16):1–45.

Centers for Disease Control and Prevention/Healthcare Infection Control Practices Advisory Committee: Infection control guidelines, available at: www.cdc.gov/ncidod/hip/Guide/guide.htm.

CDC, Infectious Disease Society of America, American Society for Blood and Marrow Transplantation. Guidelines for preventing opportunistic infections among hematopoietic stem cell transplant recipients, *MMWR Recomm Rep* 49(RR-10):1–125, 2000 [erratum 53(RR-19):396, 2004].

COID (2003). 2003 Report of the Committee on Infectious Diseases. Redbook.

Guidelines for preventing the transmission of *Mycobacterium tuberculosis* in health-care facilities, 1994 [revision in process], *MMWR Recomm Rep* 43(RR-13):1–132, 1994.

Guideline for isolation precautions in hospitals 1996 [revision in process], *Infect Control Hosp Epidemiol* 17:53–80, 1996.

Infection control in health care personnel, 1998, *Infect Control Hosp Epidemiol* 19:407–63, 1998.

Mangram AJ, Horan TC, Pearson ML, Silver LC, Jarvis WR: Guideline for the prevention of surgical site infection, Hospital Infection Control Practices Advisory Committee, *Infect Control Hosp Epidemiol* 20:250–278, 1999.

O'Grady NP, Alexander M, Dellinger EP, et al: Guidelines for prevention of intravascular catheter-related infections. Centers for Disease Control and Prevention. MMWR 51(RR-10):1–[ch29, 2002.

Recommendations for preventing transmission of infections among chronic hemodialysis patients, *MMWR Recomm Rep* 50(RR-5):1–43, 2001.

Saiman L, Siegel J: Infection control recommendations for patients with cystic fibrosis: microbiology, important pathogens, and infection control practices to prevent patient-to-patient transmission, *Infect Control Hosp Epidemiol* 24(5 suppl):S6–52, 2003.

Sehulster L, Chinn RY, CDC, HICPAC: Guideline for environmental infection control in health-care facilities 2003, recommendations of CDC and the Healthcare Infection Control Practices Advisory Committee, *MMWR Recomm Rep* 52(RR-10):1–42, 2003 [complete background information available at www.cdc.gov/ncidod/hip].

Tablan OC, Anderson LJ, Besser R, et al: Guidelines for prevention of healthcare-associated pneumonia 2003: recommendations of CDC and the Healthcare Infection Control Practices Advisory Committee, *MMWR Recomm Rep* 53(RR-3):1–36, 2004 [complete background information available at www.cdc.gov/ncidod/hip].

Copyright © 2005, Association for Professionals in Infection Control and Epidemiology, Inc.

19

Hand Hygiene

Marjorie A. Underwood, BSN, RN, CIC
Infection Control Practitioner, Three Rivers
Community Hospital
Grants Pass, Oregon

ABSTRACT

Hand hygiene is a critical component of patient and employee safety. Effective patient safety and infection control programs require that healthcare personnel be familiar with recent hand hygiene recommendations, understand the evidence behind those recommendations, and consistently adhere to the recommendations. The goal of this chapter is to provide the reader with information to successfully implement the Centers for Disease Control and Prevention (CDC) 2002 "Guideline for Hand Hygiene in Health-Care Facilities."[1]

KEY CONCEPTS

- Hands contaminated with transient bacteria are a primary means for transmission of infection.

- Hands without healthy skin are more susceptible to becoming colonized with transient bacteria, including multidrug-resistant organisms (MDROs).

- Healthcare workers need to clearly understand when and how to perform hand hygiene.

- Healthcare worker adherence to hand hygiene recommendations depends on clearly understood policies, targeted education, healthy hand skin, convenient hand hygiene products, and monitoring of performance with feedback.

- Use of alcohol-based hand rubs has increased adherence of healthcare workers to recommended hand hygiene policies.

- Improved hand hygiene practices have been associated with reduced healthcare-associated infection rates.

- Implementation of waterless hand antiseptics does not negate the need for handwashing sinks for staff.

- Patients should be offered the opportunity to clean their hands during the day.

- The Joint Commission on Accreditation of Healthcare Organizations' (JCAHO's) 2004 National Patient Safety Goal 7a[2] requires facilities to comply with the CDC's 2002 Hand Hygiene Guideline.

I.   BACKGROUND

Handwashing as a primary method of infection prevention has been a cornerstone of infection control programs since the infection control profession began in the early

Copyright © 2005, Association for Professionals in Infection Control and Epidemiology, Inc.

1970s. Although isolation practices and handwashing products have changed since then, the message that "handwashing is the single most important measure to prevent the transmission of infection" has remained the same. Unfortunately, not too many healthcare personnel were listening. Observational studies of handwashing compliance reported dismal results, with compliance rates averaging less than 40%. Reasons for poor adherence included lack of knowledge, increased demands with less time, irritated and dry hands, lack of soap and paper towels, inaccessible sinks, shortage of sinks, belief that wearing gloves obviated need for handwashing, forgetfulness, skepticism about the value of handwashing, lack of role models, lack of administrative priority for hand hygiene, and lack of administrative sanctions.

It became increasingly apparent that new approaches were needed to address these unacceptable adherence rates. In 2002, the CDC published the *Guideline for Hand Hygiene in Health-Care Settings.*[1] The authors of this guideline, John M. Boyce, MD, and Didiet Pittet, MD, extensively reviewed the scientific data to determine the following:

- Physiology of normal skin

- Evidence for transmission of pathogens on hands

- Efficacy and adverse effects of hand hygiene products

- Why healthcare workers were ignoring the evidence regarding the importance of handwashing

- Applicability of behavioral theories

- Efficacy of intervention strategies

The resulting multimodal, multidisciplinary recommendations represented a major shift in the way we think about handwashing and hand antisepsis, starting with the concepts of hand hygiene and maintaining hand skin health.

II.   BASIC PRINCIPLES

General Knowledge

Waterless, alcohol-based hand rubs are now the preferred products for routine hand hygiene in healthcare settings, unless hands are visibly soiled. The CDC guideline requires that healthcare workers be provided with a readily available alcohol-based hand rub product at the entrance to each patient care room, at the patient's bedside, or at other convenient locations. Data suggest that this recommendation will increase the frequency of healthcare worker hand hygiene and result in decreased incidence of dermatitis caused by the drying effects of soap and water and abrasive

towels. Artificial fingernails or nail extenders are prohibited for those having direct contact with patients at high risk (e.g., in intensive care units or operating rooms), but there was not enough evidence for the guideline to make a recommendation regarding jewelry and rings.

The CDC guideline clearly delineates administrative responsibility for making improved hand hygiene adherence an institutional priority and for providing appropriate administrative support and financial resources. The Joint Commission on Accreditation of Health Organizations' (JCAHO) 2004 National Patient Safety Goal 7a,[2] which requires facilities to comply with the CDC's 2002 Hand Hygiene Guideline, lends additional support for this important initiative to prevent transmission of infection and improve patient safety.

Recommendations for increased use of waterless hand hygiene products do not negate the need for handwashing sinks. The American Institute of Architects' *Guidelines for Design and Construction of Hospital and Health Care Facilities, 2001 Edition,* addressed this issue by continuing to require handwashing stations it defines as "an area providing a sink with hot and cold water supply and a faucet that facilitates easy on/off mixing capabilities. This station includes provision of cleansing agents and drying capability."[3] The 2001 American Institute of Architects' guidelines require that there be one handwashing station in the patient's bathroom for patient use and another handwashing station in the patient room, ideally near the door, for healthcare worker use.

DEFINITION OF TERMS[1]

Alcohol-based hand rub is a solution that contains 60%–95% alcohol and is designed to be applied to hands to reduce the number of viable microorganisms on the hands. Although ethyl alcohol and isopropyl alcohol are both effective against bacteria, fungi, and viruses, isopropyl alcohol has slightly greater activity against bacteria and ethyl alcohol has greater activity against viruses.

Antimicrobial soap is a soap that contains an antiseptic agent. Antiseptic agents are antimicrobial substances that are applied to the skin to reduce the number of microbial flora. Examples include alcohols, chlorhexidine, chlorine, hexachlorophene, iodine, chloroxylenol (PCMX), quaternary ammonium compounds, and triclosan. In the United States, antiseptic agents are regulated by the Food and Drug Administration (FDA).

Antiseptic hand wash is washing hands with water and soap containing an antiseptic agent. Antiseptic hand rub is applying an antiseptic hand rub product to all surfaces of the hands to reduce the number of microorganisms present, without rinsing with water. Hand

APIC Text of Infection Control and Epidemiology

Copyright © 2005, Association for Professionals in Infection Control and Epidemiology, Inc.

antisepsis refers to either antiseptic hand wash or anti-septic hand rub. Hand hygiene is a general term that applies to either handwashing, antiseptic hand rub, or surgical hand antisepsis.

Handwashing is washing hands with plain (i.e., nonanti-microbial) soap and water. Surgical hand antisepsis is an antiseptic hand wash or antiseptic hand rub per-formed preoperatively by surgical personnel to elimi-nate transient and reduce resident hand flora. Antiseptic hand wash preparations often have persis-tent antimicrobial activity.

Visibly soiled hands are hands that show visible dirt or that are visibly contaminated with proteinaceous mate-rial, blood, or other body fluids (e.g., fecal material or urine).

Waterless antiseptic agent is an antiseptic agent that does not require use of exogenous water. After applying such an agent, the hands are rubbed together until the agent has dried.

III. ROUTINE HANDWASHING AND HAND ANTISEPSIS

Handwashing

Product Selection

To improve hand hygiene adherence, facilities are required to provide an alcohol-based (60%–90% alcohol) hand rub for routine hand antisepsis "in areas in which high workloads and high intensity of patient care are anticipated."[1] In addition, for routine hand-washing and hand antisepsis, a plain lotion soap or an antimicrobial soap also needs to be available. Although the selection process may start with products covered under the facility's buying agreements, the CDC guide-line makes clear that cost should not be the primary factor influencing product selection. To maximize acceptance, it is essential that employees be involved in product trials and selection.

Alcohol-based hand rubs vary considerably in their con-sistency, odor, and added emollients. Although the rinses have been used successfully for years in Europe, gels or foams, with added emollients, seem to be selected most often in the United States. Consideration should be given to whether the dispensers drip and whether they consistently dispense an appropriate amount of product. Product replacements for dis-pensers should be packaged in unit-dose inserts to prevent "topping-off" partially empty dispensers.

Infection control professionals (ICPs) will need to review the CDC guideline carefully to determine whether their specific facilities need only plain lotion soap or only antimicrobial soap as an alternative to the waterless product or whether both plain lotion soaps

and antimicrobial soaps should be installed at sinks. The advantage of installing only an antimicrobial (e.g. 2% Chlorhexadine gluconate [CHG]) at sinks is that personnel will not have to make a choice between plain soap or an antimicrobial, ensuring that an antimi-crobial is used when indicated. Regardless, it is impor-tant to select products with a low potential for skin irritation. Part I of the CDC guideline contains an excel-lent discussion of the specific antimicrobial formula-tions, which should be reviewed prior to product selection.

Antimicrobial-impregnated wipes (towelettes) are not a substitute for an alcohol-based hand rub or an antimi-crobial soap.[1] They are also not appropriate for healthcare workers to use as an alternative to washing with plain soap and water because they may not ade-quately remove proteinaceous material. However, when placed on patients' food trays or in bedside tables, these towelettes can be a useful means for patients to clean their hands before eating.

The CDC guideline classified the use of nonalcohol-based hand rubs for hand hygiene in healthcare set-tings as an unresolved issue due to insufficient evi-dence. Therefore, ICPs will need to carefully review information about the efficacy of specific antiseptic agents in Part I of the CDC guideline, along with inde-pendent scientific studies, before considering these products. Regardless, a facility must still comply with the requirement to provide healthcare workers with an alcohol-based hand rub.

Dispenser Location

The CDC guideline recommends that dispensers for the alcohol-based product be conveniently located at the entrance to each patient room, exam room, treat-ment room, or the like. Alternatively, the dispensers can be located inside the rooms near the door or adja-cent to each bed. Individual pocket-sized containers to be carried by healthcare workers also have been sug-gested, but concerns have been expressed about the inability of keeping contaminated hands from con-tacting clothing.

Because all alcohol-based hand rubs are potentially flammable, bulk supplies should be stored in cabinets or areas approved for flammable materials. Although the CDC guideline recommends installing dispensers at the entrance to patient rooms, the 2000 edition of the National Fire Protection Association Life Safety Code prohibited installation of individual alcohol-based hand rub dispensers in egress corridors (exit corridors or areas open to exit corridors). In 2003, APIC published a position statement "The Use of Hand Sanitizers in the Healthcare Setting,"[4] recommending that alcohol-based hand rub dispensers not be placed in egress corri-dors until more definitive guidance became available.

Copyright © 2005, Association for Professionals in Infection Control and Epidemiology, Inc.

To address this issue, in 2003, a survey of 840 U.S. healthcare facilities was conducted; 95% reported use of alcohol-based hand rubs. Respondents reported a cumulative 1430 years of hand-rub use with no fires attributable to or involving a hand rub dispenser. The authors concluded that

> because increased use of alcohol-based hand rubs has been shown to improve adherence with hand hygiene among HCWs and to reduce healthcare-related infections, we believe that the potential benefits of having these products available in easily accessible areas of healthcare facilities (e.g., hallways) far outweigh the apparent low (and undocumented) potential fire hazard that may occur with their use.[5]

Also in 2003, the American Society for Healthcare Engineering (ASHE) of the American Hospital Association commissioned a fire-modeling study of how alcohol-based hand rubs will react to a fire in a typical patient care environment. The study results indicated that installing hand rub dispensers is acceptable in both corridor and suite locations. The results also showed that placing dispensers at or near each patient room entrance was not a significant risk for additional ignition and involvement of more than 1 dispenser. However, ASHE does recommend that dispensers not be installed over electrical receptacles or near other potential sources of ignition.[6]

In mid-2004, the National Fire Protection Association announced the amendment of the 2003 edition of the Life Safety Code to specifically recognize and permit the use of alcohol-based hand rub solutions in patient rooms, corridors, and suites of healthcare facilities. Adoption of this tentative interim amendment allows the installation of dispensers in corridors, provided that the following conditions are met:[7]

- The corridor width is 6 ft or greater, and dispensers are separated by at least 4 ft

- The maximum individual dispenser fluid capacity is 1.2 L for dispensers in rooms, corridors, and areas open to corridors and 2.0 L for dispensers in suites of rooms

- The dispensers are not installed over or directly adjacent to electrical outlets and switches

- In locations with carpeted floor coverings, dispensers installed directly over carpeted surfaces are permitted only in sprinklered smoke compartments.

- In addition, each smoke compartment may contain a maximum aggregate of 10 gal of alcohol-based hand rub solution in dispensers and a maximum of 5 gal in storage.

Because local or state fire code requirements may differ from national codes, facilities should check with their local authorities regarding any restrictions. Fire safety regulations related to these products are expected to change as more data become available.

Indications for Use

Use plain lotion soap and water, or antimicrobial soap and water–

- If hands are visibly soiled (important to physically remove the material)

- Before eating

- After using the restroom

- If exposure to *Bacillus anthracis* is suspected or proven

Use an alcohol-based hand rub in all other recommended situations below, unless hands are visibly soiled–

- Before and after direct patient contact

- Before donning sterile gloves

- Before inserting invasive devices

- After contact with patient's intact skin (e.g., taking pulse or blood pressure)

- After removing gloves

- After contact with objects and equipment in the patient's immediate vicinity

- When moving from a contaminated body site to a clean body site during patient care

Hand-Hygiene Technique

When using an alcohol-based hand rub, it is important to check the manufacturer's recommendation for volume of product and to adjust the dispensers accordingly. The efficacy of alcohol-based products depends on the technique of the user, as is also the case when using soap and water. If not enough product is dispensed or if the product is not applied to all parts of the hands, antimicrobial efficacy may be limited.[8] After dispensing the product, personnel also should be instructed to rub hand surfaces together until they are dry. There has been one reported occurrence of alcohol hand gel that remained "wet" on the hands and ignited after static electricity was created by removing a polyester isolation gown and then touching metal.[9]

When using soap and water, hands should be wet with water, then product should be applied per manufacturer's recommendations, and hands should be rubbed together vigorously, covering all skin surfaces and under rings, for at least 15 seconds. Hands should be rinsed thoroughly, so that no product is left, and then

APIC Text of Infection Control and Epidemiology

Copyright © 2005, Association for Professionals in Infection Control and Epidemiology, Inc.

dried with a disposable towel that is then used to turn off the water faucet. Although the CDC guideline recommends against using hot water because of increased risk of dermatitis, there was not enough evidence to make a recommendation regarding cold water.

Surgical Hand Antisepsis

Product Selection

Either an antimicrobial soap or an alcohol-based surgical hand rub *with persistent activity* may be used. Alcohol-based formulations are the most effective at immediately lowering bacterial counts. The next most effective agents, in order of decreasing activity, are CHG, iodophors, triclosan, and plain soap.[1] Persistent antimicrobial activity is another important characteristic for a surgical scrub, and the most effective are CHG (2% or 4%), triclosan, and iodophors. Alcohol has no residual antimicrobial effect. Combination formulations of 60%–90% alcohol and 0.5%–1% CHG equal or exceed the persistence of CHG alone[1] and are approved for surgical hand antisepsis. PCMX needs further studies to establish its efficacy as a surgical scrub. Hexachlorophene is absorbed into the blood after repeated use and therefore seldom used as a surgical scrub.

Users should be involved in the selection of surgical hand antiseptic products, and cost should not be the primary factor influencing product selection. Efficacy and low irritancy potential should be prime selection criteria. Product replacements for dispensers should be packaged in unit-dose inserts to prevent "topping-off" partially empty dispensers.

Technique

When using an *antimicrobial soap and water* for surgical hand antisepsis, hand and arm jewelry should be removed before the surgical scrub, and debris should be removed from underneath fingernails using a nail cleaner under running water. Artificial fingernails or nail extenders are not to be worn by personnel in operating rooms. The CDC guideline recommends that hands and forearms be scrubbed for the length of time recommended by the manufacturer, usually 2 to 6 minutes. Longer scrub times and use of a scrub brush are not necessary and may contribute to dermatitis.[1p18]

When using an *alcohol-based surgical hand rub product* (with persistent activity) for surgical hand antisepsis, hand and arm jewelry should be removed, and debris removed from underneath fingernails using a nail cleaner under running water. Artificial fingernails or nail extenders are not to be worn by personnel in operating rooms. Hands and forearms should be prewashed with a plain lotion soap and water and dried

completely. Manufacturer's instructions for use of the alcohol-based surgical hand rub product should be followed; hands and forearms must be allowed to dry completely before donning sterile gloves.

Staff Education and Effective Interventions

To improve hand hygiene adherence, healthcare personnel should be provided with evidence-based information about hand contamination, the effects of hand hygiene products on the physiology of normal skin, and the association between hand hygiene practices and transmission of infection. Because the alcohol hand rubs are relatively new in the United States, it is also important to provide healthcare workers with education about proper application technique to ensure antimicrobial effectiveness. Part I of the CDC guideline contains abundant data for the ICP to use to develop educational programs and influence adherence to hand-hygiene recommendations. The CDC Hand Hygiene website (http://www.cdc.gov/handhygiene/default.htm) has an educational slideshow available for download, along with other materials for order. The Hand Hygiene Resource Center (http://www.handhygiene.org/) established by Dr. John Boyce also has an educational program available for download at no charge.

As noted in the CDC guideline, the process of change is complex, and single interventions often fail; a multimodal, multidisciplinary strategy is necessary. To design effective interventions for improvement, potential barriers should first be identified. Elaine Larson, RN, PhD, CIC, has designed an assessment tool to identify healthcare worker attitudes and beliefs that might be barriers to guideline adherence. The tool and instructions for use are included in her article in *American Journal of Infection Control.*[10]

One of the most significant and sustained barriers to hand hygiene compliance may turn out to be healthcare workers' hand skin conditions. Frequent glove use combined with increased frequency of hand hygiene and failure to consistently use hand lotion result in dry, cracked, painful skin. Selection of hand lotions acceptable to personnel should be as much a priority as hand hygiene product selection. The CDC guideline requires that hand lotions or creams be provided to healthcare workers "to minimize the occurrence of irritant contact dermatitis associated with hand antisepsis or handwashing."[1] Consideration should be given to locating hand lotion dispensers at charting areas and in lounges as well as near handwashing sinks.

Studies have suggested that role models and the behavior of other healthcare workers significantly influence hand hygiene adherence. A recent observational

Copyright © 2005, Association for Professionals in Infection Control and Epidemiology, Inc.

study reported that the most potent effect of the role model was in negatively influencing hand hygiene behavior. In other words, if the role model (senior nurse or senior medical staff) did not perform hand hygiene, than other healthcare workers in the room were significantly less likely to perform hand hygiene.[11]

Monitoring for Adherence

The CDC guideline requires that healthcare workers' adherence to recommended hand hygiene policies be monitored and that healthcare workers be provided with information about their performance. The guideline suggests several possible performance indicators for measuring improvements in hand-hygiene adherence:

- Periodically conduct an observational study to determine the rate of adherence (number of hand hygiene episodes performed/number of hand hygiene opportunities) by ward or service. Some facilities have used "light-duty" staff or students for this purpose.

- Monitor the volume of specific hand hygiene products (e.g., soap, hand rub, hand lotion) used per 1000 patient days.

- Monitor adherence to artificial fingernail policies.

- When outbreaks occur, assess the adequacy of healthcare worker hand hygiene.

IV.   SUMMARY AND CONCLUSIONS

In-service education, distribution of information leaflets, workshops and lectures, and performance feedback on compliance rates have been associated with transient, but not sustained, improvement in hand hygiene compliance. The complex dynamic of behavioral change requires a combination of education, motivation, and system change. JCAHO's endorsement of the 2002 CDC guideline should provide impetus for facilities to invest in the multimodal, multidisciplinary programs necessary to improve hand hygiene rates, thus decreasing the risk for healthcare-associated infection. Ultimately, compliance with hand hygiene must become part of a culture of patient safety with strong administrative support.

V.   FUTURE TRENDS/RESEARCH

Given the importance of hand hygiene in the prevention of disease transmission and improving patient safety, it is important to continue to investigate ideas to increase performance and efficacy. Potential questions may include some of these unresolved issues:

- Can we improve the condition of healthcare workers' hand skin to encourage necessary hand hygiene?

- What are the benchmarks and best method(s) for monitoring adherence?

- Will we see an improvement in healthcare worker hand hygiene adherence with use of alcohol-based hand rubs?

- Are there successful behavioral, and motivational intervention programs with sustained effects?

- What is the efficacy of nonalcohol-based hand rubs in healthcare settings?

REFERENCES

1. Centers for Disease Control and Prevention: Guideline for Hand Hygiene in Health-Care Settings: Recommendations of the Healthcare Infection Control Practices Advisory Committee and the HICPAC/SHEA/APIC/IDSA Hand Hygiene Task Force. *MMWR Morb Mortal Wkly Rep* 51(No. RR-16):1–45, 2002.
2. JCAHO National Patient Safety Goals: JCHO Patient Safety Web Site, 2004 National Patient Safety Goals—FAQs . Available at: http://www.jcaho.org/accredited+organizations/patient+safety/04+npsg/04_faqs.htm#goa Accessed November 17, 2004.
3. American Institute of Architects Academy of Architecture for Health, the Facilities Guidelines Institute, with assistance from the U.S. Department of Health and Human Services: *Guidelines for design and construction of hospital and health care facilities,* Washington, DC, 2001, The American Institute of Architects.
4. APIC web site. Available at: http://www.apic.org
5. Boyce JM, Pearson ML: Low frequency of fires from alcohol-based hand rub dispensers in healthcare facilities, *Infect Control Hosp Epidemiol* 24:618–619, 2003.
6. American Society for Healthcare Engineering of the American Hospital Association: *Alcohol-based hand rub solution: fire modeling analysis report,* Chicago, 2003, Available at: http://www.hospitalconnect.com/ashe/currentevent/alcohol_based_hand_rub/Final_Report_rev1.2_Part_1_2.pdf Accessed November 17, 2004.
7. APIC web site http://www.apic.org
8. Widner AF, Dangel M: Alcohol-based handrub: evaluation of technique and microbiological efficacy with international infection control professionals, *Infect Control Hosp Epidemiol* 25:207–209, 2004.
9. Bryant KA, Pearce J, Stover B: Flash fire associated with the use of alcohol-based antiseptic agent, *Am J Infect Control* 30:256–257, 2002.
10. Larson E: A tool to assess barriers to adherence to hand hygiene guideline, *Am J Infect Control* 32:48–51, 2004.
11. Lankford MG, Zembower TR, Trick WE, Hacek DM, Noskin GA, Peterson LR: Influence of role models and hospital design on the hand hygiene of healthcare workers, *Emerg Infect Dis* 9:217–223, 2003.

SUPPLEMENTAL RESOURCES

Traditional Resources

Alcohol-based hand gels and hand hygiene in hospitals: Letters to the editor, *Lancet* 360:1509–1511, 2002.

Bottone EJ, Cheng M, Hymes S: Ineffectiveness of handwashing with lotion soap to remove nosocomial bacterial pathogens persisting on fingertips: a major link in their intrahospital spread, *Infect Control Hosp Epidemiol* 25:262–264, 2004.

Boyce JM: New insights for improving hand hygiene practices, *Infect Control Hosp Epidemiol* 25:187–189, 2004.

APIC Text of Infection Control and Epidemiology

Copyright © 2005, Association for Professionals in Infection Control and Epidemiology, Inc.

Gawande A: Notes of a surgeon: on washing hands, *N Engl J Med* 350:1283–1286, 2004.

Kramer A, Rudolph P, Kampf G, Pitter D: Limited efficacy of alcohol-based hand gels, *Lancet* 359:1489–1490,2002.

Pessoa-Silva CL, Dharan S, Hugonnet S, et al: Dynamics of bacterial hand contamination during routine neonatal care, *Infect Control Hosp Epidemiol* 25:192–197, 2004.

Pittet D, Sax H, Hugonnet S, Harvarth S: Cost implications of successful hand hygiene promotion, *Infect Control Hosp Epidemiol* 25: 264–266, 2004.

Raboud J, Saskin R, Wong K, et al: Patterns of handwashing behavior and visits to patients on a general medical ward of healthcare workers, *Infect Control Hosp Epidemiol* 25:198–202, 2004.

Wendt C, Knautz D, von Baum H: Differences in hand hygiene behavior related to the contamination risk of healthcare activities in different groups of healthcare workers, *Infect Control Hosp Epidemiol* 25:203–206, 2004.

Web-Based Hand Hygiene Resources

University of Geneva Hospitals, Geneva, Switzerland, http://www.hopisafe.ch

CDC, Atlanta, Georgia, http://www.cdc.gov/ncidod/hip

Bandolier journal, United Kingdom, http://www.jr2.ox.ac.uk/bandolier/band88/b88—8.html

University of Pennsylvania, Philadelphia, Pennsylvania, http://www.med.upenn.edu

Food and Drug Administration, Washington, D.C., http://www.fda.gov

The Hand Hygiene Resource Center of St Raphael Healthcare System, http://www.handhygiene.org

Copyright © 2005, Association for Professionals in Infection Control and Epidemiology, Inc.

Aseptic Technique

Martha G. DeCastro, RN, MS, CIC
Director, Infection Control
Tallahassee Memorial Health
Tallahassee, Florida

Pamela Iwamoto, BSN, RN, CIC
Director Epidemiology
University of New Mexico, University Hospital,
Albuquerque, New Mexico

ABSTRACT

Aseptic technique is a primary infection prevention method basic to all healthcare practice settings. Both sterile and clean techniques are elements of this infection method, although both have distinct similarities and differences.

KEY CONCEPTS

- Antiseptic agent is an antimicrobial substance applied to the skin to reduce the number of microbial flora.[1]

- Asepsis is defined as the absence of pathogenic (disease-producing) microorganisms.

- Aseptic technique is the purposeful prevention of transfer of organisms from one person to another by keeping the microbe count to an irreducible minimum. It may also be referred to as sterile technique.[2]

- Clean technique refers to practice interventions that reduce the numbers of microorganisms or prevent and reduce transmission risk from one person (or place) to another.[2]

- Hand hygiene refers to a variety of practices aimed at reducing the microbial flora on the hands. Examples include handwashing, antiseptic handwash, antiseptic hand rub, or surgical hand antisepsis.[1]

I. BACKGROUND

Microorganisms are capable of causing illness in humans and can be transmitted by direct or indirect contact. Interrupting the transmission of microorganisms from reservoir to susceptible host can prevent illnesses caused by those microorganisms.

II. BASIC PRINCIPLES

Aseptic or sterile technique is an infection prevention method that is basic to virtually all healthcare settings, and originated in the surgical setting as a means for preventing contamination of the operative field. This technique was modified for other practice settings to minimize the risk of infection transmission to patients undergoing invasive procedures or wound management.

Copyright © 2005, Association for Professionals in Infection Control and Epidemiology, Inc.

III. ASEPTIC TECHNIQUE

Sterile or aseptic technique refers to practices designed to render and maintain objects and areas maximally free from microorganisms. Sterile technique is indicated for the insertion of invasive devices, such as intravascular devices. Additional information and specific recommendations relative to the prevention of surgical site infections can be found in Chapter 23, Surgical Site Infections.

Aseptic technique involves using barriers, such as gloves, gowns, masks, and drapes, to prevent transferring microorganisms from the environment to the patient during the procedure being performed, using antiseptic agents to minimize the number of microorganisms on the skin of the patient at the time of the procedure, and appropriately cleaning and reprocessing reusable patient-care devices (see Table 20–1).

Examples of sterile practices include providing maximum reduction of skin microorganisms without damaging tissue, which is accomplished when healthcare providers decontaminate their hands using an antiseptic hand rub or antiseptic soap before donning sterile gloves,[1] prepare the patient's skins before procedure[3] by applying the hospital-approved antiseptic agent to the patient's clean skin, and remove hair only when necessary. If hair is removed, it should be removed immediately before the procedure using

clippers instead of a razor. Other sterile practices involve using single-use devices and equipment, or reusable devices and equipment that have been properly cleaned and reprocessed, using barriers to decrease the risk of transmission from practitioner or environment to the patient[3] by maintaining a sterile field with sterile drapes, gloves, and gowns as well as selecting attire to support this practice. Appropriate attire is based on the risk of the procedure and the area of the hospital where the procedure is performed. Using environmental controls to maximize the reduction of microorganisms during surgical procedures[3] is also recommended. This is done by using special treatment or operating rooms, managing activity to reduce airborne transmission if procedures are performed at the bedside, keeping doors closed during procedures, using physical barriers, such as screens, to divert traffic in open units, excluding visitors and unnecessary personnel, avoiding cleaning activities in the area during surgical procedures, and providing additional environmental controls to further reduce contamination. Higher rates of air exchanges and maintenance of positive pressure in relation to the adjacent corridors or spaces,[3] routinely cleaning and disinfecting environmental surfaces with an Environmental Protection Agency (EPA) approved hospital disinfectant detergent,[4] and using efficacious germicidal agents for cleanup of blood or body fluid spills are all examples of

Table 20-1. Examples of Suggested Techniques by Procedure

Procedure/ Intervention	Hand Hygiene Indicated	Type of Glove to Be used*	Supplies Indicated	Instrumentation
Wound cleaning	Yes	Clean exam gloves	Normal saline or prepared sterile wound cleanser. Sterile supplies such as 4 × 4 or cotton applicators.	Irrigation performed with sterile device while maintaining clean technique
Routine dressing changes without debridement	Yes	Clean exam gloves	Sterile supplies using clean technique	Sterile supplies using clean technique
Dressing change with mechanical, chemical, or enzymatic debridement	Yes	Clean exam gloves	Sterile supplies using clean technique	Sterile supplies using clean technique
Dressing change with sharp, conservative bedside debridement	Yes	Sterile gloves	Sterile supplies and sterile technique due to the potential for entering new, unaffected tissues	Sterile supplies and sterile technique
Central line dressing change	Yes	Sterile gloves for removing old dressing and new sterile gloves for dressing change procedure	Sterile dressing change kit and sterile technique Surgeon mask should be worn	Sterile supplies and sterile technique
Tracheal suctioning where the tracheal suction catheter is not within a closed sheath	Yes	Sterile gloves when suctioning	Sterile suction catheter	Sterile supplies and clean technique
Tracheostomy care or suctioning with a suction catheter within a closed sheath	Yes	Clean exam gloves	Sterile supplies using clean technique	Sterile supplies using clean technique

* The American College of Surgeons has recommended that sterile gloves be used for dressing changes performed during the first 24 hours after surgery. The use of sterile gloves should always be considered as a method for preventing the transfer of organisms to the wound site. An individual practice of the provider may include a double-gloving technique that involves removal of the gloves after the debridement before completion of dressing change.

Copyright © 2005, Association for Professionals in Infection Control and Epidemiology, Inc.

controlling the environment to reduce the risk of contamination.

Clean technique refers to practices that reduce the numbers of microorganisms and minimize the risk of transmission from personnel or environment to the patient.

Infection transmission can be reduced by reducing the numbers of skin microorganisms through proper hand hygiene, by using single-use patient devices and equipment, or reusable devices and equipment that have been properly cleaned and reprocessed, and by using barriers to reduce microbial transmission from personnel to patient, which include gloves, gowns, and hair covering. Gloves can be either sterile or nonsterile. Sterile gloves should be used for sterile dressing applications. The "no-touch" dressing technique should be used to prevent contamination of sterile dressings, depending on the type and extent of the wound care procedure.[2] The use of nonsterile versus sterile gloves for routine changing of surgical site dressings remains an unresolved issue because wounds may be colonized and, therefore, not sterile. Nonsterile gloves may be used as long as the techniques used in the dressing change prevent the transfer of new organisms to that particular patient. A clean gown should be worn to minimize contamination of clothing. Room placement should be selected for patients according to their transmission risk . The clean technique for the environment involves providing environmental controls to reduce microbial transmission, such as [4] cleaning the environment routinely, using clean equipment and supplies (mops, water, cleaning cloths), using an EPA-registered hospital detergent/disinfectant for all environmental surfaces, and using an EPA-registered germicide for cleaning up blood and body fluid spills immediately when they occur. (Most germicides recommend removing the original bioburden followed by use of the germicide to disinfect the area.)

IV.   SUMMARY AND CONCLUSIONS

The use of aseptic technique can be performed in areas of practice that have adequate as well as limited resources. Maintaining a clean environment, practicing hand hygiene, and using routine sterilization and disinfection are examples of practices that can reduce the risk of infection for both the patient and the healthcare worker.

REFERENCES

1. Centers for Disease Control and Prevention: Guideline for hand hygiene in health-care settings: recommendations of the Healthcare Infection Control Practices Advisory Committee and the HICPAC/SHEA/APIC/IDSA Hand Hygiene Task Force, *MMWR Morb Mortal Wkly Rep* 51 (No. RR-16):1–45, 2002.

2. Wooten MK, Hawkins K: Clean versus sterile: management of chronic wounds, *J Wound Ostomy Continence Nurs* 28(5): 24A–26A,2001.
3. Mangram AJ, Horan TC, Pearson ML, Silver LC, Jarvis WR: Guidelines for Prevention of Surgical Site Infection. Centers for Disease Control and Prevention (CDC) Hospital Infection Control Practices Advisory Committee. *Am J Infect Control* 27:97–132, 1999.]
4. Centers for Disease Control and Prevention: Guidelines for environmental infection control in health care facilities: recommendations of CDC and the Healthcare Infection Control Practices Advisory Committee (HICPAC), *MMWR Morb Mortal Wkly Rep* 52 (No. RR-10): 1–48, 2003.

SUPPLEMENTAL RESOURCE

Surgical Infection Prevention Project Description, available at: http://www.medqic.org/sip

Copyright © 2005, Association for Professionals in Infection Control and Epidemiology, Inc.

21

Cleaning, Disinfection, and Sterilization in Healthcare Facilities

William A. Rutala, PhD, MPH*
Hospital Epidemiology
Division of Infectious Diseases
University of North Carolina Health Care System
Chapel Hill, North Carolina

David J. Weber, MD, MPH
University of North Carolina School of Medicine
Chapel Hill, North Carolina

ABSTRACT

All invasive procedures involve contact by a medical device or surgical instrument with a patient's sterile tissue or mucous membranes. A major risk of all such procedures is the introduction of pathogenic microbes leading to infection. Failure to properly disinfect or sterilize reusable medical equipment carries a risk associated with breach of the host barriers.

The level of disinfection or sterilization is dependent on the intended use of the object: critical (items that contact sterile tissue such as surgical instruments), semicritical (items that contact mucous membrane such as endoscopes), and noncritical (devices that contact only intact skin such as stethoscopes) items require sterilization, high-level disinfection and low-level disinfection, respectively. Cleaning must always precede high-level disinfection and sterilization. Users must consider the advantages and disadvantages of specific methods when choosing a disinfection or sterilization process.

Adherence to these recommendations should improve disinfection and sterilization practices in healthcare facilities and thereby reduce infections associated with contaminated patient-care items.

I.   BACKGROUND

In the United States there were approximately 40 million inpatient surgical procedures in 2001, 31.5 million outpatient surgical procedures in 1996, and an even larger number of invasive medical procedures.[1-3] For example, there are about 5 million gastrointestinal endoscopies per year.[1] Each of these procedures involves contact by a medical device or surgical instrument with a patient's sterile tissue or mucous membranes. A major risk of all such procedures is the introduction of pathogenic microbes, which can lead to infection. For example, failure to properly disinfect or sterilize equipment may lead to person-to-person transmission via contaminated devices (e.g., bronchoscopes contaminated with *Mycobacterium tuberculosis*).

*Acknowledgments: This chapter has been extensively modified from another publication: Rutala WA, Weber DJ: Selection and use of disinfectants in health-care facilities: what clinicians should know, *Clinical Infectious Diseases*, in press.

Copyright © 2005, Association for Professionals in Infection Control and Epidemiology, Inc.

Achieving disinfection and sterilization through the use of disinfectants and sterilization practices is essential for ensuring that medical and surgical instruments do not transmit infectious pathogens to patients. Because it is not necessary to sterilize all patient-care items, healthcare policies must identify whether cleaning, disinfection, or sterilization is indicated, based primarily on each item's intended use.

Multiple studies in many countries have documented lack of compliance with established guidelines for disinfection and sterilization.[4,5] Failure to comply with scientifically based guidelines has led to numerous outbreaks.[5-9] In this chapter, a pragmatic approach to the judicious selection and proper use of disinfection and sterilization processes is presented, based on well-designed studies that assess the efficacy (via laboratory investigations) and effectiveness (via clinical studies) of disinfection and sterilization procedures.

II. BASIC PRINCIPLES

Over 35 years ago, Earle H. Spaulding[10] devised a rational approach to disinfection and sterilization of patient-care items or equipment. This classification scheme is so clear and logical that it has been retained, refined, and successfully used by infection-control professionals (ICPs) and others when planning methods for disinfection or sterilization.[11-17] Spaulding believed that the nature of disinfection could be understood more readily if instruments and items for patient care were divided into three categories based on the degree of risk of infection involved in the use of the items. The three categories he described were critical, semicritical, and noncritical. This terminology is employed by the Centers for Disease Control and Prevention's (CDC) "Guidelines for Environmental Infection Control in Healthcare Facilities"[18] and the CDC's "Guideline for Disinfection and Sterilization in Healthcare Facilities."[16]

Critical Items

Critical items involve a high risk of infection if such an item is contaminated with any microorganism, including bacterial spores. Thus, it is critical that objects that enter sterile tissue or the vascular system be sterile because any microbial contamination could result in disease transmission. This category of items includes surgical instruments, cardiac and urinary catheters, implants, and ultrasound probes used in sterile body cavities. The items in this category should be purchased sterile or be sterilized by steam sterilization if possible. If heat sensitive, the object may be treated with ethylene oxide (ETO), with hydrogen peroxide gas plasma, or with liquid chemical sterilants if other

methods are unsuitable. Tables 21–1 and 21–2 list several germicides categorized as chemical sterilants. These include > 2.4% glutaraldehyde-based formulations, 1.12% glutaraldehyde with 1.93% phenol/phenate, 7.5% stabilized hydrogen peroxide, 7.35% hydrogen peroxide with 0.23% peracetic acid, 0.2% peracetic acid, and 1.0% hydrogen peroxide with 0.08% peracetic acid. With the exception of 0.2% peracetic acid (12 minutes at 50–56°C), the indicated exposure times range from 3 to 12 hours.[19] Liquid chemical sterilants will produce sterility only if preceded by cleaning, which eliminates organic and inorganic material, and if proper guidelines of concentration, contact time, temperature, and pH are met. Another limitation to sterilizing devices with liquid chemical sterilants is that the devices cannot be wrapped during processing in a liquid chemical sterilant; thus it is impossible to maintain sterility following processing and during storage. A chemical sterilization process does provide a transport tray that aids in preventing recontamination; such trays can be used for transport, but do not allow for short- or long-term storage. Another limitation of chemical sterilization is that devices may require rinsing following exposure to the liquid chemical sterilant using water that generally is not sterile. Therefore, due to the inherent limitations of using liquid chemical sterilants in a nonautomated reprocessor, their use should be restricted to reprocessing critical devices that are heat sensitive and incompatible with other sterilization methods.

Semicritical Items

Semicritical items are those items that will contact mucous membranes or nonintact skin. Respiratory therapy and anesthesia equipment, some endoscopes, laryngoscope blades, esophageal manometry probes, anorectal manometry catheters, and diaphragm fitting rings are included in this category. These medical devices should be free of all vegetative microorganisms (i.e., mycobacteria, fungi, viruses, bacteria), although small numbers of bacterial spores may be present. Intact mucous membranes, such as those of the lungs or the gastrointestinal tract, generally are resistant to infection by common bacterial spores but susceptible to other organisms, such as bacteria, mycobacteria, and viruses. Semicritical items minimally require high-level disinfection using chemical disinfectants. Glutaraldehyde, hydrogen peroxide, ortho-phthalaldehyde, peracetic acid with hydrogen peroxide, and chlorine are cleared by the Food and Drug Administration (FDA)[19] and are dependable high-level disinfectants, provided the factors influencing germicidal procedures are met (Tables 21–1 and 21–2). The exposure time for most high-level disinfectants varies from 10 to 45 minutes at 20–25°C. Outbreaks continue to occur when ineffective disinfectants, including iodophor, alcohol, and over-

Copyright © 2005, Association for Professionals in Infection Control and Epidemiology, Inc.

Table 21–1. Methods for disinfection and sterilization of patient-care items and environmental surfaces[a]

Process	Level of Microbial Inactivation	Method	Examples (with processing times)	Healthcare Application (examples)
Sterilization	Destroys all microorganisms, including bacterial spores	High temperature	Steam (~40 min), dry heat (1–6 hr depending on temperature)	Heat-tolerant critical (surgical instruments) and semicritical patient-care items
		Low temperature	Ethylene oxide gas (~15 hr), hydrogen peroxide gas plasma (~50 min)	Heat-sensitive critical and semicritical patient-care items
		Liquid immersion	Chemical sterilants[b]: >2% glut (~10 hr); 1.12% glut and 1.93% phenol (12 hr); 7.35% HP and 0.23% PA (3 hr); 7.5% HP (6 hr); 1.0% HP and 0.08% PA (8 hr); ≥0.2% PA (~50 min)	Heat-sensitive critical and semicritical patient-care items that can be immersed
High-level disinfection (HLD)	Destroys all micro-organisms except high numbers of bacterial spores	Heat-automated	Pasteurization (~50 min)	Heat-sensitive semicritical items (respiratory therapy equipment)
		Liquid immersion	Chemical Sterilants/HLDs[b]: >2% glut (20–45 min); 0.55% OPA (12 min); 1.12% glut and 1.93% phenol (20 min); 7.35% HP and 0.23% PA (15 min); 7.5% HP (30 min); 1.0% HP and 0.08% PA (25 min); 650–675 ppm chlorine (10 min)	Heat-sensitive semicritical items (GI endoscopes, bronchoscopes)
Intermediate-level disinfection	Destroys vegetative bacteria, mycobacteria, most viruses, most fungi but not bacterial spores	Liquid contact	EPA-registered hospital disinfectant with label claim regarding tuberculocidal activity (e.g., chlorine-based products, phenolics-exposure times at least 30–60 sec)	Noncritical patient care item (blood pressure cuff) or surface with visible blood
Low-level disinfection	Destroys vegetative bacteria, some fungi and viruses but not mycobacteria or spores	Liquid contact	EPA-registered hospital disinfectant with no tuberculocidal claim (e.g., chlorine-based products, phenolics, quaternary ammonium compounds-exposure times at least 30–60 sec) or 70–90% alcohol.	Noncritical patient care item (blood pressure cuff) or surface (bedside table) with no visible blood

[a] Modified from[15,16,96]. Abbreviations: glut-glutaraldehyde; HP-hydrogen peroxide; PA-peracetic acid; OPA-ortho-phthalaldehyde; ppm-parts per million; EPA-Environmental Protection Agency; FDA-Food and Drug Administration; GI-gastrointestinal.

[b] Consult the FDA-cleared package insert for information about the cleared contact time and temperature, and see text for discussion why one product is used at a reduced exposure time (2% glutaraldehyde at 20 min, 20°C). Increasing the temperature using an automated endoscope reprocess (AER) will reduce the contact time (e.g., OPA 12 min at 20°C but 5 min at 25°C in AER). Tubing must be completely filled for high-level disinfection and liquid chemical sterilization. Material compatibility should be investigated when appropriate (e.g., HP and HP with PA will cause functional damage to endoscopes).

diluted glutaraldehyde,[7] are used for "high-level disinfection." When a disinfectant is selected for use with certain patient-care items, the chemical compatibility with the items to be disinfected also must be considered. For example, compatibility testing by Olympus America of the 7.5% hydrogen peroxide found cosmetic and functional changes with the tested endoscopes (Olympus, October 15, 1999, written communication). Similarly, Olympus does not endorse the use of the hydrogen peroxide with peracetic acid products due to cosmetic and functional damage (Olympus America, April 15, 1998 and September 13, 2000, written communication).

Semicritical items that will have contact with the mucous membranes of the respiratory tract or gastrointestinal tract should be rinsed with sterile water, filtered water, or tap water, followed by an alcohol rinse.[16,20,21] An alcohol rinse and forced-air drying markedly reduces the likelihood of contamination of the instrument (e.g., endoscope), most likely by removing the wet environment favorable for bacterial growth.[21] After rinsing, items should be dried and stored in a manner that protects them from damage or contamination. There is no recommendation for using sterile or filtered water rather than tap water for rinsing semicritical equipment that will have contact with the mucous membranes of the rectum (e.g., rectal probes, anoscope) or vagina (e.g., vaginal probes).[16]

Noncritical Items

Noncritical items are those items that contact intact skin but not mucous membranes. Intact skin acts as an effective barrier against most microorganisms; therefore, the sterility of items coming in contact with intact skin is "not critical." Examples of noncritical items are bedpans, blood pressure cuffs, crutches, bed rails, linens, bedside tables, patient furniture, and floors. In

---

Cleaning, Disinfection, and Sterilization in Healthcare Facilities

Copyright © 2005, Association for Professionals in Infection Control and Epidemiology, Inc.

Table 21–2. Summary of advantages and disadvantages of chemical agents used as chemical sterilants[1] or as highlevel disinfectants.

Sterilization Method	Advantages	Disadvantages
Peracetic Acid/Hydrogen Peroxide	• No activation required • Odor or irritation not significant	• Material compatibility concerns (lead, brass, copper, zinc) both cosmetic and functional • Limited clinical experience • Potential for eye and skin damage
Glutaraldehyde	• Numerous use studies published • Relatively inexpensive • Excellent material compatibility	• Respiratory irritation from glutaraldehyde vapor • Pungent and irritating odor • Relatively slow mycobactericidal activity • Coagulates blood and fixes tissue to surfaces • Allergic contact dermatitis
Hydrogen Peroxide	• No activation required • May enhance removal of organic matter and organisms • No disposal issues • No odor or irritation issues • Does not coagulate blood or fix tissues to surfaces • Inactivates *Cryptosporidium* • Use studies published	• Material compatibility concerns (brass, zinc, copper, and nickel/silver plating) both cosmetic and functional • Serious eye damage with contact
Ortho-phthalaldehyde	• Fast-acting high-level disinfectant • No activation required • Odor not significant • Excellent materials compatibility claimed • Does not coagulate blood or fix tissues to surfaces claimed	• Stains protein gray (e.g., skin, mucous membranes, clothing, and environmental surfaces) • Limited clinical experience • More expensive than glutaraldehyde • Eye irritation with contact • Slow sporicidal activity
Peracetic Acid	• Rapid sterilization cycle time (30–45 minutes) • Low-temperature (50–55 °C) liquid immersion sterilization • Environmental friendly by-products (acetic acid, O_2, H_2O) • Fully automated • Single-use system eliminates need for concentration testing • Standardized cycle • May enhance removal of organic material and endotoxin • No adverse health effects to operators under normal operating conditions • Compatible with many materials and instruments • Does not coagulate blood or fix tissues to surfaces • Sterilant flows through scope facilitating salt, protein, and microbe removal • Rapidly sporicidal • Provides procedure standardization (constant dilution, perfusion of channel, temperatures, exposure)	• Potential material incompatibility (e.g., aluminum anodized coating becomes dull) • Used for immersible instruments only • Biological indicator may not be suitable for routine monitoring • One scope or a small number of instruments can be processed in a cycle • More expensive (endoscope repairs, operating costs, purchase costs) than high-level disinfection • Serious eye and skin damage (concentrated solution) with contact • Point-of-use system, no sterile storage

Modified from[97].

[1] All products effective in presence of organic soil, relatively easy to use, and have a broad spectrum of antimicrobial activity (bacteria, fungi, viruses, bacterial spores, and mycobacteria). The preceding characteristics are documented in the literature; contact the manufacturer of the instrument and sterilant for additional information. All products listed in the table are FDA cleared as chemical sterilants except OPA, which is an FDA-cleared high-level disinfectant.

contrast to critical and some semicritical items, most noncritical reusable items may be decontaminated where they are used and do not need to be transported to a central processing area. There is virtually no documented risk of transmitting infectious agents to patients via noncritical items[22] when they are used as noncritical items and do not contact nonintact skin and/or mucous membranes. However, these items (e.g., bedside tables, bed rails) could potentially contribute to secondary transmission by contaminating hands of healthcare workers or by contact with medical equipment that will subsequently come in contact with

APIC Text of Infection Control and Epidemiology

Copyright © 2005, Association for Professionals in Infection Control and Epidemiology, Inc.

patients.[23] Table 21–1 lists several low-level disinfectants that may be used for noncritical items. The exposure time listed in Table 21–1 is at least 30–60 seconds.

Cleaning

Items must be cleaned using water with detergents or enzymatic cleaners[24,25] before processing. Cleaning reduces the bioburden and removes foreign material (organic residue and inorganic salts) that interferes with the sterilization process by acting as a barrier to the sterilization agent.[26-30] Precleaning in patient-care areas may be needed on items that are heavily soiled with feces, sputum, blood, and so on. Items sent to central processing without removing gross soil may be difficult to clean because of dried secretions and excretions. Cleaning and decontamination should be done as soon as possible after items have been used.

Overall, a detergent with neutral pH should be used for instrument cleaning, as these solutions generally provide the best material compatibility profile as well as good soil removal. Manual cleaning requires a nearly neutral solution and friction on the instrument surface to loosen and suspend the soil. A more alkaline detergent is generally used with mechanical equipment to compensate for the lack of friction used with manual cleaning. The manufacturers' recommendations for dilution, temperature, water hardness, and use (e.g., designed for use in washer/decontaminators, ultrasonic cleaners) should be followed.[31] Enzymes, usually proteases, are sometimes added to neutral pH detergent solutions to assist in the removal of organic material. Enzymes in these formulations attack proteins that make up a large portion of common soil (blood, pus, etc.). Cleaning solution can also contain lipases (enzymes active on fats) and amylases (enzymes active on starches). Enzymatic detergents are cleaners and not disinfectants, and disinfectants may inactivate enzymes. Like all chemicals, enzymes must be rinsed from the equipment or adverse reactions (e.g., fever) could result.[32] Neutral pH detergent solutions that contain enzymes are compatible with metals and other materials used in medical instruments and are the best choice for cleaning delicate medical instruments, especially flexible endoscopes.[27] Some data demonstrate that enzymatic detergents are more effective cleaners that neutral detergents.[24,25] A new nonenzyme, hydrogen peroxide–based formulation was as effective as enzymatic detergents in removing protein, blood, carbohydrate, and endotoxin from surface test carriers. In addition, this product was able to effect a 5-$\log_{10}$ reduction in microbial loads with a 3-minute exposure at room temperature.[33]

Although the effectiveness of high-level disinfection and sterilization mandates effective cleaning, there are currently no "real-time" tests that can be employed in a clinical setting to validate cleaning. If such testing was available, it could be used to ensure that an adequate level of cleaning has been done.[34-37] The only way to ensure adequate cleaning is to conduct reprocessing validation test (e.g., microbiologic sampling), but this is not routinely recommended. Monitoring of the cleaning processes in a laboratory setting is possible by microorganism detection, chemical detection for organic contaminants, radionuclide tagging, and chemical detection for specific ions.[26,36]

III. CURRENT ISSUES IN DISINFECTION AND STERILIZATION

Reprocessing of Endoscopes

Physicians use endoscopes to diagnose and treat numerous medical disorders. Although endoscopes represent a valuable diagnostic and therapeutic tool in modern medicine and the incidence of infection associated with use has been reported as very low (about 1 in 1.8 million procedures),[38] more healthcare-associated outbreaks have been linked to contaminated endoscopes than to any other medical device.[5-7] In order to prevent the spread of healthcare-associated infections, all heat-sensitive endoscopes (e.g., gastrointestinal endoscopes, bronchoscopes, nasopharyngoscopes) must be properly cleaned and at a minimum subjected to high-level disinfection following each use. High-level disinfection can be expected to destroy all microorganisms, although when high numbers of bacterial spores are present, a few spores may survive.

Recommendations for the cleaning and disinfection of endoscopic equipment have been published and should be strictly followed.[16,20] Unfortunately, audits have shown that personnel do not adhere to guidelines on reprocessing,[39-41] and outbreaks of infection continue to occur.[42,43] In order to ensure that reprocessing personnel are properly trained, there should be initial and annual competency testing for each individual who is involved in reprocessing endoscopic instruments.[16,20,21,44]

In general, endoscope disinfection or sterilization with a liquid chemical sterilant or high-level disinfectant involves five steps after leak testing:

1. clean—mechanically clean internal and external surfaces, including brushing internal channels and flushing each internal channel with water and a enzymatic cleaner

2. disinfect—immerse endoscope in high-level disinfectant (or chemical sterilant) and perfuse (eliminates air pockets and ensures contact of the germicide with the internal channels) disinfectant into all accessible chan-

---

Cleaning, Disinfection, and Sterilization in Healthcare Facilities

Copyright © 2005, Association for Professionals in Infection Control and Epidemiology, Inc.

nels, such as the suction/biopsy channel and air/water channel and expose for a time recommended for specific products

3. rinse—rinse the endoscope and all channels with sterile water, filtered water (commonly used with automated endoscope reprocessors), or tap water

4. dry—rinse the insertion tube and inner channels with alcohol and dry with forced air after disinfection and before storage

5. store—store the endoscope in a way that prevents recontamination and promotes drying (e.g., hung vertically)

Unfortunately, there is poor compliance with the recommendations for reprocessing endoscopes. In addition, there are rare instances in which the scientific literature and recommendations from professional organizations regarding the use of disinfectants and sterilants may differ from the manufacturer's label claim. One example is the contact time used to achieve high-level disinfection with 2% glutaraldehyde. Based on FDA requirements (FDA regulates liquid sterilants and high-level disinfectants used on critical and semicritical medical devices), manufacturers test the efficacy of their germicide formulations under worst-case conditions (i.e., minimum recommended concentration of the active ingredient) and in the presence of organic soil (typically 5% serum). The soil is used to represent the organic loading to which the device is exposed during actual use and that would remain on the device in the absence of cleaning. These stringent test conditions are designed to provide a margin of safety by ensuring that the contact conditions for the germicide provide complete elimination of the test bacteria (e.g., 10^5 to 10^6 M. tuberculosis in organic soil and dried on a scope) if inoculated into the most difficult areas for the disinfectant to penetrate and in the absence of cleaning. However, the scientific data demonstrate that M. tuberculosis levels can be reduced by at least 8-$\log_{10}$ with cleaning (4-$\log_{10}$), followed by chemical disinfection for 20 minutes at 20°C (4- to 6-$\log_{10}$).[16,17,19,20,45] Because of these data, professional organizations (at least 14 professional organizations worldwide) that have endorsed an endoscope reprocessing guideline, recommend contact conditions that differ from that of the manufacturer's label (i.e., 20 minutes at 20°C [or less than 20 minutes outside the United States] with 2% glutaraldehyde to achieve high-level disinfection).[20,46-48] It is important to emphasize that the FDA tests do not include cleaning, a critical component of the disinfection process. Therefore, when cleaning has been included in the test methodology, 2% glutaraldehyde for 20 minutes has been demonstrated to be effective in eliminating all vegetative bacteria.

Automated endoscope reprocessors (AERs) offer several advantages compared to manual reprocessing: they automate and standardize several important reprocessing steps,[49-51] reduce the likelihood that an essential reprocessing step will be skipped, and reduce personnel exposure to high-level disinfectants or chemical sterilants. Failure of AERs has been linked to outbreaks of infections[52] or colonization,[6,53] and the AER water filtration system may not be able to reliably provide bacteria-free rinse water.[54,55] It is critical that correct connectors between the AER and the device are established to ensure complete flow of disinfectants and rinse water.[6,56] In addition, some endoscopes such as the duodenoscopes (e.g., endoscopic retrograde cholangiopancreatography [ERCP]) contain features (e.g., elevator-wire channel) that require a flushing pressure that is not achieved by most AERs and must be reprocessed manually using a 2- to 5-mL syringe.

Inactivation of Creutzfeldt-Jakob Disease Agent

Creutzfeldt-Jakob disease (CJD) is a degenerative neurologic disorder of humans with an incidence in the United States of approximately 1 case/million population/year.[57] CJD is thought to be caused by a proteinaceous infectious agent or prion. CJD is related to other human transmissible spongiform encephalopathies (TSEs) that include kuru (0 incidence, now eradicated), Gerstmann-Straussler-Scheinker (GSS) syndrome (1/40 million), and fatal insomnia syndrome (FFI) (<1/40 million). The agents of CJD and other TSEs exhibit an unusual resistance to conventional chemical and physical decontamination methods. Because the CJD agent is not readily inactivated by conventional disinfection and sterilization procedures and because of the invariably fatal outcome of CJD, the procedures for disinfection and sterilization of the CJD prion have been both conservative and controversial for many years.

The current recommendations consider inactivation data but also use epidemiological studies of prion transmission, infectivity of human tissues, and efficacy of removing proteins by cleaning. On the basis of scientific data, only critical (e.g., surgical instruments) and semicritical devices contaminated with high-risk tissue (i.e., brain, spinal cord, and eye tissue) from high-risk patients (e.g., known or suspected infection with CJD or other prion disease) require special prion reprocessing. For high-risk tissues, high-risk patients, and critical or semicritical medical devices, the recommendation of the World Health Organization (WHO) is to clean the device and sterilize using a combination of sodium hydroxide and autoclaving[58] (e.g., immerse in 1N NaOH for 1 hour; remove and rinse in water, then transfer to an open pan and autoclave [121°C gravity displacement or 134°C porous or prevacuum sterilizer]

Copyright © 2005, Association for Professionals in Infection Control and Epidemiology, Inc.

for 1 hour), but other methods have also been recommended (e.g., autoclaving at 134°C for 18 minutes in a prevacuum sterilizer; at 132°C for 1 hour in a gravity displacement sterilizer).[16,59] The temperature should not exceed 134°C because under certain conditions the effectiveness of autoclaving actually declines as the temperature is increased (e.g., 136°C, 138°C).[60] Prion-contaminated medical devices that are impossible or difficult to clean should be discarded. Flash sterilization (i.e., steam sterilization of an unwrapped item at 132°C for 3 minutes) should not be used for reprocessing. To minimize environmental contamination, noncritical environmental surfaces should be covered with plastic-backed paper, and when contaminated with high-risk tissues, the paper should be properly discarded. Noncritical environmental surfaces (e.g., laboratory surfaces) contaminated with high-risk tissues should be cleaned and then spot decontaminated with a 1:10 dilution of hypochlorite solutions.[59]

Emerging Pathogens, Antibiotic-Resistant Bacteria, and Bioterrorism Agents

Emerging pathogens are of growing concern to the general public and ICPs. Relevant pathogens include *Cryptosporidium parvum, Helicobacter pylori, Escherichia coli* O157:H7, human immunodeficiency virus (HIV) , SARS coronavirus, norovirus, monkey pox, hepatitis C virus (HCV), rotavirus, multidrug-resistant *M. tuberculosis*, human papilloma virus, and nontuberculosis mycobacteria (e.g., *Mycobacterium chelonae*). Similarly, the concern about the potential for biological terrorism has been highlighted.[61] The CDC has categorized several agents as "high priority" because they can be easily disseminated or transmitted person to person, can cause high mortality, and are likely to cause public panic and social disruption.[62] These agents include *Bacillus anthracis* (anthrax), *Yersinia pestis* (plague), variola major (smallpox), *Francisella tularensis* (tularemia), filoviruses (Ebola hemorrhagic fever, Marburg hemorrhagic fever) and arenaviruses (Lassa [Lassa fever], Junin [Argentine hemorrhagic fever]), and related viruses.[62]

With rare exceptions (e.g., human papilloma virus), the susceptibility of each of these pathogens to chemical disinfectants/sterilants has been studied, and all these pathogens (or surrogate microbes such as feline-calicivirus for norovirus, vaccinia for variola,[63] and *B. atrophaeus* [formerly *B. subtilis*] for *B. anthracis*), are susceptible to currently available chemical disinfectants/sterilants.[64] Standard sterilization and disinfection procedures for patient-care equipment (as recommended in this chapter) are adequate to sterilize or disinfect instruments or devices contaminated with blood or other body fluids from persons infected with bloodborne pathogens, emerging pathogens, and bioterrorism agents, with the exception of prions (see

earlier). No changes in procedures for cleaning, disinfecting, or sterilizing need to be made.[16,17]

In addition, there are no data to show that antibiotic-resistant bacteria (methicillin-resistant *Staphylococcus aureus* [MRSA], vancomycin-resistant enterococci [VRE], multidrug-resistant *M. tuberculosis* [MDRTB]) are less sensitive to disinfectants than antibiotic-sensitive bacteria at currently used disinfectant contact conditions and concentrations.[17,65,66]

Disinfection in Ambulatory Care, Home Care, and the Home

With the advent of managed healthcare, increasing numbers of patients are now being cared for in ambulatory care and in home settings. Many patients cared for in these settings may have communicable diseases, immunocompromising conditions, or invasive devices. Therefore, adequate disinfection in these settings is necessary to provide a safe patient environment. Because the ambulatory care (outpatient facilities) setting provides the same infection risk as the hospital setting, the Spaulding classification scheme described in this guideline should be followed (Table 21–1).[15]

The home environment should be a much safer setting than hospitals or ambulatory care. Epidemics should not be a problem, and cross-infection should be rare. Among the products recommended for home disinfection use are bleach, alcohol, and hydrogen peroxide. It has been recommended that reusable objects that touch mucous membranes (e.g., tracheostomy tubes) be disinfected by immersion in a 1:2 dilution of household bleach (6.00%–6.15% sodium hypochlorite) for 1–3 min, 70% isopropyl alcohol for 5 min, or 3% hydrogen peroxide for 30 min. Noncritical items (blood pressure cuffs, crutches) can be cleaned with a detergent. Blood spills should be handled as per OSHA regulations. In general, sterilization of critical items is not practical in homes but theoretically could be accomplished by chemical sterilants or boiling. Single-use disposable items can be used or reusable items sterilized in a hospital.[67,68]

Some environmental groups advocate environmentally "safe products" as alternatives to commercial germicides in the home-care setting. These alternatives (e.g. ammonia, baking soda, vinegar, Borax, liquid detergent) are not registered with the EPA and are a poor choice for disinfecting because they are ineffective against *S. aureus*. Borax, baking soda, and detergents are not effective against *Salmonella typhi* and *E. coli*; however, undiluted vinegar and ammonia are effective against *S. typhi* and *E. coli*.[69-71] Common commercial disinfectants designed for home use have also been found effective against selected antibiotic-resistant bacteria.[70]

Copyright © 2005, Association for Professionals in Infection Control and Epidemiology, Inc.

Tonometers, Diaphragm Fitting Rings, Cryosurgical Instruments, and Endocavitary Probes

Disinfection strategies for other semicritical items (e.g., applanation tonometers, rectal/vaginal probes, cryosurgical instruments, and diaphragm fitting rings) are highly variable. For example, one study revealed that no uniform technique was in use for disinfection of applanation tonometers with disinfectant contact times varying from <15 seconds to 20 minutes.[72] In view of the potential for transmission of viruses (e.g., herpes simplex virus [HSV], adenovirus 8, HIV)[73] by tonometer tips, the CDC recommends[74] that they be wiped clean and disinfected for 5–10 minutes with either 3% hydrogen peroxide, 5000 ppm chlorine, 70% ethyl alcohol, or 70% isopropyl alcohol. Structural damage to Schiotz tonometers has been observed with a 1:10 sodium hypochlorite (6000 ppm chlorine) and 3% hydrogen peroxide.[75] After disinfection, the device should be thoroughly rinsed in tap water and dried before use. Although these disinfectants and exposure times should kill pathogens that can infect the eyes, there are no studies that provide direct support.[76,77] The guidelines of the American Academy of Ophthalmology for preventing infections in ophthalmology focus on only the potential pathogen HIV-1.[78] Because a short and simple decontamination procedure is desirable in the clinical setting, swabbing the tonometer tip with a 70% isopropyl alcohol wipe is sometimes practiced.[77] Preliminary reports suggest that wiping the tonometer tip with an alcohol swab and then allowing the alcohol to evaporate may be an effective means of eliminating HSV, HIV-1, and adenovirus.[77,79,80] However, because these studies involved only a few replicates and were conducted in a controlled laboratory setting, further studies are needed before this technique can be recommended. In addition, two reports have found that disinfection of pneumotonometer tips between uses with a 70% isopropyl alcohol wipe contributed to outbreaks of epidemic keratoconjunctivitis caused by adenovirus type 8.[81,82]

There are also limited studies that evaluated disinfection techniques for other items that contact mucous membranes such as diaphragm fitting rings, cryosurgical probes, transesophageal echocardiography probes,[83] or vaginal/rectal probes used in sonographic scanning. Lettau, Bond, and McDougal of the CDC supported a diaphragm fitting ring manufacturer's recommendation, which involved using a soap and water wash followed by a 15-minute immersion in 70% alcohol.[84] This disinfection method should be adequate to inactivate HIV-1, HBV, and HSV, even though alcohols are not classified as high-level disinfectants because their activity against picornaviruses is somewhat limited.[63] No data are available on the inactivation of human papilloma virus (HPV) by alcohol or other disinfectants because in vitro replication of complete virions has not been achieved. Thus, although alcohol for 15 minutes should kill pathogens of relevance in gynecology, there are no clinical studies that provide direct support for this practice.

Vaginal probes are used in sonographic scanning. A vaginal probe and all endocavitary probes without a probe cover are semicritical devices because they have direct contact with mucous membranes. Although one could argue that the use of the probe cover changes the category, this chapter proposes that a new condom/probe cover should be used to cover the probe for each patient and because condoms/probe covers may fail,[83,85-87] high-level disinfection of the probe should also be performed. The relevance of this recommendation is reinforced with the findings that sterile transvaginal ultrasound probe covers have a very high rate of perforations even before use (0%, 25%, and 65% perforations from three suppliers).[87] After oocyte retrieval use, Hignett and Claman found a very high rate of perforations in used endovaginal probe covers from two suppliers (75% and 81%),[87] whereas Amis and coworkers[88] and Milki and Fisch[85] demonstrated a lower rate of perforations after use of condoms (0.9% and 2.0%, respectively). Rooks and coworkers found that condoms were superior to commercially available probe covers for covering the ultrasound probe (8.3% leakage for probe covers versus 1.7% for condoms).[89] These studies underscore the need for routine probe disinfection between examinations.

Although most ultrasound manufacturers recommend the use of 2% glutaraldehyde for high-level disinfection of contaminated transvaginal transducers, the use of this agent has been questioned[90] because it shortens the life of the transducer and may have toxic effects on the gametes and embryos.[91] An alternative procedure for disinfecting the vaginal transducer has been offered by Garland and deCrespigny.[92] It involves the mechanical removal of the gel from the transducer, cleaning it in soap and water, wiping the transducer with 70% alcohol or soaking for 2 minutes in 500 ppm chlorine, and rinsing with tap water and drying. The effectiveness of this and other methods[88] has not been validated in either rigorous laboratory experiments or in clinical use. High-level disinfection, with a product that is not toxic to staff, patients, probes, and retrieved cells (e.g., hydrogen peroxide) should be used until such time as the effectiveness of alternative procedures against microbes of importance at the cavitary site is scientifically demonstrated. Other probes such as rectal, cryosurgical, and transesophageal should also be subjected to high-level disinfection between patients.

Some cryosurgical probes are not fully immersible. When reprocessing these probes, the tip of the probe

Copyright © 2005, Association for Professionals in Infection Control and Epidemiology, Inc.

should be immersed in a high-level disinfectant for the appropriate time (e.g., 20-minute exposure with 2% glutaraldehyde), and any other portion of the probe that could have mucous membrane contact could be disinfected by wrapping with a cloth soaked in a high-level disinfectant to allow the recommended contact time. After disinfection, the probe should be rinsed with tap water and dried before use. Healthcare facilities that use nonimmersible probes should replace them as soon as possible with a fully immersible probe.

As with other high-level disinfection procedures, proper cleaning of probes is also necessary to ensure the success of the subsequent high-level disinfection.[93]

Muradali and colleagues demonstrated a 3-log reduction of vegetative bacteria inoculated on vaginal ultrasound probes.[94] No information is available of the level of contamination of such probes by potential viral pathogens such as HPV that may be more resistant than vegetative bacteria to disinfection procedures. Because these pathogens may be present in vaginal and rectal secretions and contaminate probes during use, disinfection processes (i.e., high-level disinfection) likely to eliminate these agents are recommended.

Table 21–3. Summary of advantages and disadvantages of commonly used sterilization technologies.

Sterilization Method	Advantages	Disadvantages
Steam	• Nontoxic to patient, staff, environment • Cycle easy to control and monitor • Rapidly microbicidal • Least affected by organic/inorganic soils among sterilization processes listed • Rapid cycle time • Penetrates medical packing, device lumens	• Deleterious for heat-sensitive instruments • Microsurgical instruments damaged by repeated exposure • May leave instruments wet, causing them to rust • Potential for burns
Hydrogen Peroxide Gas Plasma	• Safe for the environment • Leaves no toxic residuals • Cycle time is 45–73 minutes and no aeration necessary • Used for heat- and moisture-sensitive items because process temperature < 50 °C • Simple to operate, install (208 V outlet), and monitor • Compatible with most medical devices • Only requires electrical outlet	• Cellulose (paper), linens, and liquids cannot be processed • Sterilization chamber is small, about 3.5 to 7.3 ft³ • Endoscope or medical device restrictions based on lumen internal diameter and length (see manufacturer's recommendations) • Requires synthetic packaging (polypropylene wraps, polyolefin pouches) and special container tray • Hydrogen peroxide may be toxic at levels greater than 1 ppm TWA
100% Ethylene Oxide (ETO)	• Penetrates packaging materials, device lumens • Single-dose cartridge and negative-pressure chamber minimizes the potential for gas leak and ETO exposure • Simple to operate and monitor • Compatible with most medical materials	• Requires aeration time to remove ETO residue • Sterilization chamber is small, • 4 ft³ to 8.8 ft³ • ETO is toxic, a carcinogen, and flammable • ETO emission regulated by states but catalytic cell removes 99.9% of ETO and converts it to CO_2 and H_2O • ETO cartridges should be stored in flammable liquid storage cabinet • Lengthy cycle/aeration time
ETO Mixtures 8.6% ETO/91.4% HCFC 10% ETO/90% HCFC 8.5% ETO/91.5% CO₂	• Penetrates medical packaging and many plastics • Compatible with most medical materials • Cycle easy to control and monitor	• Some states (e.g., CA, NY, MI) require ETO emission reduction of 90–99.9% • CFC (inert gas that eliminates explosion hazard) banned in 1995 • Potential hazards to staff and patients • Lengthy cycle/aeration time • ETO is toxic, a carcinogen, and flammable
Peracetic Acid	• Rapid cycle time (30–45 minutes) • Low temperature (50–55 °C) liquid immersion sterilization • Environmental friendly by-products • Sterilant flows through endoscope which facilitates salt, protein, and microbe removal	• Point-of-use system, no sterile storage • Biological indicator may not be suitable for routine monitoring • Used for immersible instruments only • Some material incompatibility (e.g., aluminium anodized coating becomes dull) • One scope or a small number of instruments processed in a cycle • Potential for serious eye and skin damage (concentrated solution) with contact • Must use connector between system and scope to ensure infusion of sterilant to all channels

Modified from[98].
Abbreviations: ETO-ethylene oxide; CFC-chlorofluorocarbon, HCFC-hydrochlorofluorocarbon.

Copyright © 2005, Association for Professionals in Infection Control and Epidemiology, Inc.

Advances in Disinfection and Sterilization Methods

In the past several years, new methods of disinfection and sterilization have been introduced in the healthcare setting. Ortho-phthalaldehyde (OPA) is a chemical sterilant that received FDA clearance in October 1999. It contains 0.55% (1;XC2-benzenedicarboxaldehyde). Studies have demonstrated excellent microbicidal activity with in vitro studies.[16,17] For example, Gregory and coworkers demonstrated that OPA has shown superior mycobactericidal activity (5-log$_{10}$ reduction in 5 minutes) compared to glutaraldehyde.[95] The advantages, disadvantages, and characteristics of ortho-phthalaldehyde are listed in Table 21-2.[17]

The FDA recently cleared a liquid high-level disinfectant (superoxidized water) that contains 650–675 ppm free chlorine and a new sterilization system using ozone. Because there are limited data in the scientific literature that assess the antimicrobial activity or material compatibility of these processes, they have not yet been integrated into clinical practice in the United States.[16]

Several methods are used to sterilize patient-care items in healthcare, including steam sterilization, ethylene oxide, hydrogen peroxide gas plasma, and a peracetic acid immersion system. The advantages and disadvantages of these systems are listed in Table 21-3.[16]

New sterilization technology based on plasma was patented in 1987 and marketed in the United States in 1993. Gas plasmas have been referred to as the fourth state of matter (i.e., liquids, solids, gases, and gas plasmas). Gas plasmas are generated in an enclosed chamber under deep vacuum using radiofrequency or microwave energy to excite the gas molecules and produce charged particles, many of which are in the form of free radicals. This process has the ability to inactivate a broad spectrum of microorganisms, including resistant bacterial spores. Studies have been conducted against vegetative bacteria (including mycobacteria), yeasts, fungi, viruses, and bacterial spores.[16] Lumen length, lumen diameter, inorganic salts, and organic materials can be used to alter the effectiveness of all sterilization processes.[16]

IV.   SUMMARY AND CONCLUSIONS

When properly used, disinfection and sterilization can ensure the safe use of invasive and noninvasive medical devices. However, current disinfection and sterilization guidelines must be strictly followed.

V.   FUTURE TRENDS/RESEARCH

The CDC and the Healthcare Infection Control Practices Advisory Committee should publish the Guideline for Disinfection and Sterilization in Health-Care Facilities in 2004. This comprehensive guideline will supersede the relevant sections contained in the 1985 CDC "Guideline for Handwashing and Environmental Control."[13]

VII.   REFERENCES AND CITATIONS

1. Centers for Disease Control. *Ambulatory and inpatient procedures in the United States,* Atlanta, GA, 1996 CDC, 1–39
2. Centers for Disease Control and Prevention. *National Center for Health Statistics-Inpatient Surgery.* Vol. www.cdc.gov/nchs/fastats/insurg.htm
3. Centers for Disease Control and Prevention. *National Center for Health Statistics-Outpatient Surgery.* Vol. www.cdc.gov/nchs/fastats/outsurg.htm
4. McCarthy GM, Koval JJ, John MA, MacDonald JK: Infection control practices across Canada: do dentists follow the recommendations? *J Can Dent Assoc* 65:506–11, 1999
5. Spach DH, Silverstein FE, Stamm WE: Transmission of infection by gastrointestinal endoscopy and bronchoscopy, *Ann Intern Med* 118:117–28, 1993
6. Weber DJ, Rutala WA: Lessons from outbreaks associated with bronchoscopy, *Infect Control Hosp Epidemiol* 22:403–8, 2001
7. Weber DJ, Rutala WA, DiMarino AJ, Jr: The prevention of infection following gastrointestinal endoscopy: the importance of prophylaxis and reprocessing. In DiMarino AJ, Jr, Benjamin SB, editors: Gastrointestinal diseases: an endoscopic approach. Thorofare, NJ, 2002, Slack Inc., pp. 87–106
8. Meyers H, Brown-Elliott BA, Moore D, et al: An outbreak of *Mycobacterium chelonae* infection following liposuction, *Clin Infect Dis* 34:1500–7, 2002
9. Lowry PW, Jarvis WR, Oberle AD, et al: *Mycobacterium chelonae* causing otitis media in an ear-nose-and-throat practice, *N Engl J Med* 319:978–82, 1988
10. Spaulding EH: Chemical disinfection of medical and surgical materials. In Lawrence C, Block SS, editors: Disinfection, sterilization, and preservation, Philadelphia, 1968, Lea & Febiger, pp. 517–31
11. Favero MS, Bond WW: Chemical disinfection of medical and surgical materials. In Block SS, editor: Disinfection, sterilization, and preservation, Philadelphia, 2001, Lippincott Williams & Wilkins, pp. 881–917
12. Simmons BP: CDC guidelines for the prevention and control of nosocomial infections. Guideline for hospital environmental control, *Am J Infect Control* 11:97–120, 1983
13. Garner JS, Favero MS: CDC guideline for handwashing and hospital environmental control, 1985, *Infect Control* 7:231–43, 1986
14. Rutala WA: APIC guideline for selection and use of disinfectants. *Am J Infect Control* 18:99–117, 1990
15. Rutala WA, 1994, 1995, and 1996 APIC Guidelines Committee: APIC guideline for selection and use of disinfectants. Association for Professionals in Infection Control and Epidemiology, Inc., *Am J Infect Control* 24:313–42, 1996
16. Rutala WA, Weber DJ, Healthcare Infection Control Practices Advisory Committee: Guideline for disinfection and sterilization in healthcare facilities: recommendations of CDC. *MMWR,* in press
17. Rutala WA, Weber DJ: Selection and use of disinfectants in healthcare. In Mayhall CG, editor: *Infection control and hospital epidemiology,* Philadelphia, in press, Lippincott Williams & Wilkins
18. Sehulster L, Chinn RYW, Healthcare Infection Control Practices Advisory Committee: Guidelines for environmental infection control in health-care facilities, *MMWR* 52:1–44, 2003
19. Food and Drug Administration: FDA-cleared sterilants and high-level disinfectants with general claims for processing reusable medical and dental devices, January 2004. www.fda.gov/cdrh/ode/germlab.html 2004

Copyright © 2005, Association for Professionals in Infection Control and Epidemiology, Inc.

20. Nelson DB, Jarvis WR, Rutala WA, et al: Multi-society guideline for reprocessing flexible gastrointestinal endoscopes, *Infect Control Hosp Epidemiol* 24:532–537, 2003
21. Gerding DN, Peterson LR, Vennes JA: Cleaning and disinfection of fiberoptic endoscopes: evaluation of glutaraldehyde exposure time and forced-air drying, *Gastroenterology* 83:613–8, 1982
22. Weber DJ, Rutala WA: Environmental issues and nosocomial infections. In Wenzel RP, editor: Prevention and control of nosocomial infections, Baltimore, 1997, Williams and Wilkins, pp. 491–514.
23. Weber DJ, Rutala WA: Role of environmental contamination in the transmission of vancomycin-resistant enterococci, *Infect Control Hosp Epidemiol* 18:306–9, 1997
24. Babb JR, Bradley CR: Endoscope decontamination: where do we go from here? *J Hosp Infect* 30:543–51, 1995
25. Merritt K, Hitchins VM, Brown SA: Safety and cleaning of medical materials and devices, *J Biomed Mater Res* 53:131–6, 2000
26. Jacobs P: Cleaning: Principles, methods and benefits. In Rutala WA, editor: *Disinfection, sterilization, and antisepsis in healthcare,* Champlain, New York, 1998, Polyscience Publications, pp. 165–81
27. Roberts CG: Studies on the bioburden on medical devices and the importance of cleaning. In Rutala WA, editor: *Disinfection, sterilization and antisepsis: principles and practices in healthcare facilities,* Washington, DC, 2001, Association for Professional in Infection Control and Epidemiology, pp. 63–9
28. Rutala WA, Gergen MF, Jones JF, Weber DJ: Levels of microbial contamination on surgical instruments, *Am J Infect Control* 26:143–5, 1998
29. Nystrom B: Disinfection of surgical instruments, *J Hosp Infect* 2:363–8, 1981
30. Chan-Myers H, McAlister D, Antonoplos P: Natural bioburden levels detected on rigid lumened medical devices before and after cleaning, *Am J Infect Control* 25:471–6, 1997
31. American Society for Healthcare Central Service Professionals: *Training manual for health care central service technicians,* Chicago, 2001, The Jossey-Bass/American Hospital Association Press Series, pp. 1–271
32. Lee CH, Cheng SM, Humar A, et al: Acute febrile reactions with hypotension temporally associated with the introduction of a concentrated bioenzyme preparation in the cleaning and sterilization process of endomyocardial bioptones, *Infect Control Hosp Epidemiol* 21:102, 2000
33. Alfa MJ, Jackson M: A new hydrogen peroxide-based medical-device detergent with germicidal properties: comparison with enzymatic cleaners, *Am J Infect Control* 29:168–77, 2001
34. Alfa MJ, DeGagne P, Olson N, Puchalski T: Comparison of ion plasma, vaporized hydrogen peroxide and 100% ethylene oxide sterilizers to the 12/88 ethylene oxide gas sterilizer, *Infect Control Hosp Epidemiol* 17:92–100, 1996
35. Alfa MJ: Flexible endoscope reprocessing, *Infect Control Steril Technol* 3:26–36, 1997
36. Alfa MJ, Degagne P, Olson N: Worst-case soiling levels for patient-used flexible endoscopes before and after cleaning, *Am J Infect Control* 27:392–401, 1999
37. Rutala WA, Weber DJ: Low-temperature sterilization technology: do we need to redefine sterilization? *Infect Control Hosp Epidemiol* 17:89–91, 1996
38. Schembre DB: Infectious complications associated with gastrointestinal endoscopy, *Gastrointest Endosc Clin N Am* 10:215–32, 2000
39. Jackson FW, Ball MD: Correction of deficiencies in flexible fiberoptic sigmoidoscope cleaning and disinfection technique in family practice and internal medicine offices, *Arch Fam Med* 6:578–82, 1997
40. Orsi GB, Filocamo A, Di Stefano L, Tittobello A: Italian National Survey of Digestive Endoscopy Disinfection Procedures, *Endoscopy* 29:732–8; quiz 739–40, 1997
41. Honeybourne D, Neumann CS: An audit of bronchoscopy practice in the United Kingdom: a survey of adherence to national guidelines, *Thorax* 52:709–13, 1997
42. Srinivasan A, Wolfenden LL, Song X, et al: An outbreak of *Pseudomonas aeruginosa* infections associated with flexible bronchoscopes, *N Engl J Med* 348:221–7, 2003
43. Cetse JC, Vanhems P: Outbreak of infection associated with bronchoscopes, *N Engl J Med* 348:2039–40, 2003
44. Food and Drug Administration, Centers for Disease Control and Prevention: *FDA and CDC public health advisory: infections from endoscopes inadequately reprocessed by an automated endoscope reprocessing system,* Rockville, MD, 1999 Food and Drug Administration,
45. Rutala WA, Weber DJ: FDA labeling requirements for disinfection of endoscopes: a counterpoint, *Infect Control Hosp Epidemiol* 16:231–5. 1995
46. Kruse A, Rey JF: Guidelines on cleaning and disinfection in GI endoscopy. Update 1999, The European Society of Gastrointestinal Endoscopy. *Endoscopy* 32:77–80, 2000
47. British Society of Gastroenterology: Cleaning and disinfection of equipment for gastrointestinal endoscopy. Report of a working party of the British Society of Gastroenterology Endoscope Committee, *Gut* 42:585–93, 1998
48. British Thoracic Society: British Thoracic Society guidelines on diagnostic flexible bronchoscopy, *Thorax* 56:1–21, 2001
49. Bradley CR, Babb JR: Endoscope decontamination: automated vs. manual, *J Hosp Infect* 30:537–42, 1995
50. Muscarella LF: Advantages and limitations of automatic flexible endoscope reprocessors, *Am J Infect Control* 24:304–9, 1996
51. Muscarella LF: Automatic flexible endoscope reprocessors, *Gastrointest Endosc Clin N Am* 10:245–57, 2000
52. Alvarado CJ, Stolz SM, Maki DG: Nosocomial infections from contaminated endoscopes: a flawed automated endoscope washer. An investigation using molecular epidemiology, *Am J Med* 91:272S–280S, 1991
53. Fraser VJ, Jones M, Murray PR, Medoff G, Zhang Y, Wallace RJ, Jr.: Contamination of flexible fiberoptic bronchoscopes with *Mycobacterium chelonae* linked to an automated bronchoscope disinfection machine, *Am Rev Respir Dis* 145:853–5, 1992
54. Cooke RP, Whymant-Morris A, Umasankar RS, Goddard SV: Bacteria-free water for automatic washer-disinfectors: an impossible dream? *J Hosp Infect* 39:63–5, 1998
55. Muscarella LF: Deja Vu|.|.|. All over again? The importance of instrument drying, *Infect Control Hosp Epidemiol* 21:628–9, 2000
56. Rutala WA, Weber DJ: Importance of lumen flow in liquid chemical sterilization, *Am J Infect Control* 20:458–9, 1999
57. Centers for Disease Control: Surveillance for Creutzfeldt-Jakob disease—United States, *MMWR* 45:665–8, 1996
58. World Health Organization: WHO infection control guidelines for transmissible spongiform encephalopathies, http://www.who/cds/csr/aph/2000.3
59. Rutala WA, Weber DJ: Creutzfeldt-Jakob disease: recommendations for disinfection and sterilization, *Clin Infect Dis* 32:1348–56, 2001
60. Taylor DM: Inactivation of prions by physical and chemical means, *J Hosp Infect* 43 (supplement):S69–S76, 1999
61. Henderson DA: The looming threat of bioterrorism, *Science* 283:1279–82, 1999
62. Centers for Disease Control: Biological and chemical terrorism: strategic plan for preparedness and response, *MMWR* 49 (no. RR-4):1–14, 2000
63. Klein M, DeForest A: The inactivation of viruses by germicides, *Chem Specialists Manuf Assoc Proc* 49:116–8, 1963
64. Rutala WA, Weber DJ: Infection control: the role of disinfection and sterilization, *J Hosp Infect* 43:S43–55, 1999
65. Rutala WA, Stiegel MM, Sarubbi FA, Weber DJ: Susceptibility of antibiotic-susceptible and antibiotic-resistant hospital bacteria to disinfectants, *Infect Control Hosp Epidemiol* 18:417–21, 1997
66. Weber DJ, Rutala WA: Use of germicides in the home and health care setting: is there a relationship between germicide use and antimicrobial resistance, *Infect Control Hosp Epidemiol,* in press
67. Rutala WA, Weber DJ: Principles of disinfecting patient-care items, In: Rutala WA, editor: *Disinfection, sterilization, and antisepsis in healthcare,* Champlain, NY, 1998, Polyscience Publications, pp. 133–49
68. Luebbert P: Home care, In: Pfeiffer JA, editor: *APIC text of infection control and epidemiology.* Vol. 1. Washington: Association for Professionals in Infection control and epidemiology, 44–7, 2000
69. Parnes CA: Efficacy of sodium hypochlorite bleach and "alternative" products in preventing transfer of bacteria to and from inanimate surfaces, *Environ Health* 59:14–20, 1997
70. Rutala WA, Barbee SL, Aguiar NC, Sobsey MD, Weber DJ: Antimicrobial activity of home disinfectants and natural products against potential human pathogens, *Infect Control Hosp Epidemiol* 21:33–8, 2000

Copyright © 2005, Association for Professionals in Infection Control and Epidemiology, Inc.

71. Karapinar M, Gonul SA: Effects of sodium bicarbonate, vinegar, acetic and citric acids on growth and survival of *Yersinia enterocolitica*, *Int J Food Microbiol* 16:343–7, 1992
72. Rutala WA, Clontz EP, Weber DJ, Hoffmann KK: Disinfection practices for endoscopes and other semicritical items, *Infect Control Hosp Epidemiol* 12:282–8, 1991
73. Weber DJ, Rutala WA: Nosocomial ocular infections, In: Mayhall CG, editor: *Infection. Control and Hospital. Epidemiology,* Philadelphia, 1999 Lippincott Williams & Wilkins, pp. 287–99
74. Centers for Disease Control: Recommendations for preventing possible transmission of human T-lymphotropic virus type III/lymphadenopathy-associated virus from tears, *MMWR* 34:533–4, 1985
75. Chronister CL: Structural damage to Schiotz tonometers after disinfection with solutions, *Optom Vis Sci* 74:164–6, 1997
76. Nagington J, Sutehall GM, Whipp P: Tonometer disinfection and viruses, *Br J Ophthalmol* 67:674–6, 1983
77. Craven ER, Butler SL, McCulley JP, Luby JP: Applanation tonometer tip sterilization for adenovirus type 8, *Ophthalmology* 94:1538–40, 1987
78. American Academy of Ophthalmology: *Updated recommendations for ophthalmic practice in relation to the human immunodeficiency virus,* San Francisco, 1988, American Academy of Ophthalmology
79. Pepose JS, Linette G, Lee SF, MacRae S: Disinfection of Goldmann tonometers against human immunodeficiency virus type 1, *Arch Ophthalmol* 107:983–5, 1989
80. Ventura LM, Dix RD: Viability of herpes simplex virus type 1 on the applanation tonometer, *Am J Ophthalmol* 103:48–52, 1987
81. Koo D, Bouvier B, Wesley M, Courtright P, Reingold A: Epidemic keratoconjunctivitis in a university medical center ophthalmology clinic: need for re-evaluation of the design and disinfection of instruments, *Infect Control Hosp Epidemiol* 10:547–52, 1989
82. Jernigan JA, Lowry BS, Hayden FG, et al: Adenovirus type 8 epidemic keratoconjunctivitis in an eye clinic: risk factors and control, *J Infect Dis* 167:1307–13, 1993
83. Fritz S, Hust MH, Ochs C, Gratwohl I, Staiger M, Braun B: Use of a latex cover sheath for transesophageal echocardiography (TEE) instead of regular disinfection of the echoscope? *Clin Cardiol* 16:737–40, 1993
84. Lettau LA, Bond WW, McDougal JS: Hepatitis and diaphragm fitting, *JAMA* 254:752, 1985
85. Milki AA, Fisch JD: Vaginal ultrasound probe cover leakage: implications for patient care, *Fertil Steril* 69:409–11, 1998
86. Storment JM, Monga M, Blanco JD: Ineffectiveness of latex condoms in preventing contamination of the transvaginal ultrasound transducer head, *South Med J* 90:206–8, 1997
87. Hignett M, Claman P: High rates of perforation are found in endovaginal ultrasound probe covers before and after oocyte retrieval for *in vitro* fertilization-embryo transfer, *J Assist Reprod Genet* 12:606–9, 1995
88. Amis S, Ruddy M, Kibbler CC, Economides DL, MacLean AB: Assessment of condoms as probe covers for transvaginal sonography, *J Clin Ultrasound* 28:295–8, 2000
89. Rooks VJ, Yancey MK, Elg SA, Brueske L: Comparison of probe sheaths for endovaginal sonography, *Obstet Gynecol* 87:27–9, 1996
90. Odwin CS, Fleischer AC, Kepple DM, Chiang DT: Probe covers and disinfectants for transvaginal transducers, *J Diagnostic Med Sonography* 6:130–5, 1990
91. Benson WG: Exposure to glutaraldehyde, *J Soc Occup Med* 34:63–4, 1984
92. Garland SM, de Crespigny L: Prevention of infection in obstetrical and gynaecological ultrasound practice, *Aust N Z J Obstet Gynaecol* 36:392–5, 1996
93. Fowler C, McCracken D: US probes: risk of cross infection and ways to reduce it—comparison of cleaning methods, *Radiology* 213:299–300, 1999
94. Muradali D, Gold WL, Phillips A, Wilson S: Can ultrasound probes and coupling gel be a source of nosocomial infection in patients undergoing sonography? An in vivo and in vitro study, *AJR Am J Roentgenol* 164:1521–4, 1995
95. Gregory AW, Schaalje GB, Smart JD, Robison RA: The mycobactericidal efficacy of ortho-phthalaldehyde and the comparative resistances of *Mycobacterium bovis, Mycobacterium terrae,* and *Mycobacterium chelonae, Infect Control Hosp Epidemiol* 20:324–30, 1999
96. Kohn WG, Collins AS, Cleveland JL, Harte JA, Eklund KJ, Malvitz DM: Guidelines for infection control in dental health-care settings—2003, *MMWR* 52 (no. RR-17):1–67, 2003
97. Rutala WA, Weber DJ: Disinfection of endoscopes: review of new chemical sterilants used for high-level disinfection, *Infect Control Hosp Epidemiol* 20:69–76, 1999
98. Rutala WA, Weber DJ: Clinical effectiveness of low-temperature sterilization technologies, *Infect Control Hosp Epidemiol* 19:798–804, 1998

SUPPLEMENTAL RESOURNCES

American Dental Association (ADA): *www.ada.org*

Association for the Advancement of Medical Instrumentation (AAMI): *www.aami.org*

ASTM International: *www.astm.org*

Centers for Disease Control and Prevention (CDC): *www.cdc.gov*

ECRI (formerly Emergency Care Research Institute): *www.ecri.org*

Medical Device Manufacturers Association (MDMA): *www.medicaldevices.org*

Society for Biomaterials: *www.biomaterials.org*

Society for Healthcare Epidemiology of America (SHEA): *www.shea-online.org*

World Health Organization (WHO): *www.who.int/en/*

SUGGESTED READING

Centers for Disease Control and Prevention Guidelines for Environmental Infection Control in Health-Care Facilities. 2003. *www.cdc.gov/ncidod/hip/enviro/guide.htm*

Copyright © 2005, Association for Professionals in Infection Control and Epidemiology, Inc.

Pneumonia

Diana Christensen, MD
Research Associate
Infection Diseases Division
University of Louisville
Louisville, Kentucky

ABSTRACT

This chapter describes the principle concepts regarding community-acquired pneumonia (CAP) and healthcare-associated pneumonia (HAP). Definitions of each type of infection, epidemiology, pathogenesis, etiology, diagnosis, measures to prevent pneumonia, quality indicators, and outcomes are included.

KEY CONCEPTS

- Importance of CAP and HAP

- Importance of host risk factors to stratify different categories of patients

- Diagnostic workup including cultures obtained prior to antibiotic administration

- Airborne isolation in patients with risk factors for tuberculosis

- Measures to prevent pneumonia

- How to improve outcomes

- How to avoid antibiotic overuse

I.   BACKGROUND

Pneumonia, indicated by an inflammatory process of the lung parenchyma and often caused by a microbial agent, remains a common and serious illness, despite the availability of potent new antimicrobials and effective vaccines. As settings for delivery of healthcare expand, the term *nosocomial,* or hospital-acquired infection, is being replaced by the term *healthcare associated.* However, as nosocomial is still used in many publications and reference materials, the term will be included in this chapter. The infection control professional should have a working knowledge of both community-acquired and healthcare-associated pneumonia. Additionally, outcome and process indicators related to these two types of respiratory infection are part of performance improvement activities as recommended by accreditation and regulatory agencies.

Copyright © 2005, Association for Professionals in Infection Control and Epidemiology, Inc.

II. BASIC PRINCIPLES

Community-acquired pneumonia (CAP) is defined as a pneumonia that was not associated with care in the hospital or other healthcare setting.

Healthcare-associated pneumonia (HAP) is defined as pneumonia that occurs in patients that reside in or have resided in a long-term care facility, acute-care facility, or other healthcare facility. HAP occurs 48 hours after admission to the hospital/healthcare facility or later.[2] Patients with a previous hospitalization, including residence in another healthcare facility such as a long-term care environment (for 72 hours or longer) within 14 days of current admission, who develop a lower respiratory tract infection also are considered HAP.

Although the clinical presentations for CAP and HAP are very similar, differences in manifestation can be related to the host and the virulence of the microorganisms. Elderly individuals with pneumonia may have vague clinical presentations and present with nonspecific symptoms (e.g., generalized weakness, decreased appetite, falls, delirium, and incontinence).

III. COMPARING AND CONTRASTING CAP AND HAP

Community-Acquired pneumonia (CAP)

Perspective of CAP

Pneumonia acquired in nonhealthcare settings is increasingly recognized among older patients and in those with comorbidities or coexisting illness.[3-7] Such contributing conditions include chronic obstructive lung disease, diabetes mellitus, renal insufficiency, congestive heart failure, coronary artery disease, malignancy, chronic neurological disease, and chronic liver disease.[4] Individuals may become infected with a variety of microbes including those traditionally recognized, emerging, or previously unrecognized pathogens.[8-11] At the same time, a number of new antimicrobial agents have become available, some with utility for pneumonia. Paralleling the improvement in our antibiotic armamentarium has been the evolution of bacterial resistance mechanisms. In the 1990s, many of the common respiratory pathogens have become resistant, in vitro, to widely used antimicrobials. Resistance, by a variety of mechanisms, is being identified with increasing frequency among *Streptococcus pneumoniae, Hemophilus influenzae, Moraxella catarrhalis,* and a number of enteric gram-negative bacteria.[12]

Concerns regarding recognition, treatment, and healthcare worker (HCW) safety have changed as new diseases have emerged. Identification of emerging microbes including the corona virus causing severe acute respiratory syndrome (SARS) as well as the H5N1 avian influenza strain have expanded the differential diagnosis and emphasizes the need to obtain an adequate history and epidemiological evaluation.

Epidemiology of CAP

CAP remains a common and serious illness, despite the availability of potent new antimicrobials and effective vaccines. In the United States pneumonia is the sixth leading cause of death and the number one cause of death from infectious diseases.[13,14] In the outpatient setting, the mortality rate of pneumonia remains low, in the range of < 1%–5%, but among patients with CAP who require hospitalization, the mortality rate averages 12% overall increasing in specific populations, such as those with bacteremia and those from nursing home settings. The mortality rates approach 40% in those who are most ill and who require admission to an intensive care unit.[15]

Pathogenesis of CAP

Pneumonia is indicated when an inflammatory process of the lung parenchyma caused by a microbial agent is present. The most common pathway for the microbial agent to reach the alveoli is by microaspiration of oropharyngeal secretions. Once the microorganisms reach the alveolar space, they can cause pneumonia by overcoming the defense mechanisms in the lungs, the alveolar macrophages. Most of the time, the alveolar macrophages phagocytize and kill the microorganism into the alveolar spaces. If alveolar macrophages are unable to control the growth of microorganisms, then, as a final protective defense mechanism, the lungs develop a local inflammatory response. This response is characterized by movement of white blood cells (granulocytes, lymphocytes, and monocytes) from the capillaries into the alveolar space.[1]

Etiology of CAP

Prospective studies evaluating the causative organisms for CAP in adults have failed to identify the cause in 40%–60% of cases. It is important to also recognize that CAP may have two or more etiologies detected in 2%–5% of cases.[16-20] This stresses the importance of following established guidelines and ensuring healthcare personnel safety in the event this duality represents both communicable and noncommunicable causative agents.

The most common etiologic agent identified in virtually all reported studies of CAP is *Streptococcus pneumoniae*, which accounts for about two-thirds of all cases of bacteremic pneumonia.[21] Other pathogens implicated include *H. influenzae* (mostly nontypeable strains), *Mycoplasma pneumoniae, Chlamydia pneu-*

Copyright © 2005, Association for Professionals in Infection Control and Epidemiology, Inc.

moniae, Staphylococcus aureus, Streptococcus pyogenes, Neisseria meningitidis, Moraxella catarrhalis, Klebsiella pneumoniae and other gram-negative rods, Legionella species, influenza viruses (depending on the season), respiratory syncytial virus, adenovirus, parainfluenza virus, and other microbes. The frequency of other etiologies is dependent on specific epidemiological factors, as with Chlamydia psittaci (psittacosis), Coxiella burnetii (Q fever), Francisella tularensis (tularemia), endemic fungi (histoplasmosis, blastomycosis, coccidioidomycosis), as well as emerging agents including SARS corona virus and avian influenza.[22]

Diagnosis of CAP

The patient with pneumonia syndrome will present with cough, sputum production, shortness of breath, pleuritic chest pain, fever, chills, tachycardia, tachypnea, rales, and signs of consolidation on physical examination.[1] Test findings include a new pulmonary infiltrate on chest x-ray and leukocytosis that may include a left shift noted in the complete blood count (CBC) differential. A left shift can be defined as the presence of bands (an immature form of neutrophils) in the circulating blood from stimulation of the immune system. The bone marrow responds by escalating the release of neutrophils into the bloodstream for subsequent migration to the tissues of the lung. This immune response may overwhelm the availability of mature cells, hence the immature forms are introduced.

The diagnosis of CAP is based on the combination of the clinical findings and the chest x-ray. Chest radiography is considered critical for establishing the diagnosis of pneumonia and for distinguishing this condition from acute bronchitis. Bronchitis treatment with antibiotics can contribute to resistant organisms, as the bronchitis is often a response from a viral cause. Other benefits of the chest x-ray include the differential diagnosis with other pathologies of the lower respiratory tract, the detection of associated pulmonary diseases, in some cases the presumption of the etiologic agent, the ability to evaluate severity, and to obtain a baseline for evaluating response to treatment. In some settings, specifically in the long-term care environment, the use of chest x-rays may be limited, thus impacting the definition of pneumonia from both a clinical and surveillance perspective. Additional information about specific surveillance definitions can be obtained in other chapters of this text or from the Centers for Disease Control and Prevention (CDC) National Healthcare Safety Network (NHSN), formerly National Nosocomial Infection Surveillance (NNIS) system.

It is important to recognize that with a good medical history and physical examination, it is possible to select patients that have very low risk for mortality without need to perform additional testing or workup. To determine if a patient with CAP has a very low risk of mortality (the mortality in this group is lower than 0.1 %) the patient needs to be less than 50 years old and not have any comorbid diseases or any significant abnormalities upon physical examination.[22]

Patients with several risk factors often require hospitalization. One score to predict the mortality risk developed by the Pneumonia Patients Outcomes Research Team (PORT) classified patients into five groups according to the presence of risk factors. For patients in group I, the predicted mortality is 0.1 %, group II 0.6 %, group III 0.9 %, group IV 9.3 %, and group V up to 27%. It is recommended that patients belonging to groups IV and V be hospitalized.[22]

According to the American Thoracic Society (ATS) guidelines and Infectious Diseases Society of America (IDSA) guidelines, it is optional to perform a sputum Gram stain and culture in patients that will be managed on an outpatient basis.[22-23]

For patients admitted to the hospital with diagnosis of CAP, in addition to the history and physical, the following workup or evaluation is suggested:

- Blood cultures (times two at least 15 minutes apart) before the administration of any antibiotic

- Performance of a sputum Gram stain and culture before the administration of any antibiotic

- Assessment of oxygen saturation

- CBC with differential

- Serum creatinine, blood urea nitrogen, glucose, electrolytes, and liver function tests

- HIV serology with informed consent should be considered, especially for persons aged 15–54 years[22] and with suspected risk factors for HIV infection or recurrent pneumonia.

Pulmonary tuberculosis (TB) caused by Mycobacterium tuberculosis can mimic CAP; therefore TB should be suspected in all patients with diagnosis of CAP that have risk factors for TB. The 25 risk factors for TB published by the CDC are included in Table 22–1.[27] In patients with cough and pulmonary infiltrate, early diagnosis of CAP due to M. tuberculosis is important for two reasons: to start treatment and to place the hospitalized patient into a special type of room with engineering controls—airborne infectious isolation (AII)—thus decreasing the risk of transmission to others. (Also refer to Chapter 18, Isolation Systems, and Chapter 93, Mycobacteria.)

Diagnostic testing procedures (e.g., bronchoscopy) or other invasive tests (e.g., lung biopsy) should be reserved for select patients. Selected patients should

Copyright © 2005, Association for Professionals in Infection Control and Epidemiology, Inc.

Table 22-1. Risk Factors for TB According to CDC

Night sweats	Hemoptysis	Weight loss
Hoarseness	HIV/AIDS	History of positive PPD
Homeless	Alcohol/drug abuse	Healthcare worker
Prior history of TB	Age > 65	Community living (e.g., prison)
Recent exposure to TB	From endemic area	Silicosis
ESRD	Gastrectomy	Cancer of GI tract
10% or < ideal body weight	Diabetes mellitus	Some hematologic disorders (e.g., leukemia)
Intestinal bypass	Other immunosuppressive state	Long-term steroids therapy

Note: Risk factors of cough and pulmonary infiltrate are not included in this table because they are inclusion criteria for CAP.

have specific microbiological studies for TB and Legionella infection. The preferred tests for detection of Legionella species are the urinary antigen assay for *Legionella pneumophila* serogroup 1 and collection of deep respiratory sputum or bronchial aspirate for culture with selective media.[22] (Also see Chapter 76, *Legionella pneumophila*.)

Measures to Prevent CAP

The population of hospitalized patients with CAP should be considered as high risk for rehospitalization related to influenza or pneumonia. Due to the mortality associated with CAP and the high recurrent rate of the disease, national organizations from multiple countries have emphasized in their pneumonia guidelines documents the importance of CAP prevention.[22-26] Most CAP guidelines recommend that all patients at risk for pneumonia be vaccinated with both the pneumococcal and influenza vaccine. Because cigarette smoking is a risk factor for development of pneumonia, smoking cessation is another important prevention strategy recommended in CAP guidelines.

Quality Indicators and Outcomes for CAP

Quality-assessment indicators for CAP that are founded on healthcare structures, processes, and outcomes have been recommended as potential audit tools to evaluate the delivery of care. The aim of these best-practice guidelines is to reduce variations in key aspects of care and, by doing so, improve the efficiency and effectiveness of healthcare.[29]

Many institutions recommend performing the vaccination against pneumococcus and influenza during the hospitalization for pneumonia. In fact, these performance measures are evaluated through both the Joint Commission on Accreditation of Healthcare Organizations (JCAHO) and Centers for Medicaid and Medicare Services (CMS) quality initiatives.

Recommendations for performance indicators in the healthcare setting include the collection of blood culture specimens before antibiotic treatment and the institution of antibiotic treatment within 4–8 hours of hospitalization, both of which are supported on the basis of evidence-based trials. Additional performance indicators recommended are laboratory tests for Legionella in patients hospitalized in the intensive care unit (ICU), demonstration of an infiltrate on chest radiographs of patients with an ICD-9 (*International Classification of Diseases,* 9th edition) code for pneumonia, and measurement of blood gases or pulse oximetry within 24 hours of admission.[22]

Healthcare Associated Pneumonia (HAP)

Perspective of HAP

Healthcare-associated pneumonia (HAP) remains an important cause of mortality and morbidity despite the introduction of potent broad-spectrum antimicrobial agents, complex supportive care modalities, and the use of preventive measures. HAP is defined as pneumonia occurring 48 hours or later after admission to the hospital/healthcare facility for most organisms and excluding any infection that is incubating at the time of admission.[30] Patients with a previous hospitalization (of 72 hours or longer) within 14 days of current admission that developed a lower respiratory tract infection also are considered HAP. Available data suggest that HAP occurs at a rate of between 5 to 10 cases per 1,000 hospital admissions, with the incidence increasing by as much as six- to 20-fold in patients who are being ventilated mechanically (ventilator-associated pneumonia, or VAP).

Pneumonia is currently the second most common nosocomial (hospital-acquired) infection in the United States but has the highest mortality and morbidity, accounting for 15% of all healthcare-acquired infections and 27% and 24% of all infections acquired in the medical intensive care unit and coronary care units, respectively.

HAP is classified as early nosocomial pneumonia (ENP) when it occurs 4–6 days after admission or late nosocomial pneumonia (LNP) when it occurs 7 days or longer

Copyright © 2005, Association for Professionals in Infection Control and Epidemiology, Inc.

after admission.[31] This is an important distinction when determining empiric therapy. Pneumonia that develops later may reflect some of the organisms typical to the given healthcare facility. Knowing the flora of the facility, often demonstrated by the facility antibiogram, provides valuable information used to initiate appropriate therapy. Initiating correct empiric antimicrobial therapy is one of the primary, if not the most important, factors that impact the patient's outcome.

Some pathogens (Legionella, Mycoplasma, Aspergillus) have longer incubation periods. Pneumonia due to one of these pathogens in a hospitalized patient should be classified nosocomial if the length of hospitalization exceeds the known incubation period.

The CDC has published guidelines for prevention of nosocomial pneumonia in 1994 and a revised guideline that addresses HAP in 2003. These guidelines should be referred to for additional background information and specific recommendations and is cited in the reference section of this chapter.

Epidemiology of HAP

HAP is the second most frequent nosocomial infection; however, it has the greatest associated mortality.[32-33] Attributable mortality is 20%–30% overall. Mortality is even higher in patients with severe (life-threatening) illness at the time pneumonia develops.[34,35] However, the risk of death can be significantly lowered by appropriate and timely antibiotic therapy.[35] Secondary modifications of an initially failing antibiotic regimen do not substantially improve the outcome for these critically ill patients. Therefore, the best approach for reducing infection-related mortality seems to be the initial institution of an adequate and broad-spectrum antibiotic regimen in severely ill patients. This broad-spectrum antibiotic regimen should be modified in a de-escalating strategy when the results from microbiologic testing become available.[36]

HAP can extend hospitalization by an average of 4 to 9 days per patient and increase the costs of hospitalization.[30] Mayhall estimates the cost per case is $5,683 with an increased average length of stay of 5.9 days.[54]

Factors associated with increased risk are generally grouped as host related, device related, or factors that increase bacterial colonization of the stomach or nasopharynx and risk factors for acquisition of a multidrug-resistant organism (MDRO) as a cause of HAP. These contributing factors include:

- Host related: age 65 years or more, underlying conditions, especially chronic lung disease, depressed level of consciousness, thoracic or chest surgery, use of paralytic agents, severe trauma, upper abdominal surgery, and recent bronchoscopy[37-40]

- Device related: tracheal intubation, continuous mechanical ventilation, orogastric or nasogastric tube placement, and frequent (e.g., every 24 hours) ventilator circuit changes[41]

- Increased colonization: admission to the intensive care unit, administration of broad-spectrum antibiotics, prophylaxis for stress ulcer bleeding with antacids or H_2 blocker, exposure to contaminated medical equipment, and inadequate hand hygiene

- MDRO (e.g., Pseudomonas, Acinetobacter, MRSA): hospitalization for more than 7 days before the diagnosis of HAP, transferred from another care facility, ventilation for more than 3 days before the diagnosis of HAP, active malignancy, AIDS, end-stage liver or renal disease, steroids (e.g., prednisone 10 mg/day or more for more than 7 days), active chemotherapy or radiotherapy, and bronchiectasis. Prior antibiotic use for more than 3 days within the previous 14 days of the diagnosis of HAP also is considered a risk factor for resistant organisms.

Inhalation of contaminated aerosols or airborne microbes can also introduce bacteria into the lower respiratory tract. This can occur during events such as utility interruptions, remodeling, or construction where infection control recommendations have not been followed. (Refer to Chapters 105 through 107 for more information.) The consequences of inadequate sterilization and disinfection have been epidemiologically demonstrated in a variety of outbreaks including those involving bronchoscopes, ventilator components, instruments, and other durable medical equipment. (Refer to Chapter 21, Cleaning, Disinfection, and Sterilization; Chapter 56, Central Services; and Chapter 102, Environmental Services.)

Pathogenesis of HAP

Aspiration of oropharyngeal bacteria is the most common initiating event. Witnessed aspiration has been found to be an independent risk factor for HAP.[41] Smaller aspiration events may also contribute to the development of pneumonia.

During hospitalization, the normal oropharyngeal flora is oftentimes altered. Aspiration of bacteria, after this colonization has occurred, can lead to proliferation of these bacteria in the lower respiratory tract.

Etiology of HAP

The reported distribution of etiologic agents that cause HAP differs between healthcare settings because of different patient populations, different flora in each institution, and different diagnostic methods employed. In general, however, bacteria have been the most frequently isolated pathogens.[42] In patients with diagnosis of early HAP (a stay of 4–6 days in the hospital), a

Copyright © 2005, Association for Professionals in Infection Control and Epidemiology, Inc.

group of core organisms are most likely responsible for infection. This includes the same pathogens (excluding atypical bacteria) that cause CAP such as *Streptococcus pneumoniae, Haemophilus influenzae, Moraxella catarrhalis, S. aureus* as well as nonresistant enteric gram-negative bacilli such as *Escherichia coli, Klebsiella spp.,* and *Proteus spp.*

In patients who developed late HAP (with a stay of 7 days or longer in the hospital), the spectrum includes the above-mentioned core organisms plus other gram-negative bacteria, including *Pseudomonas aeruginosa, Enterobacter, Acinetobacter,* and enteric gram-negative rods, which are implicated in 55% to 85% of HAP cases. Gram-positive cocci (particularly *S. aureus*) account for 20% to 30%, whereas 40% to 60% of cases are polymicrobial (mixed organisms). Methicillin-resistant *S. aureus* (MRSA), as the causative organism, has increased in frequency in the last few years. Acuity and severity of illness, duration of hospitalization, and prior antibiotic exposure are major determinants of likely pathogens. In critically ill patients requiring prolonged mechanical ventilation in ICUs, *P. aeruginosa and Acinetobacter* (e.g., *A. calcoaceticus* and *A. baumannii*), which are resistant to many antibiotics, account for 30% to 50% of HAP; these pathogens are uncommon in non-ICU settings.[36]

Anaerobes and fungi are uncommon causes of HAP even though those organisms may be identified in respiratory cultures. Identification is often indicative of colonization, not infection. Other causes in selected populations are *Pneumocystis carinii* (causing *P. carinii* pneumonia or PCP) and Cytomegalovirus (CMV). Legionella can cause HAP and is generally associated with water system colonization and subsequent transmission from ingestion (e.g., contaminated water or ice) with subsequent aspiration or through aerosol inhalation (e.g., cooling towers, ventilation systems).

Diagnosis of HAP

Diagnosis of HAP remains a major challenge for clinicians. HAP should be suspected in patients that develop a new and persistent infiltrate (as observed on the chest x-ray) and is associated with at least one of the following: (a) purulent tracheal secretions, (b) temperature $\geq$ 38°C, and (c) WBC count $\geq$ 10,000/mm^3 (cubic millimeter).

Usually a positive quantitative culture of a distal pulmonary secretion sample is required to confirm the diagnosis. Cultures of bronchoalveolar lavage (BAL) obtained by fiberoptic bronchoscopy are considered significant (threshold) with growth of at least 10^4 cfu/ml (colony forming units per milliliter) with quantitative culture. For a protected brush or catheter specimen, the significant threshold is considered 10^3 cfu/ml.[43] Quantitative cultures of tracheal aspirate are used for

the diagnosis of HAP (VAP) in ventilated patients. In patients that developed HAP without mechanical ventilation, a sputum culture is commonly required for the diagnosis. A sputum specimen is considered representative of deep respiratory secretions when there is $\leq$ 25 neutrophils and less than 10 epithelial cells on gram-stained microscopy examination.

Prior to antibiotic administration, it is important to obtain all cultures. The recommendation for patients with suspected HAP without mechanical ventilation is to obtain sputum for Gram stain and culture plus two blood cultures with those blood cultures at least 15 minutes apart. In patients with a working diagnosis of HAP and that are mechanical ventilated, a quantitative tracheal aspirate or BAL plus two blood cultures is recommended.

The signs and symptoms of pneumonia are not specific. Unfortunately, many noninfectious processes, such as congestive heart failure, pulmonary embolism, and adult respiratory distress syndrome, may be responsible for fever and new pulmonary infiltrates in hospitalized patients, and clinical approaches lead to an overestimation of the incidence of HAP. Extremely young or old patients or those who are granulocytopenic may have diminished findings.

Diagnostic criteria for bacterial pneumonia vary for many reasons, such as patient population, laboratory and clinical resources, and whether the criteria are used for surveillance or treatment.[42] No single set of criteria has been found to be fully accurate. Generally used criteria are fever, new cough, development of purulent sputum, deterioration of pulmonary functions and chest x-ray with a new or progressive infiltrate. These criteria are sensitive but not specific. Additional criteria may include isolation of a pathogen from sputum, tracheal aspirate, pleural fluid, or blood cultures.

Bronchoscopy, including collection of BAL, protected BAL (pBAL) and protected-specimen brushing (PSB), has been used to improve diagnosis, especially in ventilator patients.[42] The disadvantage is that these techniques are invasive, they may cause complications such as hypoxemia, bleeding, or arrhythmia. Reported sensitivities and specificities have ranged between 70%—100% and 60%—100%, respectively for these methods, depending on the tests and diagnostic criteria used for comparison. In addition, the sensitivity of the PSB procedure may decrease for patients receiving antibiotic therapy. Nonbronchoscopic (NB) procedures (e.g., NB-pBAL or NB-PSB) that utilize blind catheterization of the distal airways and quantitative culture of endotracheal aspirate are relatively recently developed methods. Of these, culturing of an endotracheal aspirate appears to be the most practical. The use of bronchoscopic and nonbronchoscopic diagnostic tests

Copyright © 2005, Association for Professionals in Infection Control and Epidemiology, Inc.

contribute to better defining the epidemiology of noso-comial pneumonia, especially in patients with mechani-cally assisted ventilation; further studies are needed to determine each test's applicability in daily clinical prac-tice.

New modalities of diagnosis have been recently described such as the clinical pulmonary infection score (CPIS) and soluble triggering receptor expressed on myeloid cells, both of which are under investigation. The CPIS system applies a diagnostic algorithm based on easily available clinical, radiographic, and microbio-logical criteria and could be an attractive alternative for diagnosing ventilator-associated pneumonia.[44] The trig-gering receptor expressed on myeloid cells (TREM-1) is a member of the immunoglobulin superfamily, and its expression on phagocytes is specifically stimulated by microbial cell components. The presence of soluble TREM-1 (sTREM-1) in BAL fluid from patients receiving mechanical ventilation may be an indicator of pneumonia.[45]

Legionella is generally diagnosed only if a high level of suspicion is maintained. Urinary antigen testing, sputum culture on select media, or sputum direct fluo-rescent antigen (DFA) staining or serology may confirm the diagnosis.

Nonbacterial pneumonia microbes include *Aspergillus* or *Candida spp.* with diagnosis often requiring lung biopsy and culture. *Candida* is rarely a cause of HAP but can often be isolated from cultures of respiratory specimens. Identification of this organism in sputum or tracheal aspirate specimens is likely due to colonization or oral contamination of the specimen during collec-tion. A biopsy is necessary to diagnose invasive disease; the only currently accepted criterion for the definitive diagnosis of *Candida* pneumonia is histolog-ical demonstration of the fungus in lung tissue.[22] Usually healthcare-associated infection due to *Asper-gillus spp.* and *Candida spp.* are seen in patients who are immunocompromised due to treatment associated with hematologic stem cell transplant, hematological malignancies such as acute leukemia, and chronic myeloid leukemia.[42] (Also see Chapter 15, Immuno-compromised Host, and Chapter 43, Transplants.)

Respiratory viral infections usually follow community outbreaks that occur during a particular period every year, confer only short-term immunity, affect healthy and ill persons, and have exogenous sources. A number of viruses, including adenoviruses, influenza virus, measles virus, parainfluenza viruses, respiratory syncytial virus (RSV), rhinoviruses, and varicella-zoster virus, can cause HAP. However, adenoviruses, influ-enza viruses, parainfluenza viruses, and RSV have been reported to account for most (70%) of HAPs due to viruses. In the past, diagnosis of influenza was made by virus isolation from nasopharyngeal secretions or by

serologic conversion. Recently, rapid diagnostic tests have been developed that are similar to culture with respect to sensitivity and specificity and allow for early diagnosis and treatment of cases. This also provides a basis for prompt initiation of appropriate antiviral pro-phylaxis as part of outbreak control.[46]

Pneumocystis carinii causing PCP has been described in hospital outbreaks and should be considered as a possible etiology in immunosuppressed patients; PCP is usually diagnosed by finding the organism in sputum or BAL fluid.

Measures to Prevent HAP

The optimal management of patients with HAP requires close collaboration among pulmonary and crit-ical care specialists, infectious disease practitioners, infection control professionals, radiologists, and hos-pital microbiologists. This type of collaboration will lead to early recognition and appropriate management of common source outbreaks and MDROs.[30]

Education of HCP regarding HAP pneumonias and infection prevention is very important. Because coloni-zation with hospital bacteria can be initiated with the transfer of bacteria from HCP, simple yet effective control measures of hand hygiene and appropriate use of barriers (gloves and gown use) following standard precautions should be emphasized. Immunizations (e.g., pneumococcus and influenza) for HCP and patients are recommended.[42]

Bacterial colonization of the stomach may be decreased by the use of sucralfate instead of H2 blockers plus antacids to prevent stress ulcer bleeding; the use of sucralfate has not been shown to definitely decrease the rate of HAP. The use of antibiotic regi-mens for selective decontamination is not currently rec-ommended; these regimens may decrease the rate of nosocomial pneumonia but have not improved patient mortality.[47] MDROs have been isolated more fre-quently when these regimens are used.[48]

Respiratory equipment must be properly cleaned and sterilized. Ventilator tubing must be handled appropri-ately to avoid spilling condensate into the patient's airway. Ventilator circuits should not be routinely replaced to decrease the risk of pneumonia. Rather, replace circuits if malfunctioning or if visibly contami-nated.[49] Specific instructions can be found in the CDC guidelines for preventing HAP, 2003.[42]

Measures that can decrease the risk of aspiration include positioning the patient supine with the head ele-vated 30–45 degrees, suctioning measures including continuous suctioning of subglottic secretions, and mini-mizing the use of sedating or paralytic agents.[50]

Copyright © 2005, Association for Professionals in Infection Control and Epidemiology, Inc.

Antibiotic Overuse

Selection of appropriate therapy is essential to avoid the detrimental effects of antibiotic overuse and the production of selective pressure for resistant organisms. In one study, respiratory tract infections accounted for 49% of all antibiotics prescribed in the ICU and 63% of the antibiotics used; however, they were often prescribed for clinically suspected but not proven respiratory tract infections.[51] Other studies have documented empiric antibiotic use for ICU patients with pulmonary infiltrates without pneumonia, ranging from 34% to 74%.[52]

New approaches for the treatment as short-course therapy in selected groups of patients and de-escalation antibiotic therapy, following the clinical pulmonary infection score (CPIS), have been used recently to reduce the overuse of antibiotics in this population.[53]

IV.   SUMMARY AND CONCLUSIONS

Pneumonia represents significant morbidity and mortality risks to the patient, increased healthcare costs, and potential risk to HCP. Identifying the most likely etiology of the pneumonia, targeting and streamlining antimicrobial therapy, developing and implementing strategies to prevent development of pneumonia, ensuring the safety of other patients, and HCP through immunization and environmental controls, are all components of an effective infection prevention and control program. Many of these elements are included in existing and forthcoming quality initiatives. These initiatives focus on specific processes such as timing and obtaining correct laboratory specimens, appropriate physiologic assessments such as oxygenation, timing of antimicrobial therapy administration, appropriate patient placement, smoking cessation, and immunization opportunities. Understanding that patient outcomes are becoming part of public reporting may serve as a motivator for improving both medical care and healthcare processes.

V.   FUTURE TRENDS/RESEARCH

Without respect to the significant morbidity and mortality associated with pneumonia, the trend in U.S. healthcare involves compliance with quality measures. Both JCAHO and CMS are using their influence to move actual practice toward best practice. Public reporting of compliance with best practices combined with reimbursement incentives and improving outcomes using evidence-based medicine will be the expected instead of the exception.

Identification of emerging pathogens including SARS and avian influenza has resulted in heightened concern when patients present with respiratory infection any-

where in the world. Continued emphasis on safe practice at the time of first encounter must be included in the overall care plan. This requires improved identification methods and technology, patient evaluation with appropriate placement when indicated, safer healthcare environmental settings, infection prevention measures and resources, epidemiology, and HCP health initiatives.

VI.   INTERNATIONAL PERSPECTIVES

International studies have demonstrated significant differences in empiric treatment in patients admitted with the diagnosis of CAP. Several countries do not include antibiotics that cover atypical pathogens such as *Mycoplasma pneumoniae, Chlamydia pneumoniae,* and Legionella in their empiric treatment regimen guidelines. Additional areas of research continue to define the best antibiotics for treatment of CAP.

A lack of comprehensive vaccination and smoking cessation programs continues to be a major global problem. New strategies are needed to implement vaccination in healthcare settings and to offer smoking cessation around the world.

REFERENCES

1. Ramirez J: Community-acquired pneumonia: a plan for implementing national guidelines at the local hospital level. 2003.
2. American Thoracic Society: Hospital-acquired pneumonia in adults: diagnosis, assessment of severity, initial antimicrobial therapy, and preventive strategies; a consensus statement, American Thoracic Society, November 1995. *Am J Respir Crit Care Med* 153:1711–1725, 1996
3. Niederman MS, McCombs JI, Unger AN, Kumar A, Popovian R: The cost of treating community-acquired pneumonia, *Clin Ther* 20:820–837, 1998
4. Ruiz M, Ewig S, Marcos MA, Martinez JA, Arancibia F, Mensa J, Torres A: Etiology of community-acquired pneumonia: impact of age, comorbidity, and severity, *Am J Respir Crit Care Med* 160: 397–405, 1999
5. Riquelme R, Torres A, el-Ebiary M, Mensa J, Estruch R, Ruiz M, Angrill J, Soler N: Community-acquired pneumonia in the elderly: clinical and nutritional aspects, *Am J Respir Crit Care Med* 156: 1908–1914, 1997
6. Rello J, Rodriguez R, Jubert P, Alvarez B: Severe community-acquired pneumonia in the elderly: epidemiology and prognosis, *Clin Infect Dis* 23:723–728, 1996
7. Marrie TJ: Community-acquired pneumonia, *Clin Infect Dis* 18: 501–513, 1994
8. Marrie TJ, Durant H, Yates L: Community-acquired pneumonia requiring hospitalization: a 5 year prospective study, *Rev Infect Dis* 11:586–599, 1989
9. Marston BJ, Plouffe JF, File TM Jr, Hackman BA, Salstrom SJ, Lipman HB, Kolczak MS, Breiman RF: Incidence of community-acquired pneumonia requiring hospitalization: results of a population-based active surveillance study in Ohio, The Community-Based Pneumonia Incidence Study Group, *Arch Intern Med* 157: 1709–1718, 1997
10. Lieberman D, Schlaeffer F, Boldur I, Lieberman D, Horowitz S, Friedman MG, Leiononen M, Horovitz O, Manor E, Porath A: Multiple pathogens in adult patients admitted with community-acquired pneumonia: a one year prospective study of 346 consecutive patients, *Thorax* 51:179–184, 1996
11. Porath A, Schlaeffer F, Lieberman D: The epidemiology of community acquired pneumonia among hospitalized adults, *J Infect* 34:41–48, 1997

APIC Text of Infection Control and Epidemiology

Copyright © 2005, Association for Professionals in Infection Control and Epidemiology, Inc.

12. Pallares R, Linares J, Vadillo M, Cabellos C, Manresa F, Viladrich PF, Martin R, Gudiol F: Resistance to penicillin and cephalosporin and mortality from severe pneumococcal pneumonia in Barcelona, Spain, *N Engl J Med* 333:474–480, 1995

13. Garibaldi RA: Epidemiology of community-acquired respiratory tract infections in adults: incidence, etiology, and impact, *Am J Med* 78:32S–37S, 1985

14. Niederman MS, McCombs JI, Unger AN, Kumar A, Popovian R: The cost of treating community-acquired pneumonia, *Clin Ther* 20:820–837, 1998

15. Bates JH, Campbell GD, Barron AL, McCracken GA, Morgan PN, Moses EB, Davis CM: Microbial etiology of acute pneumonia in hospitalized patients, *Chest* 101:1005–1012, 1992

16. British Thoracic Society: Guidelines for the management of community-acquired pneumonia in adults admitted to hospital, *Br J Hosp Med* 49:346–50, 1993

17. Centers for Disease Control and Prevention: Premature deaths, monthly mortality and monthly physician contacts: United States, *MMWR Morb Mortal Wkly Rep* 46:556, 1997

18. Fine MJ, Orloff JJ, Arisumi D, et al: Prognosis of patients hospitalized with community-acquired pneumonia, *Am J Med* 88:1N–8N, 1990

19. Fang GD, Fine M, Orloff J, et al: New and emerging etiologies for community-acquired pneumonia with implications for therapy: a prospective multicenter study of 359 cases, *Medicine* (Baltimore) 69:307–16, 1990

20. Mundy LM, Auwaerter PG, Oldach D, et al: Community-acquired pneumonia: impact of immune status, *Am J Respir Crit Care Med* 152:1309–15, 1995

21. Fine MJ, Smith MA, Carson CA, et al: Prognosis and outcomes of patients with community-acquired pneumonia, *JAMA* 275: 134–41, 1996

22. Fine MJ, Auble TE, Yealy DM, Hanusa BH, Weissfeld LA, Singer DE, Coley CM, Marrie TJ, Kapoor WN: A prediction rule to identify low-risk patients with community-acquired pneumonia, *N Engl J Med* 336:243–250, 1997

23. Niederman MS, Mandell LA, Anzueto A, et al: Guidelines for the management of adults with community-acquired pneumonia, American Thoracic Society, *Am J Respir Crit Care Med* 163: 1730–1754, 2001

24. Mandell LA, Bartlett JG, Dowell SF, File TM Jr, Musher DM, Whitney C: Update of practice guidelines for the management of community-acquired pneumonia in immunocompetent adults, *Clin Infect Dis* 37(11):1405–1433, 2003

25. British Thoracic Society Standards of Care Committee: BTS guidelines for the management of community acquired pneumonia in adults, *Thorax* 56 Suppl 4:IV1–64, 2001

26. Mandell LA, Marrie TJ, Grossman RF, Chow AW, Hyland RH: Canadian guidelines for the initial management of community-acquired pneumonia: an evidence-based update by the Canadian Infectious Diseases Society and the Canadian Thoracic Society. The Canadian Community-Acquired Pneumonia Working Group, *Clin Infect Dis* 31(2):383–421, 2000

27. CDC: Screening for tuberculosis and tuberculous infection in high-risk populations: recommendations of the Advisory Committee for Elimination of Tuberculosis, *MMWR* 39 (RR-8):1–7, 1990

28. Nathwani D, Williams F, Winter J, Winter J, Ogston S, Davey P: Use of indicators to evaluate the quality of community-acquired pneumonia management, *Clin Infect Dis* 34(3):318–23, 2002

29. Miller J, Petrie J: Development of practice guidelines, *Lancet* 355(9198):82–3, 2000

30. American Thoracic Society: Hospital-acquired pneumonia in adults: diagnosis, assessment of severity, initial antimicrobial therapy, and preventive strategies; a consensus statement, American Thoracic Society, November 1995, *Am J Respir Crit Care Med* 153:1711–1725, 1996

31. Brochicchio GV, Joshi M, Brochicchio K, et al: A time-dependent analysis of intensive care unit pneumonia in trauma patients, *J Trauma* 56(2):296–301, 2004

32. Gomez J, Esquinas A, Agudo MD, et al: Retrospective analysis of risk factors and prognosis in non-ventilated patients with nosocomial pneumonia, *Eur J Clin Microbiol Infect Dis* 14(3):176–81, 1995

33. National Nosocomial Infections Surveillance (NNIS) System report, data summary from January 1990–May 1999, issued June 1999, *Am J Infect Control* 27(6):520–32, 1999

34. Salemi C, Morgan J, Padilla S, Morrissey R: Association between severity of illness and mortality from nosocomial infection, *Am J Infect Control* 23(3):188–93, 1995

35. Celis R, Torres A, Gatell JM, Almela M, et al: Nosocomial pneumonia: a multivariate analysis of risk and prognosis, *Chest* 93(2): 318–24, 1988

36. Hoffken G, Niederman MS: Nosocomial pneumonia: the importance of a de-escalating strategy for antibiotic treatment of pneumonia in the ICU, *Chest* 122(6):2183–96, 2002

37. Craven DE, Steger KA: Nosocomial pneumonia in mechanically ventilated adult patients: epidemiology and prevention in 1996, *Semin Respir Infect* 11(1):32–53, 1996

38. Kollef MH, Sharpless L, Vlasnik J, et al: The impact of nosocomial infections on patient outcomes following cardiac surgery, *Chest* 112(3):666–75, 1997

39. Jarvis WR: Selected aspects of the socioeconomic impact of nosocomial infections: morbidity, mortality, cost, and prevention, *Infect Control Hosp Epidemiol* 17(8):552–7, 1996

40. George DL: Epidemiology of nosocomial pneumonia in intensive care unit patients, *Clin Chest Med* 16(1):29–44, 1995

41. McRitchie DI, Matthews JG, Fink MP: Pneumonia in patients with multiple trauma, *Clin Chest Med* 16(1):135–46, 1995

42. Guidelines for preventing health-care-associated pneumonia, *MMWR*53(RR-3);1–36, 2004

43. Chastre J, Wolff M, Fagon JY, Chevret S, et al; PneumA Trial Group: Comparison of 8 vs. 15 days of antibiotic therapy for ventilator-associated pneumonia in adults: a randomized trial, *JAMA* 290(19):2588–98, 2003

44. Schurink CA, Nieuwenhoven CA, Jacobs JA, et al: Clinical pulmonary infection score for ventilator-associated pneumonia: accuracy and inter-observer variability, *Intensive Care Med* 30(2): 217–224, 2004

45. Gibot S, Cravoisy A, Levy B, Bene MC, et al: Soluble triggering receptor expressed on myeloid cells and the diagnosis of pneumonia, *N Engl J Med* 350(5):451–8, 2004

46. Tablan OC, Anderson LJ, et al: CDC guideline for prevention of nosocomial pneumonia, Atlanta, 2002, CDC

47. Potgieter P, Hammond J: Prophylactic use of the new quinolones for prevention of nosocomial infection in the intensive care unit, *Drugs* 49:86–91, 1995

48. Bergogne-Berezin E: Treatment and prevention of nosocomial pneumonia, *Chest* 108:265–345, 1995

49. Kotilainen H, Keroack M: Cost analysis and clinical impact of weekly ventilator circuit changes in patients in intensive care unit, *Am J Infect Control* 25:117–120, 1997

50. Bressin A, Niederman M: Prevention of ventilator-associated pneumonia an attainable goal? *Clin Chest Med* 16:195–208, 1995

51. Aucar JA, Bongera M, Phillips JO, et al: Quantitative tracheal lavage versus bronchoscopic protected specimen brush for the diagnosis of nosocomial pneumonia in mechanically ventilated patients, *Am J Surg* 186(6):591–6, 2003

52. Bergmans DC, Bonten MJ, Gaillard CA, et al: Indications for antibiotic use in ICU patients: a one-year prospective surveillance, *J Antimicrob Chemother* 39(4):527–35, 1997

53. Singh N, Rogers P, Atwood CW, Wagener MM, Yu VL: Short-course empiric antibiotic therapy for patients with pulmonary infiltrates in the intensive care unit: a proposed solution for indiscriminate antibiotic prescription, *Am J Respir Crit Care Med* 162(2 Pt 1):505–11, 2000

54. Mayhall, CG: *Hospital epidemiology and infection control*, Baltimore, 2004, Williams & Wilkins, p. 319

SUPPLEMENTAL RESOURCES

Community-acquired Pneumonia Organization, a global research network team to facilitate and improve research in the area of community-acquired pneumonia—www.caposite.com

The American Thoracic Society, an independently incorporated, international, educational, and scientific society that focuses on respiratory and critical care medicine—www.thoracic.org

The Infectious Diseases Society of America (IDSA) represents physicians, scientists, and other healthcare professionals who specialize in infectious diseases. IDSA's purpose is to improve the health of individuals, communities, and society by promoting excellence in patient care, education, research, public health, and prevention relating to infectious diseases—www.idsociety.org

Copyright © 2005, Association for Professionals in Infection Control and Epidemiology, Inc.

Surgical Site Infections

Jennifer Janelle, MD
Assistant Professor of Medicine
University of Florida
Gainseville, Florida

Richard J. Howard, MD, PhD
The Robert J. and Kathleen M. Axline Professor
of Medicine
University of Florida
Gainseville, Florida

Donald Fry, MD
Professor of Surgery
University of New Mexico
Albuquerque, New Mexico

ABSTRACT

Surgical-site infections (SSIs) remain a significant cause of morbidity and mortality and account for a considerable economic burden on patients and the healthcare system as a whole. Decreasing the incidence of SSIs is a focus for all healthcare institutions, and it is critical that surgeons and committees responsible for quality improvement have information that is useful in decision-making to decrease patient risk. The risk for SSI involves several basic factors: microorganism-related factors, such as degree of contamination and virulence; patient-related factors, such as competency of the immune system; and the microenvironment of the wound. Prevention of SSIs can be achieved by better preoperative preparation of the surgical site, attention to infection control practices in the performance of surgery, and adherence to the principles for use of preventive antibiotics. New areas of attention include enhanced oxygen delivery, better core temperature control, and careful glucose control.

KEY CONCEPTS

- Pathogenesis of surgical wound infection

- Risk factors for surgical wound infection

- Surgical site infection surveillance

- Classification and risk of SSI

- Risk and Prevention of SSI

- Medical management of SSIs

I.   BACKGROUND

Surgical site infections (SSIs), formerly called surgical wound infections, have always plagued surgeons. More patients died than recovered from SSIs following amputation during the Napoleonic wars and the American Civil War. It was not until 1867, when Joseph Lister published a series on compound leg fractures treated with antiseptic placement of carbolic acid, that a dramatic advance was made in the treatment of wounds. Before Lister, amputation was the standard treatment of compound fracture. And yet even Lister did not practice asepsis until later in his career. In the later part of the nineteenth century the understanding of microbiology accelerated, and the importance of microorganisms in causing SSIs and

Copyright © 2005, Association for Professionals in Infection Control and Epidemiology, Inc.

other diseases led to rapid advances in the prevention and treatment of SSIs. The development of antibiotics was another great advancement in the treatment of SSIs, although their proper role in the prevention of SSIs after operation was not appreciated until studies done in the 1960s.

It is estimated that more than 27 million surgical procedures are performed each year in the United States.[1] SSIs are the third most frequently reported nosocomial infection among hospitalized patients[2] and account for a significant portion of healthcare-associated costs. Kirkland et al.[3] studied 255 pairs of patients with and without infection and found that SSIs added 6.5 hospital days to an infected patient's stay, with excess direct costs attributable to SSIs of $3,089. In this study, patients with SSIs were twice as likely to die and five times more likely to require readmission after initial discharge. SSIs also increased the likelihood of the patient spending time in an intensive care unit by 60%.[3] An understanding of the causes of SSIs and taking steps to prevent them are critical to the well-being of patients, as well as to improving the economic health of medicine.

II.   BASIC PRINCIPLES

PATHOGENESIS OF SURGICAL SITE INFECTIONS

Essentially every surgical site is contaminated with bacteria by the end of the procedure, but only a minority become clinically infected. The source of the pathogen for most SSIs is the endogenous flora of the patient's skin, mucous membranes, or hollow viscera. The risk of infection is primarily determined by four clinical variables: (1) inoculum of bacteria; (2) virulence of bacteria; (3) adjuvants in the microenvironment; and (4) local and systemic host defenses.

Inoculum of Bacteria: Wound Contamination

The risk of SSI is related to the number of microorganisms contaminating the wound.[4] The presence of foreign material markedly decreases the number of microorganisms required to cause an infection.[5,6]

The largest inoculum of bacteria into the wound occurs when the operation invades a body structure that is ordinarily heavily colonized with bacteria, such as the intestinal tract, female genitourinary tract, or respiratory tract.

Virulence: Microorganism-Related Risk Factors

A second variable that contributes to the risk of SSI is the virulence of the bacterial contaminant. The more virulent the microorganism, the greater the probability of infection. Coagulase-positive staphylococci (S.

aureus), group A streptococci (S. pyogenes), and Clostridium perfringens require only a small inoculum to cause severe and necrotizing infections at the surgical site. Some bacteria such as Escherichia coli can elaborate endotoxin, which can cause systemic effects. Other bacteria release exotoxins that can inhibit host defenses. An additional microbe-related factor is the possibility for microbial synergism. This is demonstrated by the enteric anaerobe Bacteroides fragilis, which has relatively low virulence in experimental models when used alone to cause infection. When part of a polymicrobial infection that includes facultative gram-negative bacteria, however, it is able to cause severe infections.[7]

Adjuvant Effects of the Microenvironment

A third important risk factor for infection at the surgical site is the microenvironment of the wound that is a consequence of the operation; this may result in clinical infection from an otherwise sub-infectious inocula of bacteria. The local environment of a surgical wound can predispose to infection in a number of ways. Hemoglobin at the surgical site in the form of a hematoma stimulates microbial proliferation by providing ferric iron with the degradation of red blood cells, potentially leading to infection.[8] The presence of necrotic tissue can provide a sanctuary for contaminants to avoid phagocytic actions of the host.[8,9] Foreign material may also harbor microbes and can significantly increase the probability of infection.[9] Thus, meticulous surgical technique is critical to the prevention of infection.

Local and Systemic Host Defenses

Finally, the integrity of host defenses is another important determinant in the risk of a SSI. Many patient-related factors have been evaluated in an attempt to determine those patients who might have risks likely to cause postoperative infectious complications. Morbid obesity, extremes of age, prolonged preoperative hospital stay, infection at other sites, low albumin, cancer, poor vascular supply in the wound, neutropenia, diabetes mellitus, nicotine use, steroid use, preoperative nasal colonization with S. aureus perioperative transfusion, and immunosuppressive therapy have all been implicated in increasing the risk of surgical site infection.[10-12]

CLASSIFICATION AND RISK OF SSI

Surgical procedures have varying risks depending on the four clinical variables outlined above. For example, cosmetic operations of the head and neck in someone who is otherwise healthy have a much lower risk of SSI than colon resection in an elderly patient with diabetes and obesity. Elective procedures carry a lower

Copyright © 2005, Association for Professionals in Infection Control and Epidemiology, Inc.

risk of postoperative infection than urgent ones. It is important to consider these factors when making decisions regarding surgical outcomes and quality improvement activities.

The traditional wound classifications system of categorizing surgeries into risk groups based on the degree of microbial contamination has been available since 1964 and for many years was used as the sole determinant of surgical risk.[13-15]

Class I, or clean wounds, are those in which no inflammation was encountered. No contaminated spaces (gastrointestinal, respiratory, genitourinary, and genital) were encountered, and the wound was primarily closed and drained if necessary with closed drains.

Class II, or clean-contaminated wounds, are those in which the respiratory, urinary, gastrointestinal, or genital tracts were involved under controlled conditions and without unusual contamination. The genitourinary and biliary tracts may be entered in the absence of infection. A minor break in surgical sterile technique in an otherwise class I procedure would also fit into this class.

Class III, or contaminated wounds, are open, fresh wounds. There may be gross spillage from the gastrointestinal tract. Entry into the genitourinary or biliary tracts in the presence of infected urine or bile or a major break in surgical technique may have occurred. Incisions in which acute, nonpurulent inflammation is present are also included in this class.

Class IV, or dirty and infected wounds, are those with retained devitalized tissue, foreign bodies, fecal contamination, or delayed treatment, or from a dirty source. A perforated viscus may be encountered. A wound with acute bacterial inflammation with pus is encountered during the operation is also included in this class.

However, as outlined previously, factors need to be taken into consideration, such as intrinsic patient risks and operation-related risk factors. In 1985, a new model was developed to stratify SSI risk.[16] This model was based on a logistic regression model of ten variables collected in the Study of the Efficacy of Nosocomial Infection Control (SENIC) project. This study showed that four variables are independently associated with SSI risk: (1) abdominal operation, (2) operation lasting more than 2 hours, (3) surgical site with wound classification of either contaminated or dirty/infected, and (4) patient with more than two discharge diagnoses. Taking these factors into consideration allows risk stratification of operations so that surveillance outcome data is more meaningful.

Taking into consideration the information gathered from the SENIC project, the Centers for Disease Control and Prevention (CDC)–sponsored National Nosocomial Infection Surveillance (NNIS) System risk index was developed. The methodology used in this NNIS index includes the traditional wound classification system described above, along with several important additional variables.[17] This simplified risk index has a range from 0 to 3 points. A point is added to the patient's risk index for each of the following three variables:

- Surgical site wound classification of contaminated or dirty (Class III or IV)

- American Society of Anesthesiology (ASA) score as rated by an anesthesiologist prior to operation of ≥3

- Procedure time over T hours, where T is the 75th percentile of the duration of surgery for the specific procedure being performed (standard T point was determined from the NNIS database)

The higher the score by this index, the greater the risk for subsequent SSI. Thus, this index takes into account the microbial burden and certain operation-specific factors, length of surgery as a surrogate marker for surgical complexity, and patient-specific factors. The ASA score allows anesthesiologists to preoperatively assess the overall physical status of a patient.[12,18] The NNIS Risk Index has become a standard format for presenting SSI data and is replacing the older wound classification system. A matrix can be constructed with wound class on one axis and risk index on the other. The risk of a SSI can then be plotted for each cell as in Table 23-1.[17] The CDC uses the data to report nationwide SSI rates and their risk factors through publication of NNIS System reports. These data provide a benchmarking scale that an individual institution can use to compare outcomes with NNIS participants for SSIs and related outcomes.

It has recently been suggested that laparoscopic surgery may change the risk of SSI so significantly in certain cases (such as cholecystectomy and colon surgery) that this may need to be considered as another variable in the calculation of SSI risks.[19]

III. CRITERIA FOR DEFINING SSIs

Clearly, purulent drainage from a wound associated with systemic signs of infection such as fever or chills signifies infection; however, in some instances infections are not quite so obvious. Also, there can be a significant difference in morbidity and mortality associated with SSIs depending on the depth of infection. In an attempt to help those performing SSI surveillance deal with these issues, the CDC has published guidelines to aid in the determination of whether an infection exists and the severity/depth of infection (see Table 23-2).[17]

Copyright © 2005, Association for Professionals in Infection Control and Epidemiology, Inc.

Table 23-1. Surgical Wound Infection Rates[a] Among 84,691 Operations by Traditional Wound Classification and NNIS Risk Index

Wound Class	Risk Category				
	0	1	2	3	All
Clean	1.0[a]	2.3	5.4	–	2.1
Clean-contaminated	2.1	4.0	9.5	–	3.3
Contaminated	–	3.4	6.8	13.2	6.4
Dirty	–	3.1	8.1	12.8	7.1
All operations	1.5	2.9	6.8	13.0	

[a] Number of surgical wound infections per 100 operations.
Adapted from Culver DH, Horan TC, Gaynes RD, et al: *Am J Surg* 91(Suppl 3B): 152S, 1991.[17]

Surgical site infections are generally divided into two categories, depending on the depth of wound involvement: incisional and organ/space. Incisional SSIs are further divided into superficial incisional SSIs, which involve only the skin or subcutaneous tissue of the incision and at least one marker of infection, and deep incisional SSIs in which infection involves the deep soft tissues of the incision. Organ/space SSIs involve any part of the anatomy other than the incision that was opened or manipulated during an operation.

While many SSIs are clear, such as when there is purulent drainage and fever or other sign of infection, occasionally there may be only subtle indications of infection. The CDC criteria for defining a SSI takes this into consideration by accepting a diagnosis of infection as determined by the attending physician or surgeon as definitive for SSI.

PREVENTION OF SSIs

An understanding of the risk factors for infection is important for the prevention of SSIs. There are many variables that can influence SSI rates and, in some instances, these can be recognized and acted on preoperatively in an attempt to prevent infection. The CDC has evaluated current methods of preventing SSIs and has published its recommendations.[12]

Reducing Bacteria at the Surgical Site

Many surgeons try to manage the site of the surgical incision even prior to the actual arrival of the patient in the operating room. Preoperative showers and scrubbing of the surgical site with antiseptic soap the evening before the procedure is often recommended in an attempt to reduce surface microbial counts, but this has not been definitely shown to reduce SSI rates.[19-22] Either chlorhexidine gluconate products or povidone-iodine can be used, but chlorhexidine gluconate reduces bacterial colony count more than povidone-iodine.[2,3]

Hair removal from the surgical site is also an important consideration. At one time, it was common to have the operative site shaved with a straight razor on the night prior to the operation. Studies, however, demonstrate that nicks and scrapes from shaving and hair removal result in colonization of the injured area with microbes, and thereby increase the risk of surgical site infection. The risk increases with increasing time from shaving to the beginning of the operation.[24-25] Therefore, shaving immediately before the operation is associated with lower infection rates compared to shaving 24 hours prior to the operation.[26] The use of depilatory agents may be associated with a hypersensitivity reaction that may increase the risk of SSI. Given this information, if hair removal is to be done, it is best to clip the surgical site just prior to skin incision. If unshaven hair is not an inconvenience for an operation, it is best not to remove it.[12]

Skin preparation in the operating room can be performed using a variety of agents. Iodophors, alcohol-containing products, and chlorhexidine gluconate (CHG) are the most commonly used agents. However, no studies have adequately compared the effects of these antiseptics on SSI risk. Due to flammability risk, isopropyl alcohol may not be desirable if electrocautery is being used, but it is an effective and rapid-acting skin antiseptic and is commonly used in Europe. Povidone-iodine, either in an aqueous or alcohol formulation, must be allowed to dry prior to skin incision. It may be inactivated by blood or serum proteins, but it will have a bacteriostatic effect as long as present on the skin.[27-28] CHG reduces skin microflora more effectively and has better residual activity than povidone-iodine after a single application.[29,30]

Preoperative hand/forearm antisepsis should be performed by all members of the surgical team who have direct contact with the sterile operative field or sterile instruments and should be performed immediately before donning sterile gown and gloves. Several choices of antiseptic agents are available including CHG, alcohol, and povidone-iodine containing prod-

APIC Text of Infection Control and Epidemiology

Copyright © 2005, Association for Professionals in Infection Control and Epidemiology, Inc.

Table 23–2. The CDC/NNIS system for definition of the three types of SSIs

Superficial Incisional SSI
Infection occurs within 30 days after the operation, and
Infection involves only the skin or subcutaneous tissue, and
At least one of the following
Purulent drainage (culture documentation not required)
Organisms isolated from fluid/tissue of superficial incision
At least one sign of inflammation (e.g., pain or tenderness, induration, erythema, local warmth of the wound)
The wound is deliberately opened by the surgeon
Surgeon or attending physician declares the wound infected
A wound is not considered a superficial site infection if:
A stitch abscess is present
Infection of episiotomy or circumcision site
Infected burn wound
Incisional SSI that extends into the fascia or muscle

Deep Incisional SSI
Infection occurs within 30 days of operation, or within one year if an implant is present, and
Infection involves deep soft tissues (e.g., fascia and/or muscle) of the incision, and
At least one of the following:
Purulent drainage from the deep incision but without organ/space involvement
Fascial dehiscence, or fascia is deliberately separated by the surgeon due to signs of inflammation
Deep abscess is identified by direct examination, or during reoperation, or by histopathology, or radiologic examination
Surgeon or attending declares that deep incisional infection is present

Organ/Space SSI
Infection occurs within 30 days after operation, or within one year if an implant is present, and
Infection involves anatomic structures not opened or manipulated by the operation, and
At least one of the following:
Purulent drainage from a drain placed by a stab wound into the organ/space
Organisms isolated from organ/space by aseptic culturing technique
Identification of abscess in the organ/space by direct examination, during reoperation, or by histopathologic or radiologic examination
Diagnosis of organ/space SSI by surgeon or attending physician

ucts. While alcohol is considered the best surgical hand antiseptic in many European countries, it is not commonly used in the United States due to concerns about flammability and skin irritation. CHG and povidone-iodine are used most commonly in U.S. operating rooms, with studies suggesting that CHG may have greater residual antimicrobial activity. [31] While issues such as the optimal duration of the surgical scrub have yet to be determined, cleaning under fingernails prior to the first case of the day, holding hands with fingertips up and arms away from the body, and the use of sterile towels for drying hands and forearms are recommended. [32-35]

Surgical hand antisepsis per the CDC *HICPAC Guideline for Hand Hygiene in Health-Care Facilities* include the following recommendations: [35]

- Remove rings, watches, and bracelets before beginning the surgical hand scrub.

- Remove debris from underneath fingernails using a nail cleaner under running water.

- Surgical hand antisepsis using either an antimicrobial soap or an alcohol-based handrub with persistent activity is recommended before donning sterile gloves when performing surgical procedures.

- When performing surgical hand antisepsis using an antimicrobial soap, scrub hands and forearms for the length of time recommended by the manufacturer, usually 2 to 6 minutes. Long scrub times (e.g., 10 minutes) are not necessary.

- When using an alcohol-based surgical hand-scrub product with persistent activity, follow the manufacturer's instructions. Before applying the alcohol solution, prewash hands and forearms with a non–antimicrobial soap and dry hands and forearms completely. After application of the alcohol-based product as recommended, allow hands and forearms to dry thoroughly before donning sterile gloves.

Antimicrobial Prophylaxis

Preoperative antibiotics can reduce the incidence of SSIs for many surgical procedures. This antimicrobial prophylaxis refers to a brief course of antibiotics initiated prior to an operation in an attempt to decrease the microbial burden of intraoperative contamination to a level that can be overcome by host defenses. The introduction of antibiotics into clinical practice after World War II raised hopes that surgical infections might be avoided. Initially, prophylactic antibiotics were given at the end of the operation, and infections persisted. Subsequent studies showed that in order to prevent infection, antibiotics needed to be present in the tissues at the time of the surgical procedure, when contamination is most likely. [36,37] It is now recommended that antibiotics given for SSI prophylaxis be given shortly before the operation. Studies in gastrointestinal surgery showed that multiple doses given preoperatively were no better than a single preoperative dose, and patients in whom antibiotics were administered only postoperatively had the same rate of SSIs as the placebo group. [38-40] Based on these and other find-

Copyright © 2005, Association for Professionals in Infection Control and Epidemiology, Inc.

ings, surgical antimicrobial prophylaxis currently is given based on the following four principles:

1. Prophylactic antibiotics should be administered when their use has been shown to reduce infection rates.

2. The antibiotic should be safe and inexpensive and should cover the most probable intraoperative contaminants for the procedure.

3. Antibiotic administration should be done at such a time as to allow a bactericidal concentration of the agent in serum and tissue at the time of the skin incision.

4. Therapeutic levels of the antibiotic should be maintained in both serum and tissue throughout the operation and at most a few hours after the operation. This may require that additional doses be given during the operative procedure, depending on its length. For the majority of surgical cases, antimicrobial prophylaxis should not be administered after the operation is complete. The exception is for caesarian section, when the antibiotic should be administered after the cord is clamped.[12]

In general, antibiotics given for the prevention of SSIs are given intravenously. The most commonly used antimicrobials in this setting are the cephalosporins, generally cefazolin, which has a narrow spectrum of activity and low cost. In some situations, for instance when there is a high incidence of infection caused by resistant organisms such as methicillin-resistant *Staphylococcus aureus* (MRSA) in a particular institution or service, agents such as vancomycin may be appropriate. In the case of colonic surgery, mechanical bowel preparation is generally recommended, with cathartics to reduce the intraluminal bacterial contents, the addition of an oral decontamination regimen, and intravenous antibiotic prophylaxis with activity against anaerobes as well as gram-positive and -negative organisms.

Indications for prophylactic antibiotics include gastrointestinal operations, operations in which foreign bodies are placed where infection might require removal of the foreign body (such as vascular, orthopedic, and cardiac procedures), open reduction and fixation of extremity fractures, hysterectomy, caesarian section, head and neck cancer surgery, ventricular-peritoneal shunt placement, and coronary artery bypass procedures.

Prevention in the Operating Room

The operating room environment is an important factor when evaluating operative risks. Proper ventilation is crucial to reducing the risk of microbial contamination of the wound. The degree of contamination also can be affected by the number of personnel moving about in the room and therefore it is recommended that personnel traffic in the room be minimized during a procedure.[41]

Operating rooms should be maintained at positive pressure with respect to corridors and other rooms, and air should be introduced at the ceiling and exhausted near the floor.[42-45] Maintain greater than 15 air changes per hour (ACH), of which greater than 3 ACH should be fresh air. All recirculated and fresh air should be filtered through filters that provide 90% efficiency (dust-spot testing) at a minimum.[45] Also refer to chapters 108, 105, and 106.

Routine microbiologic sampling of operating room air is not recommended, although it might be part of an epidemiological investigation.[45]

Sterilization

SSI outbreaks have been linked to inadequate sterilization of surgical instruments. It is important that the quality of sterilization be routinely monitored. Flash sterilization, a rapid method of sterilization for immediate use, is recommended only to reprocess an instrument inadvertently dropped during a procedure. It is not recommended for implantable devices because of the risk of serious infections.[46,47] When flash sterilization is used, certain parameters should be met: (1) the item must be decontaminated before placement in the sterilizing container; (2) exogenous contamination must be prevented during transport from the sterilizer to the patient; and (3) sterilizer function must be monitored by mechanical, chemical, and biological monitors.[47] Also refer to chapters 21 and 95.

EMERGING CONCEPTS IN SSI PREVENTION

Prevention of SSIs has traditionally focused on decreasing the inoculum of contaminants in the wound. Recently, however, there is growing interest in enhancing the host response to surgery and infection. Experimental evidence suggests that increased oxygen delivery has a positive influence on the prevention of infection.[48] It is hypothesized that increased oxygen delivery may enhance production of oxidant products that facilitate phagocytosis of microorganisms.

Temperature control of the patient also plays a role in ability of the patient to resist infection, since hypothermia is associated with an increased risk of SSI.[49]

Improved blood glucose control in patients with diabetes mellitus also has a positive effect on the reduction of SSIs, particularly in the setting of cardiothoracic surgery. Reduction of sternal wound infection rates from 2.0% to 0.8% in diabetic patients undergoing open heart surgery was demonstrated when glucose

Copyright © 2005, Association for Professionals in Infection Control and Epidemiology, Inc.

control was maintained at levels less than 200 mg/dL.[50] It is possible that better glucose control may benefit the nondiabetic patient in the intensive care unit as well.[51]

SSI SURVEILLANCE METHODS

The data obtained from SSI surveillance is useful to many persons interested in decreasing the incidence of SSIs at a particular institution. It can help determine the effectiveness of aseptic technique and the efficacy of antimicrobial prophylaxis and can also aid in the development and assessment of infection control measures. Several studies have documented the effectiveness of reporting surveillance data to surgeons and other members of the surgical team, with a subsequent reduction in SSI rate from 34% to 50%.[52,53] Surveillance was initially designed to monitor inpatients in acute care hospitals. Many operations are now performed in ambulatory surgical centers, however, and patients are discharged from the hospital much more quickly than in the past. Up to 84% of SSIs are detected after discharge and the absence of post-discharge surveillance dramatically underestimates actual SSI rates.[54,55,56] Given limits in resources, it is difficult for institutions to monitor all surgical patients. Thus it is recommended that hospitals target surveillance toward high-risk, high-volume procedures jointly chosen by infection control and surgeons.[12,57]

Inpatient SSI surveillance can consist of direct observation of the surgical site by the surgeon, trained nurse surveyor, or infection control practitioner, or indirectly through review of laboratory reports, patient records, and interactions with the patient's caregivers. There is varying sensitivity and specificity of each type of study, although direct observation of the surgical site is generally thought to provide the most accurate information.

Postdischarge surveillance can include direct examination of patients' wounds during follow-up physician visits, review of medical records of surgery clinic patients, patient surveys by mail or telephone, or surgeon surveys. At present, there is no standard method for performing SSI surveillance outside the hospital.

WOUND MANAGEMENT

The goals in treating an established surgical site infection are to: (1) control the infection; (2) promote healing; (3) minimize pain; (4) prevent further injury to or destruction of tissue; (5) prevent systemic absorption of the products of infection; and (6) prevent the spread of infection to other sites. Since treating SSIs can usually be done in an outpatient setting, ease of treatment for the patient and low cost are highly desirable.

Despite literally thousands of years of experience in treating wounds, no prospective randomized trials has yet established the optimal treatment of SSIs. Several methods of treating SSIs are acceptable as long as they achieve the goals listed above, and so much of wound care still depends on physician experience. Even so, certain principles have been established: (1) provide for adequate drainage of infected material; (2) remove necrotic tissue; (3) remove foreign material to the extent possible; and (4) minimize the growth of microorganisms.

Provide for Adequate Drainage

The majority of SSIs can be effectively treated at the bedside or in the office. When a patient develops an SSI, the wound should be adequately opened so that infected material can adequately drain. This may require opening the entire wound or opening only a small part of the wound. The wound should be initially opened at the site at which pus is draining, fluctuance is greatest, tenderness is maximal, or induration is greatest. The wound site and surrounding skin should be prepared with an antiseptic solution, and sterile towels and drapes should be used to isolate the area so that reclosure can be considered if no infection is present. The surgeon can insert a cotton-tipped swab to gauge the extent of the infection and to help determine whether the wound needs to be opened further. The same swab can be used to obtain material from the wound for culture.

A wound is opened to allow for drainage of infected material. Whether a wound must be opened along its entire length should be individualized on the basis of the extent of the infection. Opening the wound fully permits better inspection of the fascia to determine if its closure is intact and may afford better drainage and greater ease of débridement. But fully opening a wound may also increase the time required for healing. Gentle examination of the wound with a cotton-tipped applicator or a gloved finger can reveal sinus tracks and abscesses that are not obvious at first. Initially this wound exploration can cause pain. The examination should be gentle and brief, and analgesics should be used if required.

Remove Necrotic Tissue and Remove Foreign Material

Necrotic tissue should be débrided. This tissue contributes nothing to the strength of a wound and may disguise an abscess. It is usually not necessary to remove every bit of necrotic tissue at the initial débridement as long as a necrotizing soft tissue infection is not involved. The surgeon does not want to remove viable tissue. If it is unclear where the margin between necrotic and viable tissue is, further débridement can

Copyright © 2005, Association for Professionals in Infection Control and Epidemiology, Inc.

be carried out at another time. Similarly, fibrin and other protein deposition may occur in the infected wound. Removing all this protein is not required at the initial procedure, since it can be removed with subsequent dressing changes.

Minimize the Growth of Microorganisms

There is considerable controversy about the use of antibiotics to treat patients with SSIs. Many SSIs do not require antibiotic therapy. In these cases, there may be little benefit in culturing the wound except to gather epidemiological data. Indeed, there are no controlled trials addressing the proper use of antibiotics in treating SSIs. Many experts believe antibiotics generally should be given for extensive cellulitis, deep SSIs, if the patient has an implanted foreign body such as a prosthetic heart valve or joint replacement, or if the patient has systemic signs of infection such as fever or an elevated white blood cell count attributed to the SSI.

When antibiotic treatment is warranted, the type of antibiotic treatment will depend on the organisms cultured. There are no data directing the duration of therapy. Therapy need not be continued until the wound is completely healed or until the organisms are eradicated given that microbes will always be cultured from an unhealed wound. It is generally safe to stop antibiotic treatment when the cellulitis has greatly receded, the patient is afebrile, or the white blood cell count is returning to normal. If a foreign body is present, antibiotics should be continued longer.

Dressing the Wound

The wound should be irrigated with sterile saline and dressed with sterile gauze. Dressing wounds is frequently referred to as "packing"—an unfortunate term. Packing a wound implies that as much gauze as possible is placed into a wound so that it acts as a plug that inhibits drainage. Instead, the purpose of a wound dressing is to promote drainage of infected material and wound fluid. A dressing should keep the edges of the wound separated only enough to accomplish this purpose, which suggests putting as little gauze as possible into a wound. A wound dressing can promote débridement when adhering fibrin is removed during dressing changes.

Occlusive dressings are occasionally suggested for the treatment of chronic wounds to preserve a moist environment. Various dressing materials are available including foam, hydrofibers, crystalline sodium chloride gauze, calcium alginate, hydrocolloids, hydrogels, and film dressings.[58] While these materials may be helpful in treating SSIs in a limited number of circumstances, their advantage over simpler dressings is not established. Furthermore, their use increases costs and the complexity of dressing changes.

Many individuals prefer "wet-to-dry" dressings in order to prevent the wound from becoming desiccated and to promote débridement. However, a dry dressing may be all that is required. Dressings virtually never become dry between dressing changes. While wet dressings may offer an advantage early in the treatment of an SSI, they require more effort on the part of the patient if he/she changes the dressing. However, dressing removal can cause pain, especially early in the course of treatment, and wetting them shortly before dressing change facilitates removal and causes less pain.

Some surgeons soak the dressings in antiseptic solutions. Among the antiseptics placed into wounds are iodine compounds, sodium hypochlorite (Carrel-Dakin's solution), acetic acid, hydrogen peroxide, chlorhexidine, and silver compounds. There is considerable controversy about the use of these agents.[59] Their greatest use has been in acute wounds, chronic wounds, and burn wounds. There is no proof they are of any benefit in SSIs. They are more toxic to human fibroblasts in vitro than they are to bacteria.[60] We believe that the old adage that one should never place anything into a wound that you would not place into the anterior chamber of eye remains applicable.

Initially, dressings are usually changed two to four times a day. After drainage is diminished and the wound is cleaner, it is usually sufficient to change dressings only once or twice a day. Showers are encouraged because they clean the wound and aid débridement of fibrin.

The VAC System

A recent addition to the treatment of wounds is vacuum-assisted closure (VAC). This treatment uses an occlusive polyvinyl alcohol sponge connected to negative pressure pump. It increases blood flow to the wound, decreases bacterial counts, and increases the rate of granulation tissue formation. The VAC system can be used for both acute and chronic wounds.[61] While it is usually not needed for wounds due to SSIs, it can be helpful to promote healing for very large wounds, especially for those that will eventually require skin grafting. It has the disadvantages of requiring connection to a negative pressure pump and therefore limits the motility of the patient (although portable pumps are available) and of being expensive to use.

IV.   SUMMARY AND CONCLUSIONS

Surgical site infections will always be with us. The challenge to healthcare providers is to minimize the risk of SSIs to the extent possible and to provide optimal treatment when they occur. The CDC should continue to sponsor gathering of data in the United States to help determine trends in SSIs that may provide new insights

Copyright © 2005, Association for Professionals in Infection Control and Epidemiology, Inc.

into the factors associated with their cause. Continuing research also will emphasize factors associated with increasing the risk of SSIs, such as the recently demonstrated effect of body temperature and oxygenation on SSI risk. New treatment modalities can help lower risks and improve treatment, such as the VAC system for treating large open wounds. Industry has a role in developing new barriers to prevent wound contamination, although various plastic drapes that were marketed with the promise of reducing the risk of SSIs generally have not been effective when subject to carefully performed clinical trials.

The CDC has taken an important lead through its NNIS program and its advisory council by publishing important data concerning the SSIs and in suggesting preventive measures. These activities need to be continued and the guidelines for prevention periodically updated.

V.   FUTURE TRENDS/RESEARCH

We already know in detail the most important parameters associated with SSIs. Further research will refine our understanding and elaborate new factors previously thought not to contribute significantly to SSIs. A better understanding of the factors that cause SSIs will aid healthcare providers in developing techniques to reduce the risk of SSIs, although it will be impossible to completely prevent them. Current emphasis on short hospital stays and outpatient surgery make the gathering of valid SSI data a greater challenge than in previous eras. It is likely that newly identified risk factors will be shown to play only a minor role compared with known factors. Large well-controlled studies will have to be carried out in order to elucidate the relative importance of these factors in a way that is statistically valid.

Although new antibiotics may be developed that prove to be effective in prophylaxis against SSIs, it is unlikely that new antibiotics will prove more effective than those currently available, and it is highly likely that they will be more expensive. Furthermore, the studies necessary to prove that new antibiotics are more effective would have to be so large and expensive that they are unlikely to be undertaken.

VI.   INTERNATIONAL PERSPECTIVES

Surgical site infections may have different risk factors in some countries and the causative organisms may vary on occasion. For the most part, however, the same parameters associated with SSIs in the United States are also found to be important in other parts of the world. On rare occasions, SSIs may be caused by microorganisms that are found in some parts of the world but not in others, but since most SSIs are caused by the host's own endogenous flora, there is great commonality in the bacteria cultured from SSIs worldwide.

REFERENCES

1. U.S. Department of Health and Human Services, Centers for Disease Control and Prevention, National Center for Health Statistics: *Vital and Health Statistics, Detailed Diagnoses and Procedures, National Hospital Discharge Survey*, 1994, Series 13, 1997, Hyattsville, MD, DHHS Pub No. 127.
2. Emory TG, Gaynes RP: An overview of nosocomial infections, including the role of the microbiology laboratory, *Clin Microbiol Rev* 6:428–442, 1993.
3. Kirkland KB, Briggs JP, Trivette SL, et al: The impact of surgical-site infections in the 1990s: Attributable mortality, excess length of hospitalization, and extra costs, *Infect Control and Hosp Epidemiol* 20:725–730, 1999.
4. Krizek TJ, Robson MC: Evolution of quantitative bacteriology in wound management, *Am J Surg* 130:579–584, 1975.
5. Noble WC: The production of subcutaneous staphylococcal skin lesions in mice, *Br J Exper Pathol* 1965;ZS46:254–262.
6. James RC, MacLeod CJ: Induction of staphylococcal infections in mice with small inocula introduced on sutures, *Br J Exp Pathol* 42:266–277, 1961.
7. Onderdonk AB, Bartlett JG, Louie T, et al: Microbial synergy in experimental intra-abdominal abscess, *Infect Immun* 13:22–26, 1976.
8. Polk HC Jr, Miles AA: Enhancement of bacterial infection by ferric iron: kinetics, mechanisms, and surgical significance, *Surgery* 70: 71–77, 1971.
9. Elek SD, Conen PE: The virulence of Staphylococcus pyogenes for man: a study of the problem of wound infection, *Br J Exp Pathol* 38:573, 1957.
10. Society for Hospital Epidemiology of America, Association for Practitioners of Infection Control, Centers for Disease Control, Surgical Infections Society: Consensus paper on the surveillance of surgical wound infections. *Infect Control Hosp Epidemiol* 13: 599–605, 1992.
11. Lillenfeld DE, Vlahov D, Tenney JH, Mclaughlin JS: Obesity and diabetes as risk factors for postoperative wound infections after cardiac surgery, *Am J Infect Control* 16:3–6, 1988.
12. Mangram AJ, Horan TC, Pearson ML, Silver LC, Jarvis WR: The Hospital Infection Control Practices Advisory Committee. Guidelines for prevention of surgical site infection, 1999, *Infect Control Hospital Epidemiol* 20:247–280, 1999.
13. National Academy of Sciences, National Research Council, Division of Medical Sciences, Ad Hoc Committee of Trauma: Postoperative wound infection: The influence of ultraviolet irradiation of the operating room and of various other factors, *Ann Surg* 160: 1–192,1964.
14. Simmons BP: Guideline for prevention of surgical wound infections, *Infect Control* 3:188–196, 1982.
15. Garner JS: CDC guideline for prevention of surgical wound infections, 1985. Supercedes guideline for prevention of surgical wound infections published in 1982 (Originally published in 1995), Revised, *Infect Control* 7(3):193–200, 1986.
16. Haley RW, Culver DH, Morgan WM, Emori TG, et al: Identifying patients at high risk of surgical wound infection: A simple multivariate index of patient susceptibility and wound contamination, *Am J Epidemiol* 121:206–215, 1985.
17. Culver DH, Horan TC, Gaynes RP, et al: Surgical wound infection rates by wound class, operative procedure, and patient risk index, *Am J Med* 91(Suppl 3B):152S-157S, 1991.
18. Keats AS: The ASA classification of physical status: a recapitulation, *Anesthesiology* 49:233–6, 1978.
19. Gaynes RP, Culver DH, Horan TC, et al: Surgical site infection (SSI) rates in the United States, 1992–1998: The National Nosocomial Infections Surveillance System basic SSI risk index, *Clin Infect Disease* 33(Suppl 2):S69–77, 2001.
20. Rotter ML, Larsen SO, Cooke EM, et al: A comparison of the effects of preoperative whole-body bathing with detergent alone and with detergent containing chlorhexidine gluconate on the frequency of wound infection after clean surgery. The European Working Party on Control of Hospital Infections, *J Hosp Infect* 11:310–20, 1988.

Copyright © 2005, Association for Professionals in Infection Control and Epidemiology, Inc.

21. Leigh DA, Stronge JL, Marriner J, Sedgwick J: Total body bathing with 'Hibiscrub' (chlorhexidine) in surgical patients: a controlled trial, *J Hosp Infect* 4:229–35, 1983.
22. Lynch W, Favey PG, Malek M, Byrne DJ, Napier A: Cost-effectiveness analysis of the use of chlorhexidine detergent in preoperative whole-body disinfection in wound infection prophylaxis, *J Hosp Infect* 21:179–91, 1992.
23. Garibaldi RA: Prevention of intraoperative wound contamination with chlorhexidine shower and scrub, *J Hosp Infect* 11(Suppl B): 5–9, 1988.
24. Cruse PJ, Foord R: The epidemiology of wound infection: a 10-year prospective study of 62,939 wounds, *Surg Clin North Am* 60:27–40, 1980.
25. Cruse P: Wound infection surveillance, *Rev Infect Dis* 4: 734–737, 1981.
26. Seropian R, Reynolds BM: Wound infections after preoperative depilatory versus razor preparation, *Am J Surg* 121:251–254, 1971.
27. Ritter MA, French ML, Eitzen HE, Gioe TJ: The antimicrobial effectiveness of operative-site preparative agents: a microbiologic and clinical study, *J Bone Joint Surg Am* 62(5):826–828, 1980.
28. Mayhall CG: Surgical infections including burns. In: Wenzel RP, ed, *Prevention and Control of nosocomial Infections*, ed 2, Baltimore, 1993, Williams & Wilkins, pp 614–664.
29. Lowbury EJ, Lilly HA: Use of 4 percent chlorhexidine detergent solution (Hibiscrub) and other methods of skin disinfection, *Br Med J* 1:510–515, 1973.
30. Aly R, Maibach HI: Comparative antibacterial efficacy of a 2-minute surgical scrub with chlorhexidine gluconate, povidone-iodine, and chloroxylenol sponge-brushes, *Am J Infect Control* 16:173–177, 1988.
31. Wade JJ, Casewell MW: The evaluation of residual antimicrobial activity on hands and its clinical relevance, *J Hosp Infect* 18(Suppl B):23–28, 1991.
32. Committee on Control of Surgical Infections of the Committee on Pre- and Postoperative care, American College of Surgeons: *Manual on control of infection in surgical patients*, Philadelphia, 1984, J.B. Lippincott Co.
33. Larson EL: APIC guideline for handwashing and hand antisepsis in healthcare settings, *Am J Infect Control* 23:251–269, 1995.
34. Association of Operating Room Nurses: *Standards, recommended practices, guidelines*, Denver, 1999, Association of Operating Room Nurses;.
35. Boyce, J M, D Pittet, and the HICPAC: Recommendations of the Healthcare Infection Control Practices Advisory Committee and the HICPAC/SHEA/APIC/IDSA Hand Hygiene Task Force "Guideline for Hand Hygiene in Health-Care Settings." *MMWR* October 25, 2002(5/RR16):1–44 2002/51(RR1644).
36. Miles AA, Miles ES, Burke J: The value and duration of defense reactions of the skin to primary lodgment of bacteria, *Br J Exp Pathol* 38:79–96, 1957.
37. Burke JF: The effective period of preventive antibiotic action in experimental incisions and dermal lesions, *Surgery* 50:161, 1961.
38. Bernard HR, Cole WR: The prophylaxis of surgical infection: the effect of prophylactic antimicrobial drugs on the incidence of infection following potentially contaminated operations, *Surgery* 56: 151, 1964.
39. Polk HC Jr, Lopez-Mayor JF: Postoperative wound infection: a prospective study of determinant factors and prevention, *Surgery* 66:97–103, 1969.
40. Stone HH, Hooper CA, Kolb LD, et al: Antibiotic prophylaxis in gastric, biliary and colonic surgery, *Ann Surg* 184:443–452, 1976.
41. Ayliffe GA: Role of the environment of the operating suite in surgical wound infection, *Rev Infect Dis* 13(Suppl 10):S800–804, 1991.
42. Lidwell OM: Clean air at operation and subsequent sepsis in the joint, *Clin Orthop* 211:91–102, 1986.
43. Nichols RL: The operating room. In Bennet JV, Brachman PS, editors. *Hospital infections*, ed 3, Boston, 1992, Little, Brown, pp 461–473.
44. Laufman H: The operating room. In Bennet JV, Brachman PS, editors. *Hospital infections*, ed 2, Boston, 1986, Little, Brown, pp 315–323.
45. Centers for Disease Control and Prevention (CDC) and Healthcare Infection Control Practices Advisory Committee (HICPAC): *Guidelines for environmental infection control in health-care facilities: recommendations of CDC and the Healthcare Infection Control Practices Advisory Committee (HICPAC)*. Available from the CDC's Division of Healthcare Quality Promotion's Internet site at www.cdc.gov/ncidod/hip [accessed December 12, 2003].
46. Favero MS, Bond W: Sterilization, disinfection, and antisepsis in the hospital. In Balows A, Hausler WJ Jr, Herrmann KL, et al, editors, *Manual of clinical microbiology*, ed 5, Washington, DC, 1991, American Society of Microbiology, pp 183–200.
47. Rutala WA, Weber DJ: *Draft Guideline for Disinfection and Sterilization in Healthcare Facilities*, February 2002, CDC.
48. Knighton DR, Halliday B, Hunt TK: Oxygen as an antibiotic: a comparison of the effects of inspired oxygen concentration and antibiotic administration on in vivo bacterial clearance, *Arch Surg* 121:191–195, 1986.
49. Kurz A, Sessler DI, Lenhardt R: Perioperative normothermia to reduce the incidence of surgical wound infection and shorten hospitalization, *N Engl J Med* 334:1209–1215, 1996.
50. Furnary AP, Zerr KJ, Grunkemeier GL, Starr A: Continuous intravenous insulin infusion reduces the incidence of deep sternal wound infection in diabetic patients after cardiac surgical procedures, *Ann Thorac Surg* 67:352–360, 1999.
51. van den Berghe G, Wouters P, Weekers F, et al: Intensive insulin therapy in the surgical intensive care unit, *N Engl J Med* 345: 1359–1367, 2001.
52. Haley RW, Culver DH, White JW, et al: The efficacy of infection surveillance and control programs in preventing nosocomial infections in US hospitals, *Am J Epidemiol* 121:182–205, 1985.
53. Olson MM, Lee JR, Jr: Continuous 10-year wound infection surveillance results, advantages, and unanswered questions, *Arch Surg* 125:794–803, 1990.
54. Sands K, Vineyard G, Platt R: Surgical site infections occurring after hospital discharge, *J Infect Dis* 173:963–970, 1996.
55. Burns SH, Dippe SE: Postoperative wound infections detected during hospitalization and after discharge in a community hospital, *Am J Infect Control* 10:60–65, 1982.
56. Weiss CA, Statz CL, Dahms RA, et al: Six years of surgical wound infection surveillance at a tertiary care center: Review of the microbiologic and epidemiological aspects of 20,007 wounds, *Arch Surg* 134:1041–1048, 1999.
57. Lee JT: Wound infection surveillance, *Infect Dis Clin North Am* 6:643–656, 1992.
58. Schultz GS, Sibbald RG, Falanga V, et al: Wound bed preparation: a systematic approach to wound management, *Wound Repair and Regeneration* 11(No. 2 supplement):S1-S28, 2003.
59. Drosou A, Falabella A, Kirsner RS: Antiseptics on wounds: an area of controversy, *Wounds* 15:149–166, 2003.
60. Lineaweaver W, Howard R, Soucy D, et al: Topical antimicrobial toxicity, *Arch Surg* 120:267–270, 1985.
61. Patel CTC, Kinsey GC, Koperski-Moen KJ, Bungum LD: Vacuum-assisted wound closure, *Amer J Nursing* 100:46–48, 2000.

SUPPLEMENTAL RESOURCES

Association of periOperative Registered Nurses (AORN): *www.aorn.org*

Belkin NL: Use of scrubs and related apparel in health care facilities. Association of Professionals in Infection Control and Epidemiology. 1997

Centers for Disease Control and Prevention, Hospital Infections Program: Guideline for Prevention of Surgical Site Infection, 1999.

Copyright © 2005, Association for Professionals in Infection Control and Epidemiology, Inc.

Intravascular Device Infections

Christopher J. Crnich, MD
Research Fellow, Section of Infectious Diseases
University of Wisconsin Hospital and Clinics
Madison, Wisconsin

Dennis G. Maki, MD
Chairman, Section of Infectious Diseases
Professor, Department of Trauma and Life
Support
University of Wisconsin Hospital and Clinics
Madison, Wisconsin

ABSTRACT

Vascular access is associated with substantial and generally underappreciated potential for producing iatrogenic disease, particularly bloodstream infection (BSI). Intravascular-device-related (IVDR) BSIs are associated with increased length of hospitalization and excess healthcare costs. The goal must not be simply to identify and treat these infections, but rather to prevent them. Every type of IVD carries some risk of causing BSI; however, the risk varies greatly depending on the type of device. There are two major sources of IVDR BSIs: (1) colonization of the IVD (catheter-related infection) and (2) contamination of the fluid administered through the device (infusate-related infection). Contaminated infusate is the cause of most *epidemic* IVDR BSIs. In contrast, catheter-related infections are responsible for most *endemic* IVDR BSIs. Skin microorganisms account for the largest proportion of IVDR BSIs. This chapter reviews the available scientific evidence for diagnosing, preventing, and treating these infections.

KEY CONCEPTS

- The epidemiology and pathogenesis of intravascular device-related bloodstream infections

- Methods of diagnosing intravascular bloodstream infections with short-term devices, including the appropriate use of blood cultures

- New methods for diagnosing intravascular bloodstream infections with long-term devices, including delayed time-to-positivity

- Common strategies for prevention of intravascular bloodstream infections, including the choice of insertion site, choice of cutaneous antisepesis, and recommendations for maintenance of implanted intravascular devices

- The evidence demonstrating the efficacy of novel technology for prevention of intravascular device-related bloodstream infections

- The management and treatment of patients with confirmed or suspected intravascular device-related bloodstream infections

Copyright © 2005, Association for Professionals in Infection Control and Epidemiology, Inc.

I. BACKGROUND

Obtaining and maintaining reliable vascular access has become one of the most essential features of modern medical care. Unfortunately, vascular access is associated with substantial and generally underappreciated potential for producing iatrogenic disease, particularly bloodstream infection (BSI), originating from infection of the percutaneous device used for vascular access. Nearly 40% of all healthcare-associated bacteremias derive from vascular access in some form,[1] and it is estimated that more than 250,000 intravascular device-related (IVDR) BSIs occur in the United States each year.[2,3] Studies performed a decade ago found that IVDR BSIs were associated with excess attributable mortality approaching 35%;[4] however, more recent case-control studies have not consistently found excess mortality with this type of infection.[5-7] This controversy aside, every study examining the impact of IVDR BSI on patient outcomes has found that it is associated with increased length of hospitalization and excess healthcare costs.[4-7]

IVDR BSIs are largely preventable. The goal must not be simply to identify and treat these infections, but rather to prevent them. Over the past decade, much has been learned about the pathogenesis and epidemiology of infections associated with intravascular devices (IVDs). By drawing upon existent knowledge of the pathogenesis and epidemiology of intravascular IVDR BSIs, rational and effective guidelines for prevention can be formulated.

Prospective studies, in which every attempt was made to identify conclusively the presence of an IVDR BSI, show that every type of IVD carries some risk of causing BSI; however, the magnitude of risk varies greatly, depending on the type of device (Table 24–1).[8] Historically, rates of IVDR BSIs have been expressed exclusively as BSIs per 100 devices, or percent of devices studied. Currently, the CDC and the Joint Commission on Accreditation of Healthcare Organizations (JCAHO) recommend that the risk of IVDR BSIs be expressed as BSIs per 1,000 IVD days.[9,10] Table 24–1 provides the rationale as to why this method of measurement is preferable. For example, expressing the risk of IVDR BSI as a function of BSIs per 100 devices (percentage of devices infected) would lead one to conclude that surgically implanted, cuffed central venous catheters (CVCs) are more hazardous (20.9 BSIs per 100 catheters) than standard nonmedicated, noncuffed CVCs (3.3 BSIs per 100 catheters). However, when risk is expressed as BSIs per 1,000 IVD days, cuffed and tunneled catheters pose approximately one-half the risk of IVDR BSI (1.2 per 1;1000 IVD days) as standard nonmedicated, noncuffed CVCs (2.3 per 1;1000 IVD days). The importance of measuring rates of infection by BSIs per 1,000 IVD days cannot be understated, as it takes into account the cumulative risk of infection that occurs for a particular IVD over the time it remains in use. Whereas surgically implanted Hickman catheters do indeed develop more infections when taken as a percentage of devices used, they do so because they are used for much longer periods of time. Use of standard noncuffed, nontunneled CVCs in the same manner would most likely result in a much higher percentage of devices becoming infected.

The device that poses the greatest risk of IVDR BSI today is the CVC in its many forms (Table 24–1). Short-term noncuffed, single- or multi-lumen catheters inserted percutaneously into the subclavian or internal

Table 24-1. Rates of bloodstream infection (BSI) caused by various types of devices used for vascular access.*

| Device (No. prospective studies) | Rates of Device-related BSI | | | |
| | per 100 catheters | | per 1000 catheter-days | |
	Pooled Mean	95% CI	Pooled Mean	95% CI
Peripheral venous catheters (13)	0.16	0.08–0.23	0.60	0.31–0.88
Arterial catheters (17)	0.75	0.49–1.02	1.78	1.17–2.40
Short-term, nonmedicated CVCs (88)**	4.48	4.19–4.78	2.51	2.34–2.68
Pulmonary-artery catheters (15)	1.45	1.06–1.85	5.50	4.00–7.01
Hemodialysis catheters				
Noncuffed (17)	7.41	6.43–8.39	2.62	2.26–2.98
Cuffed (19)	18.48	17.13–19.82	1.81	1.67–1.96
Peripherally-inserted central catheters (14)	2.49	1.76–3.21	0.75	0.53–0.97
Long-term tunneled and cuffed CVCs (48)	21.25	20.13–22.38	1.53	1.44–1.62
Subcutaneous central venous ports (18)	3.91	3.22–4.59	0.13	0.11–0.15

* Adapted and updated from Kluger and Maki, based on 245 published prospective studies where every device was evaluated for infection.[8]

** CVCs = central venous catheters.

APIC Text of Infection Control and Epidemiology

Copyright © 2005, Association for Professionals in Infection Control and Epidemiology, Inc.

jugular vein have shown rates of catheter-related BSI in the range of 3–5% (2–3 per 1;1000 IVD days).[8] Far lower rates of infection have been encountered with surgically implanted cuffed Hickman or Broviac and subcutaneous central venous ports (1 and 0.2 per 1; 1000 IVD days, respectively).[8] Contrary to popular belief, inpatient use of peripherally inserted central catheters (PICCs) and arterial catheters is associated with a risk of catheter-related BSI that approaches that seen with noncuffed multilumen CVCs: up to 2.1[11] and 3.4[12] BSIs per 1,000 IVD days, respectively.

In recent years, the factors associated with an increased risk of IVDR BSI have become better delineated (Table 24–2). Prolonged hospitalization and severity of illness clearly influence the risk of IVDR BSI,[13] and clinical states such as underlying neutropenia,[14] acquired immunodeficiency syndrome

(AIDS),[15,16] and bone marrow transplantation[17] have been associated with 4- to 6-fold increased rates of IVDR BSI. However, the features of the IVD, its insertion, and its maintenance seem to have far greater impact on the overall risk of infection. In 289 patients, Merrer et al found that insertion of an IVD in the femoral versus the subclavian vein was associated with a greatly increased risk of infection (20.0 versus 3.7 BSIs per 1;1000 IVD days, $p = <0.001$) and thrombotic complications (21.5% versus 1.9%, $p = <0.001$).[18] Moreover, Robert et al found that patients with primary BSI were more likely to have received care during times when there was a lower nursing-to-patient ratio and a higher proportion of "float" rather than dedicated nursing staff.[19]

II.   BASIC PRINCIPLES

PATHOGENESIS OF INTRAVASCULAR DEVICE-RELATED SEPSIS

There are two major sources of IVDR BSI: 1) colonization of the IVD, *catheter-related infection* and 2) contamination of the fluid administered through the device, *infusate-related infection*.[2] Contaminated infusate is the cause of most *epidemic* IVDR BSIs. In contrast, catheter-related infections are responsible for most *endemic* IVDR BSIs.[1]

For microorganisms to cause catheter-related infection, they must first gain access to the extraluminal or intraluminal surface of the device where they can adhere and become incorporated into a biofilm that allows sustained infection and hematogenous dissemination.[20] Microorganisms gain access to the bloodstream by one of three mechanisms (Figure 24–1): (1) skin organisms invade the percutaneous tract, probably facilitated by capillary action, at the time of insertion or in the days following; (2) microorganisms contaminate the catheter hub (and lumen) when the catheter is inserted over a percutaneous guidewire or later manipulated; or (3) organisms are carried hematogenously to the implanted IVD from remote sources of local infection, such as a pneumonia.

With *short-term* IVDs (in place <10 days), such as peripheral IV catheters, arterial catheters and noncuffed, nontunneled CVCs, most device-related BSIs are of cutaneous origin, from the insertion site, and gain access extraluminally, occasionally intraluminally.[21-24] In contrast, contamination of the catheter hub and luminal fluid is the predominant mode of BSI with the *long-term* IVDs (e.g., in place >10 days), such as cuffed Hickman- and Broviac-type catheters, subcutaneous central ports, and PICCs.[25-27]

It is also important to recognize that infusate (parenteral fluid, blood products, or IV medications) administered through an IVD can also become contaminated

Table 24-2. Risk factors for intravascular device-related bloodstream infection with short-term intravascular devices.*

Risk factors (no. of studies)	Relative Risk or Odds Ratio
Underlying disease:	
AIDS (2)	4.8
Neutropenia (2)	1.0–15.1
GI disease (1)	2.4
Surgical service (1)	4.4
ICU/CCU placement (3)	0.4–6.7
Extended hospitalization (3)	1.0–6.7
Other intravascular devices (2)	1.0–3.8
Systemic antibiotics (3)	0.1–0.5
Active infection at another site (2)	8.7–9.2
High APACHE III score (1)	4.2
Mechanical ventilation (1)	2.0–2.5
Transplant patient (1)	2.6
Features of Insertion	
Difficult insertion (1)	5.4
Maximal sterile barriers (1)	0.2
Tunneling (2)	0.3–1.0
Insertion over a guidewire (8)	1.0–3.3
Insertion site:	
Internal jugular jugular vein (6)	1.0–3.3
Subclavian vein (5)	0.4–1.0
Femoral vein (2)	3.3–4.8
Defatting insertion site (1)	1.0
Use a multi-lumen catheter (8)	1.0–6.5
Catheter management	
Routine change of IV set (2)	1.0
Staffing in SICU (Nurse: Patient Ratio) (1)	
1:2.0	61.5
1:1.5	15.6
1:1.2	4.0
1:1	1.0
Inappropriate catheter usage (1)	5.3
Duration of catheterization > 7 days (5)	1.0–8.7
Colonization of catheter hub (3)	17.9–44.1
Parenteral nutrition (2)	1.0–4.8

* Adapted from Safdar et al.[13]

Intravascular Device Infections

24-3

Copyright © 2005, Association for Professionals in Infection Control and Epidemiology, Inc.

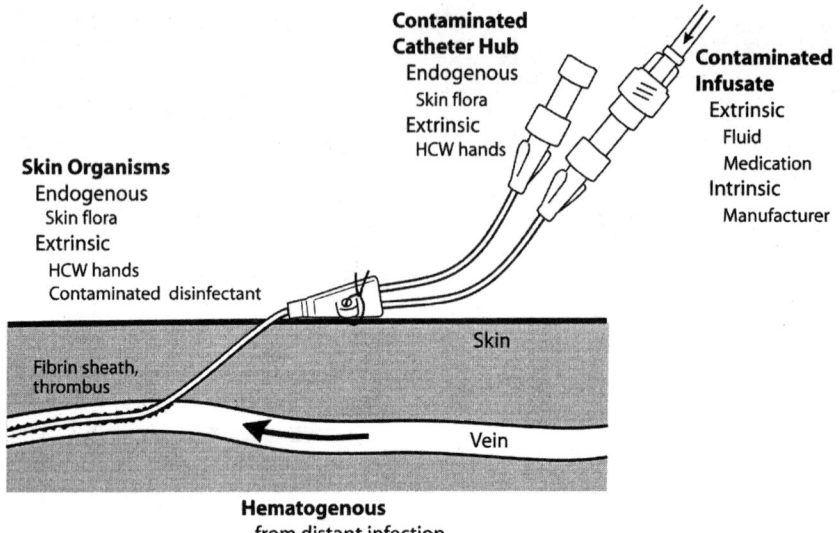

Contaminated Catheter Hub
Endogenous
  Skin flora
Extrinsic
  HCW hands

Contaminated Infusate
Extrinsic
  Fluid
  Medication
Intrinsic
  Manufacturer

Skin Organisms
Endogenous
  Skin flora
Extrinsic
  HCW hands
  Contaminated disinfectant

Skin

Fibrin sheath, thrombus

Vein

Hematogenous
from distant infection

Figure 24–1 Potential sources of infection of a percutaneous IVD: the contiguous skin flora, contamination of the catheter hub and lumen, con[chtamination of infusate, and hematogenous colonization of the IVD from distant, unrelated sites of infection. From C. J. Crnich and D. G. Maki.[20]

and produce device-related BSI. Contaminated fluid is fortunately an infrequent cause of endemic infusion-related infection with most short-term IVDs; it is, however, an important cause of BSIs with arterial catheters used for hemodynamic monitoring and long-term IVDs such as Hickman or Broviac catheters, cuffed hemodialysis CVCs, and subcutaneous central venous ports.[24,28,29]

Most nosocomial *epidemics* of infusion-related BSI, however, have been traced to contamination of infusate by gram-negative bacilli, introduced during its manufacture (intrinsic contamination) or during its preparation and administration in the hospital (extrinsic contamination).[30,31] If an epidemic is suspected, the epidemiologic approach must be methodical and thorough, yet expeditious, directed toward establishing the bona fide nature of the putative epidemic infections (i.e. ruling out "pseudoinfections")[32] and confirming the existence of an epidemic; defining the reservoirs and modes of transmission of the epidemic pathogens; and, most importantly, controlling the epidemic, quickly and completely (Table 24–3). Control measures are predicated upon accurate delineation of the epidemiology of the epidemic pathogen. The essential

steps in dealing with a suspected nosocomial outbreak have recently been reviewed.[2]

Microbiology of IVDR BSI

Figure 24–2 summarizes the microbial profile of IVDR BSI from 159 published prospective studies.[33] As might be expected from knowledge of the pathogenesis of these infections, skin microorganisms account for the largest proportion of IVDR BSIs.

Definitions for Infusion-Related Infection

IVDs are associated with both local and systemic infection. The Centers for Disease Control and Prevention (CDC) has published definitions for IVDR infection (Table 24–4).[34] These definitions are useful for the purposes of surveillance but rely heavily upon the construct, central venous catheter-associated BSI, which implicitly assumes that every primary BSI originates from a CVC. This practice results in an overestimate of the true risk of CVC-related infection because not all

Copyright © 2005, Association for Professionals in Infection Control and Epidemiology, Inc.

Table 24-3. Approach to suspected epidemic nosocomial bloodstream infections (BSIs).*

1. Administrative preparation:

a. The Infection Control Committee or a similarly designated body should be responsible for investigating a suspected epidemic.
b. When an epidemic is suspected a single person (e.g., the hospital epidemiologist) should be designated to direct the investigation.
c. The necessary disciplines, such as the involved department or departments, pharmacy, nursing, hospital administration, and employee health, should be identified and involved at the outset of the investigation.
d. All major decisions should be made in conjunction with the investigating team, attending staff, and administration.
e. All information released to the public should be cleared through the hospital epidemiologist and hospital administration.

2. Retrieve putative epidemic isolates:

a. Retrieve all available laboratory isolates of the epidemic strain(s) as soon as possible for further characterization and possible molecular subtyping.
b. Laboratory personnel should retain unusual organisms that are being encountered on an increasing basis as a matter of routine.

3. Preliminary actions:

a. Identify and characterize individual cases.
Make an epidemic-case definition.
Confirm that each suspected case-patient has true BSI and not pseudo-BSI (i.e., patient has clinical signs of infection such as fever, chills, hypotension).
Confirm the concordance of isolates from the patient's blood and IVDs or infusate (if applicable) down to the molecular level.
b. Ascertain if the situation represents an epidemic and not a pseudoepidemic by showing an increased prevalence of cases with the epidemic strain compared to baseline surveillance rates during the same interval.
c. Implement provisional measures.
Preliminary screening of case-patient's environment and those involved in their care, guided by the ecology and epidemiology of the epidemic strain. Implement preliminary control measures, based on the initial suspected source of infection (e.g., change infusion sets every 24 hours during a suspected outbreak of infusate-related BSI).
d. Intensify surveillance hospital-wide.
e. Review general infection control policies to identify any changes or breaks with these policies.
f. Determine the need for extramural assistance (i.e., local and national health authorities).

4. Epidemiologic investigations:

a. Clinical-epidemiologic studies
Identify the population at greatest risk.
Perform a retrospective case-control study to point up risk factors or potential sources.
b. Microbiologic studies
Focused studies of the inanimate environment and medical personnel, if indicated, based on the results of the case-control study.
Blind large-scale culturing of the hospital environment or medical personnel is discouraged, as it is expensive and often of limited value. Such studies are better guided by the results of the epidemiological investigation.

5. Definitive control measures:

a. Remove the probable sources or correct breaks in infection control practices.
b. If intrinsic contamination of a commercial product is suspected or, especially, proven state and local health authorities, the Food and Drug Administration, the CDC and the manufacturer should be immediately informed. Remaining supplies of the suspect product should be quarantined and retained for further investigation, possibly public health or regulatory authorities.

6. Report the findings

* Adapted from Maki.[277]

Copyright © 2005, Association for Professionals in Infection Control and Epidemiology, Inc.

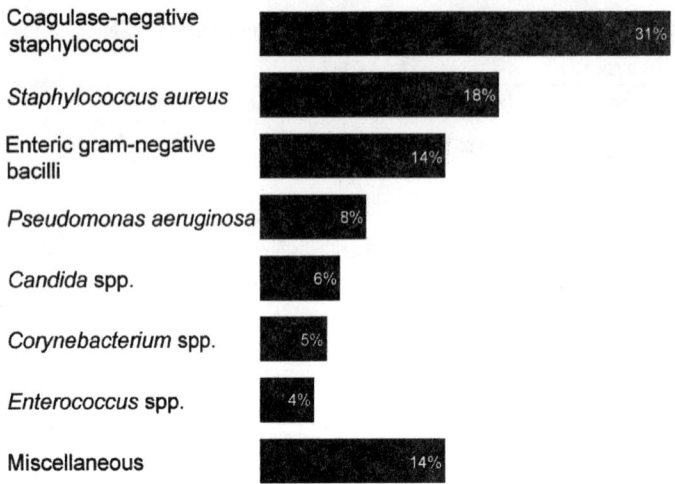

Figure 24-2 Microbial profile of intravascular device-related bloodstream infection based on an analysis 159 published prospective studies.[33]

primary BSIs originate from a central venous device; some are secondary BSIs deriving from unrecognized postoperative surgical site or intra-abdominal infections or nosocomial pneumonias, or originate from other vascular devices such as peripheral venous or, especially, arterial catheters used for hemodynamic monitoring.

By applying molecular subtyping techniques[35-37] to the results of semiquantitative or quantitative cultures of the removed IVD and hub or the results of cultures of blood drawn through the IVD and a separate peripheral blood sample, it is now possible to reliably implicate an IVD as the source of a nosocomial BSI. Using these criteria allows formulation of simple but more rigorous definitions for IVDR infection (Table 24–5), which we believe bear consideration as a standard for randomized trials and studies of risk factors for IVDR infection.

III. DIAGNOSIS, PREVENTION, AND TREATMENT OF INFUSION-RELATED SEPTICEMIA

Diagnosis

Clinical Features

Recent evidence-based guidelines provide the best current information on the evaluation of the ICU patient with fever or other signs of sepsis.[38] Before any decision regarding initiation of antimicrobial therapy or removal of an IVD, the patient must be thoroughly examined to identify *all* plausible sites of infection, including ventilator-associated pneumonia, catheter-associated urinary tract infection, surgical site infection, or antibiotic-associated colitis, as well as line sepsis.

Despite the challenge of identifying the source of a patient's signs of sepsis,[38] several clinical, epidemiologic, and microbiologic findings point strongly toward an IVD as the source of a septic episode (Table 24–6).[2,39] Patients with abrupt onset of signs and symptoms of sepsis without any other identifiable source should prompt suspicion of infection of an IVD. The presence of inflammation or purulence at the catheter insertion site is now uncommon in patients with IVDR BSI.[40] However, if purulence is seen in combination with signs and symptoms of sepsis, it is highly likely the patient has IVDR BSI and should prompt removal of the IVD. Finally, recovery of certain microorganisms in multiple blood cultures, such as staphylococci, *Corynebacterium* or *Bacillus* species, or *Candida* or *Malassezia* species, strongly suggests infection of the IVD.

Copyright © 2005, Association for Professionals in Infection Control and Epidemiology, Inc.

Table 24-4. Centers for Disease Control definitions for intravascular device-related bloodstream infection.[34]

Primary bloodstream infection*

Must meet at least one of the following criteria:

> *Criterion 1*: Recognized pathogen cultured from blood culture and the pathogen cultured is not related to an infection at another site.
>
> *Criterion 2*: One of the following signs or symptoms: fever (>38°C), chills, or hypotension combined with any one of the following:
>
> A common skin contaminant (e.g., diphtheroids, *Bacillus* sp., *Propionibacterium* sp., coagulase-negative staphylococci, or micrococci) isolated from two blood cultures on separate occasions and the organism is not related to infection at another site.
> or
> A common skin contaminant (e.g., diphtheroids, *Bacillus* sp., *Propionibacterium* sp., coagulase-negative staphylococci, or micrococci) isolated from blood culture from a patient with an intravascular device and the physician institutes appropriate antimicrobial therapy.
> or
> A positive antigen test on blood (e.g., *Candida* sp., *Haemophilus influenzae*, *Streptococcus pneumoniae*, *Neisseria meningitides* or group B streptococci) and the organism is not related to an infection at another site.
>
> *Criterion 3*: A patient ≤12 months of age who has one of the following: fever (>38°C), hypothermia (<37°C), apnea, or bradycardia combined with any of the following:
>
> A common skin contaminant (e.g., diphtheroids, *Bacillus* sp., *Propionibacterium* sp., coagulase-negative staphylococci, or micrococci) isolated from two blood cultures on separate occasions and the organism is not related to infection at another site.
> or
> A common skin contaminant (e.g., diphtheroids, *Bacillus* sp., *Propionibacterium* sp., coagulase-negative staphylococci, or micrococci) isolated from blood culture from a patient with an intravascular device and the physician institutes appropriate antimicrobial therapy.
> or
> A positive antigen test on blood (e.g., *Candida* sp., *Haemophilus influenzae*, *Streptococcus pneumoniae*, *Neisseria meningitides* or group B streptococci) and the organism is not related to an infection at another site.

Arterial or Venous infection

Must meet one of the following criterion:

> *Criterion 1*: An organism is isolated from cultures of arteries or veins removed during surgery and blood cultures not done or no organism was isolated from blood culture.
>
> *Criterion 2*: There is evidence of infection at involved vascular site seen during surgery or by histopathologic examination
>
> *Criterion 3*: One of the following is present: fever (>38°C), pain, erythema, or heat at involved vascular site and both of the following:

1) More than 15 colonies cultured from an intravascular cannula tip using semiquantitative (or quantitative) methods.

2) Blood culture not done or no organism is isolated from blood culture.

> *Criterion 4:* Purulent drainage at involved vascular site and a blood culture is not done or no organism is isolated from blood culture.
>
> *Criterion 5:* A patient ≤12 months of age and has one of the following: fever (>38°C), hypothermia (<37°C), apnea, bradycardia, lethargy, pain, erythema, or heat at involved vascular site and both of the following:

1) More than 15 colonies cultured from an intravascular cannula tip using semiquantitative (or quantitative) methods.

2) A blood culture is not done or no organism is isolated from blood culture.

* When an organism isolated from the blood culture is compatible with a related nosocomial infection at another site, the bloodstream infection is classified as a secondary bloodstream infection. Exceptions to this are intravascular device-associated bloodstream infection, all of which are classified as primary even if localized signs of infection are present at the access site.

Blood Cultures

It is indefensible to start anti-infective drugs for suspected or presumed infection in the critically-ill patient without first obtaining blood cultures from two separate sites, *at least one of which is drawn from a peripheral vein by percutaneous venipuncture*. The volume of blood cultured is essential to maximize the sensitivity of blood cultures for diagnosis of bacteremia or candidemia: in adults, obtaining at least 20 mL, ideally 30 mL, per drawing (each specimen containing 10 mL or 15 mL, inoculated into aerobic and anaerobic media),

significantly improves the yield as compared to obtaining only 5 mL at each drawing and culturing a smaller total volume.[41-44] In adults, if at least 30 mL of blood is cultured, 99% of detectable bacteremias should be identified.[41,42,45] Similar operating characteristics are achieved in the pediatric population using a weight-based graduated volume approach to blood cultures.[46] Standard blood cultures drawn through CVCs provide excellent sensitivity for diagnosis of BSI but are less specific than cultures obtained from a peripheral vein.[47-52]

Copyright © 2005, Association for Professionals in Infection Control and Epidemiology, Inc.

Table 24-5. Proposed definitions for intravascular device-related (IVDR) colonization, local infection and bloodstream infection (BSI) which are based upon microbiologic confirmation of the IVD as the source[†].

IVD colonization

	(i) A positive semiquantitative* (or quantitative**) culture of the implanted portion or portions of the IVD; (ii) absence of signs of local or systemic infection.
Local IVD infection	(i) A positive semiquantitative* (or quantitative**) culture of the removed IVD or a positive microscopic examination or culture of pus or thrombus from the cannulated vessel; (ii) clinical evidence of infection of the insertion site (i.e., erythema, induration or purulence) but; (iii) absence of systemic signs of infection and negative blood cultures, if done.
IVDR BSI	*If the IVD is removed:* (i) A positive semi-quantitative* (or quantitative**) culture of the IVD or a positive culture of the catheter hub or infusate (or positive microscopic examination or culture of pus or thrombus from the cannulated vessel) *and* one or more positive blood cultures, ideally percutaneously drawn, concordant for the same species, ideally by molecular subtyping methods; (ii) clinical and microbiologic data disclose no other clear-cut source for the BSI. *If the IVD is retained:* *(i) If quantitative blood cultures are available, cultures drawn both from the IVD and a peripheral vein (or another IVD) are both positive and show a marked step-up in quantitative positivity ($five-fold) in the IVD-drawn culture; (ii) clinical and microbiologic data disclose no other clear-cut source for the BSI.* *or* *(i) If automated monitoring of incubating blood cultures is available, blood cultures drawn concomitantly from the IVD and a peripheral vein (or another IVD) show both are positive, but the IVD-drawn blood culture turns positive more than 2 hours before the peripherally-drawn culture; (ii) clinical and microbiologic data disclose no other clear-cut source for the BSI.*

* Roll Plate of cannula segment(s) >15 colony-forming units (cfus)
** Sonication culture of cannula segment(s) $\geq 10^3$ cfus
† Adapted from Crnich and Maki.[1]

Table 24-6. Clinical, epidemiologic and microbiologic features of intravascular device-related bloodstream infection[†].

Non-Specific	Suggestive of Device-related Etiology

Fever
  Chills, shaking rigors*
  Hypotension, shock*
  Hyperventilation, respiratory failure
	Patient unlikely candidate for sepsis (e.g., young, no underlying diseases)
	Source of sepsis inapparent, no identifiable local infection

Gastrointestinal*	
Abdominal Pain	Intravascular device in place, especially central venous catheter
Vomiting	Inflammation or purulence at insertion site
Diarrhea	Abrupt onset, associated with shock
Neurologic*	
Confusion Seizures	Septicemia caused by staphylococci (especially coagulase-negative staphylococci) or *Corynebacterium, Candida, Trichophyton, Fusarium,* or *Malassezia* species** Very high-grade (.25 CFU/ml) candidemia Cluster of cryptogenic infusion-associated bloodstream infections caused by *Enterobacter cloacae, Pantoea agglomerans* or *Serratia marcescens*** Sepsis refractory to antimicrobial therapy or dramatic improvement with removal of cannula and infusion*

* Commonly seen in overwhelming gram-negative sepsis originating from contaminated infusate, peripheral suppurative phlebitis, or septic thrombosis of a central vein.
** Conversely, septicemia caused by streptococci, aerobic gram-negative bacilli or anaerobes is unlikely to derive from an intravascular device.
† Adapted from Maki and Mermel.[2]

Copyright © 2005, Association for Professionals in Infection Control and Epidemiology, Inc.

Every effort must be made to prevent introduced contamination when drawing blood cultures, as a single contaminated blood culture has been shown to prolong hospitalization by four days and increase the costs of hospitalization by $4,100–$4,400.[53,54] Tincture of iodine, isopropyl alcohol, chlorhexidine, or povidone-iodine *combined* with ethyl alcohol rather than povidone-iodine *alone* should be used for skin antisepsis prior to venipuncture for blood cultures, recognizing that studies have shown significantly reduced rates of contamination with use of these agents.[54-57] Up to 30% of blood cultures positive for coagulase-negative staphylococcus (CNS) represent true infection;[58,59] however, the majority of single positive cultures represent contamination,[59] a finding that should reemphasize the need to obtain cultures from *two* separate sites whenever BSI is suspected.

Microbiologic Analysis of Removed Intravascular Devices

Removal and direct culture of the IVD historically has been the method of choice for confirming the presence of IVDR BSI, particularly with short-term IVDs. Numerous studies have shown that culturing catheter segments semiquantitatively on solid media[21,60,61] or quantitatively in liquid media (e.g., removing the adherent organisms by sonication)[62-64] provides superior sensitivity and specificity for diagnosis of IVDR BSI, with a strong correlation between high colony counts and IVDR BSI. Growth of ≤15 CFU from a catheter segment by semiquantitative culture or growth of ≤10^3 CFU from a catheter cultured after sonication with accompanying local inflammation or signs of sepsis indicates IVDR infection. Significant growth in the absence of local or systemic inflammation suggests colonization of the device; if continued, vascular access is needed, and a new device should be placed in a *new* location rather than replacing it with a new one in the same location by guidewire exchange.

Whereas recent studies[64-66] have suggested that quantitative methods (e.g., sonication) are superior to the semiquantitative methods (e.g., roll plate), other studies have shown them to be equivalent.[67,68] Because hub contamination progressing to intraluminal colonization is the primary route of infection for long-term devices (e.g., devices in place >10 days), quantitative techniques may be superior to semiquantitative techniques in detecting infections from these types of devices because they remove organisms from both the internal and external surfaces of catheters.[26,63,69] In contrast, semiquantitative methods may be preferred over quantitative methods in cases of suspected infection related to a short-term device (e.g., devices in place <10 days) because the primary route of infection in this setting is due to extraluminal spread of skin organisms at the catheter insertion site; the semiquantitative method is

simple, less expensive, and allows identification of the infecting organisms a day earlier.

Direct and impression gram stains[21,70] or acridine orange stains[71-73] of intravascular segments of removed catheters have shown excellent correlation with quantitative techniques for culturing catheters and may permit rapid diagnosis of catheter-related infection.

A novel culture brush, which can be passed down the lumen and out the end of an implanted catheter to pick up luminal biofilm and colonized fibrin and thrombus around the tip, has been developed to diagnose infections of central venous catheters without having to remove the catheter.[74-76] A recent prospective study comparing the endoluminal brush to the semiquantitative methods found the brush to be 95% sensitive and 84% specific.[76] However, a prospective study by van Heerdan et al. calls these results into question, as they found the endoluminal brush to only be 21% sensitive, although the specificity remained high at 100%.[77] A possible explanation for this discrepancy may lie in part with the fact that the latter study used the endoluminal brush method with short-term catheters (all catheters were removed between days 5 and 7 after placement), a setting where most of the infecting organisms would be expected to have gained access extraluminally by invasion of the percutaneous insertion tract.

Quantitative skin-swab cultures of the catheter insertion site have been proposed as a simple means of detecting infection with short-term CVCs.[78-81] Studies suggest that this method is highly sensitive in identifying probable infection of the CVC, but most have not found it to be very specific. Therefore, cultures of the device insertion site can be used to rule out infection of a short-term IVD if negative, but they do not necessarily predict device infection if positive.

To rigorously identify the mechanism of IVDR BSI in prospective studies, it is necessary to culture *all* potential sources at the time of catheter removal (Figure 24–1): skin of the insertion site, each catheter hub, infusate from each lumen, and catheter segments. If the results of these cultures seem to link a BSI with microorganisms isolated from one or more portions of the device, efforts then need to be made to conclusively establish concordance, *beyond* speciation and antimicrobial susceptibility pattern, using one or more molecular subtyping systems, such as multilocus enzyme analysis, plasmid profile, or restriction-enzyme analysis of chromosomal DNA by pulsed-field electrophoresis.[36,37,43,82,83]

Copyright © 2005, Association for Professionals in Infection Control and Epidemiology, Inc.

Microbiologic Analysis of Implanted Long-Term Intravascular Devices

The methods described above require removal of the device for confirmation of IVDR BSI. This is often undesirable or difficult with surgically implanted IVDs such as Hickman and Broviac catheters, cuffed and tunneled hemodialysis catheters, and subcutaneous central venous ports. Only 15–45% of long-term IVDs that are removed for suspected infection are truly colonized or infected at the time of removal.[15,62,84-89] To avoid unnecessary removal of IVDs, methods have been developed to identify infection while allowing the device to stay in place: 1) the endoluminal brush culture described above; 2) paired quantitative blood cultures drawn from the IVD and percutaneously from a peripheral vein;[90] 3) differential time to positivity (DTP) of paired standard blood cultures, one drawn from the IVD, the second from a peripheral vein;[91-93] and 4) gram stain[94] or acridine orange staining of blood samples drawn through the IVD.[89,95,96]

If a laboratory has available an automated quantitative system for culturing blood (e.g., Isolator® lysis-centrifugation system, Wampole Laboratories, Cranbury, NJ), quantitative blood cultures drawn through the IVD *and* concomitantly by venipuncture from a peripheral vein (or another IVD) can permit the diagnosis of IVDR bacteremia or fungemia to be made with sensitivity and specificity in the range of 80–95%,[97,98] *without* removal of the catheter, *if* empiric antimicrobial therapy has not yet been initiated. With this approach, IVD-drawn cultures demonstrating 5- to 10-fold higher microorganism counts, as compared to counts of the same microorganism obtained in a culture drawn from a peripheral vein, confirm the presence of IVDR BSI.

Quantitative blood cultures are labor intensive and cost almost twice as much as standard blood cultures. It is well known that blood culture bottles inoculated with a larger number of organisms turn positive sooner than culture bottles inoculated with a lower number of organisms[91,99] and the wide availability of automated radiometric blood culture systems (e.g., BACTEC system®, manufactured by Becton Dickinson), in which blood cultures are continuously monitored for microbial growth, has led to a clever application of this system to take advantage of this phenomenon. The DTP of paired blood cultures, one drawn through the IVD and the second concomitantly from a peripheral vein, has been shown to reliably identify IVDR BSI of long-term IVDs if the blood culture drawn from the IVD turns positive 2 or more hours before the culture drawn peripherally. In studies of patients with long-term IVDs, the sensitivity and specificity of DTP ranged from 82% to 94% and 88% to 91%, respectively.[92,100-102] The performance of DTP in short-term IVDs has recently been examined with disappointing results,[103] a finding that

is not entirely unexpected given the predominant role of extraluminal infection with these devices.

A simple, rapid, and potentially cost-effective method of detecting IVDR BSI is gram stain[94] or acridine orange staining (AOS) of a sample of lysed and centrifuged blood drawn through the suspected IVD.[95,104] In a recent prospective study of 124 adult surgical patients, this method was found to be 96% sensitive and 92% specific.[95] These same authors have shown that routine use of AOS on blood aspirated from IVDs suspected to be infected can bring significant cost savings,[96] primarily as a result of reducing unnecessary IVD removal. AOS has been shown to be of limited utility in diagnosing IVDR BSI of short-term IVDs (mean duration of catheterization 6 days) where AOS failed to diagnose all 12 confirmed IVDR BSIs;[89] therefore, AOS will likely remain useful only for suspected infection of long-term IVDs.

Detection of Contaminated Infusate

To diagnose infection caused by contaminated infusate, a sample of IV fluid, aspirated from the line, should be cultured quantitatively and qualitatively;[105] concordance with positive peripheral blood cultures, without another identifiable source for the patient's BSI, definitively implicates infected infusate as the cause of the BSI. Anaerobic culture techniques are not necessary unless blood or another biologic product is involved.

STRATEGIES FOR PREVENTION OF IVDR BSI

Recommendations for the prevention of IVDR BSIs were published by the Hospital Infection Control Practices Advisory Committee (HICPAC) have recently been updated.[106] Table 24–7 summarizes the recommendations of the 2001 HICPAC guideline for the prevention of IVDR BSI and scores each recommendation based on the quality of the available scientific evidence. It must be reaffirmed that measures for prevention of any nosocomial infection must, wherever possible, be based on the best understanding of pathophysiology and epidemiology and, whenever possible, controlled clinical trials.

Choice of Catheter and Site of Device Insertion

Obviously, the choice of IVD inserted into a patient will be guided primarily by that patient's particular needs (e.g., hemodialysis versus fluid administration). However, the astute clinician can mitigate much of the risk associated with vascular access by choosing the best device for the task at hand and inserting the IVD in a location associated with the least risk of infection. Studies have shown that multilumen IVDs are associated with a higher risk of infection than single lumen

APIC Text of Infection Control and Epidemiology

Copyright © 2005, Association for Professionals in Infection Control and Epidemiology, Inc.

Table 24-7. Novel technology that has been examined in randomized clinical **trials.**

Chlorhexidine for cutaneous antisepsis
Securement device
Topical anti-infective creams or ointments

Polymyxin, neomycin, bacitracin polyantibiotic ointment
    Povidone-Iodine ointment
    Mupirocin ointment

Dressings

Transparent, polyurethane film dressings
    Hyperpermeable polyurethane dressings
    Hydrocolloid dressings
    Chlorhexidine-impregnated sponge dressings

Innovative IVD design

Cuffed and tunneled CVCs
    Subcutaneous central venous ports
    Attachable silver-impregnated cuffs
    Peripherally-inserted central venous catheters (PICCs)

Anti-infective-coated catheters

Benzalkonium chloride-impregnated catheters
    Chlorhexidine-silver sulfadiazine-coated catheters
    Cefazolin-coated catheters
    Minocycline-rifampin-coated catheters
    Silver-impregnated catheters

Anti-infective catheter hubs
Iodinated chamber   External povidone-iodine-saturated sponge cap
Anti-infective lock solutions for long-term IVDs

Vancomycin
    Vancomycin/Ciprofloxacin
    Trisodium citrate/gentamicin
    Minocycline/ethylenediaminetetraacetic acid (EDTA)
    Ethanol
    Taurolidine

Scheduled (prophylactic) thrombolysis with urokinase

Adapted from Crnich and Maki.[20,194]

catheters.[107] That said, if a particular patient has need for multiple infusions, it makes little sense to insert several single lumen IVDs in multiple locations rather than a multilumen IVD in a single location.

To date, there have been no randomized studies designed to evaluate the optimal location for placement of short-term CVCs. However, the data accumulated from numerous observational studies suggest that the lowest risk of IVDR BSI is seen with subclavian vein insertion, the highest risk of IVDR BSI is seen with femoral vein insertion, and the intermediate level of risk is associated with jugular vein insertions.[18,24,108-113]

The femoral vein is often used for central venous access, especially on nonsurgical services, because of the ease of cannulation and the lower risk of mechanical complications from insertion (i.e., bleeding or pneu-

mothorax). Unfortunately, prospective studies evaluating the risk of femoral vein device placement have shown that CVCs placed in the femoral vein are much more likely to be colonized at the time of removal than catheters placed in the internal jugular vein (RR = 4.7, CI = 2.0–8.8, p = 0.0001)[112] and are associated with an increased risk of IVDR BSI when compared to CVCs placed in the subclavian vein (4.4% versus 1.5%, p = 0.07).[18] Furthermore, recent prospective studies have found higher rates of IVDR deep vein thrombosis with femoral catheters, in the range of 6.6% to 25%.[18,114-116] In general, we believe femoral vascular access should be used only if emergent access is required, the inexperience of the operator prevents placement in the upper body, or there is a contraindication to placement in the upper body (no available sites, an extensive burn, or refractory coagulopathy). If a short-term CVC must be placed in the femoral vein or artery, we believe it is important that the catheter insertion site be located at least 2 inches (5 cm) below the inguinal crease or an intertriginous area, which is heavily colonized with bowel organisms and yeasts; this also allows a more secure protective dressing to be affixed.

In contrast to short-term CVCs, observational studies of hemodialysis catheters have not been able to confirm a lower rate of infection with IVDs inserted in the subclavian vein compared to those inserted in the internal jugular vein,[117-119] although there is still excess risk associated with femoral vein placement.[120] More importantly, prospective studies of catheters used for hemodialysis have demonstrated a significant risk of great vein thrombosis and stenosis in catheters inserted into the subclavian vein that approaches 40–50% as compared to rates of 0–10% with catheters inserted into the internal jugular vein.[121,122] Based on these data, internal jugular vein insertion is preferable to subclavian vein insertion for central access for hemodialysis.

Barrier Precautions

Hand hygiene with an antiseptic-containing preparation, either conventional handwashing with chlorhexidine (2–4%) or with a waterless alcohol rub or gel,[123] must always precede the insertion of an IVD and should also precede subsequent handling of the device or its administration set.[124] A new pair of disposable nonsterile gloves, using a "no-touch" technique, is adequate for the placement of peripheral IV catheters in most patients; however *sterile gloves* should be used during insertion in high-risk patients, such as those with granulocytopenia. Sterile gloves are strongly recommended for placement of all other types of IVDs that are associated with a 1% or higher risk of associated bacteremia, specifically arterial catheters and all types of CVCs, including PICCs.[106]

Copyright © 2005, Association for Professionals in Infection Control and Epidemiology, Inc.

Studies have shown that the use of *maximal barriers* (including a long-sleeved, sterile surgical gown, mask, cap, and large sterile drape, as well as sterile gloves) significantly reduces the risk of CVC-related BSI (0.08 BSIs with maximal barriers versus 0.5 BSIs per 1; XC000 IVD days without maximal barriers, $p = 0.02$).[125] The use of maximal barriers has further been shown to be highly cost-effective.[125] Considering that of all IVDs, CVCs are most likely to produce nosocomial BSI, a strong case can be made for *mandating* maximal barrier precautions during the insertion of *all* central IVDs.[106] They are not necessary, however, for arterial catheters used for hemodynamic monitoring, where sterile gloves and a sterile fenestrated drape will suffice.[126]

IV Teams

Good technique is also essential. Studies have shown that the use of special *IV therapy teams*, consisting of trained nurses or technicians who can assure a consistent and high level of aseptic technique during catheter insertion and in follow-up care of the catheter, have been associated with substantially lower rates of catheter-related BSI and are cost effective.[127-129] But even if an institution does not have an IV team, it can greatly reduce its rate of IVDR BSI by *formal education of nurses and physicians* and stringent adherence to IVD care protocols.[130,131]

Cutaneous Antisepsis

Given the evidence for the importance of cutaneous microorganisms in the pathogenesis of short-term IVDR infections, measures to reduce colonization of the insertion site would seem of the highest priority, particularly the choice of chemical antiseptics for disinfection of the site. In the United States, iodophors such as 10% povidone-iodine are used most widely.[132] Nine randomized, prospective trials comparing a chlorhexidine-containing antiseptic to either povidone-iodine or alcohol for preparation of the skin prior to insertion of a short-term IVD have been reported.[29,133-140] In the largest study to date, a randomized trial in 1,050 CVCs and arterial catheters placed in a university hospital ICU, cutaneous antisepsis with 1% tincture of chlorhexidine showed a highly significant reduction in IVDR BSIs compared to an iodophor (RR = 0.35, $p < 0.01$).[140] More recently, a meta-analysis that examined results from eight of the nine aforementioned studies found that use of chlorhexidine was associated with a nearly 50% reduction in the risk of IVDR compared to povidone-iodine (RR = 0.49, 95% CI = 0.28–0.88).[141]

Insertion Site Care and IVD Maintenance

IVD Dressings

IVDs can be dressed with sterile gauze and tape or with a sterile transparent, semipermeable, polyurethane film dressing. The available data suggest that the two types of dressings are equivalent in terms of their impact on IVDR BSI with peripheral IVs and short-term CVCs.[35,142-147] In contrast, results from studies of arterial catheters have found that polyurethane dressings greatly increase the risk of IVDR BSI.[144,148] As a result, polyurethane dressings should probably not be used on arterial catheters until future studies confirm their safety.

Topical Antimicrobial Ointments

In theory, application of a topical antimicrobial agent to the catheter insertion site should confer some protection against microbial invasion. Clinical trials of a topical combination antibacterial ointment containing polymyxin, neomycin, and bacitracin with peripheral IVs have shown marginal benefit,[149-151] but the use of polyantibiotic ointments has been associated with a 5-fold increased frequency of Candida infection, limiting their utility.[151,152]

The topical antibacterial, mupirocin, which is active primarily against gram-positive organisms, was shown in one study to significantly reduce colonization of internal jugular catheters without increasing colonization by *Candida* spp.,[153] and a more recent study by Sesso et al showed significant reductions in hemodialysis catheter colonization (3.17 versus 14.27 per 1; XC000 IVD days, $p = <0.001$) and *Saccharomyces aureus* IVDR BSIs (0.71 versus 8.92 BSIs per 1; XC000 IVD days, $p = <0.001$).[154] Unfortunately, resistance of *S. aureus*[155] and coagulase-negative staphylococci[156] rapidly emerges during wide-scale mupirocin use,[157] which contravenes its use as a topical agent for the prevention of IVDR BSI at this time.[106]

Three prospective studies of topical povidone-iodine ointment applied to central venous catheter sites have failed to show a statistical benefit to its use,[151,158,159] but a single comparative trial in subclavian hemodialysis catheters showed that the use of topical povidone-iodine ointment was associated with a 4-fold reduction in the incidence of IVDR *S. aureus* BSI.[160] Therefore, if a topical agent is to be used with hemodialysis catheters, an iodophor may be most desirable.

Replacement of the Device

Studies have shown that peripheral IVs may safely be left in place for up to 96 hours, if the patient and the insertion site are monitored closely.[28,161,162] Recent studies have suggested that the duration of peripheral

Copyright © 2005, Association for Professionals in Infection Control and Epidemiology, Inc.

catheterization may be prolonged even further;[163] however, after viewing recent reports of increasing nosocomial *S. aureus* bacteremias linked to prolonged peripheral venous catheterization,[164] more studies are required before this can become a standard recommendation.

Scheduled replacement of short-term, noncuffed, nontunneled CVCs has long been practiced in many centers; however, recent studies have called this practice into question.[165-167] Moreover, a meta-analysis found no benefit to routine replacement of short-term CVCs.[168] Based on these data, there seems to be no indication for scheduled replacement of short-term CVCs that are functioning well and show no clinical signs of infection.

Guidewire Exchanges of CVCs

The management of CVCs that must be replaced, either because of mechanical malfunction or suspected infection, deserves special attention. Replacement of CVCs by guidewire exchange is associated with a reduced risk of mechanical complications;[167,168] however, it is also associated with an increased risk of the newly placed CVC becoming infected and causing CVC-related BSI.[167] As result, if circumstances necessitate guidewire exchange for placement of a new catheter (e.g., the patient has limited new access sites, is morbidly obese, or is at high risk of mechanical complications because of underlying coagulopathy), the same strict aseptic technique, which includes full barrier precautions, must be used. However, the tip and/or intracutaneous segment(s) of the removed CVC should also routinely be sent for culture to determine whether the insertion tract is colonized, because if it is, the newly exchanged CVC should be promptly removed and a new CVC placed percutaneously in a new site; if the tract is not colonized, the newly exchanged CVC can remain in the old insertion site.

Although small studies have found some utility of guidewire exchange in the management of CVCs suspected of being infected,[169-172] we believe that, in the absence of randomized studies demonstrating its safety, guidewire exchange generally should not be performed if there is suspicion of IVDR BSI, especially if there are signs of local infection such as purulence or erythema at the insertion site, or signs of systemic sepsis without a source. In these cases, the old catheter should be removed and cultured, and a new catheter should be inserted in a new site.

Replacing the Delivery System

Whereas most infusion-related BSIs are caused by infection of the device used for vascular access, infusate can become contaminated and cause occasional endemic BSIs.[24,173] If an infusion runs continuously for an extended period, the cumulative risk of contamination increases, and there is further risk that contaminants can grow to concentrations that could produce BSI in the recipient of the fluid. For more than 25 years, most U.S. hospitals have routinely replaced the entire delivery system of patients' IV infusions at 24- or 48-hour intervals[174] to reduce the risk of BSI from extrinsically contaminated fluid. Prospective studies indicate that IV delivery systems need not be replaced more frequently than every 72–96 hours, including infusions used for total parenteral nutrition or any infusions in ICU patients;[162,175] extending the duration of use permits considerable cost savings to hospitals.[175]

Four clinical settings might be regarded as exceptions to using 72 hours as an interval for routine set change:[175] (1) administration of blood products or (2) lipid emulsion; and (3) arterial pressure monitoring or 4) an epidemic of infusion-related BSI is suspected. In these circumstances, it may be most prudent that administration sets be changed routinely at 24- or 48-hour intervals.

Arterial infusions used for hemodynamic monitoring seem to be more vulnerable to becoming contaminated during use and producing endemic[173] or epidemic septicemia,[176] caused by gram-negative bacilli. If the infusion for hemodynamic monitoring is set up so that the fluid flows continuously through the chamber dome, thus eliminating a blind stagnant column of fluid, extrinsic contamination seems to be greatly reduced and may even eliminate the need to replace the administration set, chamber dome, and other components of the system at frequent intervals.[177-180] If disposable transducers and chamber domes are used, there seems to be no need to replace the transducer assembly and other components of the delivery system more frequently than every 4 days,[177] and it may be safe to replace even less frequently.[178-180]

Anticoagulants and Thrombolytics

Thrombus formation on an intravascular device is associated with an increased risk of infection.[181-184] Two prospective studies have been performed to examine the efficacy of warfarin anticoagulation for reducing rates of IVDR thrombosis with long-term IVDs.[185,186] Both studies found that use of warfarin in a dose of 1 mg/day was associated with significantly reduced rates of thrombosis with long-term IVDs, although no data were provided on rates of IVDR BSI.

The use of prophylactic heparin for reducing rates of IVDR thrombosis and infection has been evaluated in a meta-analysis.[187] Evaluating a variety of different administration techniques from 14 randomized controlled studies, Randolph et al showed that heparin significantly reduced the risk of IVDR thrombosis (RR = 0.43, CI = 0.23–0.78) and device colonization (RR

Intravascular Device Infections

Copyright © 2005, Association for Professionals in Infection Control and Epidemiology, Inc.

= 0.18, CI = 0.06–0.6) but failed to show a reduction in IVDR BSIs. Heparin-bonded pulmonary artery catheters may be less prone to IVDR BSI than non-heparinized catheters.[24,188–190]

Based on the above studies, low-level anticoagulation with warfarin is warranted for long-term IVDs as long as there is no contraindication (bleeding diathesis, brain tumor, or predilection to falls) and the INR is maintained below 1.6.[185] For short-term IVDs, the use of low-dose subcutaneous heparin is more appropriate, as it is commonly given to patients with CVCs or arterial lines as part of hospital thromboembolism prophylaxis.[191]

The prophylactic installation of urokinase (5000 IU/mL) into long-term IVDs every 1–2 weeks has been shown to significantly reduce the incidence of thrombotic complications.[192] Less clear is the effect of prophylactic use of thrombolytics on risk of IVDR. One study found a reduced risk of infection with weekly urokinase;[192] however, a more recent study failed to identify any benefit.[193]

Use of Novel Technology

Despite compliance with recommended guidelines, many centers continue to have high rates of IVDR BSI. Here, novel technology holds much promise (Table 24–8). Innovative technologies designed to reduce the risk of IVDR BSI have proven not only to be effective but also reduce healthcare costs, both with short-term and long-term IVDs.[20,194]

Novel Securement Devices: Recently, a novel sutureless device for securing noncuffed vascular catheters has become available (StatLock, manufactured by Venetec International). In a randomized trial of the device, premature loss of pediatric PICCs due to accidental extrusion and PICC-associated thrombosis were significantly reduced,[195] and in two additional trials the incidence of catheter-related BSI was significantly reduced with the use of the novel securement device, both in adults and children with PICCs.[195,196]

The promise of this device for reducing infection may derive from elimination of a festering skin suture wound contiguous to the newly inserted catheter and minimizing to-and-from movement of the catheter, which may promote invasion of the tract by cutaneous microorganisms through capillary action.[197]

Novel Dressings: Studies of polyurethane dressings, which contain antiseptic such as povidone-iodine or ionized silver, have been disappointing. However, based on the demonstrated superiority of chlorhexidine for cutaneous disinfection of access sites, a novel chlorhexidine-impregnated sponge dressing has been developed (Biopatch®, manufactured by Johnson and Johnson Medical) that maintains a very high concentration of the antiseptic on the insertion site under the dressing. The largest study to date found that use of the chlorhexidine-impregnated sponge dressing was associated with a 60% reduction in catheter-related BSI (RR = 0.37, p = 0.01).[198] Whereas there were no adverse side effects associated with the use of this dressing in this trial in adults, a subsequent pediatric trial found that ~15% of low-birth-weight neonates developed local dermatotoxicity.[199]

Anti-Infective Impregnated Catheters

Intravascular devices directly coated or impregnated with antimicrobials or antiseptics have been intensively studied over the past decade. Eighteen randomized trials evaluating the efficacy of chlorhexidine-silver sulfadiazine- or minocycline-rifampin-impregnated CVCs have been published in full article or abstract form since 1994.[36,37,77,83,113,200-212]

Twelve of the 16 published studies that examined the effect of antimicrobial-impregnated CVCs on rates of CVC-related BSI found either a statistically significant reduction[36,37,83] or a strong trend toward a reduction in rates of CVC-related BSI.[200,202,203,206-210,212] Aggregate analyses of the 15 studies that compared antimicrobial-impregnated CVCs to non-impregnated CVCs,[36,37,113,200,202-212] encompassing a total of 4,250 CVCs, show that antimicrobial-impregnated CVCs are associated with a 40% reduction in CVC-related BSI (61 BSIs/2;XC129 devices versus 101 BSIs/2;XC118 devices, OR 0.60, 95% CI = 0.44–0.82, p = 0.001), a result remarkably similar to the findings of three published meta-analyses.[20,213,214]

Finally, two rigorous and sophisticated economic analyses have found that antimicrobial-impregnated CVCs are cost-effective.[215,216] Veenstra et al. showed that antimicrobial-impregnated CVCs remained cost effective even if the cost of a CVC-related BSI was as low as $687 per case; cost savings were $196 per antimicrobial-impregnated CVC when a more realistic cost of a CVC-related BSI of $9,738 was used in the analysis.[215] Shorr et al. showed that use of antimicrobial-impregnated CVCs was associated with a cost savings of $9,600 per CVC-related BSI prevented, and $165 to $280 would be saved for every patient who received an antimicrobial-impregnated CVC.[216]

On the basis of this large body of data, two national advisory panels have recommended the use of antimicrobial-impregnated CVCs *in clinical settings where, despite rigorous application of other preventative interventions, rates of IVDR remain unacceptably high* (i.e., ≥3.3 BSIs per 1,000 IVD days).[106,217]

Copyright © 2005, Association for Professionals in Infection Control and Epidemiology, Inc.

Table 24-8. Summary of CDC HICPAC Guideline for prevention of intravascular device-related bloodstream infection*.

Recommendation	Strength of Evidence**
General measures	
Educate all health care workers involved with IVD care and maintenance	IA
Ensure adequate nursing staffing levels in ICUs	IB
Surveillance	
Monitor institutional IVD infection rates of IVD-related BSI	IA
Express rates of CVC-related BSI per 1000 CVC-days	IB
At catheter insertion	
Aseptic technique:	IA
Hygienic hand care before insertion or manipulation of any IVD	IC
Clean or sterile gloves during insertion and manipulation of noncentral IVDs	IA
Maximal barrier precautions during insertion of CVCs: mask, cap, sterile gown, gloves, drapes	IA
Dedicated IVD team strongly recommended	IA
Cutaneous antisepsis: 1st choice, chlorhexidine; however, tincture of iodine, an iodophor or 70% alcohol are acceptable (no recommendations for use of chlorhexidine in infants less than 2 months, unresolved issue)	IA
In adults, other than hemodialysis catheters (jugular site preference), use a subclavian site rather than a jugular or femoral site for CVC access (in pediatric patients, no recommendations for preferred site, unresolved issue).	IA
Use of sutureless securement device	NR
Sterile gauze or a semipermeable polyurethane dressing to cover site	IA
No systemic or topical antibiotics at insertion	IA
Maintenance	
Remove IVD as soon as no longer required	IA
Monitor IVD site daily	IB
Change dressing of CVC insertion site at least weekly	II
Do not use topical antibiotic ointments	IA
Change needless IV systems at least as frequently as the administration set; replace caps no more frequently than every 3 days or per manufactures' recommendations	II
Complete lipid infusions within 12 hours	IB
Replace administration sets no more frequently than every 72 hours. When lipid-containing admixtures or blood products are given, sets should be replaced every 24 hours; with propofol, every 6–12 hours	IA
Replace peripheral IVs every 72–96 hours	IB
Do not routinely replace CVCs or PICCs solely for prevention of infection	IB
Do not remove CVCs or PICCs solely because of fever unless IVD infection is suspected but replace catheter if there is purulence at the exit site, especially if the patient is hemodynamically unstable and IVD-related BSI is suspected.	II
Technology	
Use antimicrobial-coated or antiseptic-impregnated CVC in adult patients if institutional rate of BSI is high despite consistent application of preventive measures and catheter likely to remain in place > 5 days (no data or recommendations for pediatric patients)	IB
Use chlorhexidine-impregnated sponge dressing for adolescent or adult patients with uncuffed CVCs or other catheters likely to remain in place> 5 days (no recommendation for children, do not use in neonates <7 days old or gestational age < 26 weeks)	NR
Use prophylactic antibiotic lock solution *only* in patients with long-term IVDs who have continued to experience IVD-related BSIs despite consistent application of infection control practices	II

* Adapted from the Infection Control Practice Advisory Committee (HICPAC) Guideline for the Prevention of IVD-related Infection.[106] Abbreviations: BSI-bloodstream infection; CVC-central venous catheter, IV-intravenous, IVD-intravascular device

** Taken from CDC/HICPAC system of weighting recommendations based on scientific evidence. **IA**, strongly recommended for implementation and supported by well designed experimental, clinical or epidemiological studies. **IB**, strongly recommended for implementation and supported by some experimental, clinical, or epidemiological studies and a strong theoretical rationale. **IC**, required by state or federal regulations, rules or standards. **II**, suggested for implementation and supported by suggestive clinical or epidemiological trials or a theoretical rationale. **Unresolved issue**, an unresolved issue for which evidence is insufficient or no consensus regarding efficacy exists. **NR**, no recommendation for or against at this time.

Antimicrobial Lock Solutions

Given the importance of hub contamination and intraluminal colonization in the genesis of IVDR BSI with long-term IVDs, intraluminal installation of an antibiotic or antiseptic solution has the potential to reduce the risk of BSI associated with these devices. Six randomized, prospective trials have examined a vancomycin-containing antibiotic lock solution for the prevention of IVDR BSI, the largest of which found that use of a vancomycin or vancomycin/ciprofloxacin lock solution reduced the risk of IVDR BSI nearly 80% ($p \leq$ 0.005).[183] Concern about the emergence of resistance with prophylactic antibiotic-containing lock solutions

Copyright © 2005, Association for Professionals in Infection Control and Epidemiology, Inc.

has limited their acceptance to date. However, the use of prophylactic antibiotic lock solution is considered acceptable in the HICPAC guideline if a patient with an essential long-term IVD has continued to experience recurrent IVDR BSIs despite consistent application of infection control practices.[106]

A variety of other prophylactic lock solutions have been studied as a means of preventing IVDR BSI, including trisodium citrate/gentamicin,[218] minocycline/ethylenediaminetetraacetic acid (EDTA),[219] ethanol,[220] and taurolidine containing solutions.[221,222] Concerns about increased IVD complication rates[222] and drug-related toxicity[218] associated with the use of certain types of lock solutions combined with the limited number of patients who have been studied while receiving these agents preclude their routine use at this time.

Catheter Hubs

A novel catheter hub that contains a chamber filled with iodinated alcohol has been shown to be effective in preventing colonization of IVDs in an animal model.[223] Use of this same hub model in some clinical studies has demonstrated significantly lower rates of IVD colonization compared to IVDs with control hubs.[224,225] One clinical trial has also demonstrated reduced rates of IVDR BSIs (4% versus 16%, $p = <0.01$)[224] with use of this hub. A subsequent study also showed a reduction in hub-related IVDR BSIs (1.7% versus 7%, $p < 0.049$); however, overall rates of IVDR BSIs in both groups were similar,[225] and another study was unable to find any benefit with regard to IVD colonization or IVDR BSI with use of the novel hub.[226] This device is not yet available in the United States; until further studies conclusively demonstrate its benefit, its use cannot be recommended at this time.

Prevention of IVDR BSI in Resource-Poor Countries

Many of the aforementioned technologies, including anti-infective-impregnated catheters and antimicrobial lock solutions, are not viable options for the prevention of IVDR BSIs in resource-poor countries. Despite this, a number of studies have demonstrated marked decreases in rates of IVDR BSI with simple interventions that enhance standard infection control practices such as hand washing and IVD tubing and insertion site maintenance.[227,228] The results of these and other studies suggest that a large proportion of bloodstream infections can be prevented by changes in healthcare workers' behavior; thus, significant reductions in IVDR BSIs should be achievable even in the absence of new medical technologies.

TREATMENT OF IVDR BSI

Management of the Device

Short-Term IVDs.

If a short-term vascular catheter is suspected of being infected because the patient has no obvious other source of infection to explain fever, there is inflammation at the insertion site. If cryptogenic staphylococcal bacteremia or candidemia has been documented, blood cultures should be obtained and *the catheter should be removed and cultured* (Table 24–9). Failure to remove an infected catheter puts the patient at risk of developing septic thrombophlebitis with peripheral IV catheters, septic thrombosis of a great central vein with CVCs,[229,230] or even endocarditis. Continued access, if necessary, can be established with a new catheter inserted in a new site. *A new catheter should never be placed in an old site over a guidewire if the first catheter is suspected of being infected, especially if there is purulence at the site.*

Long-Term IVDs

BSI that might have originated from a cuffed and tunneled CVC does not automatically mandate removal of the device unless there has been persistent exit site infection; the tunnel is obviously infected; there is evidence of complicating endocarditis, septic thrombosis, or septic pulmonary emboli, the infecting pathogen is *S. aureus*, *Corynebacterium* JK, a *Bacillus* species, *Stenotrophomonas* spp., *Burkholderia cepacia* and all pseudomonal species, a filamentous fungus or *Malassezia* species, or a mycobacterial species; or bacteremia or candidemia persists for more than 3 days despite adequate therapy (Table 24–9).[231]

Intravascular device-related BSI caused by *S. aureus* must always prompt removal of the IVD, even if signs of bacteremia have resolved following antimicrobial therapy, because of the significant risk of infectious endocarditis (IE) or other metastatic infection if bacteremia recurs.[232-234] Authors of several small nonrandomized studies in patients with cuffed and tunneled hemodialysis catheters that subsequently became infected with various organisms, including *S. aureus*, have reportedly been able to successfully replace infected catheters by guidewire exchange and achieve cure rates in the range of 75–82% when combined with systemic antibiotics.[170,235,236] Although this approach may allow preservation of an access site and minimize mechanical complications, randomized studies are needed to show whether guidewire exchange of infected catheters has a long-term success rate comparable to removal of the infected IVD and placement of a new catheter at another site.

Likewise, we believe that patients with IVDR candidemia should have their catheter removed in most situ-

Copyright © 2005, Association for Professionals in Infection Control and Epidemiology, Inc.

Table 24-9. Algorithm for diagnosis and management of intravascular device-related bloodstream infection.*

- Examine the patient thoroughly, to identify unrelated sources of infection.

- Carefully examine all catheter insertion sites; gram stain and culture any expressible purulence from.

- Obtain *two* 10 to 15-mL cultures:
  If standard (nonquantitative) blood cultures, draw one by *percutaneous peripheral* venipuncture and one through the suspect IVD.
  If quantitative blood culture techniques are available (e.g., the Isolator® system), catheter-drawn cultures can enhance the diagnostic specificity of blood culturing in diagnosis of line sepsis. However, a peripheral percutaneous quantitative blood culture *must* be drawn *concomitantly*.

- Option regarding a peripheral IV or arterial catheter: *remove and culture catheter.*

- Options regarding a short-term central venous catheter:
  Purulence at insertion site or no purulence, but patient *floridly septic, without obvious source:*
  Remove and culture catheter.
  Gram stain purulence.
  Re-establish access at new site.

  No purulence, patient not floridly septic:
  Leave catheter in place, pending results of blood cultures.
      or
  Remove and culture catheter, re-establish needed access at new site.

- Options regarding surgically implanted, cuffed Hickman-type catheters.
  Remove at outset if:
  Infecting organism known to be *S. aureus, Bacillus* spp., JK *Diptheroid, Mycobacterium* species or filamentous fungus.
  Refractory or progressive exit-site infection, despite antimicrobial therapy, especially with *Pseudomonas aeruginosa.*
  Tunnel infected.
  Evidence of septic thrombosis of cannulated central vein or septic pulmonary emboli.
  Evidence of endocarditis.

  Remove later on if:
  Any of the above become manifest.
  BSI persists ≥3 days, despite IV antimicrobial therapy through catheter.

- Options regarding surgically-implanted subcutaneous central ports (e.g., Portacath):
  Cellulitis without documented bacteremia: begin antimicrobial therapy, *withhold removing port.*
  Aspirate from port shows organisms on gram-stain or heavy growth in quantitative culture, or documented port related bacteremia: *remove port.*

- Decision on whether to begin antimicrobial therapy, before culture results available, based on clinical assessment and/or gram stain of exit site or the blood drawn from a long-term IVD.

- With no microbiologic data to guide antimicrobial selection in a septic patient with suspected line sepsis, consider:
  IV vancomycin and ciprofloxacin, cefepime, or imipenem/meropenem.

* Adapted from Maki.[231]

ations.[237] Several studies have reported successful treatment of IVD BSIs due to *Candida* spp. without IVD removal with prolonged courses of amphotericin B administered through the catheter;[238] however, this is in contrast to the results of other prospective studies that have found an increased duration of candidemia and mortality in patients who retain their infected IVD.[239]

Studies using 7–21 days of antibiotics infused through the infected line, primarily with BSIs caused by coagulase-negative staphylococci, have shown success rates of 60–91% without catheter removal,[230] although there was considerable variability in the clinical response, depending on the infecting microorganism. With coagulase-negative staphylococcal BSIs, the risk of recurrent bacteremia has been approximately 20%.[240]

In small, uncontrolled clinical trials of "antibiotic lock therapy" (ALT), usually in conjunction with systemic antibiotic therapy, cure rates of infected IVDs in excess of 90% have been reported.[241-253] The vast majority of IVDs reported in these studies were infected with coagulase-negative staphylococci and fermenting gram-negative bacilli; therefore, at this time, ALT cannot be recommended for the management of long-term IVDs infected by *S. aureus, Bacillus* sp., *Corynebacterium* JK, *Stenotrophomonas* spp., *B. cepacia*, all pseudomonas species, fungi, or mycobacterial species. Table 24–10 lists the types of lock solutions that have been studied most extensively, although lack of data limits recommending one solution over another. Obviously, if IVDR BSI recurs after an attempt to salvage the IVD with ALT, the device should be removed.

Intravascular Device Infections

Copyright © 2005, Association for Professionals in Infection Control and Epidemiology, Inc.

Table 24-10. Formulations of various antibiotic-containing lock solutions reported in the medical literature.*

Drug	Dosage	Dwell Time	Duration of Therapy	Stability with Heparin Solutions
Vancomycin	1–5 mg/mL	8–24 hours	7–15 days	Heparin 10 to 100 units/mL, has been shown to be safe when coadministered with low dose vancomycin (1–5 mg/mL) High dose vancomycin (83 mg/mL) has been used successfully **without** co-administration of heparin.[249]
Teicoplanin	133 mg/mL	24 hours	5–9 days	Heparin 10 units/mL
Gentamicin	1–13.3 mg/mL	8–72 hours	5–21 days	Gentamicin precipitates rapidly in heparin solutions when gentamicin doses ≥ 5 mg/mL are used. A single study has reported the stability of 1mg/mL of gentamicin in solutions with heparin concentrations as high as 2500 units/mL.[278]
Amikacin	1.5–2 mg/mL	12–24 hours	6–27 days	Most studies have not addressed the issue of stability of amikacin with heparin. A single study utilizing amikacin concentrations as high as 40 mg/mL reported no drug precipitation in heparin (100 units/mL) although formal stability studies were not performed.[244]

* Adapted, in part, from Berrington and Gould.[279]

Historically, surgically implanted subcutaneous central ports have rarely proven to be curable with medical therapy alone, especially if the device itself is clearly infected (e.g., an aspirate from the port shows heavy growth).[254-256] In vitro studies of several antibiotic lock solutions in simulated models of subcutaneous central ports raise the possibility of using ALT to preserve the use of these long-term devices when they become infected.[257,258] A recent study of patients with AIDS with surgically implanted ports who developed IVDR BSI found that ALT combined with systemic antibiotic therapy resulted in 70% of the ports being salvaged; however, long-term follow-up data on surveillance cultures of the ports were not reported.[259] The only other clinical study of the utilization of ALT in subcutaneous central port infections achieved salvage rates less than 50%.[260] Based on the marginal efficacy of ALT in these two studies and the historically poor cure rate achieved with systemic antibiotics alone, definitive treatment of infected subcutaneous central ports requires removal of the infected device.

Anti-Infective Therapy

The selection of an initial antimicrobial regimen for a septic patient in general is influenced by (1) whether the presumed infection was acquired in the community or is institutionally acquired, (2) the age of the patient, and (3) whether the patient is immunocompromised, especially granulocytopenic (<1,000 per mm³).[231]

If IVDR BSI is suspected (Table 24–6) after cultures have been obtained, the combination of IV vancomycin (for staphylococci resistant to methicillin) with a fluoroquinolone (preferably ciprofloxacin, cefepime, or imipenem/meropenem for multiresistant nosocomial

gram-negative bacilli) should prove effective against the bacterial pathogens most likely to be encountered (Figure 24–2). Initial therapy can then be modified based on the ultimate microbiologic identification and susceptibilities of the infecting organisms.

How long to treat IVDR BSI will be influenced by the infecting microorganism and by whether the patient has underlying valvular heart disease, has evidence of endocarditis or septic thrombosis, or shows evidence of metastatic infection. If endocarditis is suspected, transesophageal echocardiography offers superior sensitivity and discrimination for detecting vegetations, as compared with transthoracic echocardiography.[234] *In patients with high-grade bacteremia or fungemia, but without clinical or echocardiographic evidence of endocarditis, septic thrombosis should be suspected.*[230] Central venous thrombosis can now be diagnosed by venography,[230] ultrasonography,[261] magnetic resonance imaging,[262] or computed tomography.[263]

Although there are no prospective data to guide the optimal duration of antimicrobial therapy for IVDR BSIs, most coagulase-negative staphylococcal infections can be cured with only 5–7 days of therapy,[39,240] whereas most infections caused by other microorganisms can be adequately treated with 10–14 days of antimicrobial therapy.[39] These recommendations hold only as long as there are no complications related to the infection and the BSI clears within 72 hours of initiating therapy. Nosocomial enterococcal bacteremia deriving from an IVD is rarely associated with persistent endovascular infection, and unless there is clinical or echocardiographic evidence of endocar-

APIC Text of Infection Control and Epidemiology

Copyright © 2005, Association for Professionals in Infection Control and Epidemiology, Inc.

ditis, treatment with IV ampicillin or vancomycin alone for 7–14 days should suffice.[264]

The management of *S. aureus* device-related infection deserves special mention, as there have been no prospective studies to evaluate the optimal duration of therapy for IVDR BSIs caused by this ubiquitous human pathogen. Historically, high rates of associated IE and late complications led to a universal policy of 4–6 weeks of antimicrobial therapy for *all* patients with *S. aureus* bacteremia. Earlier diagnosis and initiation of bactericidal therapy of nosocomial *S. aureus* BSIs in recent years have been associated with lower rates of IE and metastatic complications, prompting suggestions that short-course therapy (i.e., 14 days) is effective and safe for most patients with *S. aureus* IVDR BSI, as long as the patient defervesces within 72 hours and there is no evidence of metastatic infection.[265] In a study of transesophageal echocardiography (TEE) in 103 hospitalized patients with *S. aureus* bacteremia, 69 related to an IVD, Fowler et al found a surprisingly high incidence of endocarditis, 23%, with IVDR *S. aureus* BSI.[234] In a more recent report, these authors have reported that the routine use of TEE with IVDR *S. aureus* BSI, as a means to stratify patients into short-course or long-course therapy, is cost effective.[266] However, at this time there are no prospective studies to affirm this approach. Until more data are available, short-course therapy for IVDR *S. aureus* bacteremia therapy should be approached with caution and used only when the TEE is unequivocally negative and the patient has defervesced within 72 hours of removing the IVD and starting anti-infective therapy.

We believe strongly that *all* patients with IVDR candidemia should be treated, even if the patient becomes afebrile and blood cultures spontaneously revert to negative following removal of the catheter without antifungal therapy.[237,267,268] IVDR candidemia that responds rapidly to removal of the catheter and institution of IV amphotericin B can be reliably treated with a daily dose of 0.3–0.5 mg/kg and a total dose of 3–5 mg/kg.[267] If a lipid-associated formulation of amphotericin B is being used, a daily dose of 1–2 mg/kg and total dose of 10–20 mg/kg should be sufficient in most cases.[269] If the patient has septic thrombosis of central vein, associated with high-grade candidemia and florid sepsis, a higher dose of IV amphotericin B is recommended (0.7 mg/kg/day and ≥20 mg/kg total of conventional amphotericin, and 2–3 mg/kg/day and 20–30 mg/kg total for a lipid-associated formulation).

Fluconazole (400 mg/day) has been shown to be as effective as IV amphotericin B in randomized trials in non-neutropenic patients;[270] it has further been shown to be comparable to amphotericin B in observational studies of neutropenic patients with *Candida* IVDR BSIs[269] but should not be used in IVDR BSIs associated with septic thrombosis and high-grade candidemia or BSIs caused by azole-resistant *Candida* species.

Infections caused by fluconazole-resistant organisms, such as *Candida krusei* and *Candida glabrata* have become an all too common phenomenon, with many centers reporting that >50% of their *Candida* isolates are non-albicans species that are usually resistant to azoles.[271] In these centers, fluconazole may not be the best drug to use for initial therapy of nosocomial yeast BSIs, pending identification of the infecting species. Moreover, the toxicity of amphotericin B has prompted a search for new classes of antifungals. The echinocandins are novel antifungals that inhibit the synthesis of β-1,3-glucan, a component of fungal cell walls.[272] Caspofungin, the first drug approved from this class, was recently shown to be at least as effective as IV amphotericin B in a prospective randomized double-blind trial in patients with deep candida infections, most of whom had candidemia;[273] most notably, caspofungin was associated with a greatly reduced rate of study drug withdrawal because of adverse events (2.6% versus 23.2%, $p = 0.003$). We believe that IV caspofungin, which has a low incidence of side effects and can be given once daily, can be considered a first-line drug for initial treatment of IVDR BSI caused by yeasts in centers with high rates of infection caused by non-albicans species, pending identification and susceptibility of the bloodstream isolate.

All patients with an IVDR BSI must be monitored closely for at least 6 weeks after completing therapy, especially if they have had high-grade bacteremia or candidemia, to detect late-appearing endocarditis,[230,274,275] retinitis,[274,276] or other metastatic infection such as vertebral osteomyelitis.

IV. SUMMARY AND CONCLUSIONS

In recent years, the factors associated with an increased risk of IVDR BSI have become better delineated. These include prolonged hospitalization, severity of illness, and clinical states such as underlying neutropenia, AIDS, and bone marrow transplantation. However, the features of the IVD, its insertion, and its maintenance seem to have far greater impact on the overall risk of infection. Measures for preventing IVDR BSI, and any nosocomial infection, must be based on the best understanding of pathophysiology and epidemiology and, whenever possible, controlled clinical trials.

Copyright © 2005, Association for Professionals in Infection Control and Epidemiology, Inc.

REFERENCES

1. Crnich CJ, Maki DG: The role of intravascular devices in sepsis, *Curr Infect Dis Rep* 3:497–506, 2001.
2. Maki D, Mermel L. Infections due to infusion therapy. In Bennett JV, Brachman PS, editors: *Hospital infections*, ed 4, Philadelphia, 1998, Lippincott-Raven, pp 689–724.
3. Mermel LA: Prevention of intravascular catheter-related infections, *Ann Intern Med* 132:391–402, 2000.
4. Pittet D, Tarara D, Wenzel R: Nosocomial bloodstream infection in critically ill patients: excess length of stay, extra costs, and attributable mortality, *JAMA* 271:1598–601, 1994.
5. Digiovine B, Chenoweth C, Watts C, et al: The attributable mortality and costs of primary nosocomial bloodstream infections in the intensive care unit, *Am J Respir Crit Care Med* 160: 976–81, 1999.
6. Soufir L, Timsit JF, Mahe C, et al: Attributable morbidity and mortality of catheter-related septicemia in critically ill patients: a matched, risk-adjusted, cohort study, *Infect Control Hosp Epidemiol* 20:396–401, 1999.
7. Rello J, Ochagavia A, Sabanes E, et al: Evaluation of outcome of intravenous catheter-related infections in critically ill patients, *Am J Respir Crit Care Med* 162:1027–30, 2000.
8. Kluger D, Maki D: The relative risk of intravascular device-related bloodstream infections with different types of intravascular devices in adults: a meta-analysis of 206 published studies (abstract), *Infect Control Hosp Epidemiol* 21:95–6, 2000.
9. CDC: National Nosocomial Infections Surveillance (NNIS) System report, data summary from January 1990 to May 1999, issued June 1999, *Am J Infect Control* 27:520–32, 1999.
10. Joint Commission on the Accreditation of Healthcare Organizations: Accreditation manual for hospitals. Chicago, 1994, JCAHO, pp 121–140.
11. Safdar N, Maki DG: The risk of catheter-related bloodstream infection with peripherally-inserted central venous catheters used in inpatients (abstract K-1435). *Abstracts and proceedings from the 41st international conference of antimicrobial agents and chemotherapy*, Washington, DC, 2001, ASM Press, p 428.
12. Safdar N, Maki DG: The incidence and pathogenesis of catheter-related bloodstream infection with arterial catheters (abstract K-81). *Abstracts and proceedings from the 42nd interscience conference on antimicrobial agents and chemotherapy*, Washington, DC, 2002, ASM Press, p 299.
13. Safdar N, Kluger DM, Maki DG: A review of risk factors for catheter-related bloodstream infection caused by percutaneously inserted, noncuffed central venous catheters: implications for preventive strategies, *Medicine* 81:466–79, 2002.
14. Elishoov H, Or R, Strauss N, et al: Nosocomial colonization, septicemia, and Hickman/Broviac catheter-related infections in bone marrow transplant recipients: a 5-year prospective study, *Medicine* 77:83–101, 1998.
15. Tacconelli E, Tumbarello M, Pittiruti M, et al: Central venous catheter-related sepsis in a cohort of 366 hospitalised patients, *Eur J Clin Microbiol Infect Dis* 16:203–9, 1997.
16. Astagneau P, Maugat S, Tran-Minh T, et al: Long-term central venous catheter infection in HIV-infected and cancer patients: a multicenter cohort study, *Infect Control Hosp Epidemiol* 20: 494–8, 1999.
17. Tokars JI, Cookson ST, McArthur MA, et al: Prospective evaluation of risk factors for bloodstream infection in patients receiving home infusion therapy, *Ann Intern Med* 131:340–7, 1999.
18. Merrer J, De Jonghe B, Golliot F, et al: Complications of femoral and subclavian venous catheterization in critically ill patients: a randomized controlled trial, *JAMA* 286:700–7, 2001.
19. Robert J, Fridkin SK, Blumberg HM, et al: The influence of the composition of the nursing staff on primary bloodstream infection rates in a surgical intensive care unit, *Infect Control Hosp Epidemiol* 21:12–7, 2000.
20. Crnich CJ, Maki DG: The promise of novel technology for the prevention of intravascular device-related bloodstream infection: I. pathogenesis and short-term devices, *Clin Infect Dis* 34: 1232–42, 2002.
21. Cooper GL, Hopkins CC: Rapid diagnosis of intravascular catheter-associated infection by direct Gram staining of catheter segments, *N Engl J Med* 312:1142–7, 1985.
22. Cheesbrough JS, Finch RG, Burden RP: A prospective study of the mechanisms of infection associated with hemodialysis catheters, *J Infect Dis* 154:579–89, 1986.
23. Maki DG, Cobb L, Garman JK, et al: An attachable silver-impregnated cuff for prevention of infection with central venous catheters: a prospective randomized multicenter trial, *Am J Med* 85: 307–14, 1988.
24. Mermel LA, McCormick RD, Springman SR, et al: The pathogenesis and epidemiology of catheter-related infection with pulmonary artery Swan-Ganz catheters: a prospective study utilizing molecular subtyping, *Am J Med* 91:197S—205S, 1991.
25. Linares J, Sitges-Serra A, Garau J, et al: Pathogenesis of catheter sepsis: a prospective study with quantitative and semiquantitative cultures of catheter hub and segments, *J Clin Microbiol* 21:357–60, 1985.
26. Raad I, Costerton W, Sabharwal U, et al: Ultrastructural analysis of indwelling vascular catheters: a quantitative relationship between luminal colonization and duration of placement, *J Infect Dis* 168:400–7, 1993.
27. Sitges-Serra A, Pi-Suner T, Garces JM, et al: Pathogenesis and prevention of catheter-related septicemia, *Am J Infect Control* 23:310–6, 1995.
28. Maki D, Ringer M: Prospective study of arterial catheter-related infection: incidence, sources of infection and risk factors (abstract). *Abstracts and proceedings from the 29th interscience conference on antimicrobial agents and chemotherapy*, Washington, DC, 1989, ASM Press, p 1075.
29. Maki DG, Ringer M, Alvarado CJ: Prospective randomized trial of povidone-iodine, alcohol, and chlorhexidine for prevention of infection associated with central venous and arterial catheters. *Lancet* 338:339–43, 1991.
30. Maki DG: Nosocomial bacteremia: an epidemiologic overview. *Am J Med* 70:719–32, 1981.
31. Maki D: The epidemiology and prevention of nosocomial bloodstream infections (abstract). *Programs and abstracts of the third international conference on nosocomial infections.* Washington, DC, 1990, ASM Press, p 3.
32. Maki DG: Through a glass darkly. Nosocomial pseudoepidemics and pseudobacteremias. *Arch Intern Med* 140:26–8, 1980.
33. Maki DG, Kluger DM, Crnich CJ: The microbiology of intravascular device-related (IVDR) infection in adults: 1. an analysis of 159 prospective studies; 2. implications for prevention and treatment (abstract). *Abstracts and proceedings from the 40th annual meeting of the infectious disease society of america.* Chicago, 2002, Infectious Disease Society of America.
34. Garner JS, Jarvis WR, Emori TG, et al: CDC definitions for nosocomial infections, 1988. *Am J Infect Control* 16:128–40, 1988.
35. Maki DG, Stolz SS, Wheeler S, et al: A prospective, randomized trial of gauze and two polyurethane dressings for site care of pulmonary artery catheters: implications for catheter management. *Crit Care Med* 22:1729–37, 1994.
36. Maki DG, Stolz SM, Wheeler S, et al: Prevention of central venous catheter-related bloodstream infection by use of an antiseptic-impregnated catheter: a randomized, controlled trial. *Ann Intern Med* 127:257–66, 1997.
37. Raad I, Darouiche R, Dupuis J, et al: Central venous catheters coated with minocycline and rifampin for the prevention of catheter-related colonization and bloodstream infections: a randomized, double-blind trial. *Ann Intern Med* 127:267–74, 1997.
38. O'Grady NP, Barie PS, Bartlett J, et al: Practice parameters for evaluating new fever in critically ill adult patients. *Crit Care Med* 26:392–408, 1998.
39. Mermel LA, Farr BM, Sherertz RJ, et al: Guidelines for the management of intravascular catheter-related infections. *Clin Infect Dis* 32:1249–72, 2001.
40. Safdar N, Maki DG: Inflammation at the insertion site is not predictive of catheter-related bloodstream infection with short-term, noncuffed central venous catheters. *Crit Care Med* 30:2632–5, 2002.
41. Washington JAD: Ilstrup DM. Blood cultures: issues and controversies. *Rev Infect Dis* 8:792–802, 1986.
42. Mermel LA, Maki DG: Detection of bacteremia in adults: consequences of culturing an inadequate volume of blood. *Ann Intern Med* 119:270–2, 1993.
43. Dobbins BM, Kite P, Wilcox MH: Diagnosis of central venous catheter related sepsis—a critical look inside. *J Clin Pathol* 52: 165–72, 1999.

Copyright © 2005, Association for Professionals in Infection Control and Epidemiology, Inc.

44. Lamy B, Roy P, Carret G, et al: What is the relevance of obtaining multiple blood samples for culture? A comprehensive model to optimize the strategy for diagnosing bacteremia. *Clin Infect Dis* 35:842–50, 2002.

45. Weinstein MP, Murphy JR, Reller LB, et al: The clinical significance of positive blood cultures: a comprehensive analysis of 500 episodes of bacteremia and fungemia in adults: II. clinical observations, with special reference to factors influencing prognosis. *Rev Infect Dis* 5:54–70, 1983.

46. Gaur AH, Giannini MA, Flynn PM, et al: Optimizing blood culture practices in pediatric immunocompromised patients: evaluation of media types and blood culture volume. *Pediatr Infect Dis J* 22:545–52, 2003.

47. DesJardin J, Falagas M, Ruthazer R, et al: Clinical utility of blood cultures drawn from indwelling central venous catheters in hospitalized patients with cancer. *Ann Intern Med* 131:641–7, 1999.

48. Levin PD, Hersch M, Rudensky B, et al: The use of the arterial line as a source for blood cultures. *Intensive Care Med* 26:1350–4, 2000.

49. Martinez JA, DesJardin JA, Aronoff M, et al: Clinical utility of blood cultures drawn from central venous or arterial catheters in critically ill surgical patients. *Crit Care Med* 30:7–13, 2002.

50. Norberg A, Christopher NC, Ramundo ML, et al: Contamination rates of blood cultures obtained by dedicated phlebotomy vs intravenous catheter. *JAMA* 289:726–9, 2003.

51. Beutz M, Sherman G, Mayfield J, et al: Clinical utility of blood cultures drawn from central vein catheters and peripheral venipuncture in critically ill medical patients. *Chest* 123:854–61, 2003.

52. Robinson JL: Sensitivity of a blood culture drawn through a single lumen of a multilumen, long-term, indwelling, central venous catheter in pediatric oncology patients. *J Pediatr Hematol Oncol* 24:72–4, 2002.

53. Bates DW, Goldman L, Lee TH: Contaminant blood cultures and resource utilization: the true consequences of false-positive results. *JAMA* 265:365–9, 1991.

54. Little JR, Murray PR, Traynor PS, et al: A randomized trial of povidone-iodine compared with iodine tincture for venipuncture site disinfection: effects on rates of blood culture contamination. *Am J Med* 107:119–25, 1999.

55. Strand CL, Wajsbort RR, Sturmann K: Effect of iodophor vs iodine tincture skin preparation on blood culture contamination rate. *JAMA* 269:1004–6, 1993.

56. Mimoz O, Karim A, Mercat A, et al: Chlorhexidine compared with povidone-iodine as skin preparation before blood culture: a randomized, controlled trial. *Ann Intern Med* 131:834–7, 1999.

57. Calfee DP, Farr BM: Comparison of four antiseptic preparations for skin in the prevention of contamination of percutaneously drawn blood cultures: a randomized trial. *J Clin Microbiol* 40:1660–5, 2002.

58. Herwaldt LA, Geiss M, Kao C, et al: The positive predictive value of isolating coagulase-negative staphylococci from blood cultures. *Clin Infect Dis* 22:14–20, 1996.

59. Finkelstein R, Fusman R, Oren I, et al: Clinical and epidemiologic significance of coagulase-negative staphylococci bacteremia in a tertiary care university Israeli hospital. *Am J Infect Control* 30:21–5, 2002.

60. Maki DG, Jarrett F, Sarafin HW: A semiquantitative culture method for identification of catheter-related infection in the burn patient. *J Surg Res* 22:513–20, 1977.

61. Collignon PJ, Soni N, Pearson IY, et al: Is semiquantitative culture of central vein catheter tips useful in the diagnosis of catheter-associated bacteremia? *J Clin Microbiol* 24:532–5, 1986.

62. Brun-Buisson C, Abrouk F, Legrand P, et al: Diagnosis of central venous catheter-related sepsis. Critical level of quantitative tip cultures. *Arch Intern Med* 147:873–7, 1987.

63. Sherertz RJ, Raad, II, Belani A, et al: Three-year experience with sonicated vascular catheter cultures in a clinical microbiology laboratory. *J Clin Microbiol* 28:76–82, 1990.

64. Raad, II, Sabbagh MF, Rand KH, et al: Quantitative tip culture methods and the diagnosis of central venous catheter-related infections. *Diagn Microbiol Infect Dis* 15:13–20, 1992.

65. Sherertz RJ, Heard SO, Raad II: Diagnosis of triple-lumen catheter infection: comparison of roll plate, sonication, and flushing methodologies. *J Clin Microbiol* 35:641–6, 1997.

66. Siegman-Igra Y, Anglim AM, Shapiro DE, et al: Diagnosis of vascular catheter-related bloodstream infection: a meta-analysis. *J Clin Microbiol* 35:928–36, 1997.

67. Kristinsson KG, Burnett IA, Spencer RC: Evaluation of three methods for culturing long intravascular catheters. *J Hosp Infect* 14:183–91, 1989.

68. Maki DG, Mermel LA, Martin M, et al: A prospective comparison of semiquantitative and sonication cultures of catheter segments for diagnosis of central venous catheter-related bloodstream infection (abstract). *Abstracts and proceedings from the 36th interscience conference on antimicrobial agents and chemotherapy*. Washington, DC, 1996, ASM Press, p 228.

69. Capdevila JA: Catheter-related infection: an update on diagnosis, treatment, and prevention. *Int J Infect Dis* 2:230–6, 1998.

70. Collignon P, Chan R, Munro R: Rapid diagnosis of intravascular catheter-related infection. *Arch Intern Med* 147:1609–12, 1987.

71. Coutlee F, Lemieux C, Paradis JF: Value of direct catheter staining in the diagnosis of intravascular-catheter-related infection. *J Clin Microbiol* 26:1088–90, 1988.

72. Zufferey J, Rime B, Francioli P, et al: Simple method for rapid diagnosis of catheter-associated infection by direct acridine orange staining of catheter tips. *J Clin Microbiol* 26:175–7, 1988.

73. von Baum H, Philippi P, Geiss HK: Acridine-orange leucocyte cytospin (AOLC) test as an in-situ method for the diagnosis of central venous catheter (CVC)-related sepsis in adult risk patients. *Zentralblatt fur Bakteriologie* 287:117–23, 1998.

74. Markus S, Buday S: Culturing indwelling central venous catheters in situ. *Infect Surg* 1989:157–62, 1989.

75. Tighe MJ, Kite P, Fawley WN, et al: An endoluminal brush to detect the infected central venous catheter in situ: a pilot study. *Br Med J* 313:1528–9, 1996.

76. Kite P, Dobbins BM, Wilcox MH, et al: Evaluation of a novel endoluminal brush method for in situ diagnosis of catheter related sepsis. *J Clin Pathol* 50:278–82, 1997.

77. van Heerden PV, Webb SA, Fong S, et al: Central venous catheters revisited: infection rates and an assessment of the new fibrin analysing system brush. *Anaesth Intensive Care* 24:330–3, 1996.

78. Fan S, Teoh-Chan C, Lau K, et al: Predictive value of surveillance skin and hub cultures in central venous catheters sepsis. *J Hosp Infect* 12:191–8, 1988.

79. Cercenado E, Ena J, Rodriguez-Creixems M, et al: A conservative procedure for the diagnosis of catheter-related infections. *Arch Intern Med* 150:1417–20, 1990.

80. Raad, II, Baba M, Bodey GP: Diagnosis of catheter-related infections: the role of surveillance and targeted quantitative skin cultures. *Clin Infect Dis* 20:593–7, 1995.

81. Fortun J, Perez-Molina JA, Asensio A, et al: Semiquantitative culture of subcutaneous segment for conservative diagnosis of intravascular catheter-related infection. *J Parenter Enteral Nutr* 24:210–214, 2000.

82. John JF, Jr: Molecular analysis of nosocomial epidemics. *Infect Dis Clin North Am* 3:683–700, 1989.

83. Darouiche RO, Raad II, Heard SO, et al: A comparison of two antimicrobial-impregnated central venous catheters. *N Engl J Med* 340:1–8, 1999.

84. Ryan JJ, Abel R, Abbott W, et al: Catheter complications in total parenteral nutrition: a prospective study of 200 consecutive patients. *N Engl J Med* 290:757–61, 1974.

85. Padberg FT, Jr, Ruggiero J, Blackburn GL, et al: Central venous catheterization for parenteral nutrition. *Ann Surg* 193:264–70, 1981.

86. Bjornson HS, Colley R, Bower RH, et al: Association between microorganism growth at the catheter insertion site and colonization of the catheter in patients receiving total parenteral nutrition. *Surgery* 92:720–7, 1982.

87. Sitzmann JV, Townsend TR, Siler MC, et al: Septic and technical complications of central venous catheterization: a prospective study of 200 consecutive patients. *Ann Surg* 202:766–70, 1985.

88. Porter KA, Bistrian BR, Blackburn GL: Guidewire catheter exchange with triple culture technique in the management of catheter sepsis. *J Parenter Enteral Nutr* 12:628–632, 1988.

89. Gowardman JR, Montgomery C, Thirlwell S, et al: Central venous catheter-related bloodstream infections: an analysis of incidence and risk factors in a cohort of 400 patients. *Intensive Care Med* 24:1034–9, 1998.

90. Bouza E, Burillo A, Munoz P: Catheter-related infections: diagnosis and intravascular treatment. *Clin Microbiol Infect* 8:265–74, 2002.

Intravascular Device Infections

Copyright © 2005, Association for Professionals in Infection Control and Epidemiology, Inc.

91. Rogers MS, Oppenheim BA: The use of continuous monitoring blood culture systems in the diagnosis of catheter related sepsis. *J Clin Pathol* 51:635-7, 1998.

92. Blot F, Nitenberg G, Chachaty E, et al: Diagnosis of catheter-related bacteraemia: a prospective comparison of the time to positivity of hub-blood versus peripheral-blood cultures. *Lancet* 354:1071-7, 1999.

93. Blot F, Schmidt E, Nitenberg G, et al: Earlier positivity of central-venous- versus peripheral-blood cultures is highly predictive of catheter-related sepsis. *J Clin Microbiol* 36:105-9, 1998.

94. Moonens F, el Alami S, Van Gossum A, et al: Usefulness of gram staining of blood collected from total parenteral nutrition catheter for rapid diagnosis of catheter-related sepsis. *J Clin Microbiol* 32:1578-9, 1994.

95. Kite P, Dobbins BM, Wilcox MH, et al: Rapid diagnosis of central-venous-catheter-related bloodstream infection without catheter removal. *Lancet* 354:1504-7, 1999.

96. Bong JJ, Kite P, Ammori BJ, et al: The use of a rapid in situ test in the detection of central venous catheter-related bloodstream infection: a prospective study. *J Parenter Enteral Nutr* 27:146-50, 2003.

97. Telenti A, Steckelberg JM, Stockman L, et al: Quantitative blood cultures in candidemia. *Mayo Clin Proc* 66:1120-3, 1991.

98. Douard MC, Arlet G, Longuet P, et al: Diagnosis of venous access port-related infections. *Clin Infect Dis* 29:1197-202, 1999.

99. Haimi-Cohen Y, Vellozzi EM, Rubin LG: Initial concentration of Staphylococcus epidermidis in simulated pediatric blood cultures correlates with time to positive results with the automated, continuously monitored BACTEC blood culture system. *J Clin Microbiol* 40:898-901, 2002.

100. Malgrange VB, Escande MC, Theobald S: Validity of earlier positivity of central venous blood cultures in comparison with peripheral blood cultures for diagnosing catheter-related bacteremia in cancer patients. *J Clin Microbiol* 39:274-8, 2001.

101. Gaur AH, Flynn PM, Giannini MA, et al: Difference in time to detection: a simple method to differentiate catheter-related from non-catheter-related bloodstream infection in immunocompromised pediatric patients. *Clin Infect Dis* 37:469-75, 2003.

102. Seifert H, Cornely O, Seggewiss K, et al: Bloodstream infection in neutropenic cancer patients related to short-term nontunnelled catheters determined by quantitative blood cultures, differential time to positivity, and molecular epidemiological typing with pulsed-field gel electrophoresis. *J Clin Microbiol* 41:118-23, 2003.

103. Rijnders BJ, Verwaest C, Peetermans WE, et al: Difference in time to positivity of hub-blood versus nonhub-blood cultures is not useful for the diagnosis of catheter-related bloodstream infection in critically ill patients. *Crit Care Med* 29:1399-1403, 2001.

104. Rushforth JA, Hoy CM, Kite P, et al: Rapid diagnosis of central venous catheter sepsis. *Lancet* 342:402-3, 1993.

105. Maki D: Growth properties of microorganisms in infusion fluid and methods of detection. In Phillips I, editor: *Microbiologic hazards of intravenous therapy*. Lancaster, England, 1977, MTP Press, pp 13-47.

106. O'Grady NP, Alexander M, Dellinger EP, et al: Guidelines for the prevention of intravascular catheter-related infections. *Clin Infect Dis* 35:1281-1307, 2002.

107. Dezfulian C, Lavelle J, Nallamothu BK, et al: Rates of infection for single-lumen versus multilumen central venous catheters: a meta-analysis. *Crit Care Med* 31:2385-2390, 2003.

108. Collignon P, Soni N, Pearson I, et al: Sepsis associated with central vein catheters in critically ill patients. *Intensive Care Med* 14:227-31, 1988.

109. Richet H, Hubert B, Nitemberg G, et al: Prospective multicenter study of vascular-catheter-related complications and risk factors for positive central-catheter cultures in intensive care unit patients. *J Clin Microbiol* 28:2520-5, 1990.

110. Hagley MT, Martin B, Gast P, et al: Infectious and mechanical complications of central venous catheters placed by percutaneous venipuncture and over guidewires. *Crit Care Med* 20:1426-30, 1992.

111. Charalambous C, Swoboda SM, Dick J, et al: Risk factors and clinical impact of central line infections in the surgical intensive care unit. *Arch Surg* 133:1241-6, 1998.

112. Goetz AM, Wagener MM, Miller JM, et al: Risk of infection due to central venous catheters: effect of site of placement and catheter type. *Infect Control Hosp Epidemiol* 19:842-5, 1998.

113. Heard SO, Wagle M, Vijayakumar E, et al: Influence of triple-lumen central venous catheters coated with chlorhexidine and silver sulfadiazine on the incidence of catheter-related bacteremia. *Arch Intern Med* 158:81-7, 1998.

114. Trottier SJ, Veremakis C, O'Brien J, et al: Femoral deep vein thrombosis associated with central venous catheterization: results from a prospective, randomized trial. *Crit Care Med* 23:52-9, 1995.

115. Durbec O, Viviand X, Potie F, et al: Lower extremity deep vein thrombosis: a prospective, randomized, controlled trial in comatose or sedated patients undergoing femoral vein catheterization. *Crit Care Med* 25:1982-5, 1997.

116. Durbec O, Viviand X, Potie F, et al: A prospective evaluation of the use of femoral venous catheters in critically ill adults. *Crit Care Med* 25:1986-9, 1997.

117. Uldall PR, Merchant N, Woods F, et al: Changing subclavian haemodialysis cannulas to reduce infection. *Lancet* 1:1373, 1981.

118. Dahlberg PJ, Yutuc WR, Newcomer KL: Subclavian hemodialysis catheter infections. *Am J Kidney Dis* 7:421-7, 1986.

119. Moss AH, Vasilakis C, Holley JL, et al: Use of a silicone dual-lumen catheter with a Dacron cuff as a long-term vascular access for hemodialysis patients. *Am J Kidney Dis* 16:211-5, 1990.

120. Oliver MJ, Callery SM, Thorpe KE, et al: Risk of bacteremia from temporary hemodialysis catheters by site of insertion and duration of use: a prospective study. *Kidney Int* 58:2543-5, 2000.

121. Cimochowski GE, Worley E, Rutherford WE, et al: Superiority of the internal jugular over the subclavian access for temporary dialysis. *Nephron* 54:154-61, 1990.

122. Schillinger F, Schillinger D, Montagnac R, et al: Post catheterisation vein stenosis in haemodialysis: comparative angiographic study of 50 subclavian and 50 internal jugular accesses. *Nephrol Dial Transplant* 6:722-4, 1991.

123. Boyce JM, Pittet D: Guideline for Hand Hygiene in Health-Care Settings. *Infect Control Hosp Epidemiol* 23:S3-40, 2002.

124. Hirschmann H, Fux L, Podusel J, et al: The influence of hand hygiene prior to insertion of peripheral venous catheters on the frequency of complications. *J Hosp Infect* 49:199-203, 2001.

125. Raad II, Hohn DC, Gilbreath BJ, et al: Prevention of central venous catheter-related infections by using maximal sterile barrier precautions during insertion. *Infect Control Hosp Epidemiol* 15:231-8, 1994.

126. Rijnders BJ, Van Wijngaerden E, Wilmer A, et al: Use of full sterile barrier precautions during insertion of arterial catheters: a randomized trial. *Clin Infect Dis* 36:743-8, 2003.

127. Tomford JW, Hershey CO, McLaren CE, et al: Intravenous therapy team and peripheral venous catheter-associated complications: a prospective controlled study. *Arch Intern Med* 144:1191-4, 1984.

128. Soifer N, Edlin B, Weinstein R, et al: A randomized IV team trial (abstract). *Abstracts and proceedings from the 29th interscience conference on antimicrobial agents and c hemotherapy.* Washington, DC, 1989, ASM Press, p 1076.

129. Soifer NE, Borzak S, Edlin BR, et al: Prevention of peripheral venous catheter complications with an intravenous therapy team: a randomized controlled trial. *Arch Intern Med* 158:473-7, 1998.

130. Sherertz RJ, Ely EW, Westbrook DM, et al: Education of physicians-in-training can decrease the risk for vascular catheter infection. *Ann Intern Med* 132:641-8, 2000.

131. Eggimann P, Harbarth S, Constantin M, et al: Impact of a prevention strategy targeted at vascular-access care on incidence of infections acquired in intensive care. *Lancet* 355:1864-8, 2000.

132. Clemence MA, Walker D, Farr BM: Central venous catheter practices: results of a survey. *Am J Infect Control* 23:5-12, 1995.

133. Sheehan G, Leicht K, O'Brien M, et al: Chlorhexidine versus povidone-iodine as cutaneous antisepsis for prevention of vascular-catheter infection (abstract 1616). *Abstracts and proceedings from the 33rd interscience conference on antimicrobial agents and c hemotherapy.* Washington, DC, 1993, ASM Press, p 414.

134. Garland JS, Buck RK, Maloney P, et al: Comparison of 10% povidone-iodine and 0.5% chlorhexidine gluconate for the prevention of peripheral intravenous catheter colonization in neo-

APIC Text of Infection Control and Epidemiology

Copyright © 2005, Association for Professionals in Infection Control and Epidemiology, Inc.

nates: a prospective trial. *Pediatr Infect Dis J* 14:510–6, 1995.

135. Meffre C, Girard R, Hajjar J, et al: Povidone-iodine versus alcoholic chlorhexidine for disinfection of the insertion site of peripheral venous catheters: results of a multicenter randomized trial (abstract 64). *Infect Control Hosp Epidemiol* 15:26, 1996.

136. Mimoz O, Pieroni L, Lawrence C, et al: Prospective, randomized trial of two antiseptic solutions for prevention of central venous or arterial catheter colonization and infection in intensive care unit patients. *Crit Care Med* 24:1818–23, 1996.

137. Legras A, Cattier B, Dequin PF, et al: Etude prospective randomisee pour la prevention des infections liees aux catheters: chlorhexidine alcoolique contre polyvidone iodee. *Reanimation et Urgences* 6:5–11, 1997.

138. LeBlanc A, Cobett S IV: Site infection: a prospective, randomized clinical trial comparing the efficacy of three methods of skin antisepsis. *CINA J* 15:48–50, 1999.

139. Humar A, Ostromecki A, Direnfeld J, et al: Prospective randomized trial of 10% povidone-iodine versus 0.5% tincture of chlorhexidine as cutaneous antisepsis for prevention of central venous catheter infection. *Clin Infect Dis* 31:1001–7, 2000.

140. Maki DG, Knasinski V, Narans LL, et al: A randomized trial of a novel 1% chlorhexidine-75% alcohol tincture versus 10% povidone-iodine for cutaneous disinfection with vascular catheters (abstract 142). *Abstracts and proceedings from the 31st annual society for healthcare epidemiology of America meeting.* Toronto, 2001, Society for Healthcare Epidemiology of America, p 70.

141. Chaiyakunapruk N, Veenstra DL, Lipsky BA, et al: Chlorhexidine compared with povidone-iodine solution for vascular catheter-site care: a meta-analysis. *Ann Intern Med* 136:792–801, 2002.

142. Andersen PT, Herlevsen P, Schaumburg H: A comparative study of 'op-site' and 'nobecutan gauze' dressings for central venous line care. *J Hosp Infect* 7:161–8, 1986.

143. Conly JM, Grieves K, Peters B: A prospective, randomized study comparing transparent and dry gauze dressings for central venous catheters. *J Infect Dis* 159:310–9, 1989.

144. Maki D, Will L: Colonization and infection associated with transparent dressings for central venous, arterial, and Hickman catheters: a comparative trial (abstract 1241). *Abstracts and proceedings from the 24th interscience conference on antimicrobial agents and chemotherapy.* Washington, DC, 1984, ASM Press, p 991.

145. Maki D, Mermel LA, Martin M, et al: A highly semipermeable polyurethane dressing does not increase the risk of CVC-related BSI: a prospective, multicenter, investigator-blinded trial (abstract J-64). *Abstracts and proceedings from the 36th interscience conference on antimicrobial agents and chemotherapy.* Washington, DC, 1996, ASM Press, p 230.

146. Powell CR, Traetow MJ, Fabri PJ, et al: Op-site dressing study: a prospective randomized study evaluating povidone iodine ointment and extension set changes with 7-day op-site dressings applied to total parenteral nutrition subclavian sites. *J Parenter Enteral Nutr* 9:443–446, 1985.

147. Young GP, Alexeyeff M, Russell DM, et al: Catheter sepsis during parenteral nutrition: the safety of long-term Opsite dressings. *J Parenter Enteral Nutr* 12:365–370, 1988.

148. Ricard P, Martin R, Marcoux JA: Protection on indwelling vascular catheters: incidence of bacterial contamination and catheter-related sepsis. *Crit Care Med* 13:541–543, 1985.

149. Zinner SH, Denny-Brown BC, Braun P, et al: Risk of infection with intravenous indwelling catheters: effect of application of antibiotic ointment. *J Infect Dis* 120:616–9, 1969.

150. Norden CW: Application of antibiotic ointment to the site of venous catheterization: a controlled trial. *J Infect Dis* 120:611–5, 1969.

151. Maki DG, Band JD: A comparative study of polyantibiotic and iodophor ointments in prevention of vascular catheter-related infection. *Am J Med* 70:739–44, 1981.

152. Flowers RHd, Schwenzer KJ, Kopel RF, et al: Efficacy of an attachable subcutaneous cuff for the prevention of intravascular catheter-related infection: a randomized, controlled trial. *JAMA* 261:878–83, 1989.

153. Hill RL, Fisher AP, Ware RJ, et al: Mupirocin for the reduction of colonization of internal jugular cannulae: a randomized controlled trial. *J Hosp Infect* 15:311–21, 1990.

154. Sesso R, Barbosa D, Leme IL, et al: Staphylococcus aureus prophylaxis in hemodialysis patients using central venous catheter:

effect of mupirocin ointment. *J Am Soc Nephrol* 9:1085–92, 1998.

155. Miller MA, Dascal A, Portnoy J, et al: Development of mupirocin resistance among methicillin-resistant Staphylococcus aureus after widespread use of nasal mupirocin ointment. *Infect Control Hosp Epidemiol* 17:811–3, 1996.

156. Zakrzewska-Bode A, Muytjens HL, Liem KD, et al: Mupirocin resistance in coagulase-negative staphylococci, after topical prophylaxis for the reduction of colonization of central venous catheters. *J Hosp Infect* 31:189–93, 1995.

157. Perez-Fontan M, Rosales M, Rodriguez-Carmona A, et al: Mupirocin resistance after long-term use for Staphylococcus aureus colonization in patients undergoing chronic peritoneal dialysis. *Am J Kidney Dis* 39:337–41, 2002.

158. Prager RL, Silva J: Colonization of central venous catheters. *South Med J* 77:458–461, 1984.

159. Maki D, Will L: Study of polyantibiotic and povidone-iodine ointments on central venous and arterial catheter sites dressed with gauze or polyurethane dressing (abstract). *Abstracts and proceedings from the 26th interscience conference on antimicrobial agents and chemotherapy.* Washington, DC, 1986, ASM Press, p 1041.

160. Levin A, Mason AJ, Jindal KK, et al: Prevention of hemodialysis subclavian vein catheter infections by topical povidone-iodine. *Kidney Int* 40:934–8, 1991.

161. Raad I, Umphrey J, Khan A, et al: The duration of placement as a predictor of peripheral and pulmonary arterial catheter infections. *J Hosp Infect* 23:17–26, 1993.

162. Lai KK: Safety of prolonging peripheral cannula and i.v. tubing use from 72 hours to 96 hours. *Am J Infect Control* 26:66–70, 1998.

163. Bregenzer T, Conen D, Sakmann P, et al: Is routine replacement of peripheral intravenous catheters necessary? *Arch Intern Med* 158:151–6, 1998.

164. Pujol M, Hornero A, Saballs M, et al: Clinical epidemiology of bacteremia due to peripheral vascular catheter infections (abstract K-2040). *43rd international conference on antimicrobial agents and chemotherapy.* Washington, DC, 2003, ASM Press.

165. Hilton E, Haslett TM, Borenstein MT, et al: Central catheter infections: single- versus triple-lumen catheters: influence of guide wires on infection rates when used for replacement of catheters. *Am J Med* 84:667–72, 1988.

166. Eyer S, Brummitt C, Crossley K, et al: Catheter-related sepsis: prospective, randomized study of three methods of long-term catheter maintenance. *Crit Care Med* 18:1073–9, 1990.

167. Cobb DK, High KP, Sawyer RG, et al: A controlled trial of scheduled replacement of central venous and pulmonary-artery catheters. *N Engl J Med* 327:1062–8, 1992.

168. Cook D, Randolph A, Kernerman P, et al: Central venous catheter replacement strategies: a systematic review of the literature. *Crit Care Med* 25:1417–24, 1997.

169. Duszak R, Jr., Haskal ZJ, Thomas-Hawkins C, et al: Replacement of failing tunneled hemodialysis catheters through pre-existing subcutaneous tunnels: a comparison of catheter function and infection rates for de novo placements and over-the-wire exchanges. *J Vasc Interven Radiol* 9:321–7, 1998.

170. Robinson D, Suhocki P, Schwab SJ: Treatment of infected tunneled venous access hemodialysis catheters with guidewire exchange. *Kidney Int* 53:1792–4, 1998.

171. Beathard GA: Management of bacteremia associated with tunneled-cuffed hemodialysis catheters. *J Am Soc Nephrol* 10:1045–9, 1999.

172. Martinez E, Mensa J, Rovira M, et al: Central venous catheter exchange by guidewire for treatment of catheter-related bacteremia in patients undergoing BMT or intensive chemotherapy. *Bone Marrow Transplant* 23:41–4, 1999.

173. Maki DG, Hassemer CA: Endemic rate of fluid contamination and related septicemia in arterial pressure monitoring. *Am J Med* 70:733–8, 1981.

174. Maki DG, Goldman DA, Rhame FS: Infection control in intravenous therapy. *Ann Intern Med* 79:867–87, 1973.

175. Maki DG, Botticelli JT, LeRoy ML, et al: Prospective study of replacing administration sets for intravenous therapy at 48- vs 72-hour intervals: 72 hours is safe and cost-effective. *JAMA* 258:1777–81, 1987.

176. Mermel LA, Maki DG: Epidemic bloodstream infections from hemodynamic pressure monitoring: signs of the times. *Infect Control Hosp Epidemiol* 10:47–53, 1989.

Copyright © 2005, Association for Professionals in Infection Control and Epidemiology, Inc.

177. Luskin RL, Weinstein RA, Nathan C, et al: Extended use of disposable pressure transducers: a bacteriologic evaluation. *JAMA* 255:916–920, 1986.

178. O'Malley M, Chen J, Cameron S, et al: Study of long duration placement of pressure monitoring systems (abstract). *Programs and abstracts of the third international conference of nosocomial infections.* Atlanta, 1990, Centers for Disease Control, The National Foundation for Infectious Diseases.

179. Platzner N, Marino J, Cerra F, et al: Eliminating the cul-de-sac from pressure cone infusion systems reduces fluid contamination (abstract). *Abstracts and proceedings from the 22nd interscience conference on antimicrobial agents and chemotherapy.* Washington, DC, 1982, ASM Press, p 931.

180. Shinozaki T, Deane RS, Mazuzan JE, Jr., et al: Bacterial contamination of arterial lines: a prospective study. *JAMA* 249:223–5, 1983.

181. Timsit JF, Farkas JC, Boyer JM, et al: Central vein catheter-related thrombosis in intensive care patients: incidence, risks factors, and relationship with catheter-related sepsis. *Chest* 114: 207–13, 1998.

182. Raad, II, Luna M, Khalil SA, et al: The relationship between the thrombotic and infectious complications of central venous catheters. *JAMA* 271:1014–6, 1994.

183. Henrickson KJ, Axtell RA, Hoover SM, et al: Prevention of central venous catheter-related infections and thrombotic events in immunocompromised children by the use of vancomycin/ciprofloxacin/heparin flush solution: a randomized, multicenter, double-blind trial. *J Clin Oncol* 18:1269–78, 2000.

184. Mehall JR, Saltzman DA, Jackson RJ, et al: Fibrin sheath enhances central venous catheter infection. *Crit Care Med* 30: 908–12, 2002.

185. Boraks P, Seale J, Price J, et al: Prevention of central venous catheter associated thrombosis using minidose warfarin in patients with haematological malignancies. *Br J Haematol* 101: 483–6, 1998.

186. Bern MM, Lokich JJ, Wallach SR, et al: Very low doses of warfarin can prevent thrombosis in central venous catheters: a randomized prospective trial. *Ann Intern Med* 112:423–8, 1990.

187. Randolph AG, Cook DJ, Gonzales CA, et al: Benefit of heparin in peripheral venous and arterial catheters: systematic review and meta-analysis of randomised controlled trials. *Br Med J* 316:969–75, 1998.

188. Mermel LA, Maki DG: Infectious complications of Swan-Ganz pulmonary artery catheters: pathogenesis, epidemiology, prevention, and management. *Am J Respir Crit Care Med* 149: 1020–36, 1994. Erratum: *Am J Respir Crit Care Med* 150: 290, 1994.

189. Mermel LA, Stolz SM, Maki DG: Surface antimicrobial activity of heparin-bonded and antiseptic-impregnated vascular catheters. *J Infect Dis* 167:920–4, 1993.

190. Mermel LA: Intravascular catheters impregnated with benzalkonium chloride. *J Antimicrob Chemother* 32:905–6, 1993.

191. Clagett GP, Anderson FA, Jr., Heit J, et al: Prevention of venous thromboembolism. *Chest* 108:312S–334S, 1995.

192. Ray CE, Jr., Shenoy SS, McCarthy PL, et al: Weekly prophylactic urokinase instillation in tunneled central venous access devices. *J Vasc Interv Radiol* 10:1330–4, 1999.

193. Aquino VM, Sandler ES, Mustafa MM, et al: A prospective double-blind randomized trial of urokinase flushes to prevent bacteremia resulting from luminal colonization of subcutaneous central venous catheters. *J Pediatr Hematol Oncol* 24:710–3, 2002.

194. Crnich CJ, Maki DG: The promise of novel technology for the prevention of intravascular device-related bloodstream infection: II. long-term devices. *Clin Infect Dis* 34:1362–8, 2002.

195. Schears GJ, Liebeig C, Frey AM, et al: StatLock catheter securement device significantly reduces central venous catheter complications (abstract). In *Patient safety initiative: spotlighting strategies, sharing solutions,* Chicago, 2000, Joint Commission on Accreditation of Healthcare Organizations.

196. Yamamoto AJ, Solomon JA, Soulen MC, et al: Sutureless securement device reduces complications of peripherally inserted central venous catheters (abstract). *Abstracts and proceedings from the 26th annual scientific meeting of the Society of Cardiovascular and Interventional Radiologists.* San Antonio, TX, 2001.

197. Cooper GL, Schiller AL, Hopkins CC: Possible role of capillary action in pathogenesis of experimental catheter-associated dermal tunnel infections. *J Clin Microbiol* 26:8–12, 1988.

198. Maki DG, Mermel LA, Kluger DM, et al: The efficacy of a chlorhexidine-impregnated sponge (biopatch) for the prevention of intravascular catheter-related infection: a prospective, randomized, controlled, multicenter trial (abstract 1430). *Abstracts and proceedings from the 40th interscience conference on antimicrobial agents and chemotherapy.* Washington, DC, 2000, ASM Press, p 422.

199. Garland JS, Alex CP, Mueller CD, et al: A randomized trial comparing povidone-iodine to a chlorhexidine gluconate-impregnated dressing for prevention of central venous catheter infections in neonates. *Pediatrics* 107:1431–6, 2001.

200. Ramsay J, Nolte F, Schwarzmann S: Incidence of catheter colonization and catheter-related infection with an antiseptic impregnated triple lumen catheter (abstract). *Crit Care Med* 22:A115, 1994.

201. Bach A, Bohrer H, Bottiger B, et al: Reduction of bacterial colonization of triple-lumen catheters with antiseptic bonding in septic patients (abstract). *Anesthesiology* 81:A261, 1994.

202. Trazzera S, Stern G, Rakesh B, et al: Examination of antimicrobial-coated central venous catheters in patients at high-risk for catheter related infections in a medical intensive care unit and leukemia/bone marrow transplant unit (abstract). *Crit Care Med* 23:A152, 1995.

203. Bach A, Schmidt H, Bottiger B, et al: Retention of antibacterial activity and bacterial colonization of antiseptic-bonded central venous catheters. *J Antimicrob Chemother* 37:315–22, 1996.

204. Ciresi DL, Albrecht RM, Volkers PA, et al: Failure of antiseptic bonding to prevent central venous catheter-related infection and sepsis. *Am Surg* 62:641–6, 1996.

205. Pemberton LB, Ross V, Cuddy P, et al: No difference in catheter sepsis between standard and antiseptic central venous catheters: a prospective randomized trial. *Arch Surg* 131:986–9, 1996.

206. George SJ, Vuddamalay P, Boscoe MJ: Antiseptic-impregnated central venous catheters reduce the incidence of bacterial colonization and associated infection in immunocompromised transplant patients. *Eur J Anaesthesiol* 14:428–31, 1997.

207. Logghe C, Van Ossel C, D'Hoore W, et al: Evaluation of chlorhexidine and silver-sulfadiazine impregnated central venous catheters for the prevention of bloodstream infection in leukaemic patients: a randomized controlled trial. *J Hosp Infect* 37: 145–56, 1997.

208. Tennenberg S, Lieser M, McCurdy B, et al: A prospective randomized trial of an antibiotic- and antiseptic-coated central venous catheter in the prevention of catheter-related infections. *Arch Surg* 132:1348–51, 1997.

209. Collin GR: Decreasing catheter colonization through the use of an antiseptic-impregnated catheter: a continuous quality improvement project. *Chest* 115:1632–40, 1999.

210. Hannan M, Juste RN, Umasanker S, et al: Antiseptic-bonded central venous catheters and bacterial colonisation. *Anaesthesia* 54:868–72, 1999.

211. Marik PE, Abraham G, Careau P, et al: The ex vivo antimicrobial activity and colonization rate of two antimicrobial-bonded central venous catheters. *Crit Care Med* 27:1128–31, 1999.

212. Sheng WH, Ko WJ, Wang JT, et al: Evaluation of antiseptic-impregnated central venous catheters for prevention of catheter-related infection in intensive care unit patients. *Diagn Microbiol Infect Dis* 38:1–5, 2000.

213. Veenstra DL, Saint S, Saha S, et al: Efficacy of antiseptic-impregnated central venous catheters in preventing catheter-related bloodstream infection: a meta-analysis. *JAMA* 281: 261–7, 1999.

214. Marin MG, Lee JC, Skurnick JH: Prevention of nosocomial bloodstream infections: effectiveness of antimicrobial-impregnated and heparin-bonded central venous catheters. *Crit Care Med* 28: 3332–8, 2000.

215. Veenstra DL, Saint S, Sullivan SD: Cost-effectiveness of antiseptic-impregnated central venous catheters for the prevention of catheter-related bloodstream infection. *JAMA* 282:554–60, 1999.

216. Shorr AF, Humphreys CW, Helman DL: New choices for central venous catheters. *Chest* 124:275–84, 2003.

217. Saint S: Prevention of intravascular catheter-associated infections. In Shojania KG, Duncan BW, McDonald KM and Wachter RM, editors: *Making health care safer: a critical analysis of patient safety practices.* Rockville, MD, 2001, Agency for Healthcare Research and Quality, pp 163–184.

Copyright © 2005, Association for Professionals in Infection Control and Epidemiology, Inc.

218. Dogra GK, Herson H, Hutchison B, et al: Prevention of tunneled hemodialysis catheter-related infections using catheter-restricted filling with gentamicin and citrate: a randomized controlled study. *J Am Soc Nephrol* 13:2133–9, 2002.

219. Raad I, Hachem R, Tcholakian RK, et al: Efficacy of minocycline and EDTA lock solution in preventing catheter-related bacteremia, septic phlebitis, and endocarditis in rabbits. *Antimicrob Agents Chemother* 46:327–32, 2002.

220. Maki DG, Crnich CJ, Safdar N: Successful use of a 25% alcohol lock solution for prevention of recurrent CVC-related bloodstream infection in a patient on home TNA (abstract K-671). *Abstracts and proceedings from the 42nd interscience conference on antimicrobial agents and chemotherapy.* Washington, DC, 2002, ASM Press, p 320.

221. Shah CB, Mittelman MW, Costerton JW, et al: Antimicrobial activity of a novel catheter lock solution. *Antimicrob Agents Chemother* 46:1674–9, 2002.

222. Allon M: Prophylaxis against dialysis catheter-related bacteremia with a novel antimicrobial lock solution. *Clin Infect Dis* 36:1539–44, 2003.

223. Segura M, Alia C, Valverde J, et al: Assessment of a new hub design and the semiquantitative catheter culture method using an in vivo experimental model of catheter sepsis. *J Clin Microbiol* 28:2551–4, 1990.

224. Segura M, Alvarez-Lerma F, Tellado JM, et al: A clinical trial on the prevention of catheter-related sepsis using a new hub model. *Ann Surg* 223:363–9, 1996.

225. Leon C, Alvarez-Lerma F, Ruiz-Santana S, et al: Antiseptic chamber-containing hub reduces central venous catheter-related infection: a prospective, randomized study. *Crit Care Med* 31:1318–24, 2003.

226. Luna J, Masdeu G, Perez M, et al: Clinical trial evaluating a new hub device designed to prevent catheter-related sepsis. *Eur J Clin Microbiol Infect Dis* 19:655–62, 2000.

227. Sherertz RJ, Ely EW, Westbrook DM, et al. Education of physicians-in-training can decrease the risk for vascular catheter infection. *Ann Intern Med* 132:641–8, 2000.

228. Rosenthal VD, Guzman S, Crnich CJ. Effect of an infection control program utilizing education and performance feedback on rates of intravascular device-associated bloodstream infection in intensive care units in Argentina. *Am J Infect Control* 31:405–9, 2003.

229. Strinden WD, Helgerson RB, Maki DG: Candida septic thrombosis of the great central veins associated with central catheters: clinical features and management. *Ann Surg* 202:653–8, 1985.

230. Verghese A, Widrich WC, Arbeit RD: Central venous septic thrombophlebitis: the role of medical therapy. *Medicine* 64:394–400, 1985.

231. Maki DG: Management of life-threatening infection in the intensive care unit. In Murray MJ, Coursin DB, Pearl RG and Prough DS, editors: *Critical care medicine: preoperative management.* 2nd ed. Philadelphia, 2002, Lippincott Williams & Williams, pp 616–648.

232. Dugdale DC, Ramsey PG: *Staphylococcus aureus* bacteremia in patients with Hickman catheters. *Am J Med* 89:137–41, 1990.

233. Malanoski GJ, Samore MH, Pefanis A, et al: *Staphylococcus aureus* catheter-associated bacteremia: minimal effective therapy and unusual infectious complications associated with arterial sheath catheters. *Arch Intern Med* 155:1161–6, 1995.

234. Fowler VG, Jr., Li J, Corey GR, et al: Role of echocardiography in evaluation of patients with *Staphylococcus aureus* bacteremia: experience in 103 patients. *J Am Coll Cardiol* 30:1072–8, 1997.

235. Carlisle EJ, Blake P, McCarthy F, et al: Septicemia in long-term jugular hemodialysis catheters; eradicating infection by changing the catheter over a guidewire. *Int J Artif Organs* 14:150–3, 1991.

236. Shaffer D: Catheter-related sepsis complicating long-term, tunnelled central venous dialysis catheters: management by guidewire exchange. *Am J Kidney Dis* 25:593–6, 1995.

237. Rex JH, Walsh TJ, Sobel JD: Practice guidelines for the treatment of candidiasis: Infectious Diseases Society of America. *Clin Infect Dis* 30:662–78, 2000.

238. Kulak K, Maki DG: Treatment of hickman catheter-related candidemia without removing the catheter (abstract). *Abstracts and proceedings from the 32nd interscience conference on antimicrobial agents and chemotherapy.* Washington, DC, 1992, ASM Press, p 249.

239. Nucci M, Anaisse E: Should vascualr catheters be removed from all patients with candidemia? An evidence-based review. *Clin Infect Dis* 34:591–599, 2002.

240. Raad I, Davis S, Khan A, et al: Impact of central venous catheter removal on the recurrence of catheter-related coagulase-negative staphylococcal bacteremia. *Infect Control Hosp Epidemiol* 13:215–21, 1992.

241. Messing B, Peitra-Cohen S, Debure A, et al: Antibiotic-lock technique: a new approach to optimal therapy for catheter-related sepsis in home-parenteral nutrition patients. *J Parenter Enteral Nutr* 12:185–9, 1988.

242. Messing B, Man F, Colimon R, et al: Antibiotic lock technique is an effective treatment of bacterial catheter-related sepsis during parenteral nutrition. *Clin Nutr* 9:220–224, 1990.

243. Douard MC, Arlet G, Leverger G, et al: Quantitative blood cultures for diagnosis and management of catheter-related sepsis in pediatric hematology and oncology patients. *Intensive Care Med* 17:30–5, 1991.

244. Rao JS, O'Meara A, Harvey T, et al: A new approach to the management of Broviac catheter infection. *J Hosp Infect* 22:109–16, 1992.

245. Capdevila JA, Segarra A, Planes AM, et al: Successful treatment of haemodialysis catheter-related sepsis without catheter removal. *Nephrol Dial Transplant* 8:231–4, 1993.

246. Johnson DC, Johnson FL, Goldman S: Preliminary results treating persistent central venous catheter infections with the antibiotic lock technique in pediatric patients. *Pediatr Infect Dis J* 13:930–1, 1994.

247. Benoit JL, Carandang G, Sitrin M, et al: Intraluminal antibiotic treatment of central venous catheter infections in patients receiving parenteral nutrition at home. *Clin Infect Dis* 21:1286–8, 1995.

248. Capdevila JA, Segarra A, Planes AM, et al: Long term follow-up of patients with catheter related sepsis (CRS) treated without catheter removal (abstract). *Abstracts and proceedings from the 35th interscience conference of antimicrobial agents and chemotherapy.* Washington, DC, 1995, ASM Press, p J3.

249. Krzywda EA, Andris DA, Edmiston CE, Jr., et al: Treatment of Hickman catheter sepsis using antibiotic lock technique. *Infect Control Hosp Epidemiol* 16:596–8, 1995.

250. Krzywda E, Gotoff R, Andris D, et al: Antibiotic lock treatment (ALT): impact on catheter salvage and cost savings (abstract). *Abstracts and proceedings from the 35th interscience conference of antimicrobial agents and chemotherapy.* Washington, DC, 1995, ASM Press, p J4.

251. McCarthy A, Byrne M, Breathnach F, et al: "In-situ" Teicoplanin for central venous catheter infection. *Ir J Med Sci* 164:125–7, 1995.

252. Cuntz D, Michaud L, Guimber D, et al: Local antibiotic lock for the treatment of infections related to central catheters in parenteral nutrition in children. *J Parenter Enteral Nutr* 26:104–8, 2002.

253. Guedon C, Nouvellon M, Lalaude O, et al: Efficacy of antibiotic-lock technique with teicoplanin in staphylococcus epidermidis catheter-related sepsis during long-term parenteral nutrition. *J Parenter Enteral Nutr* 26:109–13, 2002.

254. Lokich JJ, Bothe A, Jr., Benotti P, et al: Complications and management of implanted venous access catheters. *J Clin Oncol* 3:710–7, 1985.

255. Champault G: Totally implantable catheters for cancer chemotherapy: French experience on 325 cases. *Cancer Drug Deliv* 3:131–7, 1986.

256. Brothers TE, Von Moll LK, Niederhuber JE, et al: Experience with subcutaneous infusion ports in three hundred patients. *Surg Gynecol Obstet* 166:295–301, 1988.

257. Anthony TU, Rubin LG: Stability of antibiotics used for antibiotic-lock treatment of infections of implantable venous devices (ports). *Antimicrob Agents Chemother* 43:2074–6, 1999.

258. Haimi-Cohen Y, Husain N, Meenan J, et al: Vancomycin and ceftazidime bioactivities persist for at least 2 weeks in the lumen in ports: simplifying treatment of port-associated bloodstream infections by using the antibiotic lock technique. *Antimicrob Agents Chemother* 45:1565–7, 2001.

259. Domingo P, Fontanet A, Sanchez F, et al: Morbidity associated with long-term use of totally implantable ports in patients with AIDS. *Clin Infect Dis* 29:346–51, 1999.

260. Longuet P, Douard MC, Maslo C, et al: Limited efficacy of antibiotic lock techniques (ALT) in catheter related bacteremia of totally implanted ports (TIP) in HIV infected oncologic patients

(abstract). *Abstracts and proceedings from the 35th interscience conference of antimicrobial agents and chemotherapy.* Washington, DC, 1995, ASM Press, p J5.

261. Albertyn LE, Alcock MK: Diagnosis of internal jugular vein thrombosis. *Radiology* 162:505–8, 1987.

262. Braun IF, Hoffman JC, Jr., Malko JA, et al: Jugular venous thrombosis: MR imaging. *Radiology* 157:357–60, 1985.

263. Mori H, Fukuda T, Isomoto I, et al: CT diagnosis of catheter-induced septic thrombus of vena cava. *J Comput Assist Tomogr* 14:236–8, 1990.

264. Maki DG, Agger WA: Enterococcal bacteremia: clinical features, the risk of endocarditis, and management. *Medicine* 67: 248–69, 1988.

265. Raad II, Sabbagh MF: Optimal duration of therapy for catheter-related *Staphylococcus aureus* bacteremia: a study of 55 cases and review. *Clin Infect Dis* 14:75–82, 1992.

266. Rosen AB, Fowler VG, Jr., Corey GR, et al: Cost-effectiveness of transesophageal echocardiography to determine the duration of therapy for intravascular catheter-associated *Staphylococcus aureus* bacteremia. *Ann Intern Med* 130:810–20, 1999.

267. Lecciones JA, Lee JW, Navarro EE, et al: Vascular catheter-associated fungemia in patients with cancer: analysis of 155 episodes. *Clin Infect Dis* 14:875–83, 1992.

268. Wenzel RP: Nosocomial candidemia: risk factors and attributable mortality. *Clin Infect Dis* 20:1531–4, 1995.

269. Anaissie EJ, Rex JH, Uzun O, et al: Predictors of adverse outcome in cancer patients with candidemia. *Am J Med* 104: 238–45, 1998.

270. Phillips P, Shafran S, Garber G, et al: Multicenter randomized trial of fluconazole versus amphotericin B for treatment of candidemia in non-neutropenic patients. *Eur J Clin Microbiol Infect Dis* 16:337–45, 1997.

271. Colombo AL, Perfect J, DiNubile M, et al: Global distribution and outcomes for Candida species causing invasive candidiasis: results from an international randomized double-blind study of caspofungin versus amphotericin B for the treatment of invasive candidiasis. *Eur J Clin Microbiol Infect Dis* 22:470–4, 2003.

272. Letscher-Bru V, Herbrecht R: Caspofungin: the first representative of a new antifungal class. *J Antimicrob Chemother* 51: 513–21, 2003.

273. Mora-Duarte J, Betts R, Rotstein C, et al: Comparison of caspofungin and amphotericin B for invasive candidiasis. *N Engl J Med* 347:2020–9, 2002.

274. Rose HD: Venous catheter-associated candidemia. *Am J Med Sci* 275:265–9, 1978.

275. Terpenning MS, Buggy BP, Kauffman CA: Hospital-acquired infective endocarditis. *Arch Intern Med* 148:1601–3, 1988.

276. Henderson DK, Edwards JE, Jr., Montgomerie JZ: Hematogenous candida endophthalmitis in patients receiving parenteral hyperalimentation fluids. *J Infect Dis* 143:655–61, 1981.

277. Maki DG: Epidemic Nosocomial Bacteremias. In: Wenzel RP, editors: *Handbook of hospital acquired infections.* Boca Raton, FL, 1981, CRC Press, pp 371–512.

278. Krishnasami Z, Carlton D, Bimbo L, et al: Management of hemodialysis catheter-related bacteremia with an adjunctive antibiotic lock solution. *Kidney Int* 61:1136–42, 2002.

279. Berrington A, Gould FK: Use of antibiotic locks to treat colonized central venous catheters. *J Antimicrob Chemother* 48: 597–603, 2001.

Copyright © 2005, Association for Professionals in Infection Control and Epidemiology, Inc.

Urinary Tract Infections

Debra Leithauser RNC, MSN, NNP, CIC
Infection Prevention Specialist/Clinical
Performance Specialist
Henry Ford Health System
Detroit, Michigan

ABSTRACT

More than 1 million patients acquire a urinary tract infection (UTI), with catheter-associated infections being the most common type of infection. Healthcare-associated UTIs substantially contribute to morbidity, mortality, healthcare costs, antibiotic use, and other infections. In general, asymptomatic UTIs should only be treated in certain high-risk populations whereas those with clinically significant signs and/or symptoms consistent with UTI not explained by another process should be treated. Additionally, antibiotic prophylaxis is recommended for certain high-risk individuals. Acute cystitis or inflammation of the bladder in women accounts for 3.6 million medical office visits with an estimated cost of $1.6 billion annually in the United States. Certain types of urinary catheters with antimicrobial additives have shown some efficacy in preventing UTIs.

KEY CONCEPTS

- Acute lower UTIs in otherwise healthy, nonpregnant women are considered uncomplicated.

- Antimicrobial treatment of asymptomatic UTI should be avoided.

- Most healthcare-associated UTIs are asymptomatic.

- Most catheter-associated UTIs (CAUTI) are asymptomatic and do not require antibiotics.

- UTI is the most common type of healthcare-associated infection.

- Risk factors for UTI include advancing age, debilitation, urinary tract obstructive disorders, and use of spermicidal agents.

I.   BACKGROUND

Acute cystitis accounts for 3.6 million medical office visits by women in the United States annually with an estimated cost of $1.6 billion.[1,2] Urinary tract infection (UTI) is the most common type of healthcare-associated infection (HAI) in both acute and long-term care settings. Healthcare-associated UTIs substantially contribute to morbidity, mortality, healthcare costs, antibiotic use, and other HAIs (refer to Table 25–1). UTIs in hospitalized patients are estimated to cost approxi-

Copyright © 2005, Association for Professionals in Infection Control and Epidemiology, Inc.

Table 25-1. Potential Adverse Consequences of Healthcare-Associated and Catheter-Associated UTIs

Direct or Indirect	Consequence	Adverse Implications
Direct	Symptomatic localized infection	Morbidity, mortality, extended hospital stay
	Secondary bacteremia/fungemia	Morbidity, mortality, extended hospital stay
	Antimicrobial therapy (appropriate or inappropriate)	Costs, adverse effects, selection for resistance, vascular access, extended hospital stay
	Added diagnostic tests (appropriate or inappropriate)	Costs, secondary interventions, additional diagnostic tests
	Catheter obstruction	Urinary leakage/retention, sepsis, catheter replacement
	Extended hospital stay	Costs, risk for iatrogenic complications and healthcare associated infections
Indirect	Reservoir of resistant and/or virulent organisms	Infection at other site(s) in index patient, transmission to other patients

mately $600 per infection and increase length of stay by 0.4 days for asymptomatic and 2.0 days for symptomatic infections.

UTIs are commonly caused by the presence of microorganisms within the urine and/or organs and tissues of the urinary tract (i.e., urethra, bladder, ureter, kidney, perinephric tissues, prostate, and epididymis). A distinction is sometimes made between "infection" and "colonization" of the urinary tract. Individuals who are colonized do not show signs and symptoms of infection whereas infected persons generally produce host inflammatory responses and/or pathological changes attributable to the causative microorganisms. Urethritis due to sexually transmitted pathogens (e.g., herpes simplex virus and *Chlamydia trachomatis*) is customarily excluded from the designation of UTI. (Also see Chapter 101, Sexually Transmitted Diseases.) Infections of the lower urinary tract do not generally place the patient at risk for renal damage. However, an infection of the upper urinary tract puts the individual at an increased risk for pyelonephritis with resulting renal damage.[3]

II.   BASIC PRINCIPLES

Definitions and Terms

Cystitis means inflammation of the urinary bladder and may be from infectious or noninfectious causes.[4] When secondary to a UTI, it is defined clinically by the presence of bacteriuria (bacteria in the urine) and pyuria (white blood cells or pus in the urine—also see following), accompanied by voiding symptoms such as urinary frequency, urgency, and dysuria (painful or difficult urination). Noninfectious causes of cystitis include foreign bodies, drugs, and immune reactions. Typical symptoms of cystitis are uncommon in patients with healthcare-associated UTIs. In practice, localization of the infection site within the urinary tract is not always

possible. Therefore, presumed cystitis may actually involve the upper urinary tract and/or prostate.[4,5]

Emphysematous cystitis occurs when carbon dioxide is produced by gas-forming organisms in the lower urinary tract. This may occur with infection of the bladder wall or from transluminal dissection of gas. The condition is more common in women, immunocompromised individuals, and poorly controlled diabetics. Clinical manifestations range from cystitis-like symptoms to fulminating sepsis.[6-9]

Pyelonephritis is inflammation of the kidney and/or renal pelvis. Acute pyelonephritis secondary to UTI has been clinically defined by the presence of bacteriuria and pyuria. Typical signs and symptoms include: flank pain and tenderness, fever, headache, nausea, vomiting, and prostration. Various imaging studies can be used to confirm renal involvement, but in practice this is rarely necessary because treatment algorithms are based on clinical presentation alone.[10] Although patients with healthcare-associated UTI sometimes have systemic manifestations, they rarely exhibit the localizing symptoms of acute pyelonephritis.[5] Chronic (usually asymptomatic) bacteriuria associated with long-term catheter use may contribute to the morbidity and mortality of the elderly by inducing occult chronic kidney disease.[10]

Emphysematous pyelonephritis and pyelitis occur more often in diabetics. This condition is caused by gas accumulation in the genitourinary tract produced by gas-forming bacteria or fungus located within a renal abscess. Fermentation causes the release of carbon dioxide and hydrogen gases. Other causes of gas formation include iatrogenic air introduction via instrumentation including indwelling catheters. Signs and symptoms of this condition include frequency, urgency, dysuria, and less commonly gross hematuria (blood in the urine) and pneumaturia (passage of gas into the

Copyright © 2005, Association for Professionals in Infection Control and Epidemiology, Inc.

urinary tract suggesting fistula between urinary tract and bowel).[10]

Prostatitis is defined as inflammation of the prostate gland.[4] Risk factors include urologic abnormalities, bladder outlet obstruction including prostatic hyperplasia, instrumentation of the bladder, intercourse with an infectious individual, lack of circumcision, and homosexuality. Infection may progress from an asymptomatic state to a subacute or chronic pain syndrome, to an acute fulminating illness. Clinical manifestations include intense local pain, voiding symptoms, and sepsis syndrome, with or without associated bacteremia. Occult prostatic involvement is presumed to be present in men with clinical cystitis who develop recurrent bacteriuria following a course of appropriate antibiotic therapy.[10,11]

Urosepsis occurs from septic poisoning from the absorption and decomposition of urinary substances in the tissues.[4] Bloodstream infection secondary to CAUTI occurs commonly in hospitalized patients.[12]

The presence of bacteria or fungi in the urine is commonly referred to as bacteriuria and funguria respectively and may or may not be indicative of infection. Quantitative urine culture is commonly used to differentiate true or significant bladder bacteriuria from false-positive cultures related to contamination during specimen collection. The value of $\geq 10^5$ colony forming units (CFU) of bacteria per milliliter (ml) of urine was chosen because of its high specificity for diagnosis of true infection, even in asymptomatic individuals.[13] This threshold may inappropriately reject true-positive cultures from patients with lower concentrations of microorganisms who have catheter associated or symptomatic UTIs.[10] Conversely, antimicrobial therapy may be inappropriately instituted for asymptomatic UTIs with high colony counts.[14-16] Some studies have demonstrated midstream urine cultures containing $<10^5$ CFUs in acutely symptomatic women with dysuria and frequency.[17]

Pyuria is indicated by the presence of an abnormally high number of white blood cells (neutrophils) in the urine producing pus and causing inflammation within the urinary tract.[4] Pyuria is more strongly associated with infection in noncatheterized individuals than in patients with short-term indwelling catheters.[18] The degree of pyuria is predictive of subsequent symptomatic UTIs in spinal cord injured persons with indwelling catheters who previously had asymptomatic UTIs.[19] However, prophylactic therapy based on degree of pyuria in persons with asymptomatic UTI is not recommended. Comparable data are lacking for other patient populations; therefore, further study of this topic is suggested.[19]

Biofilms are surface-associated microorganisms enclosed within an extracellular polymeric substance (EPS) matrix composed primarily of polysaccharides. Noncellular materials including blood components may be contained within the matrix. Biofilms are firmly attached to a wide variety of surfaces such as living tissues, indwelling medical devices, and internal lumens of water pipes. Rougher surfaces enhance microbial colonization and biofilm development; as the surface roughens, microbial colonization and attachment to urinary catheters occur with greater ease.[20-25] (Also see Chapter 96, Biofilms.)

Hospital-Acquired Versus Community-Acquired UTI

UTI acquired or detected more than 48 hours after admission to a hospital is usually defined as hospital-acquired or nosocomial. Detection or incubating on admission or occurring in less than 48 hours postadmission is often considered a community-acquired infection. For patients who transition between various healthcare environments, true healthcare-associated versus community-acquired UTIs may be difficult to determine because urine cultures are not routinely obtained on admission to or discharge from healthcare facilities. In acute-care hospitals, UTIs are the second most frequent cause of healthcare-associated bacteremia, whereas in long-term care facilities, UTIs are the most common cause.[9] Furthermore, the majority of healthcare-associated UTIs are catheter associated.[25]

Upper UTI is associated with infection of the ureters and kidneys. Conditions associated with greater risk for upper UTI include diabetes, pregnancy, immunosuppression, previous pyelonephritis, and UTI symptoms lasting greater than 14 days or structural abnormalities of the urinary tract.[26]

III.   EPIDEMIOLOGY AND CLINICAL ASPECTS OF UTIS

Trends and Epidemiology of UTI

Neonates and Children

UTIs are a common cause of serious infection in febrile neonates and children. *Escherichia coli* have been identified as the most commonly isolated organism. Male and female neonates have an incidence of approximately 4% during the first year of life.[27] Males generally become infected by the time they are 3 months old, with uncircumcised males having a tenfold increased rate of infection. The incidence of UTI in children aged 1 to 6 years of age is approximately 0.08% in males and 3%–4% in females; females are at a higher risk for infection, most likely due to their relatively short urethras.[27,28] The majority of UTIs in this

---

Urinary Tract Infections

Copyright © 2005, Association for Professionals in Infection Control and Epidemiology, Inc.

population are caused by gastrointestinal tract microorganisms that colonize the periurethral area and ascend up the urethra.[3,29,30] The risk for infection is increased due to incomplete emptying of the bladder related to anatomical abnormalities such as grade III or greater posterior urethral valves, vesicoureteral reflux, neurogenic bladder, and voiding dysfunction especially when related to posturing. Children with urgency frequently and intentionally compress their urethras in an effort to prevent incontinence, thus termed posturing. Between ages 7 to 11 years, the incidence of reported UTIs drops substantially, most likely due to the increasing urethral length in females. Additionally, other abnormalities have most likely been diagnosed and treated.[31,32]

Adolescence and Sexual Abuse Victims

Urinary tract infection is not a common occurrence after an episode of sexual abuse. However, sexually active adolescent females have a higher incidence of infections than their celibate counterparts.[33] This increase may be related to trauma of the urethral tract that occurs with vigorous and frequent sexual encounters.[33,34] E. coli is the most common causative pathogen in adolescent females with UTI.[35]

Women

A previous history of UTI, frequent and recent sexual activity, cystoceles, urinary incontinence, and recent genitourinary surgery increase the chances of acquiring an acute uncomplicated UTI.[36,37] Estrogen deficiency that occurs in postmenopausal women may also contribute to the risk for UTI.[37] The risk for acquiring a first UTI is increased by two- to eightfold when using lubricated condoms or unlubricated condoms with spermicidal gels or creams.[34] The use of spermicidal agents increases the risk for infection from E. coli and Staphylococcus saprophyticus.[38-40] Alterations in host cell receptivity to microbial attachment may contribute to UTI risk in some female catheterized patients.[41]

More than half of all women have reported having at least one UTI during their lifetime. In the United States, these infections account for approximately 3.6 million office visits by women aged 18 to 75 years of age.[1,2] Previous history of UTI and frequent or recent sexual activity are risk factors for acute cystitis whereas celibate women rarely have cystitis.[42]

A wide range of symptoms occurs in acute uncomplicated lower UTI in healthy women. One study reported generalized symptoms including feeling unwell, weak, and tired and being irritable, restless, and hot occurred frequently. Other common symptoms include dysuria, urinary frequency, urge, pressure in the genital area, and suprapubic discomfort.[43]

Urinary reflux is a common occurrence in pregnancy due to pressure on the bladder from the enlarging uterus and ureters, placing the pregnant female at an increased risk for UTI. Asymptomatic UTI occurs in approximately 5% to 15% of pregnant women with infection usually caused by gram-negative bacilli or S. saprophyticus.[13] When untreated, progression to symptomatic infection including cystitis and pyelonephritis generally occurs in 15% to 45% of cases. A urine culture is recommended by some from all pregnant women early in the pregnancy; a small portion of those with negative cultures subsequently develop a UTI.[13,44]

Men

UTI in men is uncommon as the male urethra is longer and thus provides a protective feature. Additionally, the scrotum serves as a physical barrier protecting the urethra from the heavily colonized perianal area. The male periurethral area does not easily support bacterial growth when compared to females. Prostatic secretions contain zinc and generally inhibit bacterial growth.[17,45] Therefore, all UTIs in men are considered complicated. Older men with urologic abnormalities such as bladder outlet obstruction from prostatic hyperplasia or instrumentation of the bladder are at an increased risk for UTI. These infections occasionally occur in young men who participate in anal sex (exposure to E. coli in the rectum), who are not circumcised (increased E. coli colonization of the glans and prepuce), and whose sexual partner is colonized with uropathogens.[46]

The Elderly

An increased risk for UTI occurs with advancing age and debilitation. Catheter-associated UTI frequently occurs in the elderly living in long-term care facilities and places these individuals at risk for bacteremia.[47] Conditions associated with impaired voiding are most common. In women, anatomical and physiological alterations such as uterine prolapse, cystocele, rectocele, impaired mobility, constipation, disappearance of colonizing lactobacilli, an increase in vaginal pH, colonization with uropathogenic bacteria, and impaired hygiene and toileting significantly contribute to the increased risk for UTI in the elderly.[48,49]

Uncomplicated and Complicated UTIs

Acute lower UTIs in otherwise healthy, nonpregnant women are considered uncomplicated whereas all others should be considered complicated.[10] Complicated UTIs occur because of anatomic, functional, or pharmacologic factors that predispose an individual to persistent infection, recurrent infection, or treatment failure. These conditions include neurogenic bladder,

Copyright © 2005, Association for Professionals in Infection Control and Epidemiology, Inc.

bladder catheterization or other instrumentation of the urinary tract, urinary tract obstruction from any cause, urinary or prostatic calculi (even if not obstructing), presence of bacteria that are resistant to multiple antibiotics, diabetes mellitus, sickle cell anemia, polycystic kidney disease, and renal transplantation.[50] Old age and male gender are sometimes regarded as complicating factors, although this is not well substantiated.[51] Approximately 80% of healthcare-associated UTIs are related to the presence of indwelling catheters, hence by definition are "complicated."[25]

Catheter-Associated UTIs

Published rates for CAUTIs from surveillance systems are typically 2–8 episodes/1,000 catheter days.[52] UTI is nearly universal among chronically catheterized patients. Reported rates underestimate by nearly a factor of 10 those observed in prospective studies involving catheterized patients with rates typically between 3–5 episodes/100 catheter days.[9,25] This discrepancy is probably due to the surveillance systems used, which may rely only on cultures ordered in a non-uniform fashion based on arbitrary indications. In contrast, some research studies perform urine cultures systematically on all patients, even in the absence of clinical manifestations. Thus, only a small minority of all healthcare-associated UTIs are detected clinically and included in currently available surveillance statistics. The arbitrary approach to sampling used in clinical practice provides abundant opportunities for bias to influence apparent UTI rates, which confounds attempts to draw valid conclusions regarding differences in secular trends or institutional rates.[52] In the acute-care setting, approximately 1%–4% of CAUTI episodes result in secondary bacteremia, which is almost always due to gram-negative bacilli and has an estimated attributable mortality of 13%.[9] Because colonized collecting bags represent a potential source of cross contamination with multidrug-resistant organisms either to other anatomical sites in the same patient or to other patients, CAUTI presents an infection control challenge independent of its direct morbidity.[12]

Clinical Features of UTIs

Asymptomatic Healthcare-Associated UTIs

The great majority of healthcare-associated UTI episodes are asymptomatic. In addition to comorbid illnesses, UTIs occur relatively frequently in the elderly and are related to certain physiologic changes that occur with the aging process.[53] Treatment is generally only required for patients scheduled for invasive urological procedures, children with vesicoureteral reflux, those with urinary tract obstruction, pregnant women, recent kidney transplant recipients, and possibly

persons from whom an indwelling catheter has recently been removed.[14]

Symptomatic UTIs

Symptomatic UTI is accompanied by symptoms, signs, and/or laboratory manifestations consistent with UTI and not explained by other coexisting conditions. Typical symptoms of bladder infection (cystitis) and kidney infection (pyelonephritis), as described following, are not usually seen among patients with healthcare-associated UTI. Less-specific clinical manifestations may be encountered in patients unable to perceive or report the typical localized symptoms of cystitis and pyelonephritis. These symptoms include rigors, diaphoresis, altered mental status, pyuria, and increased autonomic dysreflexia in spinal-cord injured individuals. Healthcare-associated UTI episodes that are accompanied by unexplained voiding symptoms, fever, and/or leukocytosis usually are not the cause of such manifestations, as evidenced by the similar prevalence of these abnormalities among catheterized patients irrespective of the presence or absence of UTI.[6] However, it is customary to treat healthcare-associated UTI when it is documented in patients who have clinical manifestations consistent with UTI and who lack an alternative diagnosis.

UTI in Special Populations

Neonates born with hydronephrosis may be at an increased risk for UTI. This population exhibits more generalized signs of sepsis than do others. Clinical findings may include poor feeding, emesis, abdominal distension, irritability, weight loss, jaundice, and fever. Secondary bacteremia occurs in approximately 10% of neonates with UTI. They are also at an increased risk for dissemination of infection to the central nervous system. The clinical course of infection is generally uncomplicated when appropriate antimicrobial therapy is instituted.[27]

Clinical presentation of uncomplicated UTIs in the elderly includes urinary frequency, urgency, suprapubic discomfort, and may include a new onset of urinary incontinence. A more typical presentation including decreased appetite, delirium, confusion, and agitation is more common.[48,54] The elderly with many comorbid conditions are at a greater risk for complicated infection.

Catheter Associated UTIs (CAUTIs)

Contributing Factors

Most UTIs (66% to 86%) in the acute-care setting are caused by instrumentation of the urinary tract including indwelling bladder catheters, suprapubic catheters, and intermittent catheterization. The great majority of

---

Copyright © 2005, Association for Professionals in Infection Control and Epidemiology, Inc.

CAUTIs are not associated with symptoms and hence do not require antibiotic therapy. Moreover, a small proportion of catheterized patients with and without UTI have peripheral leukocytosis, fever, or other signs and symptoms suggesting infection.[5] These observations challenge the validity of "symptomatic CAUTI" as an identifiable clinical entity and suggest that UTI is rarely the cause of signs or symptoms of infection among catheterized patients. Whereas 10%–20% of CAUTIs are caused by the introduction of microorganisms during catheter insertion, 30%–45% are due to migration of microorganisms on the external surface of the catheter along the catheter–urethra interface to the bladder. Reflux of microorganisms up the catheter lumen to the bladder from contaminated drainage tubing or collecting bags accounts for approximately 25%–40% of infections.[55] When catheters are left in place greater than 5 days, UTIs occur in approximately half of patients.[56] Because *Serratia marcescens* and *Pseudomonas cepacia* are not common residents of the gastrointestinal tract, infection with these organisms usually suggests an iatrogenic origin.[57]

Common Pathogens

CAUTIs can be attributed to gram-negative bacilli (e.g., *E. coli, Klebsiella* spp., *Proteus* spp., *Pseudomonas* ssp., *Serratia* spp.), enterococci, staphylococci, or yeasts. Overall, the causative pathogens are divided approximately equally among gram-positive cocci, gram-negatives, and yeasts, with about 12% caused by *E. coli*.[58] Gram-positive organisms migrate predominantly along the external surface of urinary catheters whereas the gram-negative bacilli generally travel via the catheter lumen. Yeasts, however, travel by both routes.[55,59] Gram-positive organisms and susceptible gram-negative bacilli typically appear early during the period of catheterization, whereas resistant gram-negative bacilli and yeasts are more commonly seen as late pathogens.

Healthcare-Associated Candiduria

Fungal infections of the urinary tract are increasingly more common. The distinction between colonization and infection must be determined prior to deciding whether or not to treat. Diagnosis of infection is dependent on the identification of pyuria with high colony counts of yeast. Asymptomatic healthcare-associated candiduria do not often require antifungal therapy. Ascending infection from *Candida* spp. is generally uncomplicated. Oral fluconazole is very effective in eradicating uncomplicated cystitis. However, when ascending pyelonephritis occurs, a systemic agent is generally warranted.[16]

The Role of Biofilms in UTIs

As mentioned earlier, biofilms are formed when microorganisms attach to surfaces and generate a complex EPS matrix; the cells within this matrix have the ability to communicate. Such biofilms exist on surfaces of indwelling devices including urinary catheters.[20-24, 60-61] For example, *Proteus mirabilis* produces crystalline biofilms of magnesium and calcium salts that deposit on the luminal surfaces of catheters. In an in vitro study, human bladder urine was inoculated with a clinical strain of *P. mirabilis* from an encrusted catheter. When further evaluated, hydrogel-coated latex, hydrogel/silver-coated latex, and silicone elastomer-coated latex catheters became encrusted with blockage occurring within two days.[61] Bacteria can migrate from the biofilm matrix, up the catheter, and into the bladder thus causing an infection. Encrustation from biofilm may also partially or completely obstruct the catheter lumen in vivo resulting in urinary retention and/or leakage of urine around the catheter; accordingly, UTI with or without bacteremia may develop.[62] Organisms within biofilms are more resistant to antimicrobial agents than are organisms in suspension as the biofilm provides protection from the host inflammatory response and the action of antimicrobials.[20-24,60-61]

Laboratory Diagnosis

General Principles

For the purpose of diagnosing an infection, urine specimens should be collected prior to administering the first dose of antimicrobials. Appropriate sterile collection devices and aseptic technique should be employed. Specific lab criteria regarding required volumes should be followed because inadequate amounts of urine may yield false-negative results. Acute uncomplicated UTI is generally caused by a predicable array of microorganisms, and cultures are not usually obtained. However, due to the increasing prevalence of antimicrobial resistance, current recommendations are being reevaluated.

Urine Specimen Collection

- The first portion of a voided urines are appropriate for diagnosing sexually transmitted diseases and urethritis in both men and women but are not the preferred specimen for determination of UTI.

- The diagnosis of UTI in neonates involves an aggressive septic workup that may include a complete blood count, blood cultures, lumbar puncture, urinalysis, and urine culture. Urine may be obtained by the catheterization method for male neonates; however, a suprapubic tap should be performed on female neonates due to the increased risk for contamination when obtained from catheterization.[63,64]

Copyright © 2005, Association for Professionals in Infection Control and Epidemiology, Inc.

- Clean-catch midstream specimens in the noncatheterized person are recommended when there is suspicion of having complicated infections or when symptoms are not characteristic of UTI. After the perineal area has been adequately cleaned with an appropriate skin antiseptic, the individual carefully exposes the urethra with clean fingers, voids a small amount of urine (to clear the urethra of skin contaminants) before collecting the specimen from the urine stream. However, there are some reports that the cleansing procedure may not significantly change the contamination rate and therefore may be unnecessary.[65]

- For those with indwelling catheters and ileal conduits, specimens can be collected using sterile technique by aspirating urine with a sterile needle or cannula that is passed either through the catheter itself or through a special puncturable diaphragm incorporated within the collection tubing.[55] The catheter should not be disconnected to obtain specimens due to risk of introducing microorganisms into the system.[65] Urine should not be sampled from the collection bag, as the container may have been contaminated via the catheter drainage spout. The bag often contains multiplied microorganisms that are not reflective of those found in the urine collected directly from the bladder or catheter drainage tube.[55] Catheters that have been in place for extended periods of time often contain microorganisms that are different from those within the urinary tract. Therefore, specimens obtained from the collection tubing may not reflect the true microbiological status of the patient's urinary tract.[57] Additionally, when a patient is suspected of having a symptomatic UTI, the indwelling catheter should be replaced prior to the initiation of antimicrobial therapy due to the likely presence of biofilms. Therefore, when possible, urine for culture should be obtained after catheter replacement for more reliable results.[55]

- Urine in adequate amounts is difficult to collect from patients with surgically created ileal neobladders. Interpretation becomes more difficult when inadequate amounts of urine are present.[55]

- All specimens should be clearly labeled with specific patient information in addition to date, time, and method of collection (e.g., straight cath, indwelling cath, clean-catch midstream).

- After the urine is collected it should be transported to the laboratory as soon as possible. Urine specimens should be cultured within 2 hours after collection or should be refrigerated when no preservative is present.[65]

Urinalysis

Urinalysis is the examination of urine that may include macroscopic and microscopic evaluation dependent on the extent of laboratory services offered. Macroscopic examination can include appearance (color and clarity), specific gravity (concentration), and dipstick testing.

The presence of white blood cells or leukocytes may be useful in diagnosing UTI, as pyuria is indicative of inflammation within the urinary tract. Although pyuria usually occurs with acute cystitis, the absence of pyuria suggests a noninfectious cause for the symptoms. The presence of white blood cell casts with microscopic examination of spun urine sediment is indicative of an upper UTI. Microscopic evaluation of unspun urine is less sensitive but more specific but is generally not recommended for acute uncomplicated cystitis due to the difficulty of identifying low number of pathogens on wet mounts or Gram stain. The presence of red blood cells in the urine (hematuria) commonly occurs in women with UTI but is absent in women with urethritis or vaginitis. Blood may be detected in the urine during menses; presence of hematuria is not a reliable predictor for complicated infection and does not indicate the need for prolonged antimicrobial therapy.[66]

Urine dipsticks

Dipsticks are rapid test strips with reagent-impregnated tabs that can provide information about the specimen within a few seconds. For example, pH (acidity or alkalinity), protein, glucose, blood (red blood cells), leukocyte esterase (LE), and nitrites may be tested in a single strip. Different configurations are available depending on manufacturer and measures of interest by the ordering clinician and/or availability. The positive predictive value of positive nitrite and leukocyte esterase (LE) urine dipsticks in helping to diagnose asymptomatic UTI is relatively low except in institutionalized adults and diabetic women. However, an abnormal amount of LE detected is indicative of an inflammatory response.[67] UTI is generally responsible for this increase. However, other conditions such as nephropathy, stone, foreign body, genitourinary trauma, neoplasms, glomerulonephritis, vaginal contamination, or appendicitis may produce a positive LE test. This test has a sensitivity of 75% to 96% and specificity of 94% to 98% for the detection of ≥ 10 leukocytes/mm^3 of urine (approximating per high-power field microscopy). A urine culture should be performed when a positive LE is identified. Additionally, a urine culture should be performed when negative LE is obtained but the microscopic exam reveals ≥ 10 leukocytes/ml. This test, however, lacks adequate sensitivity for the detection of UTI with low colony counts in recently voided urine, or in dilute urine.[13]

Copyright © 2005, Association for Professionals in Infection Control and Epidemiology, Inc.

Imaging Studies

Patients with healthcare-associated UTI who are severely ill and have underlying conditions that predispose to infectious complications such as papillary necrosis, emphysematous pyelonephritis, and intrarenal or perinephric abscess formation (associated with obstructing nephrolithiasis) often require the use of special diagnostic tools.[50] Imaging studies, urological consultation, and urological or uroradiological interventions may be needed and should be considered, depending on the clinical context.[68,69]

Treatment Strategies

Cloudy or Foul-Smelling Urine

Cloudy or foul-smelling urine does not always necessitate a workup for UTI. However, it should be considered for patients who had previous symptomatic UTIs characterized by such changes in the urine.[66]

Asymptomatic UTIs

Antimicrobial treatment of asymptomatic UTI should be avoided. Urinalysis and urine culture should only be preformed when clinical manifestations of infection exist. When an asymptomatic patient has a urine culture that suggests UTI, antibiotic therapy is generally not indicated regardless of the organism or its susceptibility patterns and regardless of the presence or degree of associated pyuria. Exceptions include patients who fall into one of the narrowly defined risk groups for which treatment of asymptomatic UTI is indicated. Pregnant females should be treated with a 3- to 7-day course of antimicrobials.[13,66]

Symptomatic UTIs

Individuals with clinically significant signs and/or symptoms consistent with UTI not explained by another process should be treated with an antimicrobial with activity against known or likely pathogens (Table 25–2). This recommendation is made even without specific evidence of a UTI.[5] Empiric therapy can be given intravenously in the severely ill person and changed to an oral regimen once the individual has stabilized, is able to tolerate medications, and the susceptibility pattern is known. Oral antibiotics are generally given when the patient is not severely ill.[4] Existing foreign bodies such as indwelling catheters, stones, or urinary tract stents should be removed as soon as possible. For patients who require continued indwelling catheter use, catheter exchange before initiating antibiotic therapy increases the likelihood of microbiological and clinical cure if the original catheter is encrusted with biofilm.[71] A recent Cochrane review of five studies concluded there is insufficient data to recommend any specific therapy and duration for symptom-

atic pregnant women.[72] Neonates should be treated with parenteral antibiotics for 7 to 14 days due to the increased risk for bacteremia.[63,64,73]

UTI Prophylaxis

Antimicrobial prophylaxis may be recommended for women who experience two or more symptomatic UTIs in 6 months, three or more in 12 months, and for those with fewer infections but have severe discomfort. Resolution of a previous UTI should be confirmed by culture 1–2 weeks posttreatment and prior to the initiation of prophylaxis.[61] Self-treatment with low-dose antimicrobials in women with recurrent cystitis is safe and effective.[75]

Treatment Regimens

A 7-day course of oral antibiotics has been associated with cure in 94% of women. Longer courses are not more effective in eradicating or preventing recurrences and are associated with increased rates of adverse reactions. Persons with fever, chills, and flank pain may have an upper UTI; a urine culture is suggested to determine susceptibility combined with a 14-day course of appropriate antimicrobial therapy.[76]

Prevention and Infection Control Measures

Condom Catheters

Condom catheters as alternatives to indwelling catheters should be considered for use in incontinent male patients with intact voiding reflexes. However, their use may increase the risk of skin maceration and phimosis in the absence of meticulous skin care.[77] Condom catheters should be changed every few days, and careful inspection of skin should be performed.[78]

Intermittent Catheters

Although randomized comparisons have not been done, observational data suggest that intermittent catheterization (for patients with distensible bladders), and incontinence pads represent lower-risk alternatives to indwelling catheters (Table 25–2).[9]

Suprapubic Catheters

Preliminary research data suggests suprapubic catheterization may result in a decreased risk for UTI as compared to indwelling urethral catheters. However, there is a lack of controlled clinical studies supporting their use.[79,80,81] Thus, in selected patients this route may be preferable. However, making generalizations about this data report is difficult, and long-term advantages regarding infection control are not well defined.[9]

Copyright © 2005, Association for Professionals in Infection Control and Epidemiology, Inc.

Indwelling Catheters

Despite the probability that the direct morbidity, cost, and increased length of stay per episode of healthcare-associated UTI are relatively low, several considerations support that prevention deserves high priority. These include (a) the significant morbidity due to low incidence but serious complications of healthcare-associated UTI such as gram-negative bacteremia and sepsis; (b) the undefined but probably substantial contribution of the "unsuspected urinary reservoir" phenomenon to non-UTI healthcare-associated infections; and (c) the added selection process that results from unnecessary antimicrobial therapy given for asymptomatic healthcare-associated UTI (Table 25–1). Because the risk of acquiring UTI is fairly constant per day of indwelling catheter use, the cumulative risk of UTI is directly proportional to the duration of catheterization.[9] Thus, efforts to avoid catheter use altogether and to discontinue the catheter when it is no longer indicated, may prevent UTI.

Because approximately 20%–30% of patients with indwelling catheters in the acute-care setting lack an appropriate indication for catheterization, substantial reductions in total catheter days are theoretically possible.[82,83] In one study, resident and staff physicians in teaching hospitals were unaware of the presence of indwelling catheters in approximately 30% of their catheterized patients. That 30% of patients were four times more likely to lack an appropriate indication for catheterization.[31] Thus, processes that require assessment for indications for initial catheter insertion and periodic reassessment of ongoing catheter needs are essential for UTI risk reduction. For patients in whom indwelling urethral catheters are indicated, certain catheter use practices may assist in the prevention of UTI. Limiting the use of urinary catheters for specific indications is an important infection prevention measure. The following are considered legitimate indications for urinary catheterization: (1) promotion of urinary drainage in patients with urinary retention, urinary tract obstruction, and neurogenic bladder dysfunction; (2) surgery involving urological and/or contiguous structures; and (3) when monitoring of accurate urine output is necessary in critically ill patients. However, urine output monitoring in noncritically ill patients is considered a marginal indication. Specimens for diagnostic tests (i.e., urinary electrolytes) and cultures should not routinely be obtained by catheterization in an individual capable of voiding. Most importantly, urinary catheterization should never be used for care provider convenience in the incontinent patient.[82,83,84]

Areas of Controversy

A variety of research-related catheter technologies and their management have been evaluated to determine efficacy in helping to reduce the risk of UTIs.

Silicone and Hydrophilic Gel-Coated Catheters

Modern silicone and hydrophilic gel-coated catheters are more biocompatible and less receptive to microbial adherence than are traditional latex and natural rubber catheters.[9] However, whether these newer catheter materials confer a reduced risk of UTI has not been well documented or adequately studied. In contrast, numerous clinical trials have evaluated the impact of various antimicrobial coatings on the risk of CAUTI, with mixed results.

Silver-Coated Catheters

Silver oxide–coated catheters, although seemingly protective in women not receiving antibiotics, these devices yielded no overall reduction in UTI risk and are no longer marketed.[84] The most extensively studied of the available antimicrobial catheters is the silver alloy-hydrogel catheter. The early favorable results of four randomized clinical trials using this catheter were encouraging but fell short of establishing the catheter's efficacy; all four studies were conducted by the same investigators at a single Swedish hospital with unusually high rates of UTI in the control groups.[84] Cost-benefit analyses based on the results of these four trials, in conjunction with published estimates for UTI-associated costs and increased lengths of stay, have been interpreted as indicating not only cost effectiveness but cost savings.[85] However, in view of the uncertain efficacy and cost assumptions, these conclusions must be regarded as tentative.[86] In numerous trials, many performed in the United States, the apparent efficacy has been roughly inversely proportion to study quality. Studies that used a before–after design and/or a nonsystematic approach to UTI detection have yielded the most favorable results.[87,88] In contrast, the two studies that randomized patients and systematically evaluated all subjects for UTI found either no benefit or a modest benefit that lost statistical significance in a multivariate analysis limited to gram-positive bacteria.[89,90] Other investigators found nonsignificant reductions in UTIs after introducing silver-hydrogel catheters.[91,92,93] A meta-analysis including research published from 1966 to 2001 concluded additional high-quality studies are needed before the use of silver-coated catheters can be recommended.[94]

Antimicrobial Catheters

The minocycline/rifampin catheter yielded statistically significant protection against UTIs in a multicenter randomized clinical trial involving postprostatectomy

---

Copyright © 2005, Association for Professionals in Infection Control and Epidemiology, Inc.

patients.[78] However, protection was limited to gram-positive organisms, which, as noted earlier, are of less concern than gram-negative bacilli with respect to morbidity. An in vitro study involving the minocycline and rifampin catheters and uncoated catheters found the antimicrobial-coated catheter significantly impeded the migration of *E. coli, P. aeruginosa, E. faecalis,* and *C. albicans* after bacterial contamination of the catheter. Bacteruria developed at between 2 to 5 days with uncoated catheters versus 9 to 34 days with coated catheters.[91] Another reported study found bacterial migration along the catheter surface was inhibited with antimicrobial catheters.[96]

In another multiinstitution clinical trial the nitrofurazone catheter protected against UTI in a general hospital population for the first week of catheterization with the greatest effect against gram-negative bacilli.[97] Whether the apparent efficacy of the catheter remained statistically significant in a multivariate analysis has not been reported. This catheter was active against multidrug-resistant variants of normally nitrofurazone-susceptible bacterial species. However, this does not include common hospital-associated pathogens such as *P. aeruginosa, Serratia* spp., or *Proteus* spp.[98] Although the currently available antimicrobial catheters have shown some promise for UTI prevention, their true utility is not well established, and their appropriate role in routine patient care has yet to be defined.

Chlorhexidine Gluconate Catheters

Two types of catheters containing chlorhexidine gluconate (CHG) include chlorhexidine and silver sulfadiazine catheters (CSC) and chlorhexidine, silver sulfadiazine, and triclosan catheters (CSTC). In one study, the outer surfaces of these catheters demonstrated broad-spectrum, long-term resistance against microbial colonization. They also exhibited a broader antimicrobial spectrum than silver hydrogel (SH) latex and nitrofurazone-treated (NF) silicone catheters. Additionally, the CSTC catheters provided significantly longer protection from *S. aureus, S. epidermidis, E. coli,* and *P. aeruginosa* as compared with SH catheters. Silicone-containing CSTC catheters were able to resist colonization with *S. aureus* and *S. epidermidis* for significantly longer than the NF catheters.[99]

Catheter Insertion

Catheters should only be inserted and manipulated by hospital personnel, family members, and patients who are competent with insertion technique and asepsis. A no-touch, aseptic technique should be used by hospital personnel and family members. However, a clean, non-sterile technique may be used by patients who perform their own catheter insertion. To minimize urethral

trauma the smallest catheter possible should be used along with sterile equipment. Application of a sterile lubricant or anesthetic gel to the catheter tip minimizes mechanical trauma to the urethra and improves patient comfort. Additionally, catheters that are inserted emergently (i.e., trauma victims) should be removed or replaced as soon as the patient's condition permits.[9,12,84]

Catheter Care and Maintenance

- Effective hand washing should be performed immediately before and after manipulation of the catheter site or apparatus.[84]

- When not secured appropriately, catheters may move up and down in the urethra and contribute to extraluminal organism introduction into the bladder and trauma to the urethra. Additionally, the potential for kinking and bending of the catheter may exist when inadequate securement devices are used. Leg straps and circumferential Velcro fasteners have the potential to inhibit lymphatic drainage and venous return and may therefore increase the risk of deep vein thrombosis and pulmonary embolism. Therefore, it is imperative to utilize a catheter securement device that eliminates or diminishes tension on the balloon, urethral traction, in-and-out motions, and kinking or bending The device should allow for normal patient movement without compromising the catheter position.[9,12,84,100]

- Urinary flow should remain unobstructed. This may be accomplished by (1) keeping the collection bag below the level of the bladder, (2) maintaining the catheter free from kinking, (3) emptying the collection bag regularly using a separate collecting container for each patient, and (4) ensuring the drainage spigot does not come into contact with the collection container. Poorly functioning and partially obstructed catheters should be irrigated or replaced as necessary.[84]

- Standard precautions should always be incorporated when manipulating urine collection bags. Patient-specific collection containers should be used when emptying urine collection bags to reduce the risk of patient-to-patient transmission of organisms. Additionally, the catheter drainage spigot should never come into direct contact with the collection container.[9]

- Routine urine samples may be obtained through the sampling port after disinfection of the port. Irrigation may require disconnection of drainage tube, otherwise the system should remain closed.[9,12,84]

- When breaks in aseptic technique, disconnection, or leakage occur, the catheter junction should be disinfected with compatible agent per manufacturer's rec-

Copyright © 2005, Association for Professionals in Infection Control and Epidemiology, Inc.

ommendations followed by replacement of the collecting system.[9,12,84]

- Irrigation of indwelling urinary catheters should be avoided. However, when obstruction is anticipated, "closed" continuous irrigation may be useful. Intermittent irrigation may be used to dislodge clots, mucus, and other agents. The catheter-tubing junction should be disinfected before disconnection and flushed with a large-volume sterile syringe and sterile irrigant and syringes should be discarded after use. In order to maintain patency, catheters should be changed when frequent irrigation is required.[99]

- Daily meatal care with povidone-iodine solutions and cleaning with soap and water have not shown reduction in catheter-associated infections and are not endorsed by the Centers for Disease Control and Prevention.[66]

Specimen Collection and Bacteriological Monitoring

When culture is required, small volumes of urine may be removed from the sampling port when present or the distal end of the catheter. The sampling area should first be cleansed with an appropriate compatible disinfectant prior to aspiration with a sterile syringe with needle or cannula. Routine bacteriologic monitoring of catheterized patients as an infection control measure has not been established and is not recommended.[84]

Catheter Change Interval

Urinary catheters should be left in place only as long as deemed necessary and should not be routinely changed at arbitrary time intervals.[71]

Cohorting and Spatial Separation of Catheterized Patients

Because most CAUTI episodes go undetected, there is little opportunity for the cohorting of infected patients that has been proposed as an infection control measure.[11] However the risk for cross infection may be reduced through spatial separation of infected and noninfected patients with indwelling catheters. These patients should not share the same room or be in adjacent beds.[31]

Transmission-Based Precautions

In most instances of CAUTI, providers are unaware as they manipulate the infected patient's catheter system that the urine contains high concentrations of potential pathogens. Ironically, discovery of asymptomatic CAUTI often leads to unwarranted antibiotic therapy, which not only fails to benefit the index patient but also selects for more highly resistant organisms that can subsequently cause symptomatic infection in either

the index patient or other patients in the institution.[21] Thus, CAUTI may contribute more to the burden of morbidity due to healthcare-associated infections from emerging resistant microorganisms within the hospital than through its direct effects on the index patients. To avoid transferring microorganisms from one patient to another or to noncolonized sites in the same patient, healthcare workers at the bedside must observe proper infection control practices including standard precautions. Every catheterized patient must be regarded as possibly infected, even if the most recent urine culture was negative. A UTI could have been acquired subsequent to the previous specimen submission. In addition, patients known to have symptomatic or asymptomatic UTI due to organisms with special infection control implications such as MRSA or VRE must be placed in the type of isolation specified for these organisms by the institution's policies. UTI inevitably will occur in many catheterized patients despite compulsive adherence to appropriate catheter maintenance protocols.

Other Measures Without Proven Benefit

Preventive measures that increase cost without providing proven benefit include collection bag additives, antireflux valves, urine baffles, and antimicrobial inserts in the collection tubing.[25,9,101] Likewise, there is no proven role for scheduled catheter replacement as an infection-preventing measure, although this may be a desirable mechanical intervention in patients who tend to develop catheter obstruction with prolonged use.[9] Certain other measures may actually increase UTI risk and/or select for resistant organisms and are best avoided. These include daily green soap and water cleansing specifically of the urethral meatus (as opposed to routine bathing), daily or more frequent application of antimicrobial substances to the meatus, bladder irrigation (with or without antimicrobial substances), and prophylactic systemic antibiotics.[9,25,51]

IV. SUMMARY AND CONCLUSIONS

UTIs are the most commonly identified healthcare-associated infections in both acute and long-term care facilities. They significantly contribute to patient morbidity and mortality and rising healthcare costs. Among women treated for UTI, 10%–20% develop a second one within a few months, but reliable predictors of recurrence have not yet been established. Understanding the epidemiology of UTIs is important in the development of infection prevention and control strategies. Alternatives to catheterization should always be considered because indwelling urinary catheters significantly increase the risk for healthcare-associated UTI. Bedside healthcare providers must be diligent in their use of aseptic technique and hand washing. Antibiotics should be used discriminately and in general only be

Copyright © 2005, Association for Professionals in Infection Control and Epidemiology, Inc.

given to symptomatic patients. The ideal duration of antibiotic therapy remains debated and continues to be evaluated. New treatment modalities and advancing catheter technology are instrumental in the reduction of UTIs. Well-designed case-control clinical studies and trials are needed to advance current thinking and practices as they relate to UTIs.

V.   FUTURE TRENDS/RESEARCH

New Innovations in Catheter Technology

Innovations in catheter technology that are under development or remain to be fully explored include measures to block biofilm formation, incorporation of the potent gram-negative antibiotic ciprofloxacin, and catheters with a collapsible intraurethral segment.[60,102,103,104] Little or no information is available regarding the clinical efficacy of these technologies. Local delivery of an antimicrobial agent from a coated or impregnated catheter should provide much less selective pressure for resistant organisms than do systemic administration. Still, the prospect of widespread use of devices coated with ciprofloxacin, a first-line antibiotic for serious gram-negative infections, raises serious concerns that are considerably greater than those prompted by similar uses of silver, minocycline, rifampin, or nitrofurazone, none of which is particularly relevant to inpatient antimicrobial therapy.[102,103,104]

Areas of Controversy

Type and duration of antimicrobial therapy for specific patient populations remains controversial as does the use of impregnated catheters. Some researchers have supported the ingestion of cranberry juice or cranberry-derived substances for reduction and treatment of UTIs, believing it contains substances that prevent bacterial adherence (especially *E. coli*) to urinary epithelial cells and catheter surfaces, thereby controlling the formation of biofilm on urinary catheters. However, a systematic research review revealed conflicting results.[105] In women, the use of exogenous estrogen or estrogen rings may reverse genitourinary mucosal atrophy, thus restoring a more normal vaginal environment.[44,106] Using ultrasound to detect bladder volume prior to intermittent catheterization has yielded mixed results. However, one investigator found a reduction in UTIs, prevention in unnecessary catheterizations, greater patient and nurse satisfaction, and a significant cost savings.[107]

Financial Cost-Benefit Issues

Published estimates of the per-episode increases in healthcare costs and lengths of stay associated with

CAUTI in the acute-care setting vary from hundreds to thousands of dollars and from less than one day to several days. A recently published study concluded the extra direct costs associated with healthcare-associated CAUTIs were substantially lower than reported by previous investigators. The average direct cost associated with a single CAUTI was $586 per infection. Additionally, the average length of stay increased by 0.4 days for asymptomatic and 2.0 days for symptomatic CAUTIS.[3] Determining the actual cost benefit of interventions will assist infection control professionals in helping to evaluate and recommend appropriate preventative measures in a variety of healthcare settings.

Biointerference and Bladder Colonization

A novel preventive measure against symptomatic UTI that is under development is the use of an avirulent *E. coli* strain (ATCC strain 83972) to colonize the bladder of spinal cord injured patients as a way to prevent colonization with more virulent organisms.[86] This *E. coli* strain, which was originally isolated from the urine of a young woman with asymptomatic bacteriuria, is able to establish asymptomatic long-term bladder colonization in patients with neurogenic bladder, including some managed with indwelling catheters. Historically, controlled pilot data suggest a substantial reduction in the frequency of symptomatic UTI episodes among patients successfully colonized with strain 83972. Further evaluation of this and other biointerference measures is needed. Long-term bladder colonization with *E. coli* 83972 may decrease the frequency of UTI in patients with neurogenic bladder secondary to spinal cord injury.[101]

Mucosal Vaccines

In the late seventies, the presence of an antibody was discovered in the vaginal secretions of women not prone to UTI. This discovery led to research geared at developing mucosal vaccines for the prevention of UTI in certain high-risk populations.[110] Research directed at increasing the production of immunoglobulin A on the lining of the urinary tract of women is actively being conducted.[103] A whole-cell vaccine containing a mixture of heat-killed bacteria has been developed. The vaccine contains equal proportions of the following uropathogenic organisms: 6 *E. coli* strains and 1 strain each of *P. mirabilis, P. morganii, E. faecalis,* and *K. pneumonia* and is administered via vaginal suppository. In a double-blind, randomized, and placebo-controlled clinical trial, 55% of vaccinees who also received booster doses were infection free at 6 months as compared to only 22% of those who received placebo only or primary immunization only.[104] Another vaccine formulation that shows promise inhibits *E. coli* from binding to bladder cells. This

Copyright © 2005, Association for Professionals in Infection Control and Epidemiology, Inc.

vaccine acts by stimulating the production of antibodies against two key *E. coli* adhesion molecules.[110]

VI. INTERNATIONAL PERSPECTIVES

UTI occurrences and prevention remain a global issue for basic and future consideration. Evidenced-based research is essential in the development of new and improved methods of preventing, diagnosing, and treating UTIs.[72,108,109]

REFERENCES

1. Foxman B, Barlow R, D'Arey H et al: Urinary tract infection: self-reported incidence and associated costs, *Ann Epidemiol* 10: 509—515, 2000
2. Schappert SM: *Ambulatory care visits to physicians, hospital outpatient departments, and emergency departments; United States, 1997, Vital and health statistics*, Series 13, No. 143, Atlanta: National Center for Health Statistics, November 1999 [DHHS publication no. (PHS) 2000–1714.]
3. Tambylah P, Knasinski V, Maki, D: The direct costs of nosocomial catheter associated urinary tract infections in the era of managed care, *Infection Control and Hospital Epidemiology* 23(1):27—31, 2002
4. *Dorland's illustrated medical dictionary*, ed 30, Philadelphia, 2003, Saunders
5. Tambyah PA, Maki DG: Catheter associated urinary tract infection is rarely symptomatic. A prospective study of 1497 catheterized patients, *Arch Intern Med* 160:678—82, 2000
6. Decambre M, Albertson P, Rutchik S: Emphysematous cystitis: caveats of complex presentations, *Infect Urol* 15(4):19—21, 2002
7. Eggener, SE, Merrill H, Matschke MH et al: Emphysematous cystitis: review of current management, *Infect Urol* 15(2):12—14, 2002
8. Johnson JR: Pyelonephritis and abscess of the kidney. In Armstrong D, Cohen J, editors: *Infectious diseases*, vol. 1. London, 1999, Mosby, pp. 59.1–8
9. Warren J, Bakke A, Desgranchamps F, et al: Catheter associated bacteriuria and the role of biomaterial in prevention. In Naber KG, Pechere JC, Kumazawa J, Khoury S, Gerberding JL, Schaeffer AJ, editors: *Nosocomial and healthcare associated infections in urology*, Plymouth, UK, 2001, Health Publication Ltd., pp. 151–76
10. Kunin CM, VanArsdale White L, Hua TH: A reassessment of the importance of "low-count" bacteriuria in young women with acute urinary symptoms, *Ann Intern Med* 119:454—60, 1993
11. Meares EM: Prostatis, *Med Clin North Am* 75:405—24, 1991
12. Maki DG, Tambyah PA: Engineering out the risk for infection with urinary catheters, *Emerg Infect Dis* 7:342—7, 2000
13. Orenstein R, Wong ES: Urinary tract infections in adults, *American Family Physician*, March 1, 2000
14. Nicolle LE: Asymptomatic bacteriuria in the elderly, *Infect Dis Clin North Am* 11(3):647—62, 1997
15. Sobel JD, Kaufman CA, McKinsey D, et al: Candiduria: a randomized, double-blind study of treatment with fluconazole and placebo, *Clin Infect Dis* 30:19—24, 2000
16. Lundstrom T, Sobel J: Nosocomial candiduria: a review, *Clin Infect Dis* 32:1602, 2001
17. Stamm T, Hooton W: Recurrent urinary tract infection, 2002, Available at www.uptodate.com.
18. Tambyah PA, Maki DG: The relationship between pyuria and infection in patients with indwelling urinary catheters. A prospective study of 761 patients, *Arch Intern Med* 160:673, 2000
19. Cardenas DD, Hooton TM: Urinary tract infection in persons with spinal cord injury, *Arch Phys Med Rehabil* 76:272, 1995
20. Donlan RM: Biofilms: Microbial life on surfaces, *Emerging Infectious Diseases* 8(9):881–90, 2002
21. Davey ME, O'Toole GA: Microbial biofilms: from ecology to molecular genetics, *Microbiology and Molecular Biology Reviews* 64(4):847–867, 2000

22. Donlan RM, Costerton JW: Biofilms: Survival mechanisms of clinically relevant microorganisms, *Clinical Microbiology Reviews* 15(2):167–93, 2002
23. Dunne WM: Bacterial adhesion: seen any good biofilms lately? *Clinical Microbiology Reviews* 15:155–66, 2002
24. Kuhn DM, Chandra J, Mukherjee PK, et al: Comparison of biofilms formed by *Candida albicans* and *Candida parapsilosis* on bioprosthetic surfaces, *Infection and Immunity* 70:878–88, 2002
25. Warren JW: Catheter associated urinary tract infections, *Infect Dis Clin North Am* 11:609—22, 1997
26. Hooton TM: Recurrent urinary tract infection in women, *Int J Antimicrob Agents* 17:259–68, 2001
27. Roberts KB, Akintemi OB: The epidemiology and clinical presentation of urinary tract infections in children younger than 2 years of age, *Ped Ann* 28:644–9, 1999
28. Schoen EJ, Colby CJ, Ray GT: Newborn circumcision decreases incidence and costs of urinary tract infections during the first year of life, *Pediatrics* 105:789–93, 2000
29. Ashouri N, Butler J, Ofelia M, et al: Urinary tract infections in neonates: how aggressive a workup and therapy? *Infect Med* 20(2):98–102, 2003
30. Steele RW: The epidemiology and clinical presentation of urinary tract infections in children 2 years of age through adolescence, *Pediatrics Ann* 28:644–49, 1999
31. Hellerstein S: Urinary tract infections in children: pathophysiology, risk factors, and management, *Pediatrics* 19(12): 554–60, 2002
32. Klevan JL, DeJohng AR: Urinary tract symptoms and urinary tract infection, *Child Nephrol Urol* 12:62–64, 1992
33. Kunin CM: Urinary tract infections in adults. In Kunin CM, editor: *Urinary tract infections*, ed 5, Baltimore, 1997, Williams & Wilkins, pp. 128–64
34. Foxman B, Marsh J, Gillepsie B, et al: Condom use and first-time urinary tract infection, *Epidemiology* 8:637–41, 1997
35. Weir MR, Brien J: Adolescent urinary tract infections, *Adolescent Medicine* 11:293–313, 2000
36. Schles D, Hooton TM, Roberts PL, et al: Risk factors for recurrent urinary tract infection in young women, *J Infect Dis* 182: 1177–82, 2000
37. Boyko EJ, Fihn SD, Scholes D, et al: Diabetes and the risk of acute urinary tract infection among postmenopausal women, *Diabetes Care* 25:1778–83, 2002
38. Hooton TM, Scholes D, Hughes JP, et al: A prospective study of risk factors for symptomatic urinary tract infection in young women, *N Engl J Med* 335:468–74, 1996
39. Fihn SD, Boyko EJ, Normand EH, et al: Association between use of spermicide-coated condoms and *Escherichia coli* urinary tract infection in young women, *Am J Epidemiol* 144:512–20, 1996
40. Fihn SD, Boyko EJ, Chen C-L, et al: Use of spermicide-coated condoms and other risk factors for urinary tract infection caused by *Staphylococcus saprophyticus*, *Arch Intern Med* 158: 281–87, 1998
41. Daifuku R, Stamm WE: Bacterial adherence to bladder uroepithelial cells in catheter associated urinary tract infection, *New Engl J Med* 314:1208–13, 1986
42. Scholes D, Hooton TM, Roberts PL, et al: Risk factors for recurrent urinary tract infection in young women, *J of Infect Dis* 182:1177–82, 2000
43. Baerheim A, Digranes A, Jureen R, Malterud K: Generalized symptoms in adult women with acute uncomplicated lower urinary tract infection: an observational study, *Medscape General Medicine* 5(3):1, 2003
44. *Sanford guide to antimicrobial therapy*, ed 32 Hyde Park, Vermont, 2002, Antimicrobial Therapy
45. Bruce G: Diagnostic and therapeutic considerations in catheter associated bacteriuria in hospital/chronic care facility. In Cunha B, editor: *Urinary tract infections: current issues in diagnosis and treatment, Antibiotics for Clinicians* 2(suppl 2):11–16, 1998
46. Hooton TM, Stamm WE: Diagnosis and treatment of urinary tract infection, *Infect Dis Clin North Am* 11:551, 1997
47. Gromolin I, McCue J: Urinary tract infection in the elderly patient, *Infect Urol* 13(5a):s7–s13, 2000
48. Urinary Tract Infections. In Beuben D, Herr K, Pacala J, Semela T, Small G, editors: *Geriatrics at your fingertips*, Ed 5, New York, 2002, American Geriatrics Society, pp. 70–73

Copyright © 2005, Association for Professionals in Infection Control and Epidemiology, Inc.

49. McCue JD: UTIs in at-risk patients: are they "complicated"? *Infect Med* 16:522–40, 1999
50. Ronald AR, Harding GKM: Complicated urinary tract infections, *Infect Dis Clin North Am* 11:583–92, 1997
51. Lipsky BA: Prostatitis and urinary tract infection in men: what's new; what's true? *Am J Med* 106:327–34, 1999
52. Anon: National Nosocomial Infections Surveillance (NNIS) system report, data summary from January 1992–April 2000, issued June 2000, *Am J Infect Control* 28:429–48, 2000
53. Nicolle LE: Asymptomatic bacteriuria in the elderly, *Infect Dis Clin North Am* 11(3):647–62, 1997
54. Gupta K, Scholes D, Stamm W: Increasing prevalence of antimicrobial resistance among uropathogens causing acute uncomplicated cystitis in women, *JAMA* 281:736–8, 1999
55. Johnson JR, Roberts PL, Olsen R, Moyer K, Stamm WE: Prevention of catheter associated urinary tract infection with a silver oxide-coated urinary catheter: clinical and microbiological correlates, *J Infect Dis* 162:1145–50, 1990
56. Siebert JD, Thomson RB Jr, Tan JS et al: Emergence of antimicrobial resistance in gram-negative bacillus causing bacteremia during therapy, *Am J Clin Pathol* 100:47–51, 1993
57. Bergquist D, Bronnestam R, Hedelin H, et al: The relevance of urinary sampling methods in patients with indwelling Foley catheters, *Br J Urol* 52:92–95, 1997
58. Jarlier V, Fosse T, Phillippon A: Antibiotic susceptibility in aerobic gram-negative bacilli isolated in intensive care units in 39 French teaching hospitals (ICU study), *Intensive Care Med* 22:1057–65, 1996
59. Tambyah PA, Halvorson KT, Maki DG: A prospective study of pathogenesis of catheter associated urinary tract infections, *Mayo Clin Proc* 74:131–36, 1999
60. Kumon H: Pathogenesis and management of bacterial biofilms in the urinary tract, *J Infect Chemother* 2:18, 1996
61. Morris NS, Strickler DJ: Encrustation of indwelling urethral catheters by *Proteus mirabilis* biofilms growing in human urine, *Journal of Hospital Infection* 39:227–34, 1998
62. Kunin CM, Chin QP, Chambers ST: Formation of encrustations on indwelling urinary catheters in the elderly: a comparison of different types of catheter materials in "blockers" and "non-blockers," *J Urol* 138:899–902, 1987
63. Crain E, Gerschel JC: Urinary tract infections in febrile infants younger than eight week of age, *Pediatrics* 86:363–67, 1990
64. Baraff LJ: Management of febrile neonates: what to do with low risk infants, *Pediatr Infect Dis J* 13:943–45, 1994
65. Clarridge JE, Pezzlo MT: Lab diagnosis of urinary tract infections. In Weissfield AS, editor: *Cumulative techniques and procedures in clinical microbiology 2B.* Washington, DC, 1998, ASM Press, pp. 5–19
66. Fitzgerald MA: Urinary tract infection: providing the best care, *WebMD.* June 24, 2003
67. Clinical guidelines: adult urinalysis screening, *Nurse Practitioner* 20(2):55–59, 1995
68. Siegel JF, Smith A, Moldwin R: Minimally invasive treatment of renal abscess, *J Urol* 155:52–5, 1996
69. Turney JH: Renal conservation for gas-forming infections, *Lancet* 1:770–1, 2000
70. Stamm WE, Hooton TM: Management of urinary tract infections in adults, *N Engl J Med* 329:1328–34, 1993
71. Raz R, Schiller D, Nicolle LE: Chronic indwelling catheter replacement before antimicrobial therapy for symptomatic urinary tract infection, *J Urol* 164:1254–8, 2000
72. Vazquez JC, Villar J: Treatments for symptomatic urinary tract infections during pregnancy, *Cochrane Review Abstract* 4: CD0022546, 2003
73. Ferrara PC, Bartfield JM, Snyder HS: Neonatal fever: utility of the Rochester criteria in determining low risk for serious bacterial infections, *Am J Emerg Med* 15:299–302, 1997
74. Hooton TM, Stamm WE: Overview of acute cystitis in adults, *UpToDate,* 2003. Available at www.uptodate.com
75. Chew LD, Fihn SD: Recurrent cystitis in nonpregnant women, *West J Med* 170:274–78, 1999
76. Warren JW, Abrutyn E, Hebel JR, et al: Guidelines for antimicrobial treatment of uncomplicated acute bacterial cystitis and acute pyelonephritis in women, *Clin Infect Dis* 29:745–58, 1999
77. Hirsh DD, Fainstein V, Musher DM: Do condom catheter collecting systems cause urinary tract infection? *JAMA* 242:340–1, 1979
78. Esclarian De Ruz E, Garcia Leoni G, Herruzo Caberra R: Epidemiology and risk factors for urinary tract infection in patients with spinal cord injury, *Journal of Urology* 164:1285–89, 2000
79. Vandoni RE, Lironi A, Tsanchtz P: Bacteriuria during urinary tract catheterization: suprapubic versus urethral route: a prospective randomized trial, *Acta Chir Belg* 94:12–6, 1994
80. Zermann D, Wunderlich H, Derry F, Schroder S, Schubert J: Audit of early bladder management complications after spinal cord injury in first-treating hospitals, *Eur Urol* 37:156–60, 2000
81. Perrin LC, Penfold C, McLeish A: A prospective randomized controlled trial comparing suprapubic with urethral catheterization in rectal surgery, *Aust N Z J Surg* 67:554–6, 1997
82. Saint S, Wiese J, Amory JK, et al: Are physicians aware of which of their patients have indwelling urinary catheters? *Am J Med* 109:476–80, 2000
83. Jain P, Parada JP, David A, Smith LG: Overuse of the indwelling urinary tract catheter in hospitalized medical patients, *Arch Intern Med* 155:1425–9, 1995
84. Saint A, Elmore JG, Sullivan SD, Emerson SS, Koepsell TD: The efficacy of silver alloy-containing urinary catheters in preventing urinary tract infection: a meta-analysis, *Am J Med* 105:236–41, 1998
85. Saint S, Veenstra DL, Sullivan SD, Chenoweth C, Fendrick AM: The potential clinical and economic benefits of silver alloy urinary catheters in preventing urinary tract infection, *Arch Intern Med* 160:2760–675, 2000
86. Plowman R, Graves N, Esquivel J, Roberts JA: An economic model to assess the cost and benefits of the routine use of silver alloy coated urinary catheters to reduce the risk of urinary tract infections in catheterized patients, *J Hosp Infect* 48:33–42, 2001
87. Bologna RA, Tu LM, Polansky M, Fraimow HD, Gordon DA, Whitmore KE: Hydrogel/silver ion-coated urinary catheter reduces nosocomial urinary tract infection rates in intensive care unit patients: a multicenter study, *Urology* 54:982–7, 1998
88. Karchmer TB, Gianetta ET, Muto CA, Strain BA, Farr BM: A randomized crossover study of silver-coated urinary catheters in hospitalized patients, *Arch Intern Med* 160:3294–8, 2000
89. Thibon P, Coutour XL, Leroyer R, Fabry J: Randomized multicentre trial of the effects of a catheter coated with hydrogel and silver salts on the incidence of hospital-acquired urinary tract infection, *J Hosp Infect* 45:117–24, 2000
90. Maki D, Knasinski V, Halvorson K, et al: A novel silver-hydrogel-impregnated indwelling urinary catheter reduces CAUTIs: a prospective double-blind trial, *Infect Control Hosp Epidemiol* 19:682, 1998
91. Bologna R, Tu LM, Polansky M, et al: Hydrogel/silver ion-coated urinary catheter reduces nosocomial urinary tract infection rates in intensive care unit patients: a multicenter study, *Adult Urology* 54(6):982–87, 1999
92. Thibbon P, Le Contour X, Leroyer R, et al: Randomized multicentre trial of the effects of a catheter coated with hydrogel and silver salts on the incidence of hospital-acquired urinary tract infections, *Journal of Hospital Infection* 45:117–24, 2000
93. Lai KK, Fontecchio SA: Use of silver-hydrogel urinary catheters on the incidence of catheter associated urinary tract infections in hospitalized patients, *American Journal of Infection Control* 30(4);221–25, 2002
94. Neil-Weise BS, Arend SM, vanden Broek PJ: Is there evidence for recommending silver-coated urinary catheters in guidelines? *Journal of Hospital Infection* 52:81–87, 2002
95. Darouiche RO, Smith JAJ, Hanna H, et al: Efficacy of antimicrobial-impregnated bladder catheters in reducing catheter associated bacteriuria: a prospective, randomized, multicenter clinical trial, *Urol* 54:976–81, 1999
96. Darouiche RO, Hossam S, Raad II: In vitro efficacy of antimicrobial-coated bladder catheters in inhibiting bacterial migration along catheter surface, *Journal of Infectious Diseases* 176:1109–12, 1997
97. Maki DG, Knasinski V, Tambyah PA: A prospective investigator-blinded trial of a novel nitrofurazone-impregnated urinary catheter, *Infect Control Hosp Epidemiol* 18[Suppl]:P50 (Abstract M49), 1997
98. Johnson JR, Delavari P, Azar M: Activities of a nitrofurazone-containing urinary catheter and a silver hydrogel catheter against multidrug-resistant bacteria characteristic of catheter associated urinary tract infection, *Antimicrob Agents Chemother* 43:2990–5, 1999

APIC Text of Infection Control and Epidemiology

Copyright © 2005, Association for Professionals in Infection Control and Epidemiology, Inc.

99. Wong E, Hooton, TM: Guideline for prevention of catheter associated urinary tract infections. Issues in Healthcare Settings, Atlanta, 2003, Centers for Disease Control and Prevention. Division of Healthcare Quality Promotion

100. Bierman S, Carignan M: The prevention of adverse events associated with urinary tract catheterization, *Managing Infection Control* 26:43–9, 2003

101. Hull R, Rudy D, Donovan W, et al: Urinary tract infection prophylaxis using *Escherichia coli* 83972 in spinal cord injured patients, *J Urol* 163:872–7, 2000

102. Hoyle B: Colonization-resistant polymer helps battle catheter-related infections, *ASM News* 66:131–2, 2000

103. DiTizio V, Ferguson GW, Mittelman MW, Khoury AE, Bruce AW, DiCosmo F: A liposomal hydrogel for the prevention of bacterial adhesion to catheters, *Biomaterials* 19:1877–84, 1998

104. Kwok CS, Horbett TA, Ratner BD: Design of infection-resistant antibiotic-releasing polymers. II. Controlled release of antibiotics through a plasma-deposited thin film barrier, *J Controlled Release* 62:301–11, 1999

105. Jepson RG, Mihaljevic L, Craig J: Cranberries for prevention urinary tract infections, *The Cochrane Library* 3:CD001321, 2000

106. Eriksen BC: A randomized, open, parallel-group study on the preventive effect of estradiol-releasing vaginal ring (Estring) on recurrent urinary tract infections in post-menopausal women, *Am J Obstet Gynecol* 180:1072–9, 1999

107. Wagner M, Schmid M: Prevention of Urinary Tract Infections and Urinary Catheterizations by Monitoring Bladder Volumes Via the Use of a Non-invasive BladderScan™ in Neuroscience Patients, *SHEA Annual Meeting ProGram* 18(5), part 2:M51, 1997

108. Fihn SD: Acute uncomplicated urinary tract infection in women, *N Engl J Med* 349:259–66, 2003

109. Lutters M, Vogt N: Antibiotic duration for treating uncomplicated, symptomatic lower urinary tract infections in elderly women, *Cochrane Review Abstract* 4, 2003

110. Koenig S: Fim-H based vaccine for prevention of *Escherichia coli* urinary tract infections, *ProGram and abstracts of the 40th Interscience Conference on Antimicrobial Agents and Chemotherapy,* September 17–20, 2000; Toronto, Ontario, Canada. Abstract 1140

111. Uelhing DT, Hopkins WJ, Balish E, et al: Vaginal mucosal immunization for recurrent urinary tract infection: Phase II clinical trial, *Journal of Urology* 17(2):169–71, 1997

112. Hopkins WJ, Elkahwaji JE, Uehling DT, et al: Phase 2 clinical trial of a vaginal mucosal vaccine for recurrent urinary tract infections in adult women, *ProGram and abstracts of the 41st Interscience Conference of Antimicrobial Agents and Chemotherapy,* December 16–19,2001, Chicago, Illinois. Abstract UL-15

113. Trautner BW, Darouiche RO: Role of biofilm in catheter associated urinary tract infections, *Am J Infect Control* 32(3): 177–83,2004

SUPPLEMENTAL RESOURCES

Bentley D, Bradley S, High K, et al: Practice guidelines for evaluation of fever and infection in long-term care facilities, *Clin Infect Dis* 31: 640–53, 2000

Cornia P, Amory J, Fraser S, et al: Computer-based order entry decreases duration of indwelling urinary catheterization in hospitalized patients, *Am J Med* 114:404–7, 2003

Costerman J, Lewandowski S, Caldwell D, et al: Microbial biofilms, *Annu Rev Microbiol* 49:711–45, 1995

Denstedt J, Wollin T, Reid G: Biomaterials used in urology; current issues of biocompatibility, infection, and encrustation, *J Endourol* 12: 493–500, 1998

Harding G, Zhandel G, Nicolle L, Cheang M: Antimicrobial treatment in diabetic women with asymptomatic bacteruria, *N Engl J Med* 347: 1576–83, 2002

Jain P, Parada J, David A, Smith L: Overuse of the indwelling urinary tract catheter in hospitalized patients, *Arch Int Med* 155:1425–9, 1995

Nickel J, Costerton J, McClean R, Olson M: Bacterial biofilms' influence on the pathogenesis, diagnosis and treatment of urinary tract infections, *J Antimicrobial Chemother*33:31–41, 1994

Patterson T, Andrile V: Detection, significance, and therapy of bacteruria in pregnancy, *Infec Dis Clin North Am* 11:593–609, 1997

Saint S, Lipsky B, Gould S: Indwelling urinary catheters: a one point restraint? *Ann Intern Med* 137:125–8, 2002

Stewart, P: New ways to stop biofilm infections, *Lancet* 36:97, 2003

Trautner B, Drouiche R, Hull R, et al: Pre-inoculation of urinary tract catheters with *Escherichia coli* 83972 inhibits catheter colonization by *Enterococcus faecalis, J Urol* 167:375–9, 2002

Wilson ML, Gaido L: Laboratory diagnosis of urinary tract infections in adult patients, *Clin Infect Dis* 38:1150–58, 2004

Zhanel G, Harding G, Guay D: Asymptomatic bacteriuria: which patients should be treated? *Arch Intern Med* 150:1389–96, 1990

Copyright © 2005, Association for Professionals in Infection Control and Epidemiology, Inc.

Occupational Health

Sue Sebazco, RN, BS, CIC
Director of Infection Control and Employee
Health
Arlington Memorial Hospital
Arlington, Texas

ABSTRACT

This chapter will outline the infection control considerations when designing and implementing an occupational health program for a healthcare facility. Included in the content are reasons for developing an occupational health program along with the major components. Risk of transmission of infection to and from the healthcare worker is discussed. Guidelines for work restrictions for personnel with infectious diseases and exposure management are provided. There are suggestions for measuring improvement in the prevention of occupational injuries and exposures. The chapter also includes a description of workers' compensation.

KEY CONCEPTS

- Reasons for developing an occupational health program

- Elements of an occupational health program

- Transmission of infection to and from the healthcare worker

- Common infectious processes with no indications for postexposure intervention

- Work restrictions in the healthcare facility related to communicable diseases

- Measuring improvement in preventing occupational exposure

- Workers' compensation

I.   BACKGROUND

Healthcare organizations need to provide a safe environment for both patients and healthcare personnel. During the past two decades there has been an increased awareness of occupational hazards to healthcare workers. Regulatory and licensing agencies are also aware of the need to address the prevention of hazards in the healthcare workplace. The infection control professional (ICP) has a vital role within the organization in identifying risk to the patient and the worker, assessing the potential adverse outcome, implementing protective policies and procedures, and evaluating the effectiveness of measures taken. To carry out this function, the ICP needs resources that are valid and based on scientific data. Recommended practices need to be based on how infections are transmitted in a healthcare facility and should address minimizing the worker as a potential source or host. The organization

Copyright © 2005, Association for Professionals in Infection Control and Epidemiology, Inc.

needs to consider what elements should be included in its facility's program. This decision is made by recognizing the characteristics of the patient/client/resident population served and those of the worker pool. The type of facility, the services provided, the geographic location, and the diseases that are endemic in the communities served also influence the elements that need to be included.

An organizational structure may not formally include the ICP as a member of the personnel health service. However, the ICP of a healthcare organization is often called on to participate when infection control issues for a worker need to be addressed. Often the ICP is called on to provide credible references to support the policies and practices that are in place.

II.   BASIC PRINCIPLES

Infection control policies, procedures, and practices in an occupational health program in a healthcare setting are designed to interrupt the transmission of infection to and from the healthcare personnel. There are infectious processes that present a possible threat to healthcare workers and have available vaccines for preexposure intervention. There are those that pose a possible threat and have specific indications for postexposure interventions. There are some common infectious processes with no indications for postexposure intervention.

The Centers for Disease Control and Prevention (CDC) defines the term *healthcare personnel* as all paid and unpaid persons working in healthcare settings who have the potential for exposure to infectious materials, including body substances, contaminated medical supplies and equipment, contaminated environmental surfaces, or contaminated air.[1] Health Canada's Centre for Infectious Disease Prevention refers to *healthcare worker* as any individual who has the potential to acquire or transmit infectious agents during the course of his or her work in healthcare.[2] These terms include nurses, nursing assistants, physicians, technicians, therapists, pharmacists, students and trainees, contractual staff not employed by the healthcare facility, emergency medical service personnel, dental personnel, laboratory personnel, autopsy personnel, researchers, and volunteers who have direct patient care. Persons not directly involved in patient care but potentially exposed to infectious agents (e.g., clerical, dietary, housekeeping, maintenance, and volunteers) are also to be included.

Healthcare is delivered not only in acute-care hospitals and long-term care facilities, but also in freestanding surgical and outpatient centers, emergency care clinics, persons' homes, and during prehospital emergency care. Personnel who provide healthcare in any setting may acquire infections from or transmit infections to persons to whom they provide care, other personnel, household members, or other community contacts.

The healthcare organization's administration, medical staff, and other healthcare personnel need to support the infection control objectives of an occupational health program. These objectives are to (1) educate personnel about the principles of infection control and their individual responsibility for infection control, (2) collaborate with the infection control department in monitoring and investigating potentially harmful infectious exposures and outbreaks, (3) provide care to personnel for work-related illnesses or exposures, (4) identify work-related infection risks and institute appropriate preventive measures, and (5) contain costs by preventing infectious diseases that result in absenteeism and disability.[1]

There are elements that should be included when designing an occupational health service for healthcare personnel.[1] The infection control professional may be involved in many of these functions. These include the following.

- Coordination with other departments that support the infection control objectives can ensure surveillance for infection in personnel and assist with exposure investigation and implementation of preventive measures.

- Medical evaluations performed before placement can ensure that the worker will not pose a risk of infection transmission. Additionally, information gathered through this evaluation may lead to identifying a worker who may be at increased risk for infection and whose placement may need to be considered carefully. It has not been demonstrated that a physical examination is cost effective for infection control purposes. Periodic evaluations may need to be performed for job assignments or work-related problems.

- Personnel health and safety education can contribute to the workers' compliance with infection control practices through understanding of the rationale. There may be existing federal, state, and local regulations regarding requirements for employee education and training. Items to be considered are risks of a job category, preventive measures, and educational materials that are appropriate in content, vocabulary, and language.

- Immunization programs provide protection from vaccine-preventable diseases for both the workers and those under their care. The infectious diseases for which vaccines are available for preexposure intervention include hepatitis A and B, influenza, measles, mumps, rubella, tetanus, pertussis, and varicella-zoster (chickenpox).

APIC Text of Infection Control and Epidemiology

Copyright © 2005, Association for Professionals in Infection Control and Epidemiology, Inc.

Table 26-1A. Immunobiologics and schedules for health care personnel (modified from ACIP recommendations): Immunizing agents strongly recommended for health care personnel

Generic name	Primary booster dose schedule	Indications	Major precautions and contraindications	Special considerations
Hepatitis B recombinant vaccine	Two doses IM in the deltold muscle 4 wk apart; 3rd dose 5 mo after 2nd; booster doses not necessary	Health care personnel at risk of exposure to blood and body fluids	No apparent adverse effects to developing fetuses, not contraindicated in pregnancy; history of anaphylactic reaction to common baker's yeast	No therapeutic or adverse effects on HBV-infected persons; cost-effectiveness of prevaccination screening for susceptibility to HBV depends on costs of vaccination and antibody testing and prevalence of immunity in the group of potential vaccinees; health care personnel who have ongoing contact with patients or blood should be tested 1–2 mo after completing the vaccination series to determine serologic response
Influenza vaccine (inactivated whole or split virus)	Annual single-dose vaccination IM with current (either whole- or split-virus) vaccines	Health care personnel with contact with high-risk patients or working in chronic care facilities; personnel with high-risk medical conditions and/or[3] 65 yr	History of anaphylactic hypersensitivity after egg ingestion	No evidence of maternal or fetal risk when vaccine was given to pregnant women with underlying conditions that render them at high risk for serious influenza complications.
Measles live-virus vaccine	One does SC; 2nd dose at least 1 mo later	Health care personnel born in or after 1957 without documentation of (a) receipt of two doses of live vaccine or after their 1st birthday, (b) physician-diagnosed measles, or (c) laboratory evidence of immunity; vaccine should be considered for all personnel, including those born before 1957, who have no proof of immunity	Pregnancy; immuno-compromised* state; (including HIV-infected persons with severe immunosuppression) history of anaphylactic reactions after gelatin ingestion or receipt of neomycin; or recent receipt of immune globulin	MMR is the vaccine of choice if recipients are also likely to be susceptible to rubella and/or mumps; persons vaccinated between 1963 and 1967 with (a) a killed measles vaccine alone, (b) killed vaccine followed by live vaccine, or (c) a vaccine of unknown type should be revaccinated with two doses of live measles vaccine
Mumps live-virus vaccine	One dose SC; no booster	Health care personnel believed to be susceptible can be vaccinated; adults born before 1957 can be considered immune	Pregnancy; immuno-compromised* state; history of anaphylactic reaction after gelatin ingestion or receipt of neomycin	MMR is the vaccine of choice if recipients are also likely to be susceptible to measles and rubella

(continued)

Copyright © 2005, Association for Professionals in Infection Control and Epidemiology, Inc.

Table 26-1A. (Continued)

Generic name	Primary booster dose schedule	Indications	Major precautions and contraindications	Special considerations
Rubella live-virus vaccine	One dose SC; no booster	Health care personnel, both male and female, who lack documentation of receipt of live vaccine on or after their1st birthday, or of laboratory evidence of immunity; adults born before 1957 can be considered immune, except women of childbearing age	Pregnancy; immuno-compromised* state; history of anaphylactic reaction after receipt of neomycin	Women pregnant when vaccinated or who become pregnant within 3 mo of vaccination should be counseled on the theoretic risks to the fetus, the risk of rubella vaccine-associated malformations in these women is negligible; MMR is the vaccine of choice if recipients are also likely to be susceptible to measles or mumps
Varicella-zoster live-virus vaccine	Two 0.5 ml doses SC, 4–8 wk apart if[3] 13 yr	Health care personnel without reliable history of varicella or laboratory evidence of varicella immunity	Pregnancy, immuno-compromised* state, history of anaphylactic reaction after receipt of neomycin or gelatin; salicylate use should be avoided for 6 wk after vaccination	Because 71%–93% of persons without a history of varicella are immune, serologic testing before vaccination may be cost-effective

IM, Intramuscularly; SC, subcutaneously.

* Persons immunocompromised because of immune deficiencies, HIV infection, leukemia, lymphoma, generalized malignancy, or immunosuppressive therapy with corticos-teroids, alkylating drugs, antimetabolites, or radiation.

Source: Bolyard EA, Tablan OC, Williams WW, Pearson ML, Shapiro CN, Deitchman SD, and The Hospital Infection Control Practices Advisory Committee: Guideline for infection control in health care personnel, 1998, *Am J Infect Control* 26:289–354, 1998, p 294

Recommended immunization practices are addressed by the U.S. Public Health Service's Advisory Committee on Immunization Practices.[1] For vaccinations recommended for healthcare workers see Table 26.1. Immunizations are discussed in Chapter 110, Immunization in the Healthcare Worker.

- Management of job-related illnesses and exposures should also be provided for the healthcare personnel. Postexposure follow-up and medical surveillance is mandated by regulatory agencies.

- Work restrictions may be indicated for workers who present with illnesses that may be transmitted in the workplace. See Table 26.2 for summary of suggested work restrictions. The facility should have a process in place that identifies who has the authority to remove the worker from duty.

- Health counseling should be available to the worker to provide targeted information about the risk and prevention of occupationally acquired infections. The worker may need to be reassured regarding an exposure and the risks and benefits of postexposure prophylaxis regimens. Workers also need to know to report a community exposure they may have had to an infectious disease.

- Maintenance of records, data management, and confidentiality is a major requirement of the occupational health program by federal, state, and local standards. A computerized personnel database is preferred. Copies of individual records are to be made available to the worker on request.

III. OCCUPATIONAL HEALTH HAZARDS

Postexposure Interventions

There are infectious processes that present a possible threat to healthcare workers and have specific indications for postexposure intervention. Figure 26–1 provides an algorithm on how to assess an occupational exposure and when to implement an intervention.

Tuberculosis

The CDC publishes recommendations on controlling the spread of tuberculosis in healthcare facilities.[3] The Occupational Health and Safety Administration

APIC Text of Infection Control and Epidemiology

Copyright © 2005, Association for Professionals in Infection Control and Epidemiology, Inc.

Table 26-1B. Immunobiologics and schedules for healthcare personnel (modified from ACIP recommendations): Other immunizing agents available for healthcare personnel in special circumstances

Generic name	Primary/booster dose schedule	Indications	Major precautions and contraindications	Special considerations
BCG vaccine (for tuberculosis)	• One percutaneous dose of 0.3 ml • No booster dose recommended	Healthcare personnel in communities where (a) MDR-TB is prevalent, (b) strong likelihood of infection exists, and (c) full implementation of TB infection control precautions has been inadequate in controlling the spread of infection (NOTE: BCG should be used after consultation with local and/or state health department)	• Immunocompromised* state • Pregnancy	In the United States, TB control efforts are directed toward early identification and treatment of cases of active TB and toward preventive therapy with isoniazid for PPD converters
Hepatitis A vaccine	Two doses of vaccine IM, either (HAVRIX™) 6–12 mo apart or (VAQTA™) 6 mo apart	• Not routinely indicated for U.S. healthcare personnel • Persons who work with HAV-infected primates or with HAV in a laboratory setting should be vaccinated	• History of anaphylactic reaction to alum or the preservative 2-phenoxy ethanol • Vaccine safety in pregnant women has not been evaluated, risk to fetus is likely low and should be weighed against the risk of hepatitis A in women at high risk	Health care personnel who travel internationally to endemic areas should be evaluated for vaccination
Meningococcal poly saccharide (quadrivalent A, C, W135, and Y) vaccine	• One dose in volume and by route specified by manufacturer • Need for boosters is unknown	Not routinely indicated for healthcare workers in the United States	Vaccine safety in pregnant women has not been evaluated Vaccine should not be given during pregnancy unless risk of infection is high	May be useful in certain outbreak situations
Polio vaccine	• IPV, two doses SC given 4–8 wk apart • 3rd dose 6–12 mo after 2nd dose • Booster doses may be IPV or OPV	Healthcare personnel in close contact with persons who may be excreting wild virus and laboratory personnel handling specimens that may contain wild poliovirus	• History of anaphylactic reaction after receipt of streptomycin or neomycin • Because safety of vaccine has not been evaluatd in pregnant women, it should not be given during pregnancy	• Use only IPV for immunosuppressed persons or personnel who care for immuno-suppressed patients • If immediate protection against poliomyelitis is needed, OPV should be used.
Rabies vaccine	• Primary, HDCV or RVA, IM, 1.0 ml (deltoid area) one each on days 0, 7, 21, or 28 or of HDCV, ID, 1.0 ml, one each on days 0, 7, 21, and 28 • Booster, HDCV or RVA, IM, 0.1 ml (deltoid area), day 0 only, or HDCV, ID, 0.1 ml, day 0 only	Personnel who work with rabies virus or infected animals in diagnostic or research activities		Personnel who work with rabies virus or infected animals in diagnostic or research activities
Tetanus and diphtheria (Td)	• Two doses IM 4 wk apart • 3rd dose 6–12 mo after 2nd dose • Booster every 10 yr	• All adults • Tetanus prophylaxis in wound management	• First trimester of pregnancy • History of a neurologic reaction or immediate hypersensitivity reaction • Individuals with severe local (Arthus-type) reaction after previous dose of Td vaccine should not be given further routine or emergency doses of Td for 10 yr	
Typhoid vaccines: IM, SC, and oral	• One 0.5 ml dose IM; booster doses of 0.5 ml every 2 yr (Vi capsular polysaccharide) • Or two 0.5 ml doses SC, 4 or more wk apart; boosters of 0.5 ml SC or 0.1 ml ID every 3 yr if exposure continues • Or four oral doses on alternate days; (Ty21a) vaccine manufacturer's recommendation is revaccination with the entire four-dose series every 5 yr	Personnel in laboratories who frequently work with *Salmonella typhi*	• History of severe local or systemic reaction to a previous dose of typhoid vaccine • Ty21a vaccine should not be given to immunocompromised* personnel	Vaccination should not be considered as an alternative to the use of proper procedures when handling specimens and cultures in the laboratory
Vaccinia vaccine (smallpox)	• One dose administered with a bifurcated needle • Boosters every 10 yr	Personnel who directly handle cultures of or animals contaminated with recombinant vaccinia viruses or orthopox viruses (monkeypox, cowpox, vaccinia, etc.) that infect human beings	Pregnancy, presence or history of eczema, or immunocompromised* status in potential vaccinees or in their household contacts	Vaccination may be considered for healthcare personnel who have direct contact with contaminated dressings or other infectious material from volunteers in clinical studies involving recombinant vaccinia virus

HDCV, Human diploid cell rabies vaccine; RVA, rabies vaccine absorbed; IPV, inactivated poliovirus vaccine; OPV, oral poliovirus vaccine; ID, intradermally.

* Persons immunocompromised because of immune deficiencies, HIV infection, leukemia, lymphoma, generalized malignancy, or immunosuppressive therapy with corticosteroids, alkylating drugs, antimetabolites, or radiation.

Source: Bolyard EA, Tablan OC, Williams WW, Pearson ML, Shapiro CN, Deitchman SD, and The Hospital Infection Control Practices Advisory Committee: Guideline for infection control in health care personnel, 1998, *Am J Infect Control* 26: 289–354, 1998, p 295–96

Table 26-2. Summary of suggested work restrictions for health care personnel exposed to or infected with infectious diseases of importance in health care settings, in the absence of state and local regulations (modified from ACIP recommendations_g)

Disease/problem	Work restriction	Duration	Category
Conjunctivitis	Restrict from patient contact and contact with the patient's environment	Until discharge ceases	II
Cytomegalovirus infections	No restriction		II
Diarrheal diseases	Restrict from patient contact, contact with the patient's environment, or food handling	Until symptoms resolve	IB
Acute stage (diarrhea with other symptoms)			
Convalescent stage, Salmonella spp.	Restrict from care of high-risk patients	Until symptoms resolve; consult with local and state health authorities regarding need for negative stool cultures	IB
Diphtheria	Exclude from duty	Until antimicrobial therapy completed and 2 cultures obtained³ 24 hours apart are negative	IB
Enteroviral infections	Restrict from care of infants, neonates, and immuno-compromised patients and their environments	Until symptoms resolve	II
Hepatitis A	Restrict from patient contact, contact with patient's environment, and food handling	Until 7 days after onset of jaundice	IB
Hepatitis B			
Personnel with acute or chronic hepatitis B surface antigemia who do not perform exposure-prone procedures	No restriction*; refer to state regulations; standard precautions should always be observed		II
Personnel with acute or chronic hepatitis B e antigenemia who perform exposure-prone procedures	Do not perform exposure-prone invasive procedures until counsel from an expert review panel has been sought; panel should review and recommend procedures the worker can perform, taking into account specific procedure as well as skill and technique of worker; refer to state regulations	Until hepatitis B e antigen is negative	II
Hepatitis C	No recommendation		Unresolved issue
Herpes simplex			
Genital	No restriction		II
Hands (herpetic whitlow)	Restrict from patient contact and contact with the patient's environment	Until lesions heal	IA
Orofacial	Evaluate for need to restrict from care of high-risk patients		II
Human immunodeficiency virus	Do not perform exposure-prone invasive procedures until counsel from an expert review panel has been sought; panel should review and recommend procedures the worker can perform, taking into account specific procedure as well as skill and technique of the worker; standard precautions should always be observed; refer to state regulations		II
Measles			
Active	Exclude from duty	Until 7 days after the rash appears	IA
Postexposure (susceptible personnel)	Exclude from duty	From 5th day after 1st exposure through 21st day after last exposure and/or 4 days after rash appears	IB
Meningococcal infections	Exclude from duty	Until 24 hours after start of effective therapy	IA

(Continued)

APIC Text of Infection Control and Epidemiology

Copyright © 2005, Association for Professionals in Infection Control and Epidemiology, Inc.

Table 26-2. Continued

Disease/problem	Work restriction	Duration	Category
Mumps			
Active	Exclude from duty	Until 9 days after onset of parotitis	IB
Postexposure (susceptible personnel)	Exclude from duty	From 12th day after 1st exposure through 26th day after last exposure or until 9 days after onset of parotitis	II
Pediculosis	Restrict from patient contact	Until treated and observed to be free of adult and immature lice	IB
Pertussis			
Active	Exclude from duty	From beginning of catarrhal stage through 3rd wk after onset of paroxysms or until 5 days after start of effective antimicrobial therapy	IB
Postexposure (asymptomatic personnel)	No restriction, prophylaxis recommended		II
Postexposure (symptomatic personnel)	Exclude from duty	Until 5 days after start of effective antimicrobial therapy	IB
Rubella			
Active	Exclude from duty	Until 5 days after rash appears	IA
Postexposure (susceptible personnel)	Exclude from duty	From 7th day after 1st exposure through 21st day after last exposure	IB
Scabies	Restrict from patient contact	Until cleared by medical evaluation	IB
Staphylococcus aureus infection Active, draining skin lesions	Restrict from contact with patients and patient's environment or food handling	Until lesions have resolved	IB
Carrier state	No restriction, unless personnel are epidemiologically linked to transmission of the organism		IB
Streptococcal infection, group A	Restrict from patient care, contact with patient's environment, or food handling	Until 24 hours after adequate treatment started	IB
Tuberculosis			
Active disease	Exclude from duty	Until proved noninfectious	IA
PPD converter	No restriction		IA
Varicella			
Active	Exclude from duty	Until all lesions dry and crust	IA
Postexposure (susceptible personnel)	Exclude from duty	From 10th day after 1st exposure through 21st day (28th day if VZIG given) after last exposure	IA
Zoster Localized, in healthy person	Cover lesions; restrict from care of high-risk patient†	Until all lesions dry and crust	II
Generalized or localized in immunosuppressed person	Restrict from patient contact	Until all lesions dry and crust	IB
Postexposure (Susceptible personnel)	Restrict from patient contact	From 10th day after 1st exposure through 21st day (28th day if VZIG given) after last exposure or, if varicella occurs, until all lesions dry and crust	IA
Viral respiratory infections, acute febrile	Consider excluding from the care of high risk patients‡ or contact with their environment during community outbreak of RSV and influenza	Until acute symptoms resolve	IB

* Unless epidemiologically linked to transmission of infection

† Those susceptible to varicella and who are at increased risk of complications of varicella, such as neonates and immunocompromised persons of any age.

‡ High-risk patients as defined by the ACIP for complications of influenza.

Source: Bolyard EA, Tablan OC, Williams WW, Pearson ML, Shapiro CN, Deitchman SD, and The Hospital Infection Control Practices Advisory Committee: Guideline for infection control in health care personnel, 1998, *Am J Infect Control* 26:289–354, 1998, pp 299–301

Copyright © 2005, Association for Professionals in Infection Control and Epidemiology, Inc.

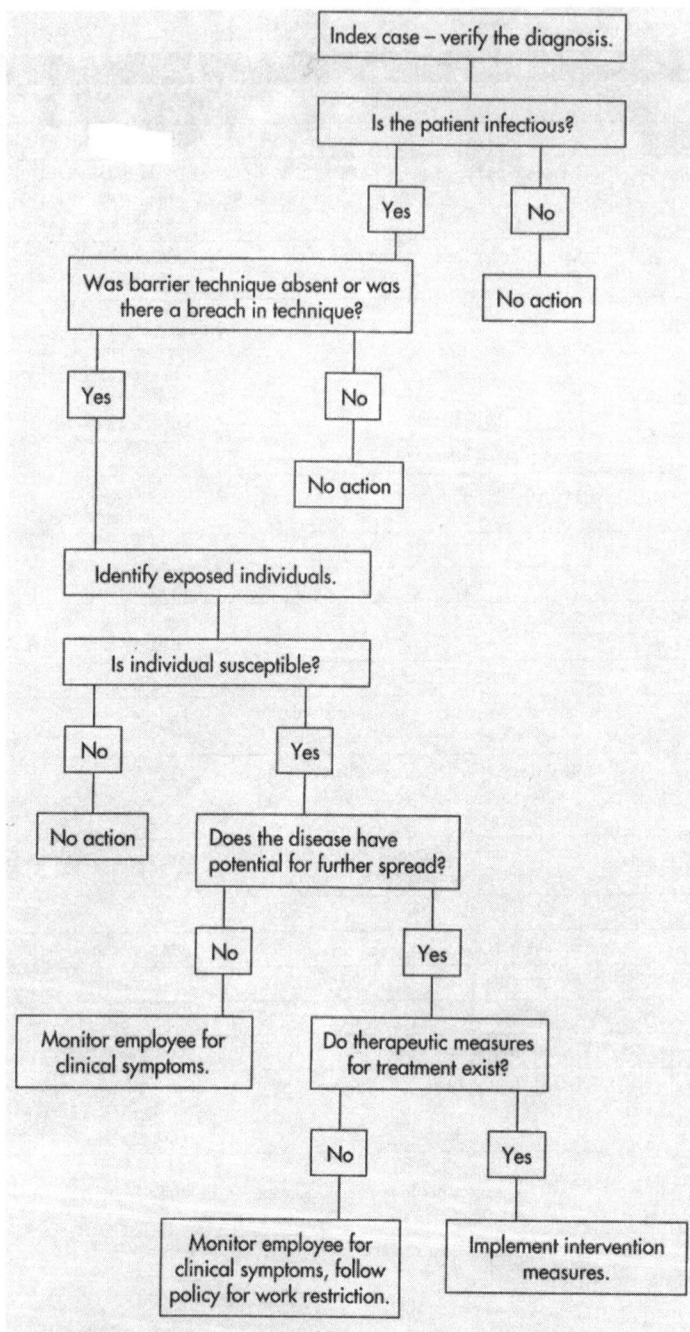

Figure 26-1 Algorithm for management of healthcare worker exposure

(OSHA) has a compliance directive addressing occupational exposure to tuberculosis[4] that focuses on the workplaces identified by CDC as those where the risk of transmission is considered the highest. This was written as a directive to their field offices to clarify the application of the General Duty Clause when inspecting facilities identified as belonging in these high hazard groups. OSHA's General Duty Clause requires each employer to provide its employees a place of employment free from recognized hazards.

An unidentified case of pulmonary or laryngeal tuberculosis can be a source of unprotected exposure to the healthcare worker. Workers should be educated about tuberculosis, how it is spread, its signs and symptoms, and preventive measures.

APIC Text of Infection Control and Epidemiology

Copyright © 2005, Association for Professionals in Infection Control and Epidemiology, Inc.

Based on a facility-specific risk assessment, a tuberculosis screening program should include all personnel with exposure potential. The purified protein derivative (PPD) skin-test program should be administered, read, and interpreted by trained personnel. Use the intracutaneous (Mantoux) method to administer the PPD skin test. Tine tests should not be used. Immunosuppressed personnel should be evaluated for anergy in conjunction with PPD testing. Two companion antigens (e.g., *Candida* antigen and tetanus toxoid A) should be administered in addition to PPD. Persons with 3 mm or more of induration to any of the skin tests (including tuberculin) are considered not anergic. Reactions of 5 mm or more to PPD are considered evidence of TB infection in HIV-infected persons regardless of the reactions to the companion antigens. If there is no reaction (i.e., less than 3 mm induration) to any of the antigens, the person being tested is considered anergic.

Baseline testing should be a component of the preemployment physical assessment. Those individuals who have a history of having received the Bacille Calmette-Guerin (BCG) vaccination should be included unless they have documentation of a previous positive reaction. A two-step should be performed when the initial PPD is negative and there is no documented negative PPD test during the preceding 12 months. Interpret the PPD test according to the CDC guidelines. See Table 26–3. The frequency of periodic follow-up PPD tests is based on the facility's risk assessment. Exempt those employees who have a positive baseline PPD or have had adequate treatment for tuberculosis.

If a worker has a positive PPD, a chest x-ray should be done promptly to check for active disease. A history of exposure should be obtained to determine if infection is occupational or community acquired. The worker should be instructed to report symptoms that are suggestive of tuberculosis. Chest x-rays do not need to be repeated unless the worker is symptomatic. If the worker is a recent converter he/she should be referred to a healthcare provider for consideration of preventive therapy.

If there has been unprotected exposure of workers to tuberculosis, PPD skin tests should be administered at the time of the exposure and repeated at 12 weeks postexposure to look for possible converters. Chest x-rays are only performed on those with prior positive PPD skin test and who are currently symptomatic. Consider retesting immunocompromised personnel at least every 6 months.

If a worker has laryngeal or pulmonary tuberculosis he/she is excluded from work until they are receiving adequate therapy, the cough has resolved, and there have been three consecutive sputum smears negative for acid-fast bacilli. The occupational health department should obtain periodic documentation from the healthcare provider. If treatment is discontinued, the worker needs to be promptly evaluated for infectiousness.

Immunocompromised personnel should be counseled regarding potential risks associated with caring for persons with tuberculosis. It may be necessary to offer reasonable accommodations for work setting.

The generally accepted respiratory protection that is used to protect the worker from a person with suspected or confirmed tuberculosis is a particulate respirator Type N95. OSHA's current interpretation requires that each worker assigned to wear a respirator must receive a fit test before the worker is required to wear the respirator in the workplace and perform a fit check with each use.[5] The fit test would need to be repeated whenever respirator design or facial changes occur that could affect the proper fit of the respirator.

Bloodborne Pathogens

The very nature of a healthcare setting will require contact between healthcare workers and the persons they serve. One of the areas of concern for these workers is bloodborne pathogens. There are many ways to prevent transmission. These include promoting the hepatitis B vaccination for the workers who have contact with blood, considering all patients as a potential source of infection, using appropriate barriers when performing tasks that require contact with blood, and preventing percutaneous injuries. Despite the evolution of a safer work environment the past few decades, occupational exposures do occur. Management of occupational exposures to hepatitis B virus (HBV), hepatitis C virus (HCV), and the human immunodeficiency virus (HIV) are outlined in the updated U.S. Public Health Service guidelines.[6]

An occupational health program in a healthcare setting should include the following elements of an effective postexposure management program: clearly stated polices and procedures that address confidentiality of exposed and source persons and how to manage the exposure; education and training of workers to alleviate misconceptions and fears; and resources for rapid access to clinical care, postexposure prophylaxis (PEP), and testing of the source person and worker. An assessment of the injury may identify ways to prevent future injuries.

OSHA's bloodborne pathogens standard[7] provides directives for employers to develop an exposure plan that includes providing the hepatitis B vaccine to employees within 10 days of employment. The standard also requires the employer to provide training on potential hazards, personal protective equipment (PPE), engineering controls, and work practices before the employee's initial assignment. An element of the

Copyright © 2005, Association for Professionals in Infection Control and Epidemiology, Inc.

Table 26-3. Summary of interpretation of purified protein derivative (PPD)-tuberculin skin-test results

1. An induration of ≥5 mm is classified as positive in:

persons who have human immunodeficiency virus (HIV) infection or risk factors for HIV infection but unknown HIV status;

persons who have had recent close contact* with persons who have active tuber-culosis (TB);

persons who have fibrotic chest radiographs (consistent with healed TB).

2. An induration of ≥10 mm is classified as positive in all persons who do not meet any of the criteria above but who have other risk factors for TB, including:

High-risk groups –

injecting-drug users known to be HIV seronegative;

persons who have other medical conditions that reportedly increase the risk for progressing from latent TB infection to active TB (e.g., silicosis; gastrectomy or jejuno-ileal bypass; being ≥10% below ideal body weight; chronic renal failure with renal dialysis; diabetes mellitus; high-dose corticosteroid or other immuno-suppressive therapy; some hematologic disorders, including malignancies such as leukemias and lymphomas; and other malignancies);

children <4 years of age.

High-prevalence groups –

persons born in countries in Asia, Africa, the Caribbean, and Latin America that have high prevalence of TB;

persons from medically underserved, low-income populations;

residents of long-term-care facilities (e.g., correctional institutions and nursing homes);

persons from high-risk populations in their communities, as determined by local public health authorities.

3. An induration of ≥15 mm is classified as positive in persons who do not meet any of the above criteria.

4. Recent converters are defined on the basis of both size of induration and age of the person being tested:

≥10 mm increase within a 2-year period is classified as a recent conversion for persons <35 years of age;

≥15 mm increase within a 2-year period is classified as a recent conversion for persons ≥35 years of age.

5. PPD skin-test results in health-care workers (HCWs)

In general, the recommendations in sections 1, 2, and 3 of this table should be fol-lowed when interpreting skin-test results in HCWs.

However, the prevalence of TB in the facility should be considered when choosing the appropriate cut-point for defining a positive PPD reaction. In facilities where there is essentially no risk for exposure to Mycobacterium tuberculosis(i.e., minimal- or very low-risk facilities [Section II.B]), an induration ≥15 mm may be a suitable cut-point for HCWs who have no other risk factors. In facilities where TB patients receive care, the cut-point for HCWs with no other risk factors may be ≥10 mm.

A recent conversion in an HCW should be defined generally as a ≥10 mm increase in size of induration within a 2-year period. For HCWs who work in facilities where exposure to TB is very unlikely (e.g., minimal-risk facilities), an increase of ≥15 mm within a 2-year period may be more appropriate for defining a recent conversion because of the lower positive-predictive value of the test in such groups.

* Recent close contact implies either household or social contact or unprotected occupational exposure similar in intensity and duration to household contact.
Source: Centers for Disease Control and Prevention. Guidelines for preventing the transmission of Mycobacterium tuberculosis in health-care facilities, 1994. MMWR 1994;43(No. RR-13), pp 62–63

revision to OSHA's bloodborne pathogen rule in 2001 was the need to maintain a sharps injury log. The log needs to protect the privacy of the injured worker and include the identification of the device, location of the incident, circumstances surrounding the incident, the procedure being performed, the body part affected, and the objects or substances involved. Another 2001 revision to the standard was the requirement of the documentation of annual consideration and implementation of appropriate engineering controls and solicitation of nonmanagerial healthcare workers in evaluating and choosing safe medical devices.

The CDC defines an occupational exposure that might place the worker at risk for HBV, HCV, or HIV infection as a percutaneous injury (e.g., a needlestick or cut with a sharp object) or contact of mucous membrane or nonintact skin (e.g., exposed skin that is chapped, abraded, or afflicted with dermatitis) with blood tissue, or other body fluids that are potentially infectious.[6]

Copyright © 2005, Association for Professionals in Infection Control and Epidemiology, Inc.

Wound care is the first element in postexposure management. The wound should be cleaned with soap and water. Mucous membranes should be flushed with water. Eyes should be flushed with eye irrigant or clean water. There is no evidence of benefit for using antiseptics or disinfectants or for squeezing the puncture site. The use of bleach or other caustic agents should be avoided.[6]

Hepatitis B Virus

The hepatitis B vaccination has contributed to the significant decrease of HBV among healthcare workers. At the time of hire, the workers' potential for exposure should be determined and their vaccine status assessed. Postvaccine screening is advised for personnel at ongoing risk for blood exposure to determine whether response to the vaccine has occurred and to determine the need for revaccination. Revaccinate nonresponders with an additional three-dose series and retest. If the worker is still a nonresponder, then test for hepatitis B surface antigen (HBSAg) to make sure the worker does not have chronic antigemia. Nonresponders in chronic dialysis centers who do not respond for HBSAg and hepatitis B surface antibody (anti-HBs) should be tested every 6 months. Risk factors for nonresponse include age, smokers, obesity, immunosuppressed, renal failure and a family history of nonresponse.[8]

An exposure to HBV is defined as the source person being HBsAg positive or his/her status is unknown. If the exposed person is vaccinated, but his/her vaccine response is unknown, then perform a baseline test for anti-HBs. Baseline testing is not necessary if the exposed person has not been vaccinated or the vaccine response is known. If the exposed person has not been vaccinated, then begin the vaccine series at the time of the exposure and administer hepatitis B immune globulin (HBIG) as soon as possible after the exposure, preferably within 24 hours.

For recommended postexposure prophylaxis for exposure to HBV see Table 26–4.

One of the frequently asked questions is whether or not booster doses of the hepatitis B vaccine are necessary. The current response is no. Maintenance of anti-HBs above 10mlU/ml is not necessary. It is believed that reliance on immunologic memory rather than booster doses will protect against breakthrough memory.[8]

Hepatitis C Virus

The average risk of transmission of Hepatitis C virus (HCV) following a percutaneous exposure is 1.8%. Transmission rarely occurs from mucosal contact with HCV-infected blood. There has been no transmission reported to a worker from intact or nonintact skin exposures to blood. Recommendations for follow-up of occupational HCV exposures include performing testing for anti-HCV for the source. For the person

Table 26-4. Recommended HIV postexposure prophylaxis for percutaneous injuries

Exposure type	HIV-Positive Class 1*	HIV-Positive Class 2*	Infection status of source Source of unknown HIV status†	Unknown source§	HIV-Negative
Less severe¶	Recommend basic 2-drug PEP	Recommend expanded 3-drug PEP	Generally, no PEP warranted; however, consider basic 2-drug PEP** for source with HIV risk factors§§	Generally, no PEP warranted; however, consider basic 2-drug PEP** in settings where exposure to HIV-infected persons is likely	No PEP warranted
More severe§§	Recommend expanded 3-drug PEP	Recommend expanded 3-drug PEP	Generally, no PEP warranted; however, consider basic 2-drug PEP** for source with HIV risk factors††	Generally, no PEP warranted; however, consider basic 2-drug PEP** in settings where exposure to HIV-infected persons is likely	No PEP warranted

* HIV-Positive, Class 1 – asymptomatic HIV infection or known low viral load (e.g., <1,500 RNA copies/mL). HIV-Positive, Class 2 – symptomatic HIV infection, AIDS, acute seroconversion, or known high viral load. If drug resistance is a concern, obtain expert consultation. Initiation of postexposure prophylaxis (PEP) should not be delayed pending expert consultation, and, because expert consultation alone cannot substitute for face-to-face counseling, resources should be available to provide immediate evaluation and follow-up care for all exposures.
† Source of unknown HIV status (e.g., deceased source person with no samples available for HIV testing).
§ Unknown source (e.g., a needle from a sharps disposal container).
¶ Less severe (e.g., solid needle and superficial injury).
** The designation "consider PEP" indicates that PEP is optional and should be based on an individualized decision between the exposed person and the treating clinician.
†† If PEP is offered and taken and the source is later determined to be HIV-negative, PEP should be discontinued.
§§ More severe (e.g., large-bore hollow needle, deep puncture, visible blood on device, or needle used in patient's artery or vein).
Source: Centers for Disease Control and Prevention. Updated U.S. Public Health Service Guidelines for the Management of Occupational Exposures to HBV, HCV, and HIV and Recommendations for Postexposure Prophylaxis. MMWR 2001;50(No. RR-11):24

Copyright © 2005, Association for Professionals in Infection Control and Epidemiology, Inc.

exposed to an HCV-positive source, perform baseline testing for anti-HCV and alanine aminotransferase (ALT) activity and follow-up testing at 4–6 months for anti-HCV and ALT activity. If earlier diagnosis of HCV infection is desired, testing for HCV-RNA may be performed at 4–6 weeks to possibly detect early infection with HCV. Confirm all anti-HCV results reported positive by enzyme immunoassay, using supplemental anti-HCV testing, such as recombinant immunoblot assay (RIBA). Immune Globulin (IG) and antiviral agents are not recommended for postexposure prophylaxis. There are no guidelines for administration of therapy during the acute phase of HCV infection. When HCV infection is identified early, the worker should be referred to a specialist knowledgeable in this area for proper management.

A worker who has been exposed to HCV should refrain from donating blood, plasma, organs, tissue, or semen. There is no need for modification of sexual practices, refraining from becoming pregnant, or special precautions to prevent secondary transmission. There are no existing recommendations regarding restricting the professional activities of a healthcare worker with HCV infection. However, discussion following a report of surgeon-to-patient transmission suggested that limitations, if any, should be determined on a case-by-case basis after consideration of factors that influence transmission. These considerations should include the worker's inability or unwillingness to comply with infection control standards.[9]

Human Immunodeficiency Virus (HIV)

Healthcare workers who sustained an exposure incident from an HIV-positive source were followed by CDC through June 2001. There were 57 workers who had documented occupationally acquired AIDS/HIV. A case control study identified risks for transmission.[10] These risk factors are a deep injury from a device with visible blood, the device was from the source person's vein or artery, and the source person died of AIDS within 60 days after the exposure incident.

The average risk of transmission of HIV by the exposure type is 0.3% for percutaneous, 0.1% for mucous membrane contact, and less than 0.1% for nonintact skin contact.

Immediately following the exposure the worker and source person should be tested to establish their HIV-AB status. HIV testing of needles or other sharps is not recommended.

If the source person is HIV-negative and has no clinical evidence of HIV infection, further testing of the exposed worker is not indicated. If the person source is HIV-positive or has clinical evidence of HIV infection or is at increased risk for HIV infection, then follow-up testing of the exposed worker is indicated. The recommended interval is baseline, 6 weeks, 12 weeks, and 6 months postexposure. It is recommended to extend the testing period to 12 months postexposure for workers who become infected with HCV following exposure to a co-infected source person. Extending the testing period to 12 months is optional in other situations.[6]

Postexposure prophylaxis (PEP) should be considered carefully weighing the risk of transmission and the risk of adverse effects. If indicated, HIV PEP should be considered an urgent medical concern and started as soon as possible after the exposure, hours rather than days. The exposed person should be reevaluated within 72 hours when additional information about the source

Table 26-5. Recommendation for postexposure prophylaxis for percutaneous or permucosal exposure to hepatitis B virus, United States

Vaccination and antibody status of exposed person	HBsAg seropositive	Treatment when source is HBsAg negative	Treatment when source is not tested or status is unknown
Unvaccinated	HBIG* ' 1 and initiate HB vaccine series	Initiate HB vaccine series	Initiate HB
Previously vaccinated			
Known responder†	No treatment	No treatment	
Known nonresponder	HBIG* ' 2 or HBIG* ' 1 and initiate revaccination	No treatment	If known high-risk source, treat as if source were HBsAg positive
Antibody response unknown	Test exposed person for anti-HBs: (1) if adequate, † no treatment; (2) if inadequate, † HBIG ' 1 and vaccine booster	No treatment	Test exposed person for anti-HBs: (1) if adequate,† no treatment; (2) if inadequate,† initiate revaccination

HBsAg, Hepatitis B surface antigen; HBIG, hepatitis B immune globulin; HB, hepatitis vaccine; anti-HBs, antibody to hepatitis B surface antigen.
* Dose 0.06 mg/kg IM.
† Responder is defined as a person with adequate serum levels of anti-HBs ($\geq$ 10 mIU/ml); inadequate vaccination defined as serum anti-HBs <10 mIU/ml.
Source: Bolyard EA, Tablan OC, Williams WW, Pearson ML, Shapiro CN, Deitchman SD, and The Hospital Infection Control Practices Advisory Committee: Guideline for infection control in health care personnel, 1998, *Am J Infect Control* 26:289–354, 1998, p 303

APIC Text of Infection Control and Epidemiology

Copyright © 2005, Association for Professionals in Infection Control and Epidemiology, Inc.

Table 26-6. Recommended HIV postexposure prophylaxis for mucous membrane exposures and nonintact skin* exposures

Exposure type	HIV-Positive Class 1†	HIV-Positive Class 2†	Infection status of source Source of unknown HIV status§	Unknown source¶	HIV-Negative
Small volume**	Consider basic 2-drug PEP††	Recommend basic 2-drug PEP	Generally, no PEP warranted; however, consider basic 2-drug PEP†† for source with HIV risk factors§§	Generally, no PEP warranted; however, consider basic 2-drug PEP†† in settings where exposure to HIV-infected persons is likely	No PEP warranted
Large volume¶¶	Recommend basic 2-drug PEP	Recommend expanded 3-drug PEP	Generally, no PEP warranted; however, consider basic 2-drug PEP†† for source with HIV risk factors§§	Generally, no PEP warranted; however, consider basic 2-drug PEP†† in settings where exposure to HIV-infected persons is likely	No PEP warranted

* For skin exposures, follow-up is indicated only if there is evidence of compromised skin integrity (e.g., dermatitis, abrasion, or open wound).
† HIV-Positive, Class 1 – asymptomatic HIV infection or known low viral load (e.g., <1,500 RNA copies/mL). HIV-Positive, Class 2 – symptomatic HIV infection, AIDS, acute seroconversion, or known high viral load. If drug resistance is a concern, obtain expert consultation. Initiation of postexposure prophylaxis (PEP) should not be delayed pending expert consultation, and, because expert consultation alone cannot substitute for face-to-face counseling, resources should be available to provide immediate evaluation and follow-up care for all exposures.
§ Source of unknown HIV status (e.g., deceased source person with no samples available for HIV testing).
¶ Unknown source (e.g., splash from inappropriately disposed blood).
** Small volume (i.e., a few drops).
†† The designation, "consider PEP," indicates that PEP is optional and should be based on an individualized decision between the exposed person and the treating clinician.
§§ If PEP is offered and taken and the source is later determined to be HIV-negative, PEP should be discontinued.
¶¶ Large volume (i.e., major blood splash).
Source: Centers for Disease Control and Prevention. Updated U.S. Public Health Service Guidelines for the Management of Occupational Exposures to HBV, HCV, and HIV and Recommendations for Postexposure Prophylaxis. MMWR 2001;50(No. RR-11): 25.

person may become available. If the source person is determined to be HIV-negative, PEP should be stopped. See Tables 26–4 and 26–6 for HIV PEP regimens per type of exposure. It is recommended that drugs be selected to which the source person's virus is unlikely to be resistant. Expert consultation is recommended in these situations.

Pregnancy is not a contraindication for PEP, but the exposed person should make an informed decision about PEP. The decision about which regimen to use is more complex and data is limited on the potential effects of antiretroviral drugs on the developing fetus or neonate. Some postexposure prophylaxis drugs are contraindicated during pregnancy. Therefore, expert consultation is warranted.

Once PEP is initiated, the exposed person should be monitored for PEP toxicity. A complete blood count and renal and hepatic profiles should be done baseline and 2 weeks after starting PEP. If the PEP regimen includes a protease inhibitor, additional follow-up testing is warranted, preferably managed by an expert.

Postexposure counseling is recommended for the HIV-exposed worker. The content should include side effects of the drugs, signs and symptoms of acute HIV infection, prevention of secondary transmission, and PEP drug risks, if breastfeeding.

Varicella

Transmission of varicella has been documented from sources from nosocomial exposures that have included patients, healthcare personnel, and visitors. In adults, a history of varicella is highly predictive of serologic immunity, and most adults who have negative or uncertain histories of varicella are also seropositive. If the worker's history is negative or uncertain, then screening prior to administering the vaccine may be cost effective. It is recommended that the varicella vaccine be administered to susceptible workers, especially those that will have contact with patients at high risk for serious complications.

If an unvaccinated susceptible worker is exposed to varicella, then exclude the worker from duty from the 10th day after exposure through the 21st day after exposure, or until all lesions are dry and crusted if varicella occurs.[1]

Serotest a vaccinated worker who is exposed to varicella immediately after exposure to assess the presence of antibody. If seronegative, exclude the worker from duty from day 10 through day 21 postexposure, or monitor daily for the development of symptoms. If fever, upper respiratory tract symptoms, or rash develop, then exclude the worker from duty.

Consider administering the vaccination for the exposed unvaccinated worker without documented immunity. The efficacy of postexposure vaccination is unknown.

Copyright © 2005, Association for Professionals in Infection Control and Epidemiology, Inc.

Therefore, workers vaccinated after exposure should be managed as previously recommended for unvaccinated persons.

Varicella zoster immune globulin (VZIG) has not been recommended for immunocompetent personnel. However, its use may be considered for immunocompromised or pregnant workers postexposure. If used, extend the time that the worker is excluded from duty from 21 days to 28 days postexposure.

Meningococcal Disease

Meningococcal disease is caused by a variety of serogroups of *Neisseria meningitidis.* Nosocomial transmission is uncommon. When proper precautions were not used, the organism has been transmitted from patient to personnel. This occurs through contact with respiratory secretions of patients that have meningococcemia, meningococcal meningitis, a lower respiratory tract infection with *N. meningitidis,* or through handling laboratory specimens.

Postexposure prophylaxis is advised for persons who have had intensive, unprotected contact with infected patients.[1] Unprotected means without wearing a mask and intensive contact would be mouth-to-mouth resuscitation, endotracheal intubation, endotracheal tube management, or close examination of the oropharynx. Prophylactic therapy should be administered immediately after the unprotected exposure. Current recommended regimens to eradicate carriage are Rifampin 600 mg orally every 12 hours for 2 days; a single dose of ciprofloxacin 500 mg orally; or a single dose of ceftriaxone 250 mg intramuscularly. Rifampin and ciprofloxacin are not recommended for pregnant women.

It is currently recommended to offer preexposure vaccination to laboratory workers who handle soluble preparations of *N. meningitidis.*[11]

Measles, Mumps, Rubella

The measles, mumps, rubella (MMR) vaccination should not be administered to a pregnant worker or one who might become pregnant within the next 28 days.[12]

Rubella

Because nosocomial transmission of rubella has occurred from both male and female personnel to susceptible personnel and patients, ensuring immunity among all healthcare personnel is the most effective way to eliminate transmission.[1] The worker should have documentation of one dose of live rubella vaccine on or after their first birthday or laboratory evidence of immunity to rubella. A dose of MMR is recommended for those healthcare personnel who were born before 1957 and who do not have laboratory evidence of immunity. Exposed personnel not immune to rubella need to be excluded from duty from the 7th day after the first exposure through the 21st day after the last exposure.

Measles

Measles transmission has occurred in healthcare facilities. Data suggests that healthcare personnel have a risk of measles 13-fold that of the general population.[1] Therefore, it is essential that all workers have documentation of measles immunity. Persons born during or after 1957 can be considered immune if they have documentation of physician-diagnosed measles, or documentation of two doses of live measles vaccine on or after their first birthday, or serologic evidence of measles immunity. Personnel who were born before 1957 can be considered immune if they have a history of previous measles disease, documentation of receipt of one dose of live measles vaccine, or serologic evidence of measles immunity. The MMR vaccination should be administered to those who cannot provide documentation of the preceding. The measles vaccine should be administered to susceptible workers who have had contact with a measles patient within 72 hours of the exposure. Personnel who are not immune to measles need to be excluded from duty 5 days after the first exposure to 21 days after the last exposure.

Mumps

Mumps can be spread in a healthcare facility. Most of mumps cases in healthcare personnel have been community acquired.[1] Personnel can be considered immune to mumps if they have documentation of physician-diagnosed mumps, documentation of receipt of one dose of live mumps vaccine on or after their first birthday, or serologic evidence of immunity. MMR vaccine should be administered to those who lack the preceding documentation. Susceptible personnel who are exposed to mumps need to be excluded from duty the 12th day after the first exposure to the 26th day after the last exposure.

Scabies and Pediculosis

Nosocomial transmission of conventional and "Norwegian" or crusted scabies has occurred in various healthcare settings. It is spread by prolonged skin-to-skin contact with an infested individual. Contact precautions can reduce spread from patient to worker. Exposed workers should be evaluated for signs and symptoms of mite infestation. Appropriate therapy should be provided for confirmed or suspected scabies.

Pediculosis is caused by infestation with any of three species of lice: human head louse, human body louse, and pubic or crab louse. Nosocomial transmission of head and body lice is unlikely, and nosocomial transmis-

Copyright © 2005, Association for Professionals in Infection Control and Epidemiology, Inc.

sion of pubic lice is very unlikely. Pediculosis treatment should be provided for exposed workers if they have evidence of infestation. Do not routinely offer prophylactic scabicides or pediculicides unless transmission has occurred.

Personnel with either scabies or pediculosis should be excluded from duty until they receive appropriate initial treatment and it is found to be effective.[1]

Pertussis

Pertussis is highly contagious and nosocomial transmission has involved both patients and personnel. Postexposure prophylaxis is indicated for personnel exposed to pertussis. The regimen used is a 14-day course of either erythromycin 500 mgm four times daily or one tablet of trimethoprim-sulfamethoxazole twice daily.[1]

Exposed personnel do not need to be excluded from duty. Personnel in whom symptoms develop (e.g., cough *lasting* 7 days or more, particularly if accompanied by paroxysms of coughing, inspiratory whoop, or posttussive vomiting) should be excluded until 5 days after the start of appropriate therapy.

Infectious Processes with No Postexposure Interventions Indicated

There are common infectious processes for which there are no indications for postexposure intervention.

Herpes Simplex Virus

Personnel with primary or recurrent orofacial herpes simplex infections should be evaluated on a case-by-case basis to assess the potential for transmission to high-risk patients. High-risk patients include neonates, intensive care unit patients, patients with severe burns or eczema, and severely immunocompromised patients. Personnel with orofacial herpes simplex should be instructed to cover and not touch infected lesions. Observing hand hygiene policies is mandatory. Precautions need to be taken to prevent the lesions from having contact with patients with dermatitis. Herpetic whitlow is a herpes simplex infection of the fingers or hands. Workers with herpetic whitlow need to be excluded from contact with patients until their lesions heal.[1]

Cytomegalovirus

The two principle reservoirs of cytomegalovirus in healthcare facilities are infants and young children and immunocompromised patients. The consistent use of standard precautions when caring for all persons should interrupt spread from the person shedding the virus to the worker. There is no need to reassign pregnant healthcare workers from caring for these patients.

The pregnant worker needs to be counseled on how transmission occurs and the importance of infection control procedures to prevent transmission.[1]

Parvovirus

Human parvovirus B19 (B19) is the cause of erythema infectiosum (fifth disease). This is a common rash illness, usually acquired in childhood. Although rare, transmission to healthcare personnel has been reported. B19 may be transmitted through contact with infected persons, fomites, or large droplets. Infected individuals are infectious before the appearance of the rash, those with infection and aplastic crisis for up to 7 days after onset of illness, and persons with chronic infection for years. Workers should be educated about risks and infection control procedures. Pregnant personnel are at no greater risk of infection. However, if acquired during the first half of pregnancy, the risk of fetal death is increased. Therefore, females of childbearing age should be instructed in risk for transmission and infection control procedures.[1]

Respiratory Syncytial Virus

Respiratory syncytial virus (RSV) can be transmitted directly through large droplets during close contact with infected individuals. Although RSV is most common in infants and children, outbreaks have been reported in bone-marrow transplant units, intensive care units, and long-term care facilities. Transmission is greatest during the early winter months. RSV can occur simultaneously with other respiratory viruses and may go unrecognized. It may not be possible to restrict workers with viral respiratory illness during the winter. Personnel with acute respiratory infections should be excluded from caring for high-risk patients.[1]

Staphylococcal Infection or Carriage

Personnel with a draining lesion suspected to be caused by *Staphylococcus aureus* need to be excluded from patient care or food handling until appropriate culture results have ruled out infection or adequate therapy has resulted in resolution of their infection. Only those workers who are epidemiologically linked to disseminating the organism should be cultured. Culture surveys of workers can detect carriers, but do not indicate when carriers are likely to disseminate organisms.[1]

Emerging Pathogens

Vaccinia (Smallpox)

In 1980 smallpox was eradicated as a naturally occurring disease. It is feared that this disease may be brought back as a biological weapon. For this reason, communities have been asked to form smallpox prepar-

Copyright © 2005, Association for Professionals in Infection Control and Epidemiology, Inc.

edness teams who would be vaccinated and ready to care for infected patients if there was a smallpox attack. Smallpox vaccine is made from vaccinia virus. The vaccinia virus is similar to smallpox virus, but is less harmful and will protect against smallpox. There is a usual progression of the vaccination site and special precautions that the vaccinee needs to follow so as not to self-inoculate or spread to close household contacts or persons to whom they provide care.[13]

Severe Acute Respiratory Syndrome

Severe acute respiratory syndrome (SARS) has been transmitted within a healthcare facility, and most often the source of transmission has been an unidentified case or failure to don and remove PPE appropriately. Occupational acquisition of SARS has been documented. Therefore, the occupational health program in a healthcare facility that could possibly care for a SARS patient has to include elements that address worker issues associated with SARS.[14]

Healthcare personnel should be informed that they are expected to comply with all infection control and public health recommendations. They should also be made aware that those recommendations may change as a SARS outbreak progresses.

An exposure reporting process needs to be established. This process should include methods for identifying exposed personnel (e.g., self-reporting by employees and logs of personnel entering SARS patient rooms). Measures should be developed for symptom monitoring in accordance with public health recommendations. Systems need to be developed for healthcare worker follow-up and possible work restrictions after unprotected exposures to SARS patients. The workers need to be instructed to notify each facility at which they work if any one of those facilities is providing care to SARS patients. Quarantine may be used as an exposure management tool, and appropriate measures need to be developed to help the workers comply with restriction.

Healthcare workers will need to have access to mental health professionals to help them cope with the emotional strain of managing a SARS outbreak.

Workers' Compensation

The ICP may be asked to help assess a situation to determine if a worker has experienced occupational acquisition of an infectious agent or disease. ICPs should be familiar with the workers' compensation system in place within their country.

The workers' compensation system is a wage-replacement system of disability insurance for the individual who sustains an illness or injury in the course of employment. Most expenses related to the illness or injury, including medical and other costs associated with the rehabilitation, are covered. These programs vary from state to state. The laws are designed to relieve employers of liability from common-law suits involving negligence and are based on employer–employee relationship instead of theory of negligence. The laws hold that the employers insure costs of occupational disabilities without regard to any fault involved. Most jurisdictions require employers to obtain insurance or prove financial ability to carry their own risk (e.g., self-insured). In some states the employees may choose between accepting compensation provided by law or instituting a lawsuit against the employer.[15-19]

The components of a workers' compensation program may include medical benefits, weekly compensation benefits, safety and rehabilitation programs charged to study the cause of accidents and promote prevention, and retraining of workers who are unable to return to their pre-injury status.

All states in the United States recognize responsibility for specific provisions for occupational diseases. Disease that results from occupational exposure usually is eligible for compensation if: the occupational exposure is the sole cause of disease; the occupational exposure is one of several causes of the disease; the occupational exposure aggravates a preexisting disease (e.g., asthma); or the occupational exposure hastens the onset of disability. The burden of proving that disease was occupationally acquired lies with the workers. Most states do not provide compensation for a disease that is an ordinary disease of life (e.g., stroke, heart attack).

Measuring Improvement in Preventing Occupational Exposure

When applied to occupational health and safety, surveillance involves collection, analysis, and dissemination of data on hazards that have or may endanger the healthcare worker. The current emphasis is on protecting healthcare workers from occupational acquisition of disease. There is a need to evaluate interventions and practices for effectiveness.

An epidemiologic approach can be taken to manage occupational exposures.[20] Reductions or increases in injuries and exposures are monitored over time. The causes of the injuries and exposures are then identified. Variations that occur are analyzed. Prevention strategies are designed and implemented. The effectiveness of prevention strategies is tracked by comparing injury and exposure rates to previous rates. Feedback is then provided to the workers involved in the effectiveness of the prevention strategies.

Copyright © 2005, Association for Professionals in Infection Control and Epidemiology, Inc.

The rates of reported injuries and exposures for measuring performance improvement are calculated in the following ways.[21]

1. The average daily census of occupied beds in the institution for the same year can be used as the denominator that can be compared with other institutions. For example,

   • Total number of needlesticks reported in 1 year

   • Total number of occupied beds/average daily census

   • Equals the number of needlesticks per bed per year

2. The rates can be identified per occupational category. For example,

   • Total number of needlesticks reported by nurses in 1 year

   • Number of full-time equivalent nurses employed in that year

   • Equals the rate of needlesticks per full-time equivalent nurse per year

3. A device-based rate can be used to compare needlestick risk from different devices and to evaluate the effectiveness of the product design. The type of needle must be identified when each needlestick is reported. For example,

   • Number of needlesticks from device type in 1 year

   • Number of that device type used or purchased in same year

   • Equals the number of needlesticks per device type in 1 year

IV.   SUMMARY AND CONCLUSIONS

The role of the ICP in an occupational health program in a healthcare facility is to provide reassurance to the worker concerned with issues relating to infectious agents that may be encountered in the workplace. The ICP may also participate in designing plans that address emerging pathogens and possible bioterrorism agents. The ICP's knowledge of the principles of how infectious agents are spread and proven control measures can be invaluable when an organization is faced with the need to address an emergent situation.

V.   FUTURE TRENDS/RESEARCH

In 2001, the QuantiFERON-TB Test (QFT) (manufactured by Cellestis Limited) was approved by the Food and Drug Administration (FDA) as an aid for detecting latent *Mycobacterium tuberculosis* infection. This test is an in vitro diagnostic aid that measures a component of cell-mediated immune reactivity to *M. tuberculosis*. Compared with tuberculin skin testing (TST), QFT results are less subject to reader bias and error. This diagnostic test requires phlebotomy and can be accomplished after a single patient visit. The blood needs to be processed in 12 hours after collection. Presently, there is limited laboratory and clinical experience with this assay. Also, predicting the progression to active tuberculosis has not been evaluated. As second and third generations of this test are developed, it may replace the traditional use of TST in detecting *M. tuberculosis* infections among certain populations.[22]

The potential of emerging pathogens yet to be identified is real. The ICP plays a vital role in ongoing education of the worker population and as an advisor to administration when planning for an event. Healthcare personnel need to recognize the importance of hand hygiene practices, standard precautions, respiratory hygiene, and transmission-based precautions to reduce the risk of transmission within the healthcare facility and into the community.

VI.   INTERNATIONAL PERSPECTIVES

The SARS outbreak of 2003 began in one country and spread to other continents by way of international travel. This present-day epidemic demonstrated the need for all countries to be vigilant about the incidence of infectious diseases worldwide. The literature has reported the spread of vaccine-preventable diseases introduced into a previously vaccinated but waning population from individuals who traveled from areas where vaccinations were not as prevalent or readily available.

When planning an occupational health program for a healthcare facility, consideration needs to be made for the incidence of infectious diseases identified in the community that may be introduced into the worker pool. The infectious diseases may differ from country to country and from areas within a country.

REFERENCES

1. CDC: Guidelines for infection control in healthcare personnel, 1998, *Am J Infect Control* 26:289–354, 1998.
2. Division of nosocomial and occupational infections. Bureau of infectious diseases. Centre for infectious disease prevention and control. Health Canada: Prevention and control of occupational infections in health care. Infection control guidelines. Ottawa, Ontario, 2002. 28S1.
3. CDC: Guidelines for preventing the transmission of *Mycobacterium tuberculosis* in health-care facilities, *MMWR* 43(No. RR-13), 1994.
4. U.S. Department of Labor. *Enforcement policy and procedures for occupational exposure to tuberculosis,* OSHA instruction. October 8, 1993.
5. Fairfax RE: Frequency of fit-testing for respirators to protect against *M. tuberculosis* exposure, *U.S. Department of Labor. Standard Interpretation,* April 12, 1999.

Copyright © 2005, Association for Professionals in Infection Control and Epidemiology, Inc.

6. CDC: Updated U.S. public health service guidelines for the management of occupational exposures to HBV, HCV, and HIV and recommendations for postexposure prophylaxis, *MMWR*50:RR-11, 2001.
7. U.S. Department of Labor: 29 CFR Part 1910.1030. Occupational exposure to bloodborne pathogens; Final rule. *Federal Register* 56(235), 1991.
8. Poland GA: Presentation: New vaccines and policies: an update, APIC annual conference, June 21, 2000.
9. Surgeons-to-patient HCV infections raise questions, *Hospital Employee Health* 21(8):88–90, 2000.
10. Cardo DM, et al: A case study of HIV seroconversion in health care workers after percutaneous exposure, *N Engl J Med* 337(21):1485–1498, 1997.
11. Laboratory-acquired meningococcal disease—United States, 2000, *MMWR* 51:7, 2002.
12. ACIP: Notice to readers: Revised ACIP recommendations for avoiding pregnancy after receiving a Rubella-containing vaccine, *MMWR* 50(49):117, 2001.
13. CDC: Smallpox vaccination and adverse reactions. Guidance for clinicians, *MMWR* 52:RR-4, 2003.
14. CDC: Infection control precautions for aerosol-generating procedures on patients with severe acute respiratory syndrome (SARS). www.cdc.gov/ncidod/sars/aerosolinfection control.htm.
15. US Chamber of Commerce: Analysis of workers' compensation laws, Washington, DC, 1993, US Government Printing Office.
16. Felton JS: The injured worker and learned helplessness, *Occup Environ Med Report* 8:45–48, 1994.
17. Martin JM: Stress-related workers' compensation claims, *American Association of Occupational Health News Journal* 40(B):370–375, 1992.
18. Boden LI: Workers' compensation. In Levy BS, Wegeman A, editors: *Occupational health: recognizing and preventing work-related diseases.* Boston, 1995, Little, Brown.
19. Pozgar GDS: Labor relations. In *Legal aspects of healthcare administration,* ed 5, Gaithersburg, MD, 1993, Aspen, pp. 449–76.
20. Levy BS: The role of surveillance in occupational health: an update, *OEM Report* 6(9):67–68, 1992.
21. Jagger J: Calculating needlestick rates. In *BD safety compliance initiative exposure prevention information network,* Franklin Lakes, NJ, 1992, Becton Dickinson (instruction manual).
22. CDC: Guidelines for using the QuantiFERON-TB test for diagnosing latent *mycobacterium tuberculosis* infection, *MMWR* 52(RR-2):15–18, 2003.

SUPPLEMENTAL RESOURCES

Web Sites:

Centers for Disease Control and Prevention, www.cdc.gov

Occupational Safety and Health Administration, www.osha.gov

Association for Professionals in Infection Control and Epidemiology, Inc. www.apic.org

Society of Healthcare Epidemiologists of America, www.sheahq.talley.com

Health Canada Centre for Infectious Disease Prevention and Control, www.hc-sc.ca

International Federation of Infection Control, www.ific.narod.ru/manual/occup.htm

Copyright © 2005, Association for Professionals in Infection Control and Epidemiology, Inc.

Occupational Exposure

Elise M. Beltrami, MD, MPH
DeKalb County Board of Health
Decatur, Georgia

Adelisa L. Panlilio, MD, MPH
Division of Healthcare Quality Promotion
Centers for Disease Control and Prevention
Atlanta, Georgia

ABSTRACT

Preventing transmission of bloodborne viruses in healthcare settings requires a multifaceted approach, including promoting hepatitis B vaccination of all healthcare personnel who may have contact with blood or body fluids, considering all patients as potentially infectious, using appropriate barriers to prevent blood and body fluid contact, and preventing percutaneous injuries by eliminating unnecessary needle use, implementing devices with safety features, using safe work practices when handling needles and other sharp devices, and safely disposing sharps and blood-contaminated materials. Postexposure management is also an integral component of a complete program to prevent infection following blood-borne pathogen exposure and an important element of workplace safety. This chapter will focus on the risk and management of occupational blood exposures.

KEY CONCEPTS

- Prevention of occupational blood exposures is the primary way to reduce transmission of hepatitis B virus, hepatitis C virus, and HIV in healthcare settings.

- Healthcare personnel who may come into contact with body fluids should be vaccinated against hepatitis B.

- The risk of hepatitis B virus seroconversion after a percutaneous injury ranges from 5% to 35% depending on the hepatitis B e antigen (HBeAg) status of the source person.

- The average risk of seroconversion after a percutaneous injury involving blood infected with hepatitis C virus is approximately 1.8%.

- The average risk of seroconversion after a percutaneous injury involving blood infected with HIV is approximately 0.3%.

- All healthcare personnel taking HIV postexposure prophylaxis should be evaluated within 48–72 hours after exposure and monitored for drug toxicity for at least 2 weeks.

- Healthcare organizations and facilities should set up programs to prevent exposure to blood-borne viruses and to manage cases of exposure should they occur.

Copyright © 2005, Association for Professionals in Infection Control and Epidemiology, Inc.

I. BACKGROUND

Exposure to bloodborne pathogens poses a serious risk to healthcare personnel. Avoiding occupational blood exposures through the use of appropriate barriers to prevent blood and body fluid contact and preventing percutaneous injuries by eliminating unnecessary needle use, implementing devices with safety features, using safe work practices when handling needles and other sharp devices, and safely disposing sharps and blood-contaminated materials is the primary way to prevent transmission of hepatitis B virus (HBV), hepatitis C virus (HCV), and human immunodeficiency virus (HIV) in healthcare settings. Despite improved methods of preventing exposure, occupational exposures will continue to occur. In this chapter, we provide information about HBV, HCV, and HIV infection and review the risk and management of occupational blood exposure, including recommendations for postexposure prophylaxis.

II. BASIC PRINCIPLES

Definition of Healthcare Personnel and Exposure

Healthcare personnel (HCP) are defined as persons (e.g., employees, students, contractors, attending clinicians, public-safety workers, or volunteers) whose activities involve contact with patients or with blood or other body fluids from patients in a healthcare, laboratory, or public safety setting.[1]

An exposure that might place HCP at risk for HBV, HCV, or HIV infection is defined as a percutaneous injury (e.g., a needlestick or cut with a sharp object) or contact of mucous membrane or nonintact skin (e.g., exposed skin that is chapped, abraded, or afflicted with dermatitis) with blood, tissue, or other body fluids that are potentially infectious.[1,2]

In addition to blood and body fluids containing visible blood, semen and vaginal secretions are also considered potentially infectious. Although semen and vaginal secretions have been implicated in the sexual transmission of HBV, HCV, and HIV, they have not been implicated in occupational transmission from patients to HCP. The following fluids also are considered potentially infectious: cerebrospinal fluid, synovial fluid, pleural fluid, peritoneal fluid, pericardial fluid, and amniotic fluid. The risk for transmission of HBV, HCV, and HIV infection from these fluids is unknown; the potential risk to the HCP from occupational exposures to these fluids has not been assessed by epidemiologic studies in healthcare settings. Feces, nasal secretions, saliva, sputum, sweat, tears, urine, and vomitus are not considered potentially infectious unless they contain blood. The risk for transmission of HBV, HCV, and HIV infection from these fluids and materials is extremely low.

Any direct contact (i.e., contact without barrier protection) to concentrated virus in a research laboratory or production facility is considered an exposure that requires clinical evaluation. For human bites, the clinical evaluation must include the possibility that both the person bitten and the person who inflicted the bite were exposed to blood-borne pathogens. Transmission of HBV or HIV infection has rarely been reported by this route.[3-5]

III. BLOODBORNE PATHOGENS AND OCCUPATIONAL EXPOSURE

Hepatitis B Virus

Epidemiology

Hepatitis B virus (HBV) is transmitted by direct exposure to blood and other infected body fluids. HBV is a relatively hardy virus capable of surviving on environmental surfaces and fomites. Transmission in households is well documented and may, in part, be attributable to mucosal contact with fomites contaminated with secretions or blood from infected persons. HCP and others at risk for occupational blood exposure through percutaneous, mucosal, or dermal routes can acquire HBV infection. The risk associated with accidental needlestick inoculation of infected blood to susceptible HCP varies between 5% to 35%, depending on the hepatitis B e antigen (HBeAg) status, and hence the viral titer, of the source.

Clinical Features

HBV infection results in clinically apparent hepatitis in about one-third of acutely infected adults. Clinical hepatitis may be preceded by a prodrome of fever, malaise, urticarial or maculopapular rash, and arthralgias for several days. Fever usually resolves before the onset of jaundice. Jaundice, dark urine, and scleral icterus usually are present by the time patients seek medical attention. Right upper quadrant tenderness, mild hepatic enlargement, and, occasionally, splenomegaly are signs that should suggest the diagnosis. The most striking laboratory findings are extreme elevations in the serum aminotransferase levels. Alanine aminotransferase (ALT) and aspartate aminotransferase (AST) levels may be elevated to more than 10 times the normal levels, whereas the alkaline phosphatase levels are increased to a much lesser extent.

Fulminant liver involvement occurs in about 1% of adults and may be complicated by more serious abnormalities, including hypoglycemia, coagulopathy, and hypoalbuminemia. About 2%–6% of adults with acute HBV infection proceed to chronic HBV infection and

Copyright © 2005, Association for Professionals in Infection Control and Epidemiology, Inc.

are at risk for chronic hepatitis, cirrhosis, and primary hepatocellular carcinoma.

Patients with asymptomatic primary HBV infection are at higher risk for chronic infection than are those with symptomatic infection. Chronic infection may result in chronic persistent hepatitis, a benign illness of little clinical consequence except for the potential for HBV transmission to susceptible persons or for chronic active hepatitis, which eventually may produce cirrhosis, liver failure, and hepatoma.

Laboratory Diagnosis

Hepatitis B is differentiated from other causes of hepatitis by serologic assays (Table 27–1).[6] Several well-defined antigen-antibody systems are associated with HBV infection, including HBsAg and antibody to hepatitis B surface antigen (anti-HBs); hepatitis B core antigen (HBcAg) and anti-HBc; and hepatitis B e antigen (HBeAg) and antibody to HBeAg (anti-HBe). Serologic assays are commercially available for all of these except HBcAg because no free HBcAg circulates in blood. These markers of HBV infection change over time, with different patterns seen in patients with acute infection that resolve and patients with chronic infection (Table 27–1).

The presence of HBsAg is indicative of ongoing HBV infection and potential infectiousness. In newly infected persons, HBsAg is present in serum 30–60 days after exposure to HBV and persists for variable periods. Anti-HBc develops in all HBV infections, appearing at onset of symptoms or liver test abnormalities in acute HBV infection, rising rapidly to high levels, and persisting for life. Acute or recently acquired infection can be distinguished by the presence of the IgM class of anti-HBc, which persists for approximately 6 months.

In persons who recover from HBV infection, HBsAg is eliminated from the blood, usually in 2 to 3 months, and anti-HBs develops during convalescence. The presence of anti-HBs indicates immunity from HBV infection. After recovery from natural infection, most persons will be positive for both anti-HBs and anti-HBc, whereas only anti-HBs develops in persons who are successfully vaccinated against hepatitis B. Persons who do not recover from HBV infection and become chronically infected remain positive for HBsAg (and anti-HBc), although a small proportion (0.3% per year) eventually clear HBsAg and might develop anti-HBs.[7] The persistence of HBsAg for 6 months after the diagnosis of acute HBV is indicative of progression to chronic HBV infection.

HBeAg can be detected in serum of persons with acute or chronic HBV infection. The presence of HBeAg correlates with viral replication and high levels of virus (i.e., high infectivity). Anti-HBe correlates with the loss of replicating virus and with lower levels of virus. However, all HBsAg-positive persons should be considered potentially infectious, regardless of their HBeAg or anti-HBe status.

HBV infection can be detected using qualitative or quantitative tests for HBV DNA. These tests are not U.S. Food and Drug Administration (FDA) approved and are most commonly used for patients being managed with antiviral therapy.

Table 27-1. Interpretation of Patterns of Hepatitis B Virus Serologic Markers

Serologic Markers				
HBsAg*	Total Anti-HBc[H]	IgM[ꞌ] Anti-HBc	Anti-HBs[¶]	Interpretation
−	−	−	−	Susceptible, never infected
+	−	−	−	Acute infection, early incubation**
+	+	+	−	Acute resolving infection
−	+	+	−	Acute resolving infection
−	+	−	+	Past infection, recovered and immune
+	+	−	−	Chronic infection
−	+	−	−	False positive (i.e., susceptible), past infection, or "low-level" chronic infection
−	−	−	+	Immune if titer is ≥10 mIU/mL

* HBsAg – Hepatitis B surface antigen.
[H] Anti-HBc – Antibody to hepatitis B core antigen. The total anti-HBc assay detects both IgM and IgG antibody.
[ꞌ] Immunoglobulin M
[¶] Anti-HBs – Antibody to hepatitis B surface antigen.
** Transient HBsAg positivity (lasting 18 days or less) might be detected in some patients during vaccination.
+, Positive; −, Negative
Adapted from Table 1 Centers for Disease Control and Prevention. Recommendations for preventing transmission of infections among chronic hemodialysis patients. *MMWR* 50(No. RR-5):1–43, 2000.

Copyright © 2005, Association for Professionals in Infection Control and Epidemiology, Inc.

Treatment, Prevention, and Control

Initial evaluation of patients with chronic HBV infection includes biochemical tests for liver disease (e.g., ALT and AST for the extent of liver disease), and status of HBV replication (e.g., HBeAg, anti-HBe, and HBV DNA). Alpha interferon, lamivudine, or adefovir dipivoxil are approved by the FDA for treatment of chronic hepatitis B.[7] Therapy can be appropriate for patients who have abnormal levels of liver enzymes, active virus replication (HBeAg-positive or high levels of HBV DNA), and a liver biopsy indicating presence of moderate disease activity and fibrosis.[7]

Treatment with interferon, administered by injection 3 times/week, substantially decreases HBV DNA levels and clears HBeAg among more than 50% of patients with ALT levels greater than 6 times the upper limit of normal, and among 2%–35% of patients with ALT levels 2–5 times the upper limit of normal. Among patients with ALT levels less than 2 times the upper limit of normal, response is poor and therapy should be deferred. Long-term follow-up of treated patients indicates that remission of chronic hepatitis induced by alpha interferon is of long duration.[7] Patient characteristics associated with positive response to interferon therapy include low pretherapy HBV DNA levels, high pretherapy ALT levels, short duration of infection, acquisition of disease in adulthood, and histology indicative of active inflammation.

Lamivudine, administered orally daily, has been as effective as interferon at clearing HBeAg. Although a majority of patients taking lamivudine demonstrate improved liver histology, development of lamivudine-resistant HBV mutants is common, especially with prolonged use, and diminishes the effectiveness of treatment. Studies of lamivudine in combination with interferon have not been demonstrated to be superior to monotherapy.[7]

The newest therapy to be approved is adefovir, which also is administered orally daily. Patients treated with adefovir exhibited substantial improvements in liver histology and decreased levels of HBV DNA; however, durability of the response has not been determined.[8] Adefovir has been demonstrated to be effective in patients with chronic hepatitis B who have developed resistance to lamivudine.[8]

Persons identified with chronic HBV infection can benefit from counseling regarding ways to prevent transmitting HBV infection to others. Vaccination of sexual and household contacts is recommended to prevent transmission.[9]

HBV infection is largely preventable through vaccination. Hepatitis B vaccine provides both pre- and postexposure protection against HBV infection. The currently available vaccines in the United States are produced by recombinant DNA technology. Three intramuscular doses of hepatitis B vaccine induce a protective antibody response in more than 90% of healthy recipients. Adults who develop a protective antibody response are protected from clinical disease and chronic infection. The duration of vaccine protection is under investigation. HCP at ongoing risk for percutaneous injuries should be tested 1 to 2 months after completion of the 3-dose vaccination series for anti-HBs.[10] Factors associated with a lack of response include improper vaccination (e.g., improperly stored vaccine, gluteal inoculation, subcutaneous injection, improperly timed dosing), obesity, older age, and smoking. Persons who do not respond to the primary vaccine series should receive a second 3-dose series or be evaluated for HBsAg positivity. Booster doses of hepatitis B vaccine are not necessary, and periodic serologic testing to monitor antibody concentrations after completion of the vaccine series is not recommended.

Since 1982, substantial progress has been made toward reducing the risk for HBV infection in adults.[11] The Occupational Safety and Health Administration's (OSHA's) Bloodborne Pathogen Standard mandates provision of hepatitis B vaccine at no cost to all HCPs and others at occupational risk for blood exposure.[12] Substantial declines in the incidence of acute hepatitis B have occurred among highly vaccinated populations, such as HCPs.

Postexposure Prophylaxis

The need for prophylaxis for persons sustaining accidental percutaneous or mucosal exposures to blood should be based on several factors, including the HBsAg status of the source and the hepatitis B vaccination and vaccine-response status of the exposed person. Such exposures usually involve persons for whom hepatitis B vaccination is recommended. Any blood or body fluid exposure to an unvaccinated person should lead to initiation of the hepatitis B vaccine series. Table 27–2 summarizes recommendations for prophylaxis after percutaneous or mucosal exposure to blood according to the HBsAg status of the exposure source and the vaccination and vaccine-response status of the exposed person.[10]

When hepatitis B immune globulin (HBIG) is indicated, it should be administered as soon as possible after exposure (preferably within 24 hours). The effectiveness of HBIG when administered later than 7 days after exposure is unknown. When hepatitis B vaccine is indicated, it should also be administered as soon as possible (preferably within 24 hours) and can be administered simultaneously with HBIG at a separate site (vaccine should always be administered in the deltoid muscle).

Copyright © 2005, Association for Professionals in Infection Control and Epidemiology, Inc.

Table 27-2. Recommended Postexposure Prophylaxis for Exposure to Hepatitis B Virus

Vaccination and antibody response status of exposed healthcare personnel*	Treatment		
	Source HBsAg[†] positive	Source HBsAg[†] negative	Source unknown or not available for testing
Unvaccinated **Previously vaccinated**	HBIG§ × 1 and initiate hepatitis B vaccine series	Initiate hepatitis B vaccine series	Initiate hepatitis B vaccine series
Known responder¶	No treatment	No treatment	No treatment
Known nonresponder**	HBIG × 1 and initiate revaccination or HBIG × 2[††]	No treatment	If known high-risk source, treat as if source were HBsAg positive
Antibody response unknown	Test exposed person for anti-HBs§§ 1. If adequate,¶ no treatment is necessary 2. If inadequate,** HBIG × 1 and vaccine booster	No treatment	Test exposed person for anti-HBs: 1. If adequate, no treatment is necessary 2. If inadequate, administer vaccine booster and recheck titer in 1–2 months

* Persons who have previously been infected with HBV are immune to reinfection and do not require postexposure prophylaxis.
† Hepatitis B surface antigen.
§ Hepatitis B immune globulin; dose is 0.06 mL/kg intramuscularly.
¶ A responder is a person with adequate levels of serum antibody to HBsAg (i.e., anti-HBs ≥10 mIU/mL).
** A nonresponder is a person with inadequate response to vaccination (i.e., serum anti-HBS <10 mIU/mL).
†† The option of giving one dose of HBIG and reinitiating the vaccine series is preferred for nonresponders who have not completed a second 3-dose vaccine series. For persons who previously completed a second vaccine series but failed to respond, two doses of HBIG are preferred.
§§ Antibody to HBsAg.

For exposed persons who are in the process of being vaccinated but have not completed the vaccination series, vaccination should be completed as scheduled, and HBIG should be added as indicated (Table 27–2). Persons exposed to HBsAg-positive blood or body fluids that are known not to have responded to a primary vaccine series should receive a single dose of HBIG and should reinitiate the hepatitis B vaccine series with the first dose of the hepatitis B vaccine as soon as possible after exposure. Alternatively, they should receive two doses of HBIG, one dose as soon as possible after exposure, and the second dose 1 month later. The option of administering one dose of HBIG and reinitiating the vaccine series is preferred for nonresponders who did not complete a second 3-dose vaccine series. For persons who previously completed a second vaccine series but failed to respond, two doses of HBIG are preferred.[10]

Hepatitis C Virus

Epidemiology

Hepatitis C virus (HCV) infection is the most common chronic blood-borne infection in the United States, affecting an estimated 1.3%.[13] HCV-associated end-stage liver disease is the most frequent indication for liver transplantation among U.S. adults.[13]

The incubation period for acute HCV infection ranges from 2 to 24 weeks (averaging 6 to 7 weeks). HCV transmission occurs primarily through exposure to infected blood and injection drug use, but also through transfusion and solid organ transplantation from infected donors, unsafe medical practices, occupational exposure to infected blood, birth from an infected mother, and sex with an infected partner.

HCV is not transmitted efficiently through occupational exposures to blood. HCPs who are exposed to infected blood through needlestick injuries may acquire HCV infection, but the magnitude of risk (approximately 1.8%) is less than that associated with HBV exposure. One epidemiologic study indicated that transmission occurred only from hollow-bore needles compared with other sharps.[14] Transmission rarely occurs from mucous membrane exposures to blood, and, more rarely, has been documented from nonintact skin exposures to blood.[15]

Data are limited on survival of HCV in the environment. Degradation of HCV occurs when serum containing HCV is left at room temperature. Specific animal infectivity studies have shown survival up to 16 hours, but not longer than 4 days.[16] The potential for environmental survival of HCV suggests that environmental contamination with blood containing HCV could pose a risk for transmission in the healthcare setting. The risk for transmission from exposure to fluids or tissues other than HCV-infected blood has not been quantified, but is expected to be low. HCV is not known to be transmissible through the airborne route, through casual contact in the workplace, or by fomites.

Clinical Features

HCV infection produces a spectrum of clinical illness similar to that of HBV infection and is indistinguishable from other forms of viral hepatitis based on clinical symptoms alone. Serologic tests are necessary to estab-

Copyright © 2005, Association for Professionals in Infection Control and Epidemiology, Inc.

lish a specific diagnosis of hepatitis C. Most adults acutely infected with HCV are asymptomatic. After acute infection, 15% to 25% of persons appear to resolve their infection without sequelae, as defined by sustained absence of HCV RNA in serum and normalization of ALT levels.[13] Chronic HCV infection develops in most (75% to 85%) people; 60% to 70% of these chronically infected people have persistent or fluctuating ALT elevations, indicating active liver disease. Except for age, no clinical or epidemiologic features among patients with acute infection have been predictive of either persistent infection or chronic liver disease. Limited data suggest that lower rates of chronic infection and disease develop in persons infected as children or young adults. Various ALT patterns have been observed in these patients during follow-up, and patients might have prolonged periods (greater than or equal to 12 months) of normal ALT activity even though they have histologic-confirmed chronic hepatitis. Thus, a single ALT determination cannot be used to exclude ongoing hepatic injury, and long-term follow-up of patients with HCV infection is required to determine their clinical outcome or prognosis.

The course of chronic liver disease is usually insidious, progressing slowly without symptoms or physical signs in the majority of patients during the first two or more decades after infection. Chronic hepatitis C frequently is not recognized until asymptomatic persons are identified as HCV-positive during blood-donor screening, or elevated ALT levels are detected during routine physical examinations. Most studies have reported that cirrhosis develops in 10% to 20% of persons with chronic hepatitis C over a period of 20 to 30 years, and hepatocellular carcinoma in 1% to 5%, with striking geographic variations in rates of this disease. However, when cirrhosis is established, the rate of development of hepatocellular carcinoma might be as high as 1% to 4% per year.

Laboratory Diagnosis

Laboratory testing is necessary to establish a specific diagnosis of hepatitis C.[6,17] The two major types of tests available for the laboratory diagnosis of HCV infections are serologic assays for antibodies to HCV (anti-HCV) and nucleic acid tests (NAT) to detect HCV RNA. Testing for anti-HCV is recommended for initially identifying persons with HCV infection and includes initial screening with an immunoassay, and, if positive, confirmation by an additional more specific assay.[17] Anti-HCV may be detected within 5 to 6 weeks after the onset of infection, but it is not possible to determine if someone has acute, chronic, or past infection with an anti-HCV test. HCV RNA may be detected within 1 to 2 weeks of exposure to the virus

and several weeks before elevations of ALT and detection of anti-HCV.

Treatment, Prevention, and Control

HCV-positive persons benefit from evaluation for the presence and severity of chronic liver disease. Antiviral therapy is recommended for persons with persistently elevated ALT levels, detectable HCV RNA, and a liver biopsy that indicates either portal or bridging fibrosis or moderate degrees of inflammation and necrosis. No clear consensus exists on whether to treat patients with persistently normal serum transaminases. The FDA has approved three antiviral therapies for treatment of chronic hepatitis C in persons aged older than 18 years: alpha interferon, pegylated interferon, and alpha or pegylated interferon in combination with ribavirin.[18] All are administered for less than 52 weeks. Among persons with HCV genotype 1, the most common genotype in the United States, the response rate to either of the interferons administered alone is less than 20%, but the response rate to the combination of alpha interferon and ribavirin is 30% to 40%, and, to pegylated interferon and ribavirin, 40% to 50%. Both the alpha and pegylated interferons are administered by injection; ribavirin is taken orally. All of these drug regimens have side effects, some of which can be serious. Successful treatment eliminates viremia and the potentials for HCV transmission and further chronic liver disease.[18,19]

Postexposure Management

For persons exposed to an HCV-positive source, testing for anti-HCV by immunoassay and ALT activity is recommended 4 to 6 months after the exposure to detect infection; testing for HCV-RNA may be performed 4 to 6 weeks after exposure if earlier detection of infection is desired.[10] No clinical trials have been conducted to assess postexposure use of antiviral agents (e.g., interferon with or without ribavirin) to prevent HCV infection, and antivirals are not FDA-approved for this indication. Available data suggest that an established infection might need to be present before interferon can be an effective treatment.[10,18]

Because there is currently no postexposure prophylaxis for HCV, the intent of recommendations for postexposure management is to achieve early identification of chronic disease and, if present, referral for evaluation of treatment options. In addition, no guidelines exist for administration of therapy during the acute phase of HCV infection. However, limited data indicate that antiviral therapy might be beneficial when started early in the course of HCV infection. When HCV infection is identified early, the person should be referred to a specialist knowledgeable in this area for medical management.[10] At present, avoidance of exposure to blood,

Copyright © 2005, Association for Professionals in Infection Control and Epidemiology, Inc.

primarily through percutaneous injury, is the only available strategy for preventing HCV infection.

Human Immunodeficiency Virus

Epidemiology

It is estimated that more than 60 million people worldwide were infected by HIV, and that 40 million of these were living with HIV/AIDS by the end of 2000.[20] In the United States, almost 1 million people are infected with HIV.[20] The primary means of acquiring infection among adults involves the exchange of body fluids through unprotected sexual intercourse with an infected partner involving and injection drug use using shared needles and syringes. The virus also is perinatally transmitted to approximately 20% to 40% of children born to infected mothers. Since 1985, all donated blood in the United States is screened for HIV. The risk of HIV infection due to transfusion of screened blood products screened is estimated to be 2 per million units transfused.[21] Screening does not completely eliminate the potential for a seronegative but infected unit from a recently infected donor to escape detection.

HIV is not transmitted by the airborne route, household or workplace contact with infected persons; exposure to contaminated environmental surfaces; or insect vectors. The virus is easily inactivated by most common disinfectants, including household bleach (diluted 1:10 to 1:100).[1]

Groups of workers at risk for acquiring HIV infection occupationally are HCPs and other workers in contact with blood or other body fluids who sustain accidental percutaneous or mucosal inoculations with HIV-infected material. The magnitude of risk depends on the severity of exposure, but, on the average, is about 0.3% after percutaneous injury. The risk for infection following mucosal exposures is estimated to be lower, at approximately 0.09%. In the absence of direct exposure, HCPs are not at occupational risk for HIV infection. In the United States, through December 2002, 57 HCPs have been documented as having seroconverted to HIV following occupational exposures.[22] In addition, 139 other cases of HIV infection or AIDS have occurred among HCPs who have not reported other risk factors for HIV infection and who report a history of occupational exposure to blood, body fluids, or HIV-infected laboratory material, but for whom seroconversion after exposure was not documented. The number of these workers who acquired their infection through occupational exposures is unknown.

Clinical Features and Laboratory Diagnosis

The clinical course of HIV infection is variable and changing with the advent of antiretroviral therapy and treatment and prophylaxis for infectious complications. Early after infection, within a few weeks to months, an acute febrile illness characterized by malaise, pharyngitis, lymphadenopathy, maculopapular rash, and headache may occur. At initial presentation of such patients, HIV antibody screening tests (EIA) may be negative, but viral antigen (p24 antigen) and serologic reactivity to one or more viral components (Western blot test) allow the diagnosis to be established at this stage.

Following initial infection, most persons have generalized asymptomatic lymphadenopathy and appear well. However, laboratory tests document a gradual decline in the number of circulating T-helper lymphocytes (CD4 cells) beginning soon after infection and continuing over the next several years. T-helper cells are essential components of the immune system and mediate aspects of both cellular and humoral immunity.

In the absence of therapy, symptoms, signs, and illness suggestive of mild–to-moderate immunodeficiency appear after about 5 years, when CD4 cells decrease by about 50%, to less than 500 cells/dL. Intermittent fever, oral thrush, bacterial pneumonia, enteric infections, and reactivated tuberculosis (TB) are typically diagnosed at this time. When CD4 cell counts fall below 200, serious opportunistic infections can be anticipated. *Pneumocystis carinii* pneumonia (PCP) was the most common index diagnosis in the first 5 years of the epidemic, but the advent of effective prophylaxis has decreased the incidence of PCP. Other opportunistic infections and malignancies, including Kaposi's sarcoma, lymphoma, disseminated TB, toxoplasmosis, and cryptococcal meningitis, now account for the majority of index HIV diagnoses.

With the exception of TB, the infectious complications of HIV infection generally are not transmissible to healthy persons and pose no risk in the workplace. Indeed, the causative organisms of these complications (e.g., candida and toxoplasmosis) are ubiquitous, and most adults have already been exposed. Opportunistic infections in HIV-infected patients usually represent reactivation of dormant organisms when the immune system can no longer keep them inactive.

Treatment, Prevention, and Control

Treatment should be offered to all patients with symptoms ascribed to HIV infection.[23] Recommendations for offering antiretroviral therapy in asymptomatic patients requires analysis of many real and potential risks and benefits. Information regarding treatment of acute HIV infection from clinical trials is very limited. Ongoing clinical trials are addressing the question of the long-term clinical benefit of potent treatment regimens for primary infection. In general, treatment

Copyright © 2005, Association for Professionals in Infection Control and Epidemiology, Inc.

should be offered to persons with fewer than 350 CD4 T cells/mm or plasma HIV RNA levels exceeding 55,000 copies/mL (by polymerase chain reaction [PCR] or branched DNA assay). If antiretroviral therapy is initiated, the goals of therapy should include maximal and durable suppression of viral load, restoration and/or preservation of immunologic function, improvement of quality of life, and reduction of HIV-related morbidity and mortality.[23]

People at risk for direct contact with blood and other potentially infected materials should receive specific instruction in Standard Precautions, as recommended by the Centers for Disease Control and Prevention (CDC)[1,2,24] and mandated by OSHA.[12] For most environments outside of healthcare settings, common sense and attention to personal hygiene are adequate to protect workers. Gloves should be worn to clean up sites of visible blood contamination. Environmental surfaces can then be decontaminated with disinfectant solutions or household bleach (diluted 1:10 to 1:100).[1]

Postexposure Prophylaxis

Workers sustaining accidental parenteral exposures to HIV should be counseled to undergo baseline and follow-up testing for 6 months after exposure (e.g., 6 weeks, 3 months, and 6 months) to diagnose infection. Since 1996, the U.S. Public Health Service has recommended postexposure chemoprophylaxis with antiretroviral agents after certain exposures to HIV-infected sources that pose a risk of infection transmission, such as needlesticks, mucous membrane exposures, and nonintact skin exposures (Tables 27–3 and 27–4).[10] Most HIV exposures will warrant a two-drug regimen using two nucleoside analogues (e.g., zidovudine and lamivudine [3TC]; or 3TC and stavudine [d4T]; or d4T and didanosine [ddl]). The addition of a third drug should be considered for exposures that pose an increased risk for transmission. Updated guidelines that include additional antiretrovirals, such as boosted protease inhibitors, for HIV PEP are being developed. Selection of the postexposure prophylaxis (PEP) regimen should consider the comparative risk represented by the exposure and information about the exposure source, including history of and response to antiretroviral therapy based on clinical response, CD4+ T-cell counts, viral load measurements, and current disease stage. Data from animal models of prophylaxis with these agents suggest that antiviral activity is diminished when treatment is delayed for more than 24 hours. For this reason, immediate reporting and access to chemoprophylaxis is recommended.

In addition to follow-up serologic testing, monitoring for PEP toxicity is needed if PEP is taken. A complete blood count and renal and hepatic profiles should be done at baseline and 2 weeks after starting PEP. If the PEP regimen includes a protease inhibitor, the exposed person also should be monitored for hypoglycemia, crystalluria, hematuria, hemolytic anemia, and hepatitis. The PEP regimen should be discontinued or modified and expert consultation obtained if PEP toxicity develops.

Occupational exposure to HIV can be a frightening experience. Consultation with clinicians knowledgeable about HIV transmission risks who can provide supportive counseling to the worker is essential during the follow-up interval. CDC recommends that occupationally exposed workers refrain from unsafe sexual prac-

Table 27-3. Recommended HIV Postexposure Prophylaxis for Percutaneous Injuries

Exposure type	HIV Positive, Class 1*	HIV Positive, Class 2*	Infection Status of Source Known Source, Unknown HIV Status†	Unknown Source§	HIV Negative
Less severe¶	Recommend basic two-drug PEP	Recommend expanded three-drug PEP	Generally, no PEP warranted; however, consider basic two-drug PEP** for source with HIV risk factors†	Generally, no PEP warranted; however, consider basic two-drug PEP** in settings where exposure to HIV-infected persons is likely	No PEP warranted
More severe§§	Recommend expanded three-drug PEP	Recommend expanded three-drug PEP	Generally, no PEP warranted; however, consider basic two-drug PEP** for source with HIV risk factors†	Generally, no PEP warranted; however, consider basic two-drug PEP** in settings where exposure to HIV-infected persons is likely	No PEP warranted

* HIV positive, Class 1—asymptomatic HIV infection or known low viral load (e.g., <1,500 RNA copies/mL). HIV positive, Class 2—symptomatic HIV infection, AIDS, acute seroconversion, or known high viral load. If drug resistance is a concern, obtain expert consultation. Initiation of postexposure prophylaxis (PEP) should not be delayed pending expert consultation, and, because expert consultation alone cannot substitute for face-to-face counseling, resources should be available to provide immediate evaluation and follow-up care for all exposures.
† Source of unknown HIV status (e.g., deceased source person with no samples available for HIV testing).
§ Unknown source (e.g., a needle from a sharps disposal container).
¶ Less severe (e.g., solid needle and superficial injury).
** The designation, "consider PEP," indicates that PEP is optional and should be based on an individualized decision between the exposed person and the treating clinician.
‡ If PEP is offered and taken, and the source is later determined to be HIV negative, PEP should be discontinued.
§§ More severe (e.g., large-bore hollow needle, deep puncture, visible blood on device, or needle used in patient's artery or vein).

APIC Text of Infection Control and Epidemiology

Copyright © 2005, Association for Professionals in Infection Control and Epidemiology, Inc.

Table 27-4. Recommended HIV Postexposure Prophylaxis for Mucous Membrane Exposures and Nonintact Skin* Exposures

Exposure Type	HIV Positive, Class 1†	HIV Positive, Class 2†	Infection Status of Source — Source Known, Unknown HIV Status§	Unknown Source¶	HIV Negative
Small volume**	Consider basic two-drug PEP†	Recommend basic two-drug PEP	Generally, no PEP warranted; however, consider basic two-drug PEP‡ for source with HIV risk factors§§	Generally, no PEP warranted; however, consider basic two-drug PEP‡ in settings where exposure to HIV-infected persons is likely	No PEP warranted
Large Volume¶¶	Recommend basic two-drug PEP	Recommend expanded three-drug PEP	Generally, no PEP warranted; however, consider basic two-drug PEP† for source with HIV risk factors§§	Generally, no PEP warranted; however, consider basic two-drug PEP‡ in settings where exposure to HIV-infected persons is likely	No PEP warranted

* For skin exposures, follow-up is indicated only if there is evidence of compromised skin integrity (e.g., dermatitis, abrasion, or open wound).
† HIV Positive, Class 1—asymptomatic HIV infection or known low viral load (e.g., <1,500 RNA copies/mL). HIV Positive, Class 2—symptomatic HIV infection, AIDS, acute seroconversion, or known high viral load. If drug resistance is a concern, obtain expert consultation. Initiation of postexposure prophylaxis (PEP) should not be delayed pending expert consultation, and, because expert consultation alone cannot substitute for face-to-face counseling, resources should be available to provide immediate evaluation and follow-up care for all exposures.
§ Source of unknown HIV status (e.g., deceased source person with no samples available for HIV testing).
¶ Unknown source (e.g., splash from inappropriately disposed blood).
** Small volume (i.e., a few drops).
† The designation, "consider PEP," indicates that PEP is optional and should be based on an individualized decision between the exposed person and the treating clinician.
§§ If PEP is offered and taken, and the source is later determined to be HIV negative, PEP should be discontinued.
¶¶ Large volume (i.e., major blood splash).

tices, pregnancy, breastfeeding, and blood and organ donation for 6 months after exposure.

IV.   SUMMARY AND CONCLUSIONS

Exposure to blood-borne viruses is a serious concern to HCPs. Prevention of transmission of HBV, HCV, and HIV infection in healthcare settings requires a multifaceted approach, including promoting hepatitis B vaccination of all HCPs who may have contact with blood or body fluids, practicing Standard Precautions, and preventing percutaneous injuries. Postexposure management also is an integral component of a complete program to prevent blood-borne virus transmission.

Recommendations for HBV postexposure management include initiation of the hepatitis B vaccine series to any susceptible, unvaccinated person who sustains an occupational blood or body fluid exposure. PEP with HBIG and/or hepatitis B vaccine series should be considered for occupational exposures after evaluation of the HBsAg status of the source and the vaccination and vaccine-response status of the exposed person. Table 27–2 provides guidance for selecting the appropriate HBV PEP.

Immune globulin and antiviral agents (e.g., interferon with or without ribavirin) are not recommended for PEP of HCV exposure. For HCV postexposure management, the HCV status of the source and exposed person should be determined, and for HCP exposed to an HCV positive source, follow-up HCV testing should be performed to determine if infection develops.

Recommendations for HIV PEP include a basic 4-week regimen of two drugs (zidovudine and 3TC; 3TC and d4T; or ddI and d4T) for most HIV exposures, and an expanded regimen that includes the addition of a third drug for HIV exposures that pose an increased risk for transmission (Tables 27–3 and 27–4). When the source person's virus is known or suspected to be resistant to one or more of the drugs considered for the PEP regimen, the selection of drugs to which the source person's virus is unlikely to be resistant is recommended.

Occupational exposures should be considered urgent medical concerns to ensure timely postexposure management and administration of HBIG, hepatitis B vaccine, and/or HIV PEP.

V.   FUTURE TRENDS

Future directions in the area of management of occupational blood exposures include more systematic (e.g., Internet-based) surveillance of occupationally acquired HBV, HCV, and HIV infection; better definition of the epidemiology of blood contact and the efficacy of preventive measures; development and evaluation of new safety devices and protective barriers; modification/improvement of HIV PEP regimens; and development and evaluation of vaccines for HIV and HCV.

VI.   INTERNATIONAL PERSPECTIVES

In the international arena, the same risk factors and prevention strategies apply to occupational blood exposures and blood-borne virus transmission. However,

Copyright © 2005, Association for Professionals in Infection Control and Epidemiology, Inc.

countries with the highest prevalence of HBV, HCV, and HIV infection often have limited resources for infection control, sterile supplies, personal protective equipment, occupational exposure management, and postexposure prophylaxis. This may result in greater opportunity for occupational exposures and infection transmission.

Preventive strategies for international HCP are important because the likelihood that these workers will interact with patients with HBV, HCV, and HIV infection is high. As in the United States, strategies for prevention of occupational blood-borne virus infection include: (1) routine use of barriers such as gloves, gowns, and eye protection; (2) careful handling of sharp instruments; and (3) provision of exposure management, including postexposure prophylaxis, as appropriate.

A number of special challenges exist in international settings. Scarce resources influence which prevention strategies will be adopted in healthcare settings. Strategies for changing behaviors of HCPs to handle and dispose of sharps safely and use barrier precautions need to be culturally appropriate. Finally, the stigma of blood-borne virus infection, particularly HIV infection, influences the willingness of HCPs to be tested after occupational exposure and complete follow-up for occupational exposure management.

REFERENCES

1. Centers for Disease Control. Recommendations for prevention of HIV transmission in health-care settings. *MMWR* 43(No. RR-11), 1994.
2. Centers for Disease Control. Update: universal precautions for prevention of transmission of human immunodeficiency virus, hepatitis B virus, and other bloodborne pathogens in health-care settings. *MMWR* 37:377–382,387–388, 1988.
3. Shapiro CN, McCaig LF, Gensheimer KF, et al. Hepatitis B virus transmission between children in day care. *Pediatr Infect Dis J* 8:870–875, 1989.
4. Richman KM, Rickman LS. The potential for transmission of human immunodeficiency virus through human bites. *J Acquir Immune Defic Syndr* 6:402–406, 1993.
5. Vidmar L, Poljak M, Tomazic J, et al. Transmission of HIV-1 by human bite [Letter]. *Lancet* 347:1762–1763, 1996.
6. Beltrami EM, Williams IT, Shapiro CN, et al. Risk and management of bloodborne infections in health care workers. *Clin Micro Rev* 13:385–407, 2000.
7. Lok AS, McMahon BJ. Chronic hepatitis B. *Hepatology* 34: 1225–1241, 2001.
8. Marcellin P, Chang TT, Lim SG, et al. Baseline ALT predicts histologic and serologic response in patients with HBeAg + chronic hepatitis B treated with Adefovir Dipivoxil (ADV) [Abstract]. In the 37th Annual Meeting of the European Association for the Study of the Liver, Madrid, Spain, 2002
9. Centers for Disease Control and Prevention. Hepatitis B virus: a comprehensive strategy for eliminating transmission in the United States through universal childhood vaccination—recommendations of the Immunization Practices Advisory Committee (ACIP). *MMWR* 40(RR-13):1–25, 1991
10. Centers for Disease Control and Prevention. Updated U.S. Public Health Service guidelines for the management of occupational exposures to HBV, HCV, and HIV and recommendations for postexposure prophylaxis. *MMWR* 50(RR-11):1–52, 2001.
11. Centers for Disease Control and Prevention. Achievements in public health: hepatitis B vaccination—United States, 1982—2002. *MMWR* 51:549–552,563, 2002.
12. Occupational Safety and Health Administration, Department of Labor. 29 CFR Part 1910.1030, Occupational exposure to bloodborne pathogens; final rule. *Federal Register* 56: 64004–64182, 1991.
13. Centers for Disease Control and Prevention. Recommendations for prevention and control of hepatitis C virus (HCV) infection and HCV-related chronic disease. *MMWR* 47(RR-19):1–39, 1998
14. Puro V, Petrosillo N, Ippolito G, Italian Study Group on occupational risk of HIV and other bloodborne infections. Risk of hepatitis C seroconversion after occupational exposure in health care workers. *Am J Infect Control* 23:273–277, 1995.
15. Beltrami EM, Kozak A, Williams IT, et al. Transmission of HIV and hepatitis C virus from a nursing home patient to a health care worker. *Am J Infect Control* 31:168–175, 2003.
16. Krawczynski K, Alter MJ, Robertson BH, et al. Environmental stability of hepatitis C virus (HCV): Viability of dried/stored HCV in chimpanzee infectivity studies. *Hepatology* 38(Suppl. 1): 428A, 2003.
17. Centers for Disease Control and Prevention. Guidelines for laboratory testing and result reporting of antibody to hepatitis C virus. *MMWR* 52(RR-3):1–15, 2003.
18. National Institutes of Health Consensus Development Conference Panel Statement. Management of Hepatitis C. *Hepatology* 36: S3–S20, 2002
19. Fried MW, Shiffman ML, Reddy KR, et al. Peginterferon alfa-2a plus ribavirin for chronic hepatitis C viruss infection. *N Engl J Med* 347:975–982, 2002
20. DeCock KM, Janssen RS. An unequal epidemic in an unequal world. *JAMA* 288:236–238, 2002.
21. Schreiber GB, Busch MP, Kleinman SH, et al. The risk of transfusion-transmitted viral infections. *N Engl J Med* 334:1685–1690, 1996
22. Centers for Disease Control and Prevention. Surveillance of healthcare personnel with HIV/AIDS, as of December 2001. Fact sheet. Available at: http://www.cdc.gov/ncidod/hip/BLOOD/hivpersonnel.htm (accessed August 5, 2003).
23. U.S. Public Health Service. Guidelines for the use of antiretroviral agents in HIV-infected adults and adolescents. Updated February 4, 2002. Available at: http://www.hivatis.org/trtgdlns.html#Adult (accessed September 10, 2002).
24. Garner JS, Hospital Infection Control Practices Advisory Comitee. Guideline for isolation precautions in hospitals. *Infect Control Hosp Epidemiol* 17:53–80, 1996, and *Am J Infect Control* 24:24–52, 1996.
25. Centers for Disease Control and Prevention. Targeted tuberculin testing and treatment of latent tuberculosis infection. *MMWR* 49(RR-6):1–54, 2000.

SUPPLEMENTAL RESOURCES

Division of Healthcare Quality Promotion, Centers for Disease Control and Prevention

Phone: 800-893-0485

http://www.cdc.gov/ncidod/hip/

Division of Viral Hepatitis, Centers for Disease Control and Prevention

Phone: 888-443-7232

http://www.cdc.gov/ncidod/diseases/hepatitis/index.htm

Needlestick!

http://www.needlestick.mednet.ucla.edu

National Institute for Occupational Safety and Health, Centers for Disease Control and

Prevention—bloodborne pathogens website

http://www.cdc.gov/niosh/topics/bbp/

Occupational Safety and Health Administration—bloodborne pathogens website

http://www.osha-slc.gov/SLTC/bloodbornepathogens/indes.html

PEPline (National Clinicians' Postexposure Prophylaxis Hotline)

Phone: 888-448-4911 (24 hours/7 days a week)

http://www.ucsf.edu/hivcntr/PEPline/

Copyright © 2005, Association for Professionals in Infection Control and Epidemiology, Inc.